Advances in Nd:YAG Laser Surgery

Stephen N. Joffe and Yanao Oguro
Editors

Advances in Nd:YAG Laser Surgery

With 230 Figures

Springer-Verlag
New York Berlin Heidelberg
London Paris Tokyo

Stephen N. Joffe, M.D., F.A.C.S., F.R.C.S.
Professor of Surgery
University of Cincinnati Medical Center
Cincinnati, Ohio, USA

Yanao Oguro, M.D.
Head, Department of Internal Medicine
National Cancer Center Hospital
Tsukiji, Chuo-ku, Tokyo, Japan

Library of Congress Cataloging-in-Publication Data
Advances in Nd-YAG laser surgery.
Includes bibliographies and index.
1. Lasers in surgery. 2. Nd-YAG lasers.
I. Joffe, Stephen N. II. Oguro, Yanao. [DNLM:
1. Laser Surgery. WO 500 A244]
RD73.L3A38 1987 617'.05 87-20703
ISBN-13: 978-1-4612-8322-5

Softcover reprint of the hardcover 1st edition 1988

Typeset by David A. Seham Associates, Metuchen, New Jersey.

9 8 7 6 5 4 3 2 1

ISBN-13: 978-1-4612-8322-5 e-ISBN-13: 978-1-4612-3728-0
DOI: 10.1007/978-1-4612-3728-0

Preface

The Nd:YAG laser has finally become the multidisciplinary and multispecialty tool of the 1980s. Primarily developed for gastrointestinal applications for controlling bleeding, at present it is also used for endoscopic treatment of gastrointestinal tumors, endobronchial cancer, and bladder and gynecological lesions and finding applications in otorhinolaryngology and neurosurgery. Development of laser scalpels and focusing head-pieces has now allowed the Nd:YAG laser to be used for open surgical procedures in general and plastic surgery, head and neck surgery, urology, gynecology, dermatology, and neurosurgery.

The rapid development in ceramic technology has led to contact surgery allowing physicians a choice of excision, vaporization, coagulation, incision, or combinations thereof by easily changing probes rather than having to select new laser wavelengths. This technology is rapidly replacing the carbon dioxide laser which currently has no adequate flexible waveguide for fiberoptic endoscopy, cannot be used in a water medium (e.g., bladder), and has poor coagulation properties when compared to the Nd:YAG laser.

Future developments may see the Nd:YAG laser even replacing electrocautery in the operating room due to its greater safety and efficacy. Local hyperthermia (laserthermia) with computer control, photodynamic therapy, and ophthalmic applications make the Nd:YAG laser the most exciting technological advancement in medicine and surgery for the 1980s.

Cost containment, DRGs (Diagnosis Related Groups), alternative health care delivery systems, rising costs, decreasing revenue, medical malpractice, inflation, and unemployment are forcing physicians and hospitals to cut health care costs. No economy can afford to spend over one billion dollars per day on health care. Lasers lower the cost of patient treatment, improve the quality of care, and significantly reduce the morbidity and mortality associated with surgical procedures. The era of outpatient minimally invasive surgery is with us and the Nd:YAG laser now provides the tool to accomplish these objectives.

Stephen N. Joffe and Yanao Oguro

Contents

Contributors

R. Yuta Amemiya, M.D., F.C.C.P., Senior Instructor, Department of Surgery, Tokyo Medical College, Nishi-shinjuku, Shinjuku, Tokyo, Japan

J.P. Ancelin, M.D., University of Lille, Centre Multidisciplinaire de Traitment par Laser, Hôpital Regional, Lille, France

Fumitaka Ando, M.D., National Nagoya Hospital, San-No-Maru, Naka-Ku, Nagoya, Japan

Jun Aoki, M.D., Department of Internal Medicine, Tokai University, School of Medicine, Boseidai, Isehara-shi, Kanagawa, Japan

David B. Apfelberg, M.D., Director, Comprehensive Laser Center, Palo Alto Medical Foundation, Palo Alto, California, USA

K. Arai, M.D., National Defense Medical College, Namiki, Tokorozawa-shi, Saitama-ken, Japan

Tsunenori Arai, Ph.D., Assistant Professor, Department of Medical Engineering, National Defense Medical College, Namiki, Tokorizawa-shi, Saitama-ken, Japan

Peter Wolf Ascher, M.D., Department of Neurosurgery, University of Graz, Graz, Austria

Kazuhiko Atsumi, M.D., Professor, Institute of Medical Electronics, Faculty of Medicine, University of Tokyo, Hongo, Bunkyo-ku, Tokyo, Japan

Arthur A. Bertolero, Director of Marketing, Surgical Laser Technologies, One Great Valley Parkway, Malvern, Pennsylvania, USA

Kim A. Brackett, Ph.D., Research Associate Professor of Surgery, Department of Surgery M.L. SSB, University of Cincinnati College of Medicine, Cincinnati, Ohio, USA

Jean-Marc Brunetaud, M.D., Associate Professor of Medicine, and Chief, Laser Center, University Hospital, Lille, France

D. Cochelard, M.D., Biomathematics Laboratory, School of Pharmacy, University of Lille, Lille, France

A. Cortot, M.D., University of Lille, Gastroenterology Department, Hôpital Regional, Lille, France

Norio Daikuzono, M.Sc., Surgical Laser Technologies, Japan Co., Ltd., Iidabashi, Chiyoda-ku, Tokyo, Japan

J.F. Dumon, M.D., Service d'Endoscopie Thoracique, Hôpital Salvator, Marseille, France

Richard M. Dwyer, M.D., Associate Clinical Professor, Harbor UCLA Medical Center, Los Angeles, California, USA

Victor Aldo Fasano, M.D., Ph.D., Director, Institute of Neurosurgery, University of Turin, Torino, Italy

Jay L. Federman, M.D., Co-Director Research, Research Department, Wills Eye Hospital, Philadelphia, Pennsylvania, USA

John C. Fisher, Sc.D., Heart and Lung Institute of Wisconsin, and St. Luke's Hospital, Milwaukee; Consultant in Laser Medicine and Surgery, Bradenton, Florida, USA

David E. Fleischer, M.D., Chief, Endoscopy Unit, Division of Gastroenterology, Georgetown University, Washington, DC, USA

John Foster, M.D., Resident in Surgery, University of San Francisco, San Francisco, California, USA

Frank Frank, Ph.D., MBB Medizintechnik, GmbH Application and Research Munich, FRG

Shigeru Furuta, M.D., Assistant Professor, Department of Otolaryngology, Faculty of Medicine, Kagoshima University, Usuki-cho, Kagoshima, Japan

Kazumichi Harada, M.D., The Third Department of Internal Medicine, Asahikawa Medical College, Nishi-kagura, Asahikawa-shi, Hokkaido, Japan

Yoshiki Hiki, M.D., Kitazato University, Kitazato, Sagamihara-shi, Kanagawa, Japan

Prof, Dr. med. A.G. Hofstetter, Director, Urology Clinic, Medical University of Lubeck, Lubeck, FRG

Issei Ichimiya, M.D., Department of Otolaryngology, Medical College of Oita, Hazama-cho, Oita, Japan

Satoshi Iwabuchi, M.D., Department of Neurosurgery, Ohashi Hospital, Toho University, School of Medicine, Ohashi, Meguro-ku, Tokyo, Japan

Stephen N. Joffe, M.D., F.A.C.S., F.R.C.S., Professor of Surgery, University of Cincinnati Medical Center, Cincinnati, Ohio, USA

Tetsuro Karasawa, M.D., Department of Obstetrics and Gynecology, Nagoya National Hospital, Sannomaru, Naka-ku, Nagoya-shi, Aichi, Japan

Teruo Kayano, Department of Oral Pathology, Faculty of Dentistry, Tokyo Medical and Dental University, Yushima, Bunkyo-ku, Tokyo, Japan

Makoto Kikuchi, Ph.D., Professor, Department of Medical Engineering, National Defense Medical College, Namiki, Tokorozawa-shi, Saitama-ken, Japan

Teruo Kouzu, M.D., Assistant Professor, Second Department of Surgery, Chiba University, School of Medicine, Inohana, Chiba-shi, Chiba Pref., Japan

Yuichi Kurono, M.D., Department of Otolaryngology, Oita Medical College, Hazama-cho, Oita-gun, Japan

Jack M. Lomano, M.D., Director for Educational Development and Co-Director of Grant Laser Center, Grant Hospital Medical Center; and Clinical Assistant Professor, The Ohio State University, Columbus, Ohio, USA

Carolyn J. Mackety, R.N., M.A., Vice President, Laser Centers of America, Inc., Columbia Plaza, Cincinnati, Ohio, USA

V. Maunoury, M.D., University of Lille, Centre Multidisciplinaire de Traitment par Laser, Hôpital Regional, Lille, France

B. Meric, M.D., Service d'Endoscopie Thoracique, Hopital Salvator, Marseille, France

Takeshi Miwa, M.D., Department of Internal Medicine, School of Medicine, Tokai University, Bohseidai, Isehara, Kanagawa, Japan

Goro Mogi, M.D., Professor and Chairman, Department of Otolaryngology, Medical College of Oita, Hazama-cho, Oita, Japan

Kevin C. Moore, M.B., Ch.B., F.F.A.R.C.S., D.A., Consultant Anesthetist, Department of Anesthesiology, Oldham General Hospital, Rochdale Road, Oldham, Lancashire, UK

Akinori Nagasawa, M.D., Department of Oral Surgery, Metropolitan Hiroo General Hospital, Tokyo, Ebisu, Shibuya-ku, Tokyo, Japan

Masayoshi Namiki, M.D., The Third Department of Internal Medicine, Asahikawa Medical College, Nishi-kagura, Asahikawa-Shi, Hokkaido, Japan

Takuo Nobori, M.D., Associate Professor, Department of Otolaryngology, Faculty of Medicine, Kagoshima University, Usuki-cho, Kagoshima, Japan

Yanao Oguro, M.D., Head, Department of Internal Medicine, National Cancer Center Hospital, Tsukiji, Chuo-tau, Tokyo, Japan

Kenkichi Oho, F.C.C.P., Professor, Department of Surgery, Tokyo Medical College, Nishishinjuku, Shinjuku-ku, Tokyo, Japan

Masaru Ohyama, M.D., Professor and Chairman, Department of Otolaryngology, Faculty of Medicine, Kagoshima University, Usuki-cho, Kagoshima, Japan

J.C. Paris, M.D., University of Lille, Gastroenterology Department, Hôpital Regional, Lille, France

Carmen A. Puliafito, M.D., Director, Laser Research Laboratory, Massachusetts Eye and Ear Infirmary; Assistant Professor of Ophthalmology, Department of Ophthalmology, Harvard Medical School, Boston, Massachusetts, USA

Richard C. Ranard, M.D., Gastroenterologist in Private Practice, McLean, Virginia, USA

R. James Rockwell, Jr., President, Rockwell Associates, Inc. Cincinnati, Ohio, USA

Hirotsugo Samejima, M.D., Department of Neurosurgery, Ohashi Hospital, Toho University, School of Medicine, Ohashi, Meguro-ku, Tokyo, Japan

M.Y. Sankar, M.D., F.R.C.S., Assistant Professor of Surgery, Department of Surgery, University of Cincinnati Medical Center, Cincinnati, Ohio, USA

T. Sato, M.D., National Defense Medical College, Namiki, Tokorozawa-shi, Saitama-ken, Japan

Tom Schröder, M.D., Ph.D., Associate Professor, Fourth Department of Surgery, University of Helsinki, Kasarminkatu, Helsinki, Finland

Stanley M. Shapshay, M.D., F.A.C.S., Chairman, Department of Otolaryngology-Head and Neck Surgery and Director, Eleanor Naylon Dana Laser Research Laboratory, Lahey Clinic Medical Center, Burlington, Massachusetts, USA

Hitoshi Shimao, M.D., Kitazato University, Kitazato, Sagamihara-shi, Kanagawa, Japan

Teruko Smith, P.A.C., R.N., Laser Specialist, Palo Alto Medical Foundation, Department of Plastic and Reconstructive Surgery and Comprehensive Laser Center, Palo Alto, California, USA

Roger F. Steinert, M.D., Assistant Clinical Professor, Harvard Medical School, Associate Surgeon in Ophthalmology, Massachusetts Eye and Ear Infirmary, Laser Research Laboratory, Boston, Massachusetts, USA

Soutaro Suzuki, M.D., Instructor, Gastrointestinal Endoscopy, Department of Internal Medicine, School of Medicine, Tokai University, Bohseidai, Isehara, Kanagawa, Japan

Yozo Suzuoki, M.D., Department of Obstetrics and Gynecology, Nagoya National Hospital, Sannomaru, Naka-tu, Nagoya-shi, Aichi, Japan

Hisao Tajiri, M.D., Medical Staff of the National Cancer Center, Department of Internal Medicine, National Cancer Center Hospital, Tsukiji, Chuo-ku, Tokyo, Japan

John M. Tew, Jr., M.D., Professor and Chairman, Department of Neurosurgery, University of Cincinnati, College of Medicine, Cincinnati, Ohio, USA

William D. Tobler, M.D., Assistant Professor, Department of Neurosurgery, University of Cincinnati, College of Medicine, Cincinnati, Ohio, USA

Ryozo Totani, M.D., Department of Obstetrics and Gynecology, Nagoya National Hospital, Sannomaru, Naku-ku, Nagoya-shi, Aichi, Japan

Hiroshi Tsunekawa, Meitetsu Hospital, Japan

K. Tsutsumiuchi, M.D., Department of Otolaryngology, Kanazawa Medical College, Uchinada, Ishikawa, Japan

Hiroto Washida, M.D., Chief Doctor of Urology, Department of Urology, Anjo Kosei Hospital, Miyukihonmachi, Anjo, Japan

Hajime Yamamoto, M.D., Department of Oral Pathology, Faculty of Dentistry, Tokyo Medical and Dental University, Yushima, Bunkyo-ku, Tokyo, Japan

Tetsuhiko Yamao, M.D., Kitazato University, Kitazato, Sagamihara-shi, Kanagawa, Japan

Kouchi Yamashita, M.D., Department of Otolaryngology, Kanazawa Medical College, Uchinada, Ishikawa, Japan

Yoshikazu Yamazaki, M.D., Second Department of Surgery, Chiba University, School of Medicine, Inohana, Chiba-shi, Chiba, Japan

Nobuo Yoshii, M.D., Department of Neurosurgery, Ohasi Hospital, Toho University, School of Medicine, Ohashi, Meguro-ku, Tokyo, Japan

Theresa Zumwalt, M.D., Assistant Clinical Professor, Department of Obstetrics and Gynecology, University of California at Irvine, Irvine, California, USA

1
Recent Advances in Laser Medicine and Surgery in Japan

Kazuhiko Atsumi

The emission of a "laser" beam—first successfully achieved using a synthetic ruby by T.H. Maiman in 1960—is one of the greatest discoveries of this century.

Unlike ordinary light, a laser beam is coherent, monochromatic, focusable, and directable.

Since 1961, when the ruby laser was first used to photocoagulate a detached retina, laser medicine has become firmly established, with successful applications in many clinical specialties and basic research, including plastic surgery, neurosurgery, otolaryngology, gynecology, and other fields.

At the present time, the field of laser surgery can be divided into five levels according to their maturity—from the veteran ophthalmology to the fledgling cardiovascular surgery (Figure 1.1).

In 1975, the First International Symposium on Laser Surgery was organized by Dr. I. Kaplan in Tel Aviv. Since then, the International Society of Laser Medicine and Surgery has organized an international symposium biannually; so far, these symposia have been held in Dallas, Graz, Tokyo, Detroit, Jerusalem, and Munich (see Table 1.1). At the same time, many international symposia and conferences concerned with laser medicine and surgery were organized by physicians and engineers for the exchange of information on laser technology, medical applications, education, and so on.

Many kinds of lasers have been used in medicine, but, at present, the three used most often are carbon dioxide, Nd:YAG, and argon lasers. These laser applications require the use of high power to attain the desired thermal effects on biologic tissues. Recently, however, the tendency of laser applications in medicine has been changing toward the use of low energy and short pulses (Figure 1.2).

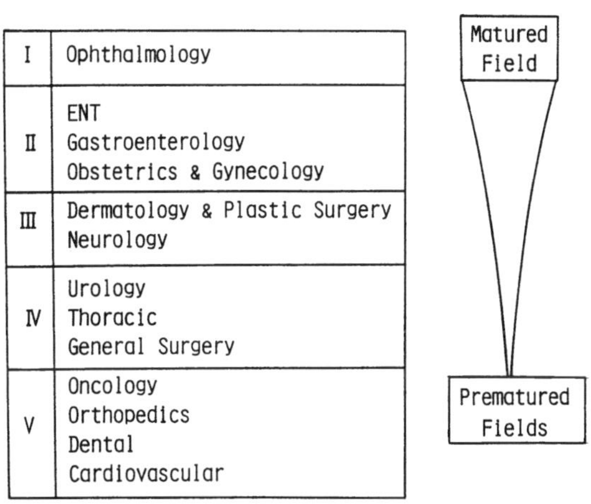

FIGURE 1.1. Maturity of laser surgery.

Current Status of Laser Surgery and Medicine in Japan

In 1965, a ruby laser unit for medical use was developed at the University of Tokyo, and the first clinical case of skin cancer was treated in 1967.

Since 1970, scientific meetings on laser medicine were organized annually by Japanese research groups, and in 1980 the Japanese Society of Laser Medicine and Surgery was formally organized. At the present time, 800 members are registered with the Society, covering various clinical fields as well as basic medical research and engineering.[1] By October 1984, 500 lasers were installed in medical facilities in Japan. This

TABLE 1.1. Symposia and Congresses of the International Society for Laser Medicine and Surgery

Date	Symposium or Congress	President	Place	No. of Participants	No. of Papers
1975 (Nov. 5–6)	1st International Symposium on Laser Surgery	Dr. I. Kaplan	Tel Aviv (Israel)	150	34
1977 (Oct. 23–26)	2nd International Symposium on Laser Surgery	Dr. B. Aronoff	Dallas (USA)	250	37
1979 (Sep. 24–26)	3rd International Congress on Laser Surgery	Dr. F. Heppner	Graz (Austria)	350	138
1981 (Nov. 25–27)	4th Congress of the International Society for Laser Surgery	Dr. K. Atsumi	Tokyo (Japan)	800	292
1983 (Oct.7–9)	5th International Congress of Laser Medicine and Surgery	Dr. T. Fuller	Detroit (USA)	850	318
1985 (Oct. 13–18)	6th Congress of the International Society for Laser Medicine and Surgery	Dr. I. Kaplan	Jerusalem (Israel)	700	334
1987 (June 22–26)	7th Congress of the International Society for Laser Medicine and Surgery	Dr. W. Waidelich	Munich (West Germany)	476	302

included 180 CO_2, 180 Nd:YAG, 40 argon, and 25 argon-dye lasers.

Figure 1.3 shows the classification of the lasers used in medicine, as reported at the annual meetings from 1983 to 1985. The Nd:YAG laser was used most often, followed by the CO_2. Argon-dye and diode lasers have been used increasingly each year for photodynamic therapy and for low-energy applications.

Figure 1.4 shows the medical areas in which lasers are applied most frequently, in the following order: Photodynamic therapy, gastrointestinal endoscopy, dentistry, biostimulation, and medical diagnosis.

Recent Developments in Medical Laser Instruments

Many of the medical lasers were developed in Japan. For example, the world's smallest portable CO_2 laser scalpel of 10 W, and nontoxic halide fibers to deliver the CO_2 laser beam, were developed in Japan, and also the widely used contact Nd:YAG laser. The recent advancements in medical laser instruments in Japan are shown in Table 1.2.

The wavelength of the carbon monoxide laser beam, 5 μm, is half that of the carbon dioxide

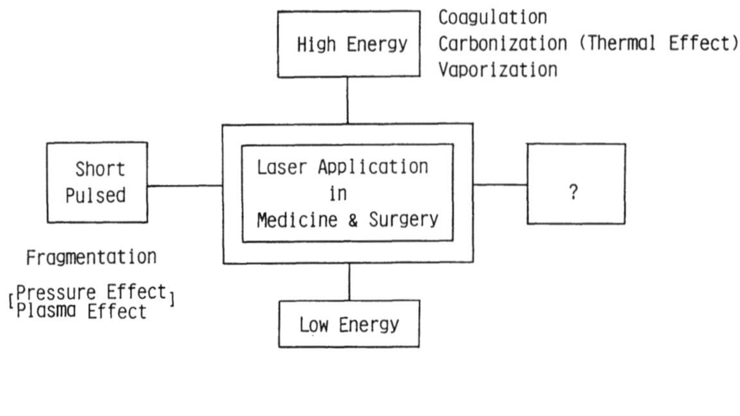

FIGURE 1.2. Biostimulation (nonthermal effect).

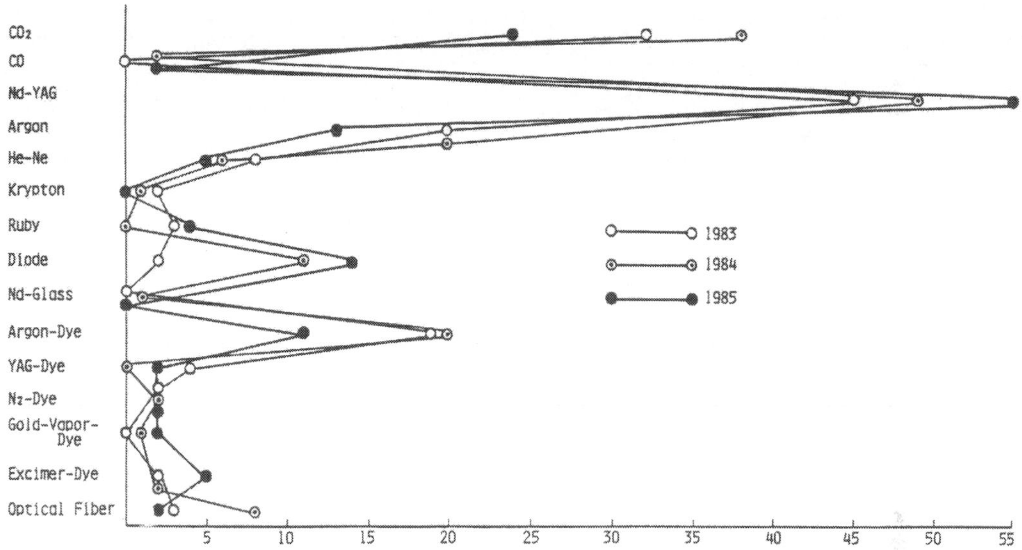

FIGURE 1.3. Classification of laser use. (From the papers presented at the annual meeting of the Japan Society for Laser Surgery and Medicine, 1983–1985.)

laser. Therefore the CO laser beam is more easily delivered through an optical fiber as compared to the CO_2 laser beam. The CO laser surgical unit was constructed by Dr. Kikuchi and an As_2S_3 fiber was used as the delivery system.

The application of argon-dye, N_2, and gold-vapor lasers in clinical photodynamic therapy for cancer cases is increasing. Argon-dye lasers were manufactured in Japan and first used there for the diagnosis and treatment of cancer.

Recently, MITI started a national project to develop cancer diagnostic and treatment sys-

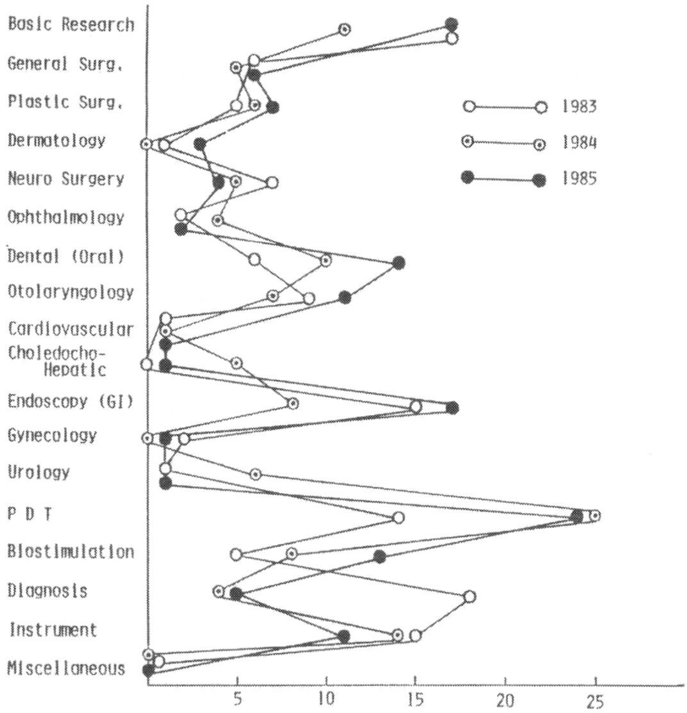

FIGURE 1.4. Frequency of use of lasers by medical specialty. (From papers presented at the annual meeting of the Japan Society for Laser Surgery and Medicine, 1983–1985.)

TABLE 1.2. Recent developments in medical laser instruments in Japan

CO laser surgical scalpel
1.32-μm Nd:YAG laser
Photodynamic therapy with N_2-dye laser
Photodynamic therapy with gold-vapor laser
Cancer diagnostics and treatment with argon-dye laser
Cancer diagnostics and treatment with excimer-dye laser
Semiconductor Ga-Al-As laser

TABLE 1.4. The 6th International Congress of Laser Surgery and Medicine (Jerusalem, October 13–18, 1985)

Fields	No. of applications	Lasers used	No. lase
Basic research	2	CO_2	165
General surgery	25	Helium-neon	10
Neurosurgery	29	Nd:YAG	72
Ophthalmology	21	Argon	45
Otolaryngology	28	Argon-dye	22
Dental and oral surgery	13	Diode	9
Thoracic surgery	5	Excimer	1
Cardiovascular surgery	29	Krypton	2
Plastic surgery	9	Gold-vapor	2
Dermatology	20	Copper-vapor	
Gynecology	33	Ruby	2
Urology	11	Optical fiber	5
Orthopedics	3	Miscellaneous	0
Endoscopy	13		359
Photodynamic therapy	24		
Low-energy laser	24		
Instrument	16		
Miscellaneous	29		
	334		

tems using the excimer laser. In these systems, a tunable excimer laser is used—405 nm for diagnosis and 630 nm for cancer treatment.

Diode lasers for biostimulation were also developed.

Recent Advancement in Laser Therapeutics

Recent advancements in laser therapeutics are shown in Table 1.3. Microvascular anastomosis has been achieved by using a special low-energy, 5–80 mW, CO_2 laser developed by Dr. Hayashi.

Choledocholithotripsy has been performed with excellent results by use of the contact Nd:YAG laser with a new ceramic endoscopic tip attachment designed by Dr. Kouzu. With this technique he succeeded in destroying stones in 92% of the cases, but in only 66% were successfully removed without the laser.

Low-energy laser applications is one of the main investigations in laser medicine and surgery. The 6th International Congress of Laser Surgery and Medicine was held in Jerusalem in October 1985. Table 1.4 shows the applied fields and lasers used by the participants at the congress. Low-energy laser applications was one session among the major applications in medicine. This included use in wound healing, biostimulation, pain relief, and vascular anastomosis (Figure 1.5).

With this background, the First International Symposium on Low Energy Laser Surgery and Medicine was held in Tokyo in June 1986.

The definition of low laser energy has not yet been clarified; however, there are some general agreements.

A low-energy laser has a power output of less than 100 mW and an energy density of less than 50 mW/cm^2. The biologic effects of the low-energy laser are considered to be as follows: activation of biochemical substances, stimulation of biologic tissues, and denaturation of biologic proteins, as shown in Figure 1.6.

In our laboratory, in cooperation with Dr. Ohshiro, the low-energy diode laser, with a wavelength of 830 nm and a power output of 60 mW, has been used for pain relief. The clinical data for our study of pain were obtained by the patients' responses in a double-blind test and by the use of thermographic imaging. In 70% of patients there was relief of pain, with diode laser treatment, although 40% obtained similar pain relief (placebo) without laser irradiation. Further studies are therefore necessary to analyze the pain relief mechanisms induced by laser stimulation.

TABLE 1.3. Recent advancements in laser therapeutics

Microvascular anastomosis by CO_2 laser
Choledocholithotripsy by contact Nd:YAG laser with new ceramic probes
Ureterolithotripsy by contact Nd:YAG laser with new ceramic probes
Pain relief by semiconductor laser
Laser endoscopy treatment for ectopic pregnancy
Selective vagotomy by CO_2 laser

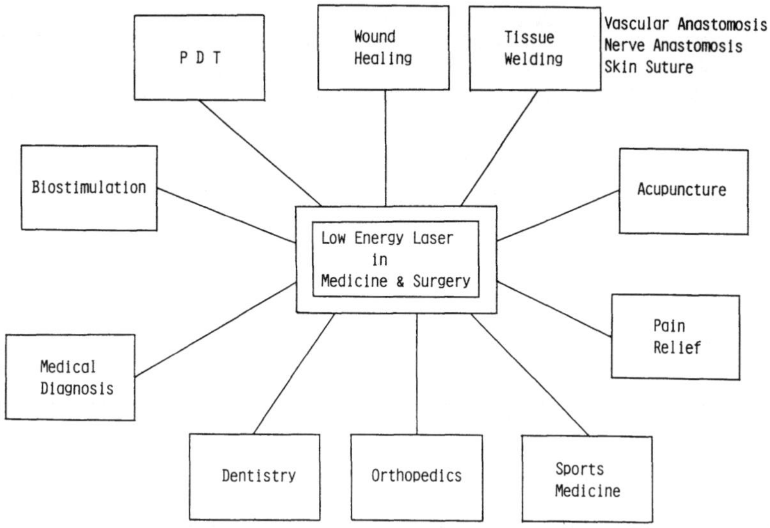

FIGURE 1.5. Applications of the low-energy laser in medicine and surgery.

Recent studies are seeking how to use short-pulsed lasers effectively for highly precise removal of small volumes of tissue and their fragmentation. An example of the short-pulsed laser is the excimer laser, which has a promising future in cardiovascular surgery for laser angioplasty or in combination with balloon angioplasty. Research is also being carried out on the very short pulse excimer pumped-dye laser with metal—copper and gold—vapors and on the long-pulsed flash-lamp pumped-dye lasers. The longer pulsed laser can be used in the fragmentation of kidney stones.

Education and the Laser Hospital

In consequence of the rapid progress of laser medicine and surgery, educational problems are increasing for doctors, nurses, and technicians. For this purpose, educational curricula, teachers, and facilities are required.

To meet the requirements of the researchers and clinical users of laser medicine, the first Laser Hospital in the world—Nanasato High-Tech Medical Center—was built in Omiya City, 30 miles north of Tokyo, and opened in 1985.

In this hospital, the laser instruments—Nd:YAG, argon, argon-dye—are installed in a central room. The laser beams are delivered through optical fibers into the two surgical operation rooms and the seven outpatient rooms. The laser selection, output, and time are controlled by a central computer (Figure 1.7). Over 100 cases have to date been treated. The laser hospital will be expected to contribute not only to the community's care but also to the edu-

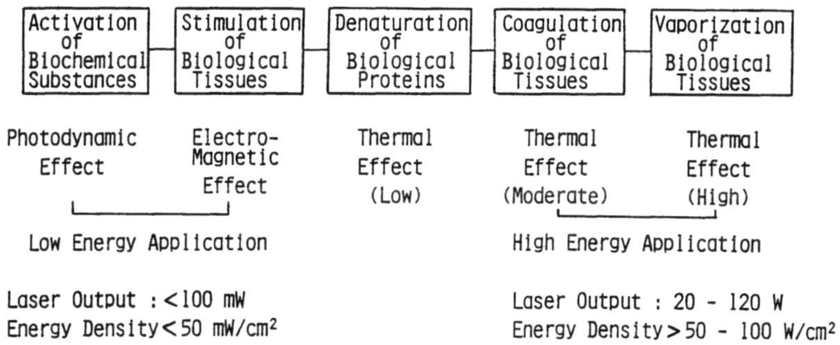

FIGURE 1.6. Biologic effects of laser energy irradiation.

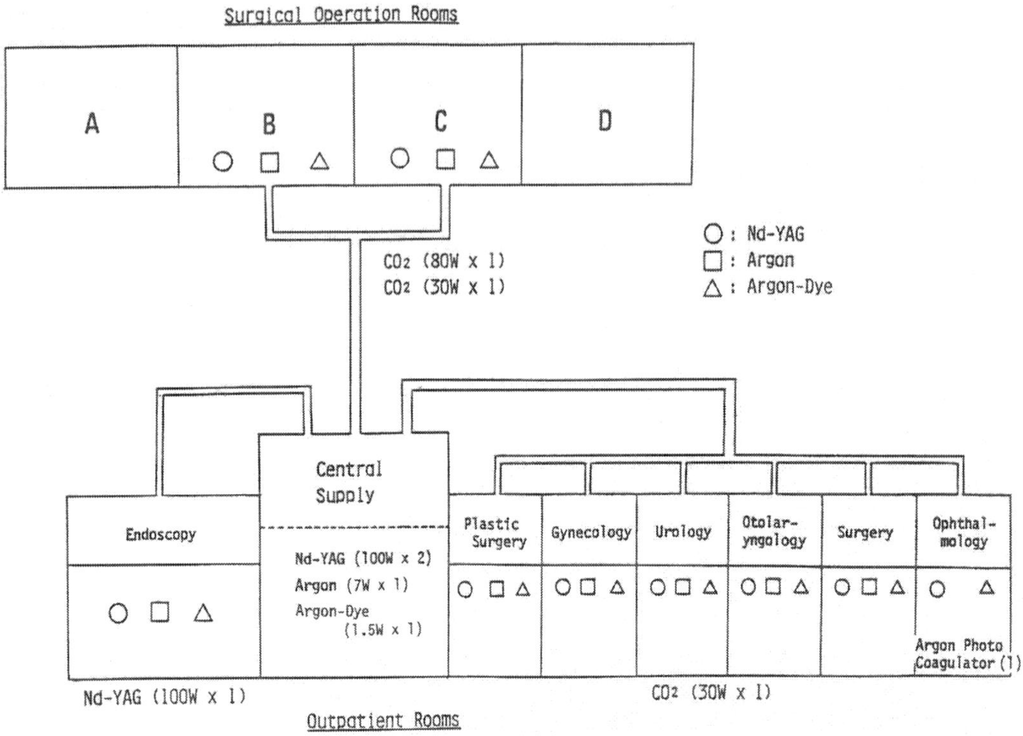

FIGURE 1.7. Arrangement of the medical laser system in the Nanasato High-Tech Medical Center (Japan).

cation of laser surgeons and technicians, as well as provide international information on developments in laser medicine.[2,3]

The Future of Laser Medicine

In the future, the diagnostic and therapeutic options not previously available will include:

1. Noninvasive, bloodless surgery
2. Precise diagnostic and selective treatment of cancer
3. Ultramicrosurgery
4. Laser genetic engineering
5. Specific diagnosis by laser immunology
6. Subcellular biomedical research
7. Sensitive diagnosis by laser doppler flowmetry
8. Online, three-dimensional imaging of the whole body by x-ray holography
9. Medical data processing by optical fibers
10. Medical data bank and networking by laser communication

Laser medicine will mark a revolutionary change in traditional medical and surgical procedures leading to new medical research and new horizons in the treatment of patients.

References

1. Atsumi K: Overall research and development of laser medicine and surgery in Japan. New Frontiers Laser Med Surg 13:19–38, 1983.
2. Atsumi K: New designed, central supplied laser hospital. Abstracts, 6th Congress of the International Society of Laser Surgery and Medicine, Jerusalem, 1985.
3. Atsumi K, et al: The new laser hospital. Technological and clinical aspects. Lasers Surg Med 6(2):213, 1986.

2
A Brief History of the Nd:YAG Laser

John C. Fisher

The successful operation of the first working laser by Theodore Maiman[1] in 1960 was like the key to a locked chest full of other types of laser, just waiting to be discovered. Only six years later, working prototypes of gas, liquid, solid, and semiconductor lasers had been constructed by several groups of investigators, spurred on by Maiman's achievement. By the end of that decade, hundreds of materials had been found capable of laser action.

In December of 1961, Elias Snitzer[2] reported achieving laser action in barium crown glass doped with neodymium ions. His work undoubtedly stimulated Geusic, Marcos, and Van Uitert[3] to pursue the development of the Nd:YAG laser, which they announced in 1964, together with laser action in other neodymium-doped garnets.

All of these scientists, of course, were the ultimate intellectual beneficiaries of the legacy of Albert Einstein,[4] whose 76-year lifespan ended in 1955, just five years too soon for him to see the fulfillment of his inspired prediction, in 1917, of the possibility of stimulated emission of radiation. However, he did survive long enough to witness the construction of the first masers by Gordon, Zeiger, and Townes[5] in the United States, and by Bassov and Prokhorov[6] in the Soviet Union, in the year 1954.

The early medical experimenters who saw potential value in lasers as surgical tools began their trials, often haphazard and unscientific, not long after Maiman's first firing of the ruby laser. Perhaps prophetically, G. Meyer-Schwickerath[7] in Germany had reported the first surgical use of light in 1954, the year of the maser, to prevent retinal separation.

Bessis and his associates[8] in France in 1962 described the use of the ruby laser to irradiate the constituents of living cells. In that same year, Koester, Snitzer et al.[9] wrote of experimental retinal coagulation by ruby laser. In 1965, Minton, Zelen, and Ketcham[10] described the use of ruby and pulsed Nd:glass laser lasers on the Cloudman S 91 mouse melanoma. In 1971, James Fidler[11] in Cincinnati reported his use of a 100-W Nd:YAG laser with a Nath fiber to incise canine livers, and in that same year, Mussigang and Katsaros[12] in West Germany used a 25 W Nd:YAG laser to study its effects on excised tissues.

The first clinically significant application of the Nd:YAG laser to surgery was Peter Kiefhaber's[13] use of it in West Germany to control massive gastrointestinal bleeding in humans. In 1978, Alfons Hofstetter and Karlheinz Rothenberger[14] tried coagulation of tumors of the bladder wall, transmitting the laser beam through an optical fiber inserted via the urethra. In 1979, L. Toty et al.[15] in France reported the endoscopic treatment of tracheobronchial lesions by the Nd:YAG laser. In the hands of Jean-Francois Dumon and his colleagues[16] in Marseille, by 1983 the Nd:YAG laser had become the preferred modality for palliative treatment of obstructing malignant tumors of the airway.

In 1973, in Paris, Daniele Aron-Rosa[17] had begun her long search for an ultrashort-pulsed laser to do intraocular surgery, which culminated in 1980 in the use of a mode-locked, picosecond-pulsed Nd:YAG laser to cut vitreous strands. Concurrently, Franz Fankhauser[18] in Bern was developing the ophthalmic applications of the Q-switched, nanosecond-pulsed Nd:YAG laser in collaboration with the firm Lasag, A.G. of Thun, Switzerland. By 1978 he had performed iridectomies in 102 eyes, using the multimode Lasag Microrupter 1 laser. At this writing, short-pulsed Nd:YAG lasers have become standard tools of the ophthalmologist, performing posterior capsulotomies and other precise intraocular procedures that are difficult or impossible to do by means of the argon-ion laser or other modalities.

In 1984, in Cincinnati, Stephen Joffe and his associates[19] introduced sapphire tips for quartz optical fibers to the United States, following a collaborative development with Norio Daikuzono and his associates in Japan. These shaped waveguides, attached to the standard quartz fibers used for transmission of Nd:YAG laser beams, are placed in contact with the surgical target, and permit precise cutting of soft tissue with excellent first-pass hemostasis of transected vessels, but without the extensive thermal damage characteristic of Nd:YAG beams delivered by noncontacting fibers. I was a scientific reviewer of Joffe's paper for the journal *Medical Instrumentation,* and I was impressed by the elegant simplicity of this concept, which has opened the whole field of thoracic and abdominal surgery to the Nd:YAG laser, formerly thought to be useless for precise cutting and vaporization.

Today the Nd:YAG laser has become a standard instrument in general laser surgery, complementing the CO_2, which originally dominated the field. Its applications extend to bronchology, gastroenterology, dermatology, gynecology, ophthalmology, neurosurgery, urology, and vascular surgery. There is probably no part of the human body that cannot be surgically treated in an effective manner by the Nd:YAG laser in one form or another.

With the use of nonlinear optical materials, such as potassium titanyl phosphate and others, it may be possible in the near future to build a frequency-quadrupled Nd:YAG laser to produce a wavelength of 266 nm for the precise surgery now being done experimentally with various excimer lasers. Perhaps the most important applications of all will be in the field of biostimulation, where Abergel and his associates[20] have demonstrated the ability of rays at 1064 nm to lyse collagen in keloids. Uses of this kind may well overshadow the purely surgical applications of the Nd:YAG laser in the next decade.

References

1. Maiman TH: Report in Phys Rev Lett 4:564, 1960.
2. Snitzer E: Optical maser action of Nd^{3+} in barium crown glass. Phys Rev Lett 7:444–446, 1961.
3. Geusic JE, Marcos HW, Van Uitert LG: Laser oscillations in Nd-doped yttrium aluminum, yttrium gallium, and gadolinium garnets. Appl Phys Lett 4:182, 1964.
4. Einstein A: On the quantum theory of radiation. Phys Z 18:121, 1917.
5. Gordon JP, Zeiger HJ, Townes CH: Molecular microwave oscillator and new hyperfine structure in microwave spectrum of NH_3. Phys Rev 95:282–284, 1954.
6. Bassov NG, Prokhorov AM: Article in J Exp Theor Phys (USSR) 27:431, 1954.
7. Meyer-Schwickerath G: Lichtkoagulation: Eine Methode zur Behandlung und Verhutung der Netzhautablosung. Graefes Arch Ophthalmol 156:2, 1954.
8. Bessis M, Gires F, Mayer G, Nomarski G: Irradiation des organites cellulaires à l'aide d'un laser à rubis. Compt Rend Acad Sci 225:1010, 1962.
9. Koester CJ, Snitzer E, Campbell CJ, Ritter MC: Experimental laser retinal coagulation. J Opt Soc Am 52:607, 1962.
10. Minton JP, Zelen M, Ketcham AS: Experimental results from exposure of Cloudman S-91 mouse melanoma in the CDBA/2F hybrid mouse to neodymium or ruby laser radiation. Ann N Y Acad Sci 122:758, 1965.
11. Fidler JP: Personal communication to Stanley Stellar et al., 1971.
12. Mussigang H, Katsaros W: Lasers in operative surgery with possibilities of transmission by flexible light conductors. Bruns Beitr Klin Chir 218(8):746–763, 1971.
13. Kiefhaber P, Nath G, Moritz K: Endoscopic control of massive gastrointestinal hemorrhage by irradiation with a high power neodymium:YAG laser. Prog Surg 15:140–145, 1977.
14. Hofstetter A, Rothenberger K, Keiditsch E, et al: The efficiency of the neodymium:YAG laser in urinary bladder treatment. Proceedings of the 4th Congress of the International Society for Laser Surgery, 1981. Laser Tokyo 10:18–20, 1981.
15. Toty L, et al: Utilisation d'un faiscean laser YAG à conduction souple pour le traitement endoscopique des certaines lésions tracheo-bronchiques. Rev Fr Mal Respir 87:57–69, 1979.

16. Dumon JF, Meric B: Handbook of Endobronchial YAG Laser Surgery, Marseille. Privately published by Dumon & Meric, 1983.
17. Aron-Rosa D, Griesemann JC: Pulsed ultrarapid YAG neodymium laser. Section of vitreous strands and cyclitic membranes in the management of retinal detachment. Conferenza Internaz sul Distaco di Retina, Rome, 29 Sept–1 Oct, 1980.
18. Fankhauser F: The Q-switched laser: Principles and clinical results. In Trokel SL (ed): YAG Laser OphthalmicMicrosurgery. Appleton-Century-Crofts, Norwalk, CT, 1983, pp 101–146.
19. Joffe S, Daikuzono N: Artificial sapphire probe for contact photocoagulation and tissue vaporization with the Nd:YAG laser. Med Instrum 19:173–178, 1985.
20. Abergel RP, Meeker CA, Thomas SL, et al: Control of connective tissue metabolism by lasers: Recent developments and future prospects. J Am Acad Dermatol 11(6):1142–1150, 1984.

3
Noncontact Delivery Systems and Accessories for the Application of the Nd:YAG Laser in Endoscopy and Surgery

Frank Frank

The almost explosive development of numerous laser systems has led to a wide spectrum of applications. Among the earliest suggested applications were those employed in material processing, such as cutting, drilling, and welding, and applications in medicine. The properties of the laser beam, such as monochromaticity and coherence, are utilized primarily in the field of medical diagnosis. The small divergence of laser light or, rather, the resulting possibility of concentrating a very high light intensity at the focal point of a lens, is of fundamental importance for therapeutic purposes. All applications in surgery and associated fields utilize the conversion of laser light into heat within the tissue, and the reactions thus produced, for cutting and coagulating tissue.

The Nd:YAG laser has become a coagulation instrument, which has found acceptance in interdisciplinary surgery. Due to the low absorption and high scattering in tissue, the radiation of the Nd:YAG laser leads to a deep and homogeneous coagulation effect. The noncontact treatment and the fact that blood and lymphatic vessels are coagulated and closed have led to successful applications, especially with regard to tumor surgery.

Biophysical Considerations

For a consideration of the interactions between the laser light and biomolecules, for example, in cells and tissue, the parameters of the biologic objects must be related to the physical parameters of laser radiation.

For surgical applications, the thermal interaction is of primary importance. The degree and extent of the thermal effect depend on the optical and the thermal properties of the tissue, the geometry of the laser beam, and the energy of the incident light.

The most important optical parameter is the wavelength-dependent absorption of the laser light by biomolecules. The transitions of the biomolecules are equivalent to the wavelengths shorter than about 280 nm. In this region, only few, mostly low-power, lasers are available at present.

The much more molecule-specific vibrational and rotational absorption bands are all within the range of wavelengths larger than 1000 nm. With a few exceptions, visible radiation is virtually not absorbed by biologic objects. Among the major exceptions to this rule are the hemoglobin in the red blood cells, and the pigment melanin. Here, marked absorption in the green visible spectrum occurs.

The high water content of most tissues leads to a very marked absorption of infrared radiation. This leads to an extremely efficient conversion of energy, and heating of tissue when irradiating with lasers employing these wavelengths.

Apart from absorption, a further important optical tissue parameter that has to be considered is scattering. Biologic tissue is highly structured, so that a beam of light directed into it undergoes a considerable change in spatial distribution owing to reflection, refraction, and diffusion effects. Scattering occurs mainly when absorption is low.

The thermal properties of tissue are its thermal capacity and thermal conductivity. This is often thought to be equivalent to water. This assumption is incorrect as it is often difficult to estimate the transmission of energy by thermal conduction, when layers of tissue of highly differing structure and complicated geometry are involved. For example, the wall of the stomach, the retina, the wall of the bladder—or in the presence of blood vessels, with usually irregular blood flow through them leads to a very heterogeneous dissipation of energy. Furthermore, during irradiation, phase transitions, such as vaporization or carbonization, which alter the optical and thermal properties of the tissue, frequently occur.

Effect of Nd:YAG Laser Light on Tissue

The Nd:YAG laser emits light in the near-infrared range at 1064 and 1318 nm. At 1064 nm absorption in tissue is very low. Optical scattering is therefore very pronounced, resulting in uniform distribution of the radiation in tissue.

Slow heating of a large tissue volume around the point of impingement of radiation occurs, followed by a deep, slowly progressing coagulation.

The tissue volume covered by the laser light is heated, which results in delayed destruction of the tissue, with no noticeable structural damage. The low absorption leads to coagulation depths of down to 6 mm. Finally, protoplasm vaporizes at the tissue surface, leading to marked shrinking, although the tissue surface itself is hardly damaged. The surface of the tissue is covered with only a thin layer of fibrin.[1] Particularly in multilayered tissue, for example, the wall of the stomach, the depth of the necrosis depends on the blood circulation.

The effects at the surface of the tissue are, for the most part, influenced by the power density applied on irradiation. The focused Nd:YAG laser beam, 1064 nm, power density approximately 10 kW/cm^2, ruptures the tissue surface and leads to a wide, conical coagulation lesion. Defocused delivery—power density approximately 200 W/cm^2—leads to a shallow coagulation effect, with sealing of the vessels under the surface. Blood vessels are sealed by the combined effect of shrinkage and uniform coagulation of tissue. Arteries of up to 2 mm and veins of up to 3 mm in diameter can be closed rapidly and reliably.[2]

Also of importance for the form and nature of tissue damage by Nd:YAG laser is surface cooling. The main advantage of the Nd:YAG laser is the possibility of coagulating without vaporization. When the surface of the tissue is cooled with gas, the extent of the necrosis is clearly marked on the surface. With water cooling, which is possible only at the 1064-nm wavelength, a deep, drop-shaped necrosis develops, the surface of the tissue hardly being injured. Initially, the coagulation volume expands with increasing irradiance, but is then limited by backscatter from the blanched surface. If carbonization occurs on the surface, absorption increases and the tissue is vaporized. If the surface of the tissue is cooled with water, the blanching effect is delayed, carbonization avoided, with the result that deep coagulation occurs.[3]

A comparison of the coagulation effect of electrocautery and Nd:YAG laser light reveals marked differences. This difference is particularly noticeable in multilayered tissue such as the wall of the bladder. With comparable surface necrosis, the coagulation zone produced by electrocoagulation is shallow, with rough, irregular lateral and deep boundaries. Nd:YAG lasing results in a laterally sharply delineated necrosis involving all the layers of the bladder wall. In parenchymatous organs, such as, liver tissue, the coagulation effect of an electric current is much shallower than that of the Nd:YAG laser.[4,5]

The deep coagulation effect of the Nd:YAG laser also leads to the temporary sealing of lymph vessels. This effect can be clearly demonstrated experimentally. Dye is injected into the apex of a rat bladder. If a transmural necrosis is produced by laser irradiation around the resulting weal, it can be seen that the lymph flow stops at the lasered zone for 3 to 4 weeks. After electrocoagulation, however, dye is deposited in the lymph nodes—proof enough that the lymph vessels are not properly closed by electrocautery.[6]

The absorption coefficient of water and saline is approximately 10 times higher at the Nd:YAG laser wavelength of 1318 nm than at 1064 nm. This results in more efficient conversion of energy into heat in tissue at 1318 nm. The extinction coefficient in blood at 1318 nm is only one-third of that at 1064 nm.[7] This results in less heat dissipation by blood and deeper penetration in tissue at 1318 nm.

Especially in tissue with a high water content, a marked loosening of the necrotic tissue is obtained with laser light of 1318-nm wavelength with ablation. However, it is by no means to be compared with the well-known precise incision obtained with a 10,600-nm CO_2 laser. Unlike the CO_2 laser incision, tissue ablation with the Nd:YAG laser at 1318 nm is distinguished by a clear and effective coagulation zone along the borders of the incision.[8,9]

Nd:YAG Laser Systems and Accessories

Through use of targeted noncontact irradiation with the Nd:YAG laser pathological tissue can be destroyed. The marked depth effect results in the occlusion of blood and lymph vessels.[9]

The first continuous wave Nd:YAG laser, working on the 1064-nm wavelength, was introduced in the medical field in 1973. Since then a number of different systems with power ranges from 40 to 120 W have been developed (Table 3.1, Figure 3.1). All these instruments have similar construction characteristics. The essential component is the laser head, which accommodates all the optical elements of the Nd:YAG laser: crystal, pump lamps, and resonator mirrors, as well as a pilot laser within the visible spectrum. The pilot light is emitted by a helium-neon laser in the milliwatt range, and is concentric with the main invisible Nd:YAG laser beam. Both are transmitted to the operative field via a flexible quartz fiber light guide. The pilot light marks the target point of the therapeutic beam.

Early in the development of the medical Nd:YAG laser, it became apparent that laser

TABLE 3.1. Commercial continuous wave Nd:YAG laser systems for endoscopic and surgical use with date of clinical introduction

Company	Model	Power (on tissue)	Launched (year)
Aloka	LMY 1001	100 W	1985
Cilas	YM 575	50 W	1980
	YM 100	100 W (quasi-cw)	1981
	YM 101	85 W	1985
Cooper Laser Sonics (Molectron Medical)	8000	100 W	1978
	4000	50 W	1985
	6000	80 W	1986
	8900	120 W	1986
	ML 880	100 W (1.06 μm), 45 W (10.6 μm)	1984
Fujinon	FYL M1	100 W	1984
Laser Industries	2100	100 W	1986
MBB-Medizintechnik (MBB-AT)	mediLas	100 W	1973
	mediLas 2	120 W	1979
	mediLas 40 N	40 W	1986
	mediLas 60 N	60 W	1987
NIIC	130YZ	100 W (1.06 μm), 30 W (10.6 μm)	1983
	IS 101	100 W	1986
Olympus	MYL-1	100 W	1984
Osada	Nd:YAG	60 W	1985
Pentax	SLY-1	100 W	1984
Pilkington Medical (Barr & Stroud)	Fiberlase 100	100 W	1982
Surgical Laser Technologies	SLT CL60	60 W	1986

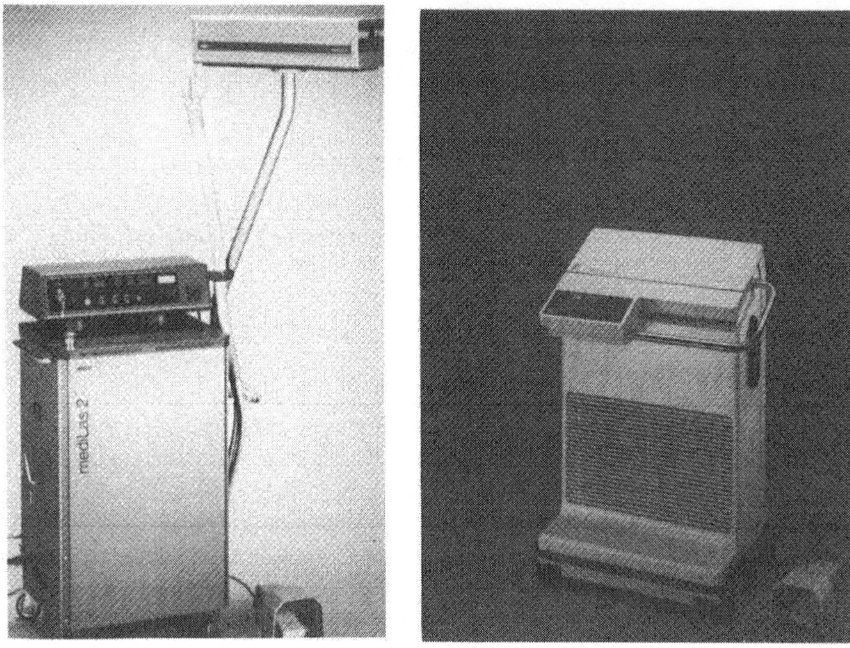

FIGURE 3.1. Examples of clinical Nd:YAG laser systems. Model mediLas 2 (120 W) with separate laser head and model mediLas 40 N (40 W) with integrated laser (MBB-Medizintechnik GmbH).

radiation is only as useful as the available accessory instruments. The surgeon needs appropriate instruments to take full advantage of the efficient properties of the Nd:YAG laser. Various instruments have been developed for routine clinical use, following the philosophy that they should be as similar as possible to instruments that are already familiar to the user.

Flexible Laser Light Guides

Transmission of the laser beam via flexible light guides is based on the total reflection occurring at the interface between two media with different refractive indices. The light is propagated within the optically denser medium. The light wave being repeatedly totally reflected along the length of the light guide. The transmission takes place in quartz glass fibers.

Commercially available quartz optical fibers with a strong Teflon covering (fiber diameter 0.2–0.6 mm) fulfill all the requirements relating to mechanical stability and high flexibility. Laser light is introduced at the proximal end by means of lens systems whose focal point is adjusted to the fiber core diameter. The transmission efficiency of these fiber systems is 90%. The exit divergence ranges from 6° to 24° and can be compensated by adjusting the irradiation distance or by the use of appropriate lenses.

Gas-cooled or liquid-flushed light guide systems are available. The gas is introduced into the light guide at the optical coupling. A suitable nozzle at the distal end provides efficient irrigation and cooling. The rinsing solution is either introduced in the same way or more often directly connected to the endoscope or handpiece, which is used together with the light guide. The fiber tip can easily be repaired if damaged. Systems from 1 to 2.6 mm in diameter are available.

Instrumentation for Endoscopic Application

Of the various indications for the use of the Nd:YAG laser in medicine, applications in the endoscopic field have reached essential importance. For the well-known endoscopic indications in gastroenterology, pulmonology, and urology, the common instrumentation has been modified for laser use.[10–28] New endoscopic techniques for special endourologic interventions, gynecology, ENT, and neurosurgery have led to developments of suitable systems.[29–38] In this section a choice of typical endoscopic systems using different technical principles are described (Figure 3.2).

In gastroenterology all routine diagnostic instruments are used without any modification. The light guide is passed directly through the working channel and can be advanced distally as far as desired.

The noncontact application of the Nd:YAG laser in gastroenterology is suitable for stanching bleedings from esophageal varices, ulcers, and Mallory–Weiss tears. The treatment of tumors in the upper and lower gastrointestinal tract, palliative elimination of stenosing tumors, curative radiation of sessile neoplastic polyps and benign intestinal and esophageal stenoses, are additional indications, which are rapidly becoming more important than hemostasis.

With the endoscopic application of the Nd:YAG laser in gastroenterology a triconical quartz-glass fiber was used initially. The substantially lower 4° divergence of this fiber makes the power density at the site of exposure largely independent of variations in the irradiation distance. An operating distance of up to several centimeters is possible without any appreciable reduction in the power density required for coagulation. The 0.3- or 0.2-mm quartz glass fiber is loosely mounted in a Teflon tube, which makes it extremely susceptible to mechanical damage. The use of this light guide requires modified gastroscopes. The operating channel is sealed at the distal end by a window. If the tip is damaged, the whole light guide must be replaced.

Because of the exceptionally good vision it affords, some operators use a rigid endoscope in the treatment of esophageal varices. The light guide, together with the telescope, is introduced into the shaft, which is provided with an aspiration channel. By angulating the light guide it is possible to irradiate the esophageal wall perpendicularly. The instrument has a diameter of 14 mm, which limits its application.

Also in pulmonology, all routine flexible diagnostic instruments can be applied. Two-channel instruments have the advantage that one channel is available for aspiration while the fiber is in place. Most of the interventions to recanalize endobronchial and endotracheal stenoses are performed under outpatient conditions.

In complicated cases of bronchial tumor resection, an operating technique is required in which aspiration and ventilation can be performed simultaneously. For this purpose a multichannel rigid bronchoscope is available. The light guide is introduced, together with the telescope, through the sheath containing the aspiration and ventilation channels. By angulating the light guide, it is possible to irradiate the bronchial wall perpendicularly. The instrument has a diameter of 13 mm, which limits its application (Figure 3.2).

In another multichannel rigid bronchoscope, a diameter of 11 mm has been obtained by omitting the angulation mechanism. The channels for the aspiration catheter and the light guide are identical, adjacent, and interchangeable. The smoke generated during tissue vaporization can be aspirated through another channel to ensure

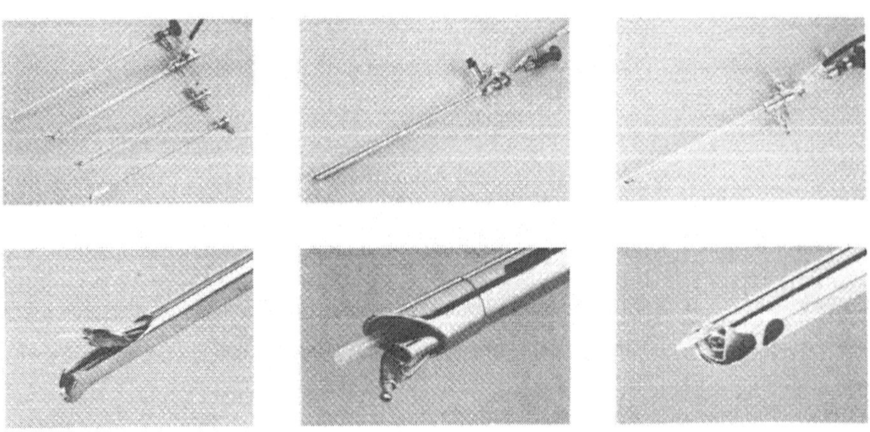

FIGURE 3.2. Examples of different rigid laser endoscopes for noncontact application of the Nd:YAG laser: cystoscope, bronchoscope, neurosurgical endoscope (Karl Storz , GmbH & Co.).

good vision. The rotatable anesthetic attachment ensures optimal irradiation conditions with simple operation.

For treating tumors in the genitourinary system, such as multicentric tumors or colonizing tumors of the urethral, vesical, and ureteral mucosa, and tumors in the pyolocaliceal area, several endoscopic laser instruments are available.

The standard laser cystoscope for outpatient treatment of small bladder tumors, stage TIS and T1, consists of a conventional cystoscope sheath of 19–21 French, an observation telescope with variable viewing angles, and a special laser cystoscope insert, similar to a normal Albarran insert. The light guide is passed through the working channel. The distal end of the light guide can be flexed to up to 80° with the aid of the modified Albarran lever. In addition, the fiber tip can be moved distally to permit exact adjustment of the distance from the area to be irradiated (Figure 3.2). A rinsing solution is introduced onto the attachment and led to the distal end, so that, with circulating rinsing, the volume can easily be kept constant. Practically all regions of the bladder can be irradiated perpendicularly.

For clinical interventions on larger tumors and for laser irradiation of the tumor bed after electroresection, a 24 French resection sheath with an oblique tip and a central cock is used instead of the sheath described above. The greater rinsing effect that can be achieved with this arrangement permits efficient laser irradiation even when bleeding occurs.

For the combined treatment of electroresection and laser irradiation in one session, the light guide is attached directly to the electrotome but the distal fiber end cannot be bent.

Interventions within the urethra, in the treatment of urethral carcinomas and condylomas, allow the use of a system with a modified sheath of 20 French and an additional overall reflux sheath. There is no need for the Albarran lever, since the fiber is passed directly through the laser insert with the observation optic. Any possible damage to the urethral mucosa is thus avoided.

A ureterorenoscope of 9 French has been designed for tumor treatment within the lower part of the ureter. An inspection insert with a bougie channel facilitates the introduction of the instrument. Fiber and telescope are inserted into the part of the system that will be introduced into the ureter.

For the irradiation of tumors in the pelvis and the calices of the kidney, a flexible endoscope with an outer diameter of only 4 mm can be used. The light guide and rinsing fluid are passed through the working channel.

Owing to the homogeneous coagulation effect the Nd:YAG laser is also successfully applied to tubal sterilization in the gynecologic field. The laparoscopic sterilization by partial coagulation of the oviducts improves the chances of future refertilization. This laparoscope insert is equipped with distal forceps to ensure a permanent obturation of the ovular tuba. The gas-cooled light guide is combined with the forceps insert. The forceps are so constructed that the laser beam always remains within the branches. This prevents damage to the surrounding tissue.

For laparoscopic application of the Nd:YAG laser in gynecology, such as in the treatment of endometriosis, the laser light guide with a coaxial gas flow can be adapted to the routine operation laparoscopes using a special laser insert. The distal flexibility permits exact and safe irradiation of the area to be treated.

A laser hysteroscope is applied for the en doscopic treatment of uterine hemorrhage and coagulation of tumors and lesions in the uterus. The rigid optic permits laser treatment under direct visual control. The mobility of the distal fiber end guarantees efficient irradiation. The continuous irrigation system ensures adequate cooling.

A laser laryngoscope as well as a laser tracheoscope operate on the same principles as the bronchoscopes described previously. Distal illumination and the flexible gas-cooled light guide allow optimal, targeted irradiation.

New neurosurgical indications for the endoscopic noncontact application of the Nd:YAG laser are the treatments in cases of hydrocephalus, cystic brain tumors, or massive bleeding. A laser encephaloscope that permits controlled movement of the distal end of the flexible fiber has been created for the endoscopic Nd:YAG laser interventions in the ventricle system, for perforating brain cysts and vaporizing the neoplastic tissue in the cyst wall. With the special viewing obturator, the 15 French sheath can be introduced under visual control. Rinsing and fiber movement is done in the same manner as with the urologic endoscopes.

For the atraumatic aspiration of hematomas in the cervicocranial region the laser neurosurgical endoscope with a simultaneous rinsing and suction mechanism is available. The integrated light guide allows a directed microcoagulation of bleeding vessels (Figure 3.2).

Instrumentation for Open Surgery

For all external applications in dermatology, urology, and gynecology, and for interventions on exposed areas in neurosurgery or in general surgery[39–45]—with or without the operating microscope—various handpieces have been designed for unrestricted, free-hand manipulation (Figure 3.3).

The focusing handpiece is equipped with an interchangeable optic. Focus points as small as 0.4 mm diameter can be achieved. By altering the irradiation distance, both the power density and the diameter of the treated area can be varied (Figure 3.3).

For operations that have to be performed under microscopic control, hand applicators of various designs have been developed that permit free, three-dimensional working. Both gas-cooled and liquid-flushed systems are used. The small, 3 mm, diameter of these instruments, does not impair vision (Figure 3.3). In addition to the standard shapes, such hand applicators with flexible tubes enable the surgeon to reach otherwise inaccessible regions.

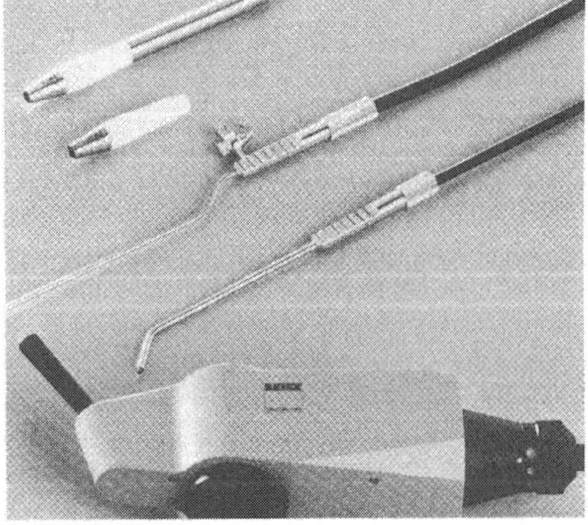

FIGURE 3.3. Examples of hand-held devices for noncontact application of the Nd:YAG laser (MBB-Medizintechnik GmbH) and an operating microscope adapter for Nd:YAG laser (Manufactured by Carl Zeiss, West Germany.)

Integration with the Microscope

For operations in extremely restricted access areas, such as in neurosurgery and ENT, or for microsurgical laser-assisted anastomosis in connection with the 1318-nm Nd:YAG system,[46,47] an operating microscope adapter is available.

The optical elements of the micromanipulator are the fiber coupler, the main optics, and a movable mirror, controlled by a joystick. A safety filter at the top protects the eyes against reflected radiation. A window at the bottom protects the optics against dust and smoke. The micromanipulator is mounted on the operating microscope firmly by a dovetail joint. The diameter of the laser beam can be adjusted on the micromanipulator between 0.9 and 5.0 mm. The aiming beam and the high-power Nd:YAG beam are guided coaxially through the optics of the microscope, so that the focal plane coincides with the focal plane of the microscope. The beam can be moved within the operating field precisely by the joystick. The sensitivity of the joystick is adjustable to the size of the visual field, determined by the magnification setting of the microscope. It is limited exactly to the diameter of the visual field, avoiding any accidental pointing of the laser beam outside the operative field[48] (Figure 3.3).

Conclusions

Apart from many and various Nd:YAG laser applications in medicine, approved and established, there is a definite perspective of other successful laser applications, especially in the field of tumor surgery. The laser is a valuable supplement to other auxiliary tools in modern medicine. Consequently, its application is justified whenever the therapeutic outcome achieved with this technology is superior to that obtained using other methods.

The endoscopic applicability of the Nd:YAG laser warrants special mentioning, as it leads to considerably less morbidity on the patient, as well as reduction of prolonged hospitalization and subsequent expenditures.

The applicability and the value of contact Nd:YAG laser surgery is currently under investigation. Experimental and clinical results indicate that for special indications contact surgery is feasible. Similar to the initial areas of application in Nd:YAG laser surgery, an analysis and optimization for this new method will be necessary before routine clinical practice.

References

1. Hofstetter A, Frank F [unter Mitarbeit von Bülow H] Halldorsson Th, Keiditsch E: Der Neodym-YAG-Laser in der Urologie. Editiones Roches, Basel, 1979.
2. Beck OJ, Wilske J, Schönberger JL, Gorisch W: Tissue changes following application of lasers to the rabbit brain. Results with CO_2 and Nd:YAG lasers. Neurosurg Rev 1:31–36, 1979.
3. Landthaler M, Brunner R, Haina D, et al: The neodymium-YAG laser in dermatology. MMW 126:1108–1112, 1984.
4. Keiditsch E, Maiwald H, Hofstetter AG, et al: Comparison of the effects of the neodymium-YAG laser and electrocoagulation in experimental animal research. In Kaplan I (ed): Laser Surgery III, Part II. Tel Aviv, 1979, pp 185–193.
5. Keiditsch E, Hofstetter AG, Rothenberger K, et al: Comparative morphological investigations of the effects of the neodymium-YAG laser and electro-coagulation in experimental animal research. In Bellina JH (ed): Gynecological Laser Surgery. Plenum, New York and London, 1981, pp 327–336.
6. Zimmermann I, Stern J, Frank F, et al: Interception of lymphatic drainage by Nd:YAG laser irradiation in rat urinary bladder. Lasers Surg Med 4:167–172, 1984.
7. Stokes LF, Auth DC, Tanaka D, et al: Biomedical utility of 1.34 μm Nd:YAG laser radiation. IEEE Trans Biomed Eng BME-28:297–299, 1981.
8. Beck OJ, Frank F, Keiditsch E, Wondrazek F: Klinische und experimentelle Untersuchungen zur Erweiterung der Nd:YAG-Laseranwendung in der Neurochirurgie. Laser 1:13–18, 1985.
9. Frank F, Beck OJ, Hessel S, Keiditsch E: Comparative investigations of the effects of the Nd:YAG laser at 1.06 μm and 1.32 μm on tissue. Lasers Surg Med 6:546–551, 1986.
10. Kiefhaber P, Nath G, Moritz K: Endoscopical control of massive gastrointestinal hemorrhage by irradiation with a high-power neodymium-YAG laser. Prog Surg 15:140–155, 1977.
11. Sander R, Pösl H, Spuhler A, Frank F: Neodym-YAG-Laser mit CO_2-jet-stream Erfahrungsbericht. Fortschr Gastroenterol Endosk Vol. 11:105–108, 1979.
12. Sander P, Pösl H, Spuhler A, Hitzler H: Der Neodym-YAG Laser: Ein effektives Instrument für die Stillung lebensbedrohlicher Gastrointestinalblutungen. Leber Magen Darm 11:31–36, 1981.
13. Hochberger J, Ell Ch, Lux G: Protective tips for endoscopes used in laser therapy. Endoscopy 18:163, 1986.
14. Dumon J-F, Reboud E, Garbe L, et al: Treatment of tracheobronchial lesions by laser photoresection. Chest 81:278–284, 1982.
15. Dumon J-F, Shapshay S, Bourcereau J, et al: Principles for safety in application of neodymium-YAG laser bronchology. Chest 86:163–168, 1984.
16. Dierkesmann R, Huzly A: Technik der endobronchialen Laser-Behandlung. Prax Klin Pneumol 6:211–256, 1983.
17. Staehler G, Hofstetter AG, Schmiedt E, et al: Zerstörung von Blasentumoren durch endoskopische Laser-Bestrahlung. Dtsch Ärztebl 75:681–686, 1978.
18. Hofstetter AG, Frank F: Ein neues Laser-Endoskop zur Bestrahlung von Blasentumoren. Fortschr Med 97:232–234, 1979.
19. Frank F, Hofstetter AG, Böwering R, Keiditsch E: Endoscopic application of the Nd:YAG laser in urology. Biophysical fundamentals and instrumentation. SPIE Proc 211:36–40, 1979.
20. Rothenberger K, Pensel J, Hofstetter AG, et al: Transurethral laser coagulation for treatment of urinary bladder tumors. Lasers Surg Med 2:255–260, 1983.
21. Frank F, Bailer P, Beck OJ, et al: Instrumentation for the surgical application of the Nd:YAG laser. SPIE Proc 405:105–109, 1983.
22. Frank F, Bailer P, Beck OJ, et al: Instrumente für die chirurgische Anwendung des Nd:YAG Lasers. In Waidelich W (ed): Optoelektronik in der Medizin. Springer-Verlag, Berlin, 1984, pp. 39–45.
23. Frank F: Multidisciplinary use of the Nd:YAG laser. SPIE Proc 658: , 1986.
24. Hofstetter AG, Frank F, Keiditsch E: Laser treatment of the bladder: Experimental and clinical results. In Smith JA (ed): Lasers in Urologic Surgery. Year Book, Chicago and London, 1985, pp 63–81.
25. Frank F: Biophysical fundamentals, technical prerequisites, and safety aspects for the application of the neodymium-YAG laser in urology. Eur Urol 12:3–11, 1986.
26. Frank F: Technical prerequisites and safety considerations for the use of the Nd:YAG laser in

gastroenterology. Endoscopy 18(Suppl 1):6–9, 1986.
27. Frank F: Biophysical aspects, instruments and safety in the use of the Nd:YAG laser in pulmonology. Tumor Diagn Ther 7:5–9, 1986.
28. Malloy TR: Urologic neodymium:YAG laser surgery. Surg Clin North Am 64:905, 1981.
29. Hofstetter AG, Böwering R, Keiditsch E, Frank F: Zerstörung von Uretertumoren mit dem Neodym-YAG-Laser. Fortschr Med 101(14):619–664, 1983.
30. Hofstetter AG, Böwering R, Keiditsch E, Frank F: Zerstörung von Uretertumoren mit dem Neodym-YAG-Laser. Verhandlungsber Dtsch Ges Lasermed 1:136–138, 1982.
31. Malloy TR, Schultz RE, Wein AJ, Carpiniello VL: Renal preservation utilizing neodymium:YAG laser. Urology 27:99–103, 1986.
32. Bailer P: Tubensterilisation durch Laser-Koagulation. Fortschr Med 43:1977, 1983.
33. Lomano JM: Photocoagulation of early pelvic endometriosis with the Nd:YAG laser through the laparoscope. Reprod Med 30:77–81, 1985.
34. Karduck A, Richter H-G: Lasermikrochirurgische Behandlung gutartiger Stimmlippenveränderungen und ihre funktionellen Ergebnisse. Laryngol Rhinol Otol 58:764–769, 1979.
35. Beck OJ, Gorisch W, Frank F: Endoskopische selektive Plexuskoagulation mittels Laser, ein denkbarer Weg zur Behandlung des Hydrocephalus? In Kaplan I (ed): Laser Surgery III, Part II. Tel Aviv, 1979, 75–78.
36. Auer LM, Ascher, PW, Holzer P: Endoscopic evacuation of intracerebral haemorrhage. High-Tech Surgical Treatment—A New Approach to the Problem? 1st International Symposium on Lasers in Cardiovascular Diseases, Baden/Vienna, 26–28 June, 1986.
37. Frank F, Hofstetter AG, Keiditsch E: Experimental investigation and new instrumentation for Nd:YAG laser treatment in urology. In Bellina JH (ed): Gynecologic Laser Surgery. Plenum Press, New York and London, 1981, pp 345–356.
38. Frank F, Halldorsson Th, Hofstetter AG, et al: Neue Instrumente und Sicherheitsuntersuchungen zur Anwendung des Neodym-YAG-Lasers. Verhandlungsber Dtsch Ges Lasermed 1:165–176, 1982.
39. Hofstetter AG, Staehler G, Keiditsch E, Frank F: Lokale Laser-Bestrahlung eines Peniskarzinoms. Fortschr Med 96:369–371, 1978.
40. Frank F, Bailer P, Beck OJ, et al: Instrumentation and safety aspects for the surgical application of the Nd:YAG laser. In Joffe SN, Muckerheid M, Goldman L (eds): Neodymium-YAG Laser in Medicine and Surgery. Elsevier, New York, 1983, 205–214.
41. Beck OJ, Frank F: ND-YAG-Laser in der Neurochirurgie. Münch Med Wochenschr (or) MMW 126:109–113, 1984.
42. Oeckler RCT, Beck OJ, Frank F: Erfahrungen mit dem Nd-YAG-Laser in der chirurgischen Behandlung intra- und suprasellärer Tumoren. Fortschr Med 102:218–220, 1984.
43. Frank F: Biophysical basis and technical requisites for the use of the Nd-YAG laser in neurosurgery. Neurosurg Rev 7:145–150, 1984.
44. Beck OJ, Frank F: The use of the Nd-YAG laser in neurosurgery. Lasers Surg Med 5:345–356, 1984.
45. Landthaler M, Brunner R, Haina D, et al: First experiences with the Nd:YAG laser in dermatology. In Joffe SN, Muckerheid M, Goldman L (eds): Neodymium-YAG Laser in Medicine and Surgery. Elsevier, New York, 1983, pp 175–183.
46. Ulrich F, Bock WJ, Schober R, Wechsler W: Repair of the carotid artery of the rat with the Nd:YAG laser. First Congress of LANSI, Fuschl, 26–30 September, 1984.
47. Schober R, Ulrich F, Sander T, et al: Laser-induced alteration of collagen substructure allows microsurgical tissue welding. Science 232:1421–1422, 1986.
48. Ulrich F, Nicola N, Bock WJ, et al: A micromanipulator to aid microsurgical removal of intracranial tumours with the Nd-YAG laser. Lasers Med Sci 1:131–133, 1986.

4
Contact Delivery Systems and Accessories

Norio Daikuzono

Contact Laser Probes offer a completely new method of delivering Nd:YAG energy to tissue, and overcome many of the limitations encountered with the conventional noncontact medical laser systems. Using less than 25 W of power, Contact Laser Probes will cut, coagulate, vaporize, or administer low levels of interstitial irradiation. They can be attached to a variety of handles for use in open surgical procedures, or can be affixed to a standard optical fiber and passed through any rigid or flexible endoscope for use in an ever-increasing range of endoscopic applications.

SLT Contact Laser Probes®[1] are made of a specially selected, physiologically neutral synthetic sapphire crystal with great mechanical strength, low thermal conductivity, and a high melting temperature (2030 to 2050°C) (Table 4.1). They are used in direct contact with tissue, which allows precisely controlled manipulations and restores the tactile feedback that was lost in conventional laser techniques. Due to the optical properties and geometric design of each probe, SLT Contact Laser Probes® shape the power density to deliver the optimal laser energy intensity and distribution for each type of procedure. By selecting the appropriate probe and laser power, not only can the user determine the precise spot size and power density, but he can also control the shape and volume of thermal effect. This is not possible with any noncontact laser or with other thermal techniques (Table 4.2). A conventional, noncontact YAG laser delivery system emits a diverging beam of gradually increasing size and diminishing power density. Approximately 30 to 40% of the beam energy can be lost to backscatter, and a portion of the rest is expended on nontargeted healthy tissue due to inaccurate focusing and beam scattering. SLT Contact Laser Probes® create a well-defined localized region of high-power density right at the tip of the probe, which is placed precisely against the target tissue. The problem of focusing is completely eliminated. Spot size and power density are under accurate and precise control. Energy loss to backscatter is cut to less than 5%, and the overall laser output power needed to achieve a given therapeutic effect is 75 to 90% lower than would be needed in a noncontact procedure. Since less total energy is delivered to the site, damage to healthy neighboring tissue is greatly reduced (Figure 4.1).

The Nd:YAG laser is ideally suited for use with SLT Contact Laser Probes®. The YAG is not limited by its absorption spectrum to any particular tissue type. It is the best available thermal coagulator, has good penetration, and its drawbacks in the noncontact mode—poor cutting, excessive backscatter, inaccuracy, and excessive tissue damage—are precisely eliminated by SLT Contact Laser Probes®. Since 25 W is the maximum power used with SLT Contact Laser Probes® in any therapeutic situation, a compact, low-cost Nd:YAG laser unit will meet every procedural requirement. A single portable laser system can be used in inpatient or outpatient operating rooms, the endoscopy suite, or the physician's office, providing an extremely versatile and cost-effective addition to any hospital or clinic (Table 4.3).

TABLE 4.1. Comparison of single crystal synthetic sapphire and quartz crystal

Property	Sapphire	Quartz
Melting point	2030–2050°C	1600°C
Thermal conductivity (g•cal•cm^2•sec) at 40°C	0.0016–0.0034	9.0158–0.0299
Coefficient of thermal expansion ($10^{-7} \times$ cm/°C)	50–67	80
Elastic coefficient ($10^{-6} \times$ kg/cm^2)	5.0	0.78
Specific gravity	4.0	2.2
Hardness (mho)	9	7
Compressive strength (kg/cm^2)	28,000	2000
Tensile strength	2000	900–1200
Refraction index	1.76	1.54
Absorption of water	0.00	0.00
Chemical characteristics	Acid- and base-proof	Acid- and base-proof
Appearance	Clear	Clear
Crystal form	Hexagonal	Hexagonal
Transmission of Nd:YAG laser	>90%	>90%

Clinical Evaluations

Both experimental and clinical studies with SLT Contact Laser Probes® have produced remarkable results.[2] Resection of rat liver could be accomplished at 5 W with a Contact Laser Scalpel, whereas noncontact Nd:YAG laser powers below 20 W invariably resulted in fatal bleeding complications. The resection was performed much more quickly with the low-power contact probe than was possible with a noncontact YAG beam (Figure 4.2).

Blood loss was significantly less in the contact surgery group because of the SLT. Laser Scalpel's® unique ability to control the balance between cutting and coagulation. The noncontact Nd:YAG laser beam produced excessive smoke at high powers, requiring evacuation, whereas smoke was not a problem at any of the powers needed in the contact situation. Most significant, however, is the difference in tissue necrosis between the two techniques. The noncontact resection caused up to 3 mm of lateral necrosis, depending upon the laser power. The contact procedure, on the other hand, did not cause liver necrosis of more than 0.5 mm under any circumstance. This was true both immediately postoperatively and at 15 days after surgery, implying more rapid healing following contact laser surgery (Figures 4.3 and 4.4).

In clinical applications SLT Contact Laser Probes® demonstrate parallel advantages: Contact procedures are better controlled and less traumatic than conventional noncontact laser techniques. In endoscopic procedures in particular, SLT Contact Laser Probes® have proved to be dramatically effective, and so versatile that they lend themselves to treatments never possible with noncontact lasers or with any other techniques. Damage to adjacent healthy tissue is reduced by up to 75%, and there is consequently much less sloughing of necrotic tissue and less incidence of subsequent infection. The depth of the thermal effect is carefully controlled, which lowers the risk of perforation when working in hollow viscera, and reduces pain because the thermal effects do not penetrate through to the serosal surface (Figure 4.5).

TABLE 4.2. Comparison of power densities: Contact vs noncontact Nd:YAG laser

Laser power (W) required to achieve given power density at the tissue surface		
Contact Nd:YAG	Noncontact Nd:YAG	Power density (W/cm^2)
1	12	700
5	62	3,500
10	124	7,000
15	185	10,500
20	247	14,000
25	309	17,500

Assumes typical noncontact Nd:YAG laser spot size of 1.5 mm and 0.4 mm diameter SLT Contact Laser Scalpel.® Power indicated is that detected after exiting fiberoptic.

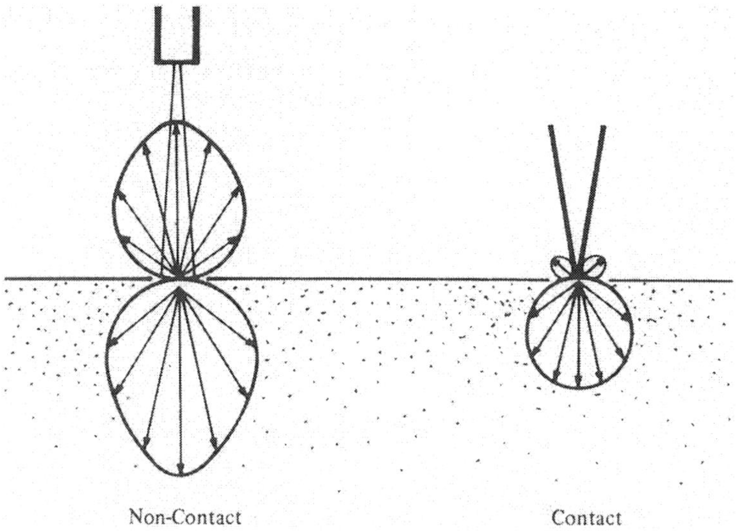

FIGURE 4.1. Nd:YAG laser energy distribution in tissue and loss through backscatter.

Contact Probes

SLT (Surgical Laser Technologies) Contact Laser Probes® are designed to serve four general medical functions: cutting, vaporization, coagulation, and delivery of interstitial irradiation (Figure 4.6). Each of these functions results from the induction of a thermal effect of given intensity in a certain tissue volume. Cutting requires intense, highly localized heat to vaporize small tissue volumes rapidly, creating a controlled incision with little damage to adjacent areas. For vaporization of fairly large tissue volumes, an intense but broader thermal effect is needed. Coagulation requires milder temperatures in yet larger volumes. For interstitial irradiation, where a probe is inserted into the tissue, one needs a fairly mild effect that is homogeneously distributed laterally as well as along the vertical axis.

SLT Contact Delivery Systems®

SLT Contact Laser Probes® can be used not only with gas delivery but also with water, which can bring several advantages to clinical application, for example, cooling adjacent normal tissue, reducing fumes, and eliminating gaseous distension of the stomach. The SLT Contact Laser® can deliver water by the simple control of a foot switch. SLT Contact Laser Probes® are designed in a variety of configurations that produce power density distributions well suited to these specific therapeutic tasks. The synthetic sapphire probes are available in two formats:

TABLE 4.3. Comparison of surgical laser system features

Feature	CO_2	Argon	Nd:YAG Noncontact	Nd:YAG Contact
Beam easily deliverable to any part of the body	No	Yes	Yes	Yes
Beam transmissible through fluids	No	Yes	Yes	Yes
Convenience in providing any required power density	Moderate	Low	Moderate	High
Precisely controllable focal point	No	No	No	Yes
Degree of damage to healthy tissue	Low	Moderate	High	Low
Smoke generation	High	Moderate	High	Low
Tactile feedback	No	No	No	Yes
Laser power requirements	High	High	High	Low
Laser maintenance requirments	Moderate	High	Low	Low
Delivery system maintenance requirements	Moderate	High	High	Low

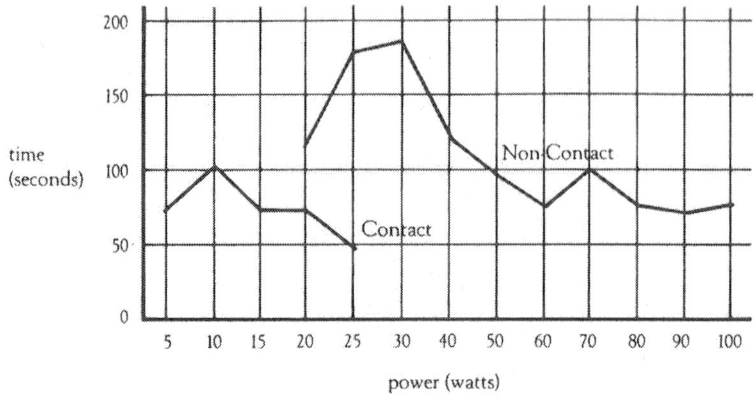

FIGURE 4.2. Time required for rat liver resection as a function of laser power

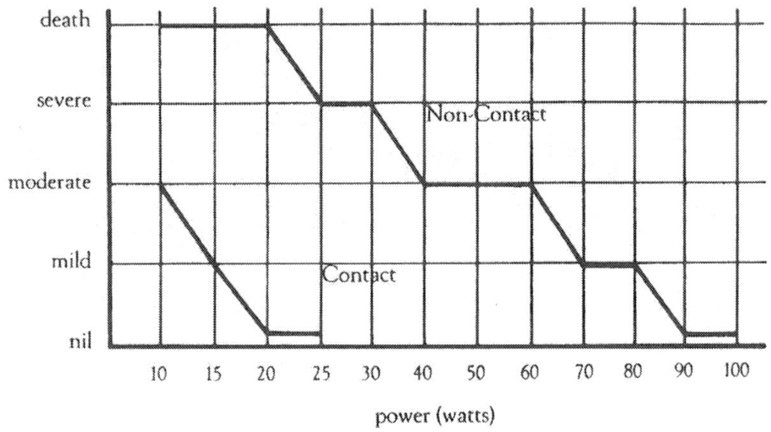

FIGURE 4.3. Blood loss as a function of laser power.

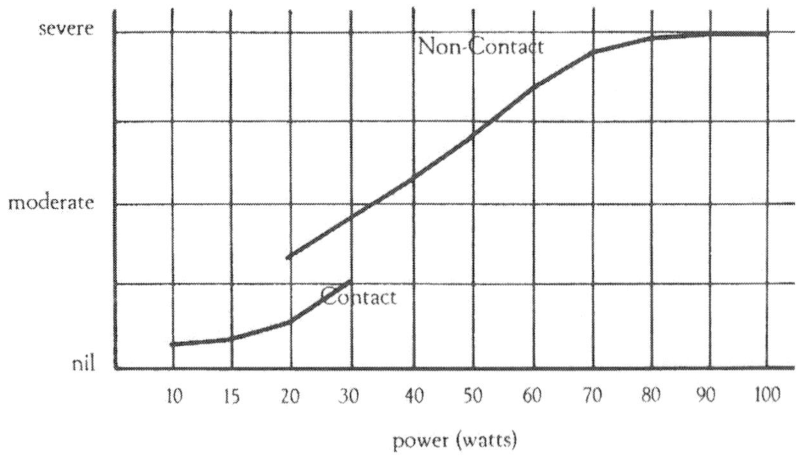

FIGURE 4.4. Amount of smoke as a function of laser power.

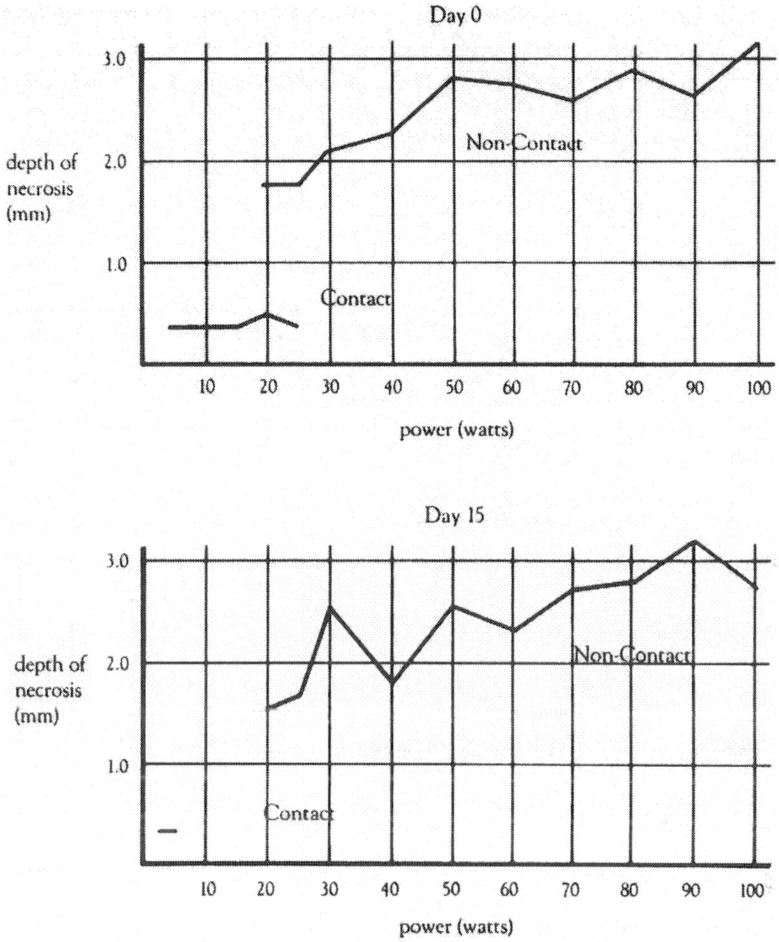

FIGURE 4.5. Depth of tissue necrosis as a function of laser power.

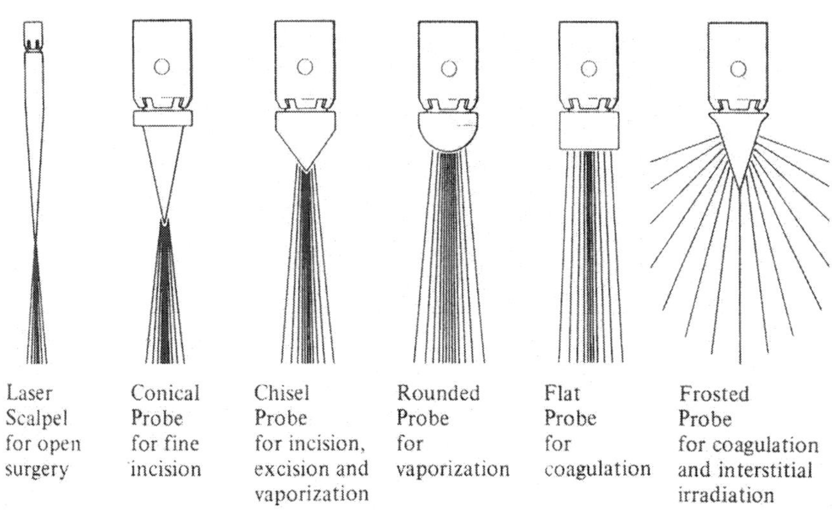

FIGURE 4.6. Contact Laser Probes and their energy distribution patterns.

(1) incising probes, called SLT Laser Scalpels®, used exclusively as hand-held instruments in open surgery for many specialties; and (2) various small SLT Contact Laser Probes® used predominantly in endoscopic applications, but which can also be used in open procedures connected with hand-held instruments (Figure 4.7). All SLT Contact Laser Probes®, handpieces, and optical fiber for endoscopy can be used with stable Nd:YAG lasers at low output powers, such as the SLT Contact Laser® (Figure 4.8). The selection of interchangeable SLT Laser Scalpels® have distal tip diameters ranging from 0.2 to 1.2 mm, and screw into a variety of handles that fit directly on the end of standard optical quartz fibers (Figure 4.9). SLT Laser Scalpels® are used with the Nd:YAG laser at powers below 25 W, and in some applications at power as low as 2–3 W. It transforms the Nd:YAG into a multidisciplinary, multipurpose surgical laser that cuts as cleanly and precisely as the CO_2 laser, yet retains the coagulative properties of the noncontact Nd:YAG.

SLT Contact Laser Probes® are designed primarily for use in endoscopic procedures. They screw onto a metal Universal Connector that fastens to 1.8 or 2.2 mm OD optical quartz fiber (Figure 4.10), and will pass through rigid endoscopes or the biopsy channel of any standard flexible fiberoptic endoscope. Different probe geometries shape the laser energy distribution into appropriate configurations for vaporization, coagulation, cutting, or interstitial irradiation. The user can, if desired, change

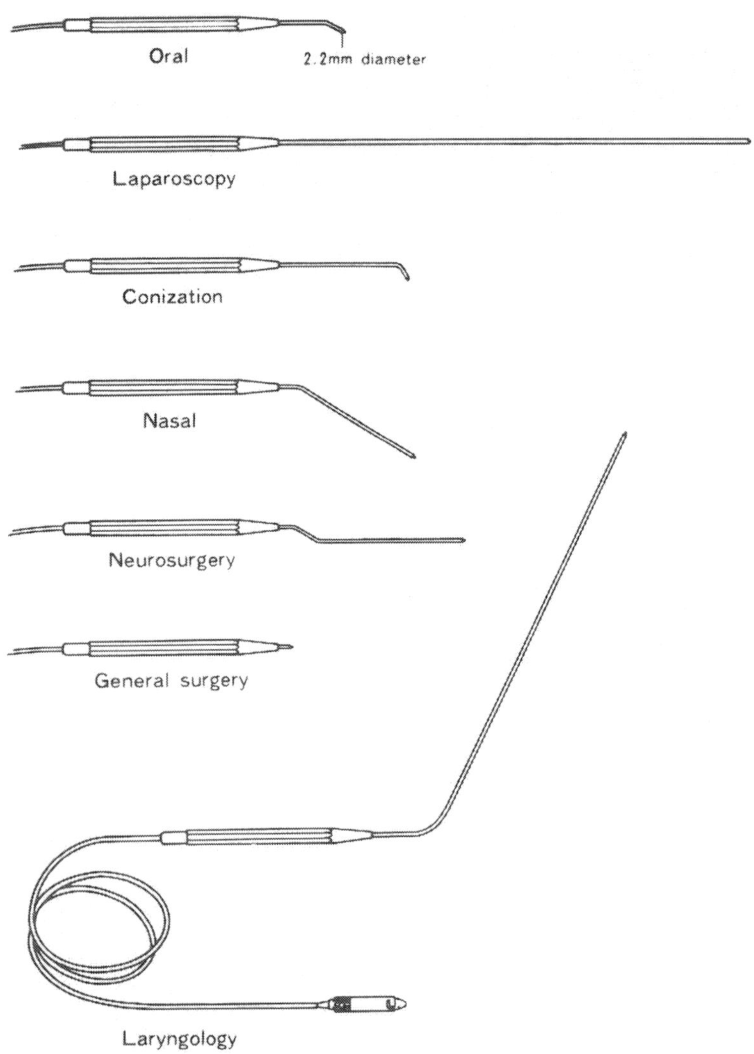

FIGURE 4.7. Optical fibers with handle.

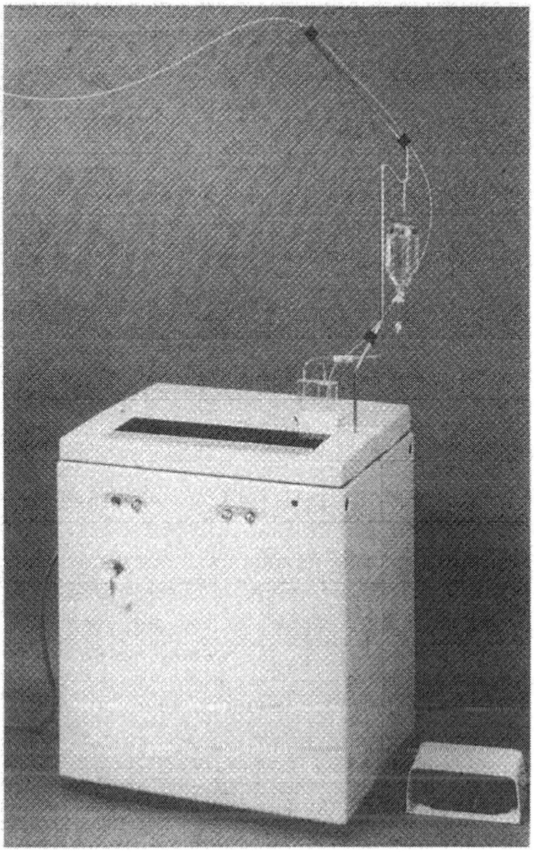

FIGURE 4.8. SLT Contact Laser.

probes during a procedure simply by withdrawing the fiber from the endoscope, unscrewing one probe, and screwing on another (Figure 4.11).

SLT Contact Laser Probes® are used with the Nd:YAG laser at powers under 25 W. The YAG beam is effective in water or at sites of active bleeding, and provides exceptional coagulative abilities. SLT Contact Laser Probes® give complete control of energy penetration and dispersion, minimizing unwanted damage to healthy tissue. Since very low laser powers are used, there is minimal backscatter and virtually no smoke. Significantly less heat is generated around the target tissue. SLT Contact Laser Probes® are designed to be either gas- or water-cooled, and in most applications coaxial water cooling can be used, eliminating the discomfort and dangers of gaseous distension of the patient. Due to the physical characteristics of the synthetic sapphire crystal, SLT Contact Laser Probes® can be used in direct contact with tissue or blood without danger of melting. Once the Universal Connector® has been affixed to the fiber, there is no need for subsequent recleaving or polishing. The direct contact technique makes possible more accurate targeting of the laser effect, even on moving tissues, and permits coaptation of bleeding vessels for simpler and more rapid hemostasis.

General Medical Functions

Cutting with the SLT Laser Scalpel® and the Conical® and Chisel Probes®

SLT incision probes provide simultaneous cutting and coagulation, while causing minimal damage to adjacent healthy tissue. Cutting can be accomplished with any of the SLT Laser Scalpels® in open surgery or with the SLT Chisel® and SLT Conical Probes® in endoscopic procedures. The geometric and optical properties of the synthetic sapphire probes are such that the YAG beam is brought to a tight focus and very high-power density exactly at the tip of the probe. Power density then drops off rapidly at short distances from the tip, giving an extremely localized and accurately controlled thermal effect (Figure 4.12). In other words, "what you see is what you get." Cutting takes place at the tip, not in adjacent tissue. When the probe is removed from the tissue, cutting ceases. This is not the case with the noncontact YAG beam. Moreover, since the thermal effects in contact cutting are so carefully circumscribed, the invisible subsurface tissue damage that can occur in noncontact YAG procedures is reduced by over 80%.

The diameter of the distal tip of the SLT Laser Scalpel® defines the spot size of the laser beam when the Scalpel is in contact with tissue. Dif-

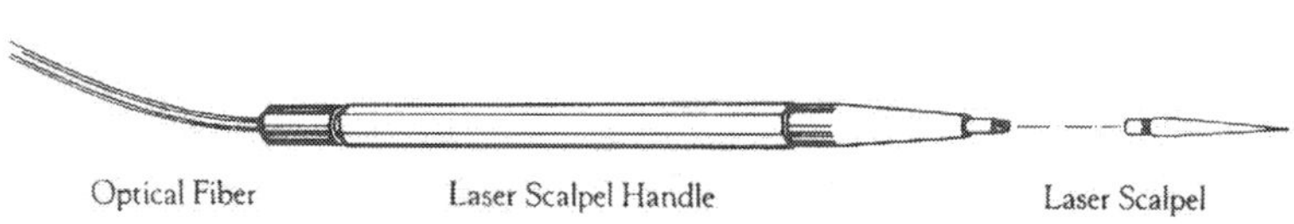

FIGURE 4.9. Contact Laser Scalpel.

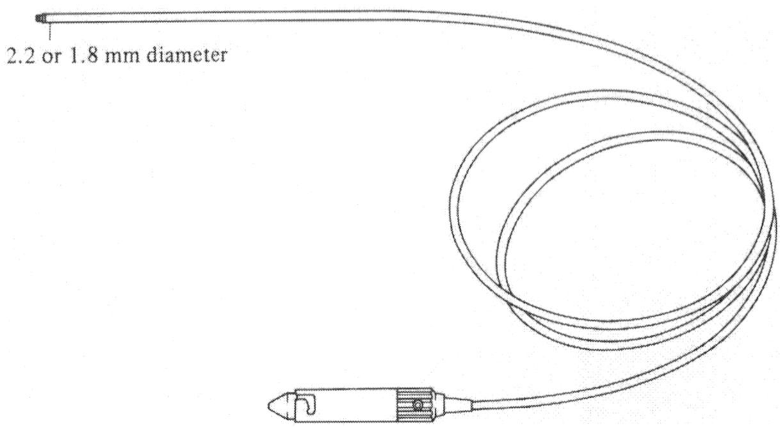

FIGURE 4.10. Optical fiber for endoscopy.

ferent Laser Scalpel tip diameters give the surgeon the ability to select either greater cutting or greater coagulation. The choice of scalpels depends upon the tissue texture and vascularity. Smaller tip diameters, for example, can be used for an initial clean incision, whereas when working with soft, highly vascular tissue such as the liver or spleen, larger tip diameters provide better hemostasis. The maximum power required is 25 W, though precise cutting can be achieved at substantially lower power levels. In general, the smaller the tip diameter, the lower the power level needed to produce a given tissue effect. The SLT Laser Scalpels® screw easily onto the various handles, and the surgeon can quickly change tips as circumstances require. While holding the tissue under tension, the SLT Laser Scalpel® should be drawn lightly across the surface of tissue, not used mechanically to separate or tear. It is the laser energy rather than physical pressure of the probe that is creating the incision. Incision depth is determined by a combination of tip diameter, laser power, and the speed of movement across the tissue.

The SLT Laser Scalpel® should be held in a comfortable and natural position, much as one would hold a pencil, although at a slightly steeper angle to the tissue surface. Since the SLT Laser Scalpel crystal® channels beam energy directly along its longitudinal axis, with virtually no lateral irradiation, the cutting effect is somewhat greater as the orientation approaches perpendicular. At the initial incision, the Laser Scalpel® may appear to cut more slowly than a steel scalpel or the CO_2 beam. Over the course of an entire procedure, however, the Laser Scalpel is considerably quicker, since it efficiently cauterizes as it cuts. When working with highly vascular tissue, there is no need to stop to ligate or clip most bleeding vessels. Vessels with the almost same diameter as the tip of the scalpel can be cut and sealed simply by moving the Laser Scalpel® slowly across them. If necessary, one can go back and coagulate bleeding spots, without changing instruments, by dabbing lightly at the area with the scalpel. For larger vessels, light dabbing or stroking with the Laser Scalpel® along each side of the vessel will create edema, after which the vessel can be cut. The Laser Scalpel uses power levels 75–90% lower than those needed by noncontact lasers to accomplish a given surgical effect. There is minimal backscatter, a constant and well-defined spot size, and less energy is put into the tissue. The result is far less damage to adjacent healthy tissue, as seen from histologic studies of incision sites. Operating time and blood loss are greatly reduced, resulting in an overall decrease in postoperative complications.

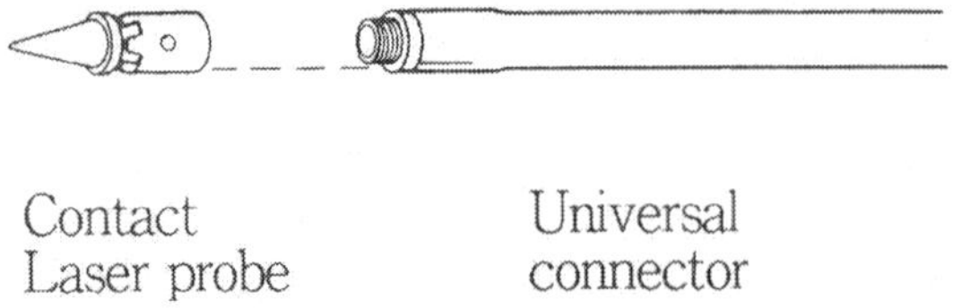

FIGURE 4.11. Contact Laser Probe.

Two different SLT Contact Laser Probes® offer a choice of endoscopic cutting styles. Powers below 15 W are sufficient for most therapeutic situations, and some operations can be performed at much lower powers. Users should realize, however, that recommended power set-

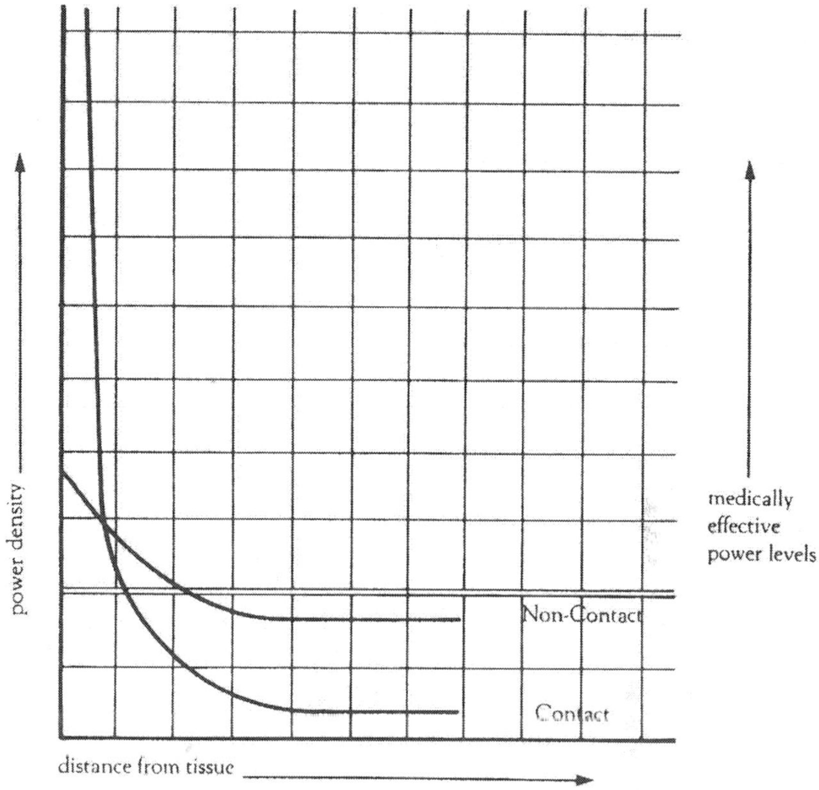

FIGURE 4.12. Power density vs distance from tissue.

tings are of less importance than the actual observed tissue effects, and changes in the tissue texture and color are the only reliable indications of the laser effect. The SLT Conical Probe® provides a power density distribution pattern very similar to that of the SLT Laser Scalpel® and is used in much the same way to create fine incisions. Since the tip of the SLT Conical Probe® should ideally be moved laterally across the tissue surface, rather than pressed against it, the use of a rigid endoscope offers certain advantages, since once the probe has been oriented against the tissue, the entire delivery system can be gently shifted to guide the incision. The SLT Chisel Probe® will cut directly through tissue, although its primary use, as its shape and name suggest, is to shave off thin layers of tissue. The SLT Chisel Probe® vaporizes and coagulates as it cuts, providing a clean and bloodless site. Used with a rigid or flexible fiberoptic endoscope, this probe can be pressed to the tissue surface and pushed lightly across it. It is ideal for recanalization of a totally or partially obstructing carcinoma of the esophagus, bronchus, or colon. It removes tissue more rapidly than vaporization with the SLT Rounded Probe®, and is effective for quick preliminary work when there is no danger of perforation. To achieve optimal cutting and greatest depth control, the SLT Chisel Probe® should be held with one of the flat faces nearly parallel to the tissue.

Coagulation with SLT Flat®, Frosted®, and Hollow Probes®

Hemostasis is accomplished by heating tissue sufficiently to produce edema and protein coagulation. For this purpose one needs a power density distribution that creates a milder, broader, and deeper thermal effect than is required for cutting or vaporization. The Nd:YAG laser is generally the instrument of choice for coagulation because its beam penetrates fluid and tissue to a depth sufficient to seal, rather than merely cap, bleeding vessels. The noncontact YAG requires 60–100 W of power for coagulation, however, which causes a certain degree of uncontrolled tissue damage and occasionally precipitates severe bleeding as a result. SLT Contact Laser Probes®, on the other hand, safely and effectively seal vessels up to 3 mm in diameter using powers below 10 W.

All SLT Contact Laser Probes® provide a certain measure of coagulative ability, but the physical shape and power density distributions of the SLT Flat® and Frosted Probes® are best suited to this purpose. The Flat Probe is the instrument most often used for general coagulation. At power settings between 8 and 10 W it provides much more rapid hemostasis than other laser or thermal methods, with minimal necrosis in adjacent tissue. The Frosted Probe, which was designed primarily for use in interstitial irradiation, can also be used for deep coagulation. By pressing this probe into mucosal tissue up to its flange, and using very low power and longer durations, less than 7 W and 9 seconds, it provides effective coagulation of vessels several millimeters below the tissue surface. Because the power is low and the probe is embedded in the tissue, neither air nor water cooling is needed with this technique.

Vaporization with the SLT Rounded Probe®

Vaporization requires higher power density and temperature than coagulation, and a broader energy delivery than is needed for cutting. The SLT Rounded Probe® allows rapid removal of thin layers of tissue for controlled debulking of large tissue volumes. The SLT Chisel Probe®, as described in the previous section on "cutting," can also be used for a cruder and quicker combination of shaving and vaporization in areas where there is little risk of perforation. When the Nd:YAG laser is used in the noncontact mode, vaporization is generally performed at 70–100 W and produces a mixed effect of coagulation and vaporization with significant bleeding and subsurface tissue damage. In endoscopic application, where the precise distance of the fiber from the target tissue and the angle of beam incidence are difficult to control, the power density and thermal effect at and below the tissue surface vary greatly and unpredictably. The SLT Rounded Probe®, on the other hand, delivers approximately the same power density as an 8o-W noncontact YAG beam using only 15 W of power, and produces true vaporization with minimal subsurface effects yet with sufficient coagulation to limit bleeding. Vaporization takes place only when the probe is in direct contact with the tissue. There are many advantages to the true vaporization delivered by the SLT Rounded Probe®. For endoscopic esophageal cancer removal, for example, the conventional noncontact technique involves coagulating to some depth below the surface, causing necrosis, waiting 48–72 hours for the blanched layer to slough off, and then repeating the process as necessary until the tumor has been removed. Until sloughing has taken place, it is not clear how deep tissue damage extends, and one must therefore proceed cautiously, layer by layer, over the course of three to eight treatment sessions. The results still may not be altogether satisfactory, since the procedure is limited by the danger of thermal or necrotic perforation. The SLT Rounded Probe®, on the other hand, actually removes layers of cells, and can vaporize tissue to an arbitrary depth in the course of one or two sessions. The probe is simply dabbed, stroked or painted across the target site, and vaporization is indicated by a slight darkening of the tissue. Because the power density is localized at the rounded surface of the probe, there is less danger of immediate thermal perforation or of later complications due to necrosis of underlying tissue, and one can confidently work closer to the mucosal wall. Water delivery is sufficient to cool the probe during endoscopic vaporization, which eliminates the discomfort and danges of patient distension, and further reduces the small quantities of smoke generated by debulking procedures. Since there is less uncontrolled heating of deep tissue layers, contact vaporization is also less painful to the patient.

Interstitial Irradiation

The primary present function of the SLT Frosted Probe® is to provide deep coagulation, but its chief future application will be in the administration of local hyperthermia and photodynamic therapy. The SLT Frosted Probe® is pushed into the tissue up to its flange and delivers YAG power density and thermal energy in a hemispherical volume of 2 to 3 cm radius. With powers of 5–7 W the SLT Frosted Probe® coagulates, but at powers in the 1- to 3-W range it provides local hyperthermia. For the treatment of areas more than 2 to 3 cm in size, multiple probes can be implanted. A feedback system for temperature, using a computer, probes connected with multiple distribution delivery systems, and thermocouples, allows far more accurate control of treatment sites than current methods.

Safety Precautions

When employing SLT Laser Scalpels® and Contact Laser Probes®, observe all regulations and safety guidelines governing the Nd:YAG laser. Though the use of lower power levels and the reduction in backscattered energy make the contact method safer than conventional noncontact techniques, any medical laser can cause harm if improperly handled. Warning notices must be posted at all entrances to any room where the laser will be used, and precautions should be taken to avoid accidental entry while the laser is in operation. Access should be restricted to personnel who have been suitably informed about the relevant safety measures. Protective eyewear, equipped with sideguards and rated as suitable for use with the Nd:YAG laser, must be worn by all personnel present in the room during a laser operation, and appropriate protective eyepieces must be used when performing endoscopic procedures. The patient should be given complete protection. Care should be taken to avoid the use of combustible gases or inflammable materials in the vicinity of the laser. Use nonreflective instruments and equipment to avoid specular reflection of the laser beam. Above all, even with SLT Contact Laser Probes® the power density of the beam drops off very quickly at short distances from the probe, the laser should be activated only when the probe is directed at the surgical site. These recommendations are not to be taken as a definitive list of safety precautions. Refer to the manual of the particular laser being employed.

References

1. Daikuzono N, Joffe SN: Artificial sapphire probe for contact photocoagulation and tissue vaporization with the Nd:YAG laser. Med Instrum 19(4):Jul–Aug, 1985.
2. Joffe SN, et al. Liver resection with the Neodymium:YAG laser. Surg Gynecol Obstet 163:437–442, 1986.

5
Clinical Applications in Gastrointestinal Bleeding

Stephen N. Joffe and Richard M. Dwyer

As recently as 1981, fewer than 12 medical centers in the United States were using lasers in the treatment of gastrointestinal (GI) disease. By 1984, 200 hospitals were using lasers for this purpose,[1] and by the end of 1986,[2] there were approximately 1,000. The reasons for such proliferation include increased applications of the use of lasers in GI problems, the relative ease with which they can be used, and the recent ruling by the Food and Drug Administration that the Nd:YAG laser is safe and effective and is therefore no longer considered to be an investigational device. Furthermore, lasers provide a multidisciplinary and multispecialty modality as well as therapeutic options where such choices did not exist or were limited previously.[3] More importantly, they have been found to be safe, efficient, and cost-effective in most cases.

Experimental Studies

In 1979 Goodale et al.[4] first reported control of bleeding from gastric erosions using a CO_2 laser with a rigid gastroscope. In 1973 Nath et al.[5] described the transmission of a laser beam through a fiberoptic flexible gastroscope, and in 1975 Dwyer[6] reported laser-induced hemostasis in an animal model. In 1979 Silverstein et al.[7] and Waitman et al.[8] compared the effects of the argon laser to the Nd:YAG laser in the treatment of experimentally induced bleeding in canine gastric ulcers. Each came to the conclusion that both types of lasers were effective in achieving hemostasis, and, since argon produced less tissue damage, it was considered safer. In the same year Dixon et al.[9] published their results of the acute and chronic studies of photocoagulation, penetration, and perforation of the Nd:YAG laser in the treatment of experimental canine gastric bleeding. According to their study, Nd:YAG laser photocoagulation was an effective method of controlling experimental bleeding. Energy densities (W/cm^2) three times that required to achieve control of bleeding were necessary to cause the serious complication of perforation. Johnston et al.[10] compared efficacy and histologic damage caused by monopolar and bipolar electrocoagulation to that of argon and Nd:YAG laser photocoagulation when applied endoscopically to control bleeding from standard canine gastric ulcers. They indicated that more energy and greater power was required with each method to treat bleeding ulcers efficiently through endoscopy than at laparotomy. They concluded that each method was 93% effective in stopping the bleeding, but the lasers were easier to use. Furthermore, the argon laser and bipolar electrocoagulation caused less tissue injury.

Laser-related tissue injury was generally predictable and correlated with total energy administered and gastric distension. A quantifiable arterial bleeding gastric ulcer was produced in dogs by McLeod et al.,[11] by suturing the splenic artery to the base of the ulcer. The main artery blood flow rate varied from 50 to 120 ml/min. The Nd:YAG laser, via the flexible endoscope, successfully arrested bleeding in all dogs. It was noted that coaxial CO_2 allowed adequate visualization of the spurting blood vessel and that the helium-neon laser provided a satisfactory aiming beam.

The histologic changes following Nd:YAG

laser photocoagulation of canine gastric mucosa were studied by Kelly et al.,[12] who concluded that exposure of the dog stomach to Nd:YAG laser produced tissue changes varying from mild mucosal edema to cell vaporization. Thermal contraction was the primary hemostatic mechanism, with thrombosis occurring only as a secondary effect.

The effect on gastric acid secretion following intragastric Nd:YAG laser application to the lesser curve and the pyloric mucosa of the stomachs of rats has been studied. This technique of intragastric vagolysis produced a statistical reduction in acid secretion maintained over several weeks.[13]

Endoscopic Applications of Lasers

Upper gastrointestinal (UGI) hemorrhage accounts for approximately 200,000 admissions to acute-care hospitals annually, making it a major health issue. Fiberoptic endoscopes can help to determine the precise cause of the bleeding in more than 90% of cases. Duodenal ulcers (24%), gastric erosions (23%), and esophageal varices (10%) account for the bleeding in the vast majority of cases.

Therapeutic endoscopy, using the laser, requires a change in approach to GI bleeding. To become a therapeutic laser endoscopist requires changing from a simple diagnostic procedure into a new therapeutic arena under emergency and often adverse circumstances. By using the laser, the amount of blood transfused and the overall morbidity and mortality of GI bleeding can be decreased. It is important to have a well-trained team to achieve the goals of early endoscopic diagnosis and laser therapy, especially in the management of critically ill patients.

The application of lasers to the problem of GI bleeding was first conceived by the University of Washington group, Silverstein and Rubin, Kiefhaber of the University of Munich, Dwyer and the Los Angeles group, and the Joffe group at the University of Glasgow. Therapeutic endoscopy developed because of a lack of any consistently effective alternate method between the extreme of ice water lavage through a nasogastric tube and laparotomy with an overall mortality rate of 10%. Widespread availability of flexible fiberoptic endoscopy in the early 1970s provided adequate visualization of the bleeding site, and the door was opened for the possibility of endoscopically controlling such a situation. In an effort to achieve this goal, many techniques were tried, including electrocoagulation, injection of vasoactive substances and sclerosant solutions, tissue adhesives, heater probes, and thrombotic sprays (Table 5.1). With technical advances represented by coupling lasers to flexible fiberoptic endoscopes, the next priority was the development of a technique for safe photocoagulation of the large variety and number of bleeding lesions found in the gastrointestinal tract. Of all the endoscopic modalities for treating UGI bleeding, the greatest amount of information is available about lasers. Tens of thousands of patients have now been treated. With the exception of injection sclerotherapy, the Nd:YAG laser is the only device used to treat both variceal and nonvariceal lesions.[14]

The clinical applications of lasers for GI bleeding are shown in Table 5.2 and refer primarily to use of the continuous wave Nd:YAG laser with a fiberoptic delivery system.

TABLE 5.1. Endoscopic methods of treating GI bleeding

Injection therapy
Variceal sclerosants
Ethanol
Topical therapy
Tissue adhesives
Clotting factors
Collagen
Ferromagnetic tamponade
Mechanical therapy
Sutures
Balloons
Hemoclips
Thermal therapy
Electrocoagulation
Monpolar
Electrohydrothermal
Bipolar (multipolar)
Heater probe
Laser
Argon
Nd:YAG
Noncontact (air fiber)
Contact (sapphire)

TABLE 5.2. GI endoscopic applications of the Nd:YAG laser

Coagulation
Acute hemorrhage
Active bleeding
Recent bleeding (e.g., visible vessel, fresh blood clot)
Stigmata of recent hemorrhage (SRH)
Potential bleeding
Angiodysplasia
Varices
Hemorrhoids
Vaporization
Neoplastic disease
Palliation
Curative
Ancillary (e.g., placement of esophageal prosthesis)
Benign stricture or web
Biliary disease
Strictures
Fracturing gallstones
Cutting
Tumor excision (polyps)
Sphincteroplasty
Stricture
Cyst drainage

Laser Fiberoptic Delivery Systems

Present fiber delivery systems are composed of fibers with a quartz core surrounded by a silicone rubber cladding and a Teflon cover. The quartz core, cladding, and Teflon cover are enclosed within a polyethylene catheter. The catheter provides protection for the fiber, permitting gas or water to flow between the fiber and catheter to cool and clean the fiber tip and the treatment site. Fibers can range from 50 to 1000 μm in diameter; the production size is 400 to 600 μm. The divergence angle of the laser beam at the tip of the catheter is typically between 8° and 12°.

Fibers are flexible and can be used in conjunction with endoscopes or attached to microscopes. Flexible fibers are easily inserted into commercial endoscopes. The endoscope manufacturers such as Olympus, Fujinon, Pentax, and ACMI provide endoscopes with biopsy channels that accept the fiber without modifications being required.

Current delivery systems have major limitations: they cannot be sterilized adequately, noncontact surgery is often difficult and imprecise, tips burn out if they touch blood or tissue, and fibers break and are expensive. If the quartz tip touches tissue or blood, it absorbs heat and melts. Then the delivery system must be removed, the polyethylene catheter and Teflon cover cut back, the quartz fiber cleaved and polished, and a new metal tip inserted. This can take 10 to 30 minutes and may have to be repeated during a procedure. Contact endoscopic surgery with endoprobes made of synthetic sapphires allow direct surgery with greater precision and safety.[15]

A Laser Endoscopy Suite

The small examining room that is usually available for diagnostic endoscopy purposes may be inadequate. The room should be sufficiently large to house a procedure table, a cart with materials for resuscitation, cardiac monitoring devices, and suction.

The laser equipment requires proper electric supply sources with special wiring, running-water facilities for cooling the high-powered lasers, and space for the stretcher. The room preferably should not have multiple entry doors, and a warning light with laser signs should be installed outside. Patients being considered for laser photocoagulation invariably have considerable blood loss and may be actively bleeding. These patients are at risk of aspiration and may require longer periods of endoscopy. Protective glass filters can be fixed to the viewing end of the flexible endoscope to prevent eye damage when the laser is activated. Videoendoscopy now allows a totally closed system for laser utilization, and, with the fiber placed into the endoscope, no eye protection is required.

In patients with UGI bleeding, gastric lavage with saline or water is initially carried out with a larger bore tube until the effluent is clear. Alternatively, if not contraindicated, vasopressin is given intravenously; this assists in causing gastric emptying and may diminish the bleeding, which aids proper visualization of the bleeding sites during endoscopy. A forward- or end-viewing endoscope with two- or single-channel endoscopes can be used. With the latter, it is preferable to use a separate polyethylene tube of adequate size with distal side holes attached to the endoscope for proper evacuation of coaxial gas and smoke known as "laser plume," which is produced during noncontact laser surgery. Coaxial water with the contact endoprobes avoid this problem and prevent gaseous abdominal distension. Endoscopy is performed using a local anesthetic and an adequate amount of intravenous Demerol and diazepam. General anesthesia is administered only when patients are uncooperative and when proper airway control is required.

The power and duration, as well as the coaxial gas or water flow, are adjusted on the laser machine, and the laser fiber is inserted through the biopsy channel of the endoscope. If the laser fiber is kept 0.5 to 1.5 cm away from the mucosa, it is known as noncontact or air–fiber photocoagulation. Touching tissue or blood with the bare quartz fiber when the laser is activated causes damage to the tip of the fiber, which will subsequently melt. In the same way, the fiber tip should be kept well outside the distal end of the endoscope; otherwise it will damage the endoscope when the laser is activated. There are several methods of treating the bleeding lesion, including peripherally, circumferentially, or Z-pattern photocoagulation.

Clinical Results in Upper GI Hemorrhage Treated with Noncontact (Air-Fiber) Nd:YAG Laser Technique

Uncontrolled Studies

In 1973 in Munich, Nath and Kiefhaber[5] first described the passage of Nd:YAG laser radiation down an endoscopic waveguide. Two years later, the first patients with gastrointestinal bleeding were treated by this group with the Nd:YAG laser, and, by 1979, Kiefhaber[16] reported treating 459 patients with 94% permanent hemostasis. Subsequently, the number of unselected patients treated by Kiefhaber[17,18] increased to 852. Bleeding was treated successfully in 92% of the 1092 acute bleeding episodes. In bleeding esophageal varices, the mortality was reduced from 70% to 36% by using sclerotherapy following laser photocoagulation. Comparing the results of laser treatment versus surgery, the mortality rate from bleeding acute ulcers was reduced from 58% with gastric resection to 23% using the laser, and from 15% for vagotomy to 0% using the laser.[18] Reasons for failure include coagulopathies, especially those associated with platelet abnormalities and technical difficulties, which included a bleeding site inaccessible to the laser beam.

Many centers in the United States and Europe are now using the Nd:YAG laser for the treatment of GI bleeding. Results are variable, depending on multiple factors, not least of which is the training and learning experience of the users of these endoscopic methods and their ability to undertake emergency endoscopy efficiently, safely, and with accuracy in determining the bleeding lesion before the laser is even used. Use of the argon laser has virtually been discontinued for treatment of GI bleeding, as it appears adequate only in stopping superficial lesions such as erosions.[19–21]

Controlled Studies

The efficacy and safety of laser therapy for GI hemorrhage have been evaluated in controlled trials[22–30] and reviews published.[31] Although scientific evaluation of any new modality requires a randomized and controlled study to resolve uncertainty, variations in design, size of study populations, and interpretations of data may prevent a definitive answer. Studies need to be precisely assessed with regard to which bleeding patients were studied. To date, nine studies have been performed using the Nd:YAG laser with the noncontact technique, of which eight relate to nonvariceal bleeding.[22–29]

The following sections summarize details of these controlled randomized clinical trials performed to evaluate safety and effectiveness of the Nd:YAG laser in the treatment of UGI hemorrhage. In each of these studies, patients presenting with acute UGI bleeding were allocated to either a control or a laser-treatment group.

London Study

In the London multicenter Nd:YAG study[25,32] recently completed, 527 consecutive patients were admitted with UGI hemorrhage. At emergency endoscopy, the 260 patients with peptic ulcer and the 138 cases of stigmata of recent hemorrhage (SRH) were included in the trial as

TABLE 5.3. London study of Nd:YAG laser in upper GI bleeding

Treatment group	Total	Rebleed	Surgery	Died
Laser	70	7	7	1
Contol	68	27	24	8
		$p < 0.001$	$p < 0.005$	$p < 0.05$

being accessible to laser therapy. Of this group, 26 patients had inaccessible lesions for laser treatment and 97 had no SRH. The laser-treated patients had a significant reduction in rebleeding ($p < 0.001$), requirement for emergency surgery ($p < 0.05$), and mortality ($p < 0.05$). Notably, only 10% of the laser-treated patients required emergency surgery, compared to 35% in the control group, of whom 33% died postoperatively (Table 5.3).

Stratification of the different endoscopic appearances of the bleeding lesions showed the importance of treating visible vessels with the laser ($p < 0.01$) (Table 5.4).

Glasgow Study

The criteria for entry into the Glasgow single-blind controlled study[26] were a major UGI bleed (at least 3 pints of blood, hemoglobin < 10 g/dl, shock or postural hypotension), and at the time of emergency endoscopy a lesion had to be visualized. From a consecutive pool of 698 patients admitted with acute nonvariceal UGI hemorrhage, 184 patients were found to have gastric or duodenal ulceration as a cause for the bleeding; 16 patients were found to have a visible vessel, either bleeding or not bleeding, and were subsequently randomized to active laser treatment or to act as a control. Only those patients who would have been considered for emergency surgery were included.

This study, which was the first prospective randomized investigation into the therapeutic effect of the Nd:YAG laser, also showed a reduction in bleeding and in the requirement for emergency surgery. No perforations were reported, and the mortality rate following surgery was a high, but commonly reported, 25% in the non-laser-treated patients (Table 5.5).

Belgium Study

In the Belgium study,[22] 388 consecutive cases with bleeding peptic ulcers were admitted. Of these, 152 patients were included in the trial (129 ulcers). Patients were divided into two bleeding groups: patients who had active arterial bleeding and patients who had active, but nonpulsatile, bleeding at the time of endoscopy. The results in the ulcer group combine recurrent and continued bleeding as rebleeding (Table 5.6).

The rebleeding rate in Group 2 was significantly reduced ($p < 0.005$) in the laser-treated group. This trial had a major disadvantage, in that the ethical committee refused to allow randomization of the highest-risk patients with spurting vessels to a control group.

In the first group, although the initial hemostasis achieved with the Nd:YAG laser was 87%, there were episodes of rebleeding, thereby lowering the figures of permanent hemostasis to 45%. In the second group, the initial hemostasis was achieved in 100% and an incidence of 5% rebleeding was noted.

Other Studies

In four additional studies[23,24,27,28] it was concluded that the laser-treated group did no better than the control groups with regard to continued bleeding, need for surgery, or mortality. In the study of Rohde et al.[27] only active bleeders were included, and the authors did not believe laser therapy was of value. In two other studies[23,24] the features of the design may have made it difficult to ascertain a laser benefit, if one actually existed.

Krejs[28] recently assessed the Nd:YAG laser

TABLE 5.4. Lesions found on emergency endoscopy

Treatment group	Visible vessel		SRH		Overlying clots	
	No.	Rebleeding	No.	Rebleeding	No.	Rebleeding
Laser	39	6	17	0	13	1
Control	43	23	13	1	11	2
		$p < 0.01$		NS		NS

SRH, stigmata of recent hemorrhage; NS, not significant.

TABLE 5.5. Glasgow study of Nd:YAG in upper GI bleeding

Treatment group	Total	Rebleed	Surgery	Died
Laser	8	2	1	0
Contol	8	8	8	2
		$p < 0.001$	$p < 0.001$	NS

NS, not significant.

in a 30-month randomized, controlled trial. Actively bleeding patients (18 laser, 15 control) and patients who had recently bled and stopped but had stigmata of recent hemorrhage (64 laser, 69 control) were studied. The laser conferred no benefit to either group. The study must be faulted, as the most severely ill patients, those who could not be transported to the laser, were excluded. Furthermore, the laser treatment was often carried out by rotating residents in training who probably did not have sufficient skill or experience.

Trudeau et al.[29] evaluated the Nd:YAG laser for patients with endoscopic stigmata of recent bleeding with visible vessels. In the 33 patients studied, the Nd:YAG laser reduced the number of rebleeding episodes, reduced the need for urgent surgery, and improved survival.

A point to be noted is that there was not a single perforation in any of these eight studies where the laser was used to treat nonvariceal bleeding in severely ill patients. The evidence is thus overwhelming in the truly scientifically performed studies that the Nd:YAG laser is effective in UGI bleeding, and there can be no argument regarding its safety.

The study of Fleischer[30,31] randomized patients with active esophageal variceal bleeding into a laser-treatment group and a control group. In this small study, initial hemostasis was significantly greater in the laser-treated group, but the variceal incidence of rebleeding was high. Laser therapy may be useful for acute variceal bleeding and may be of interim benefit, but it does not represent definitive therapy. A similar conclusion was reached by Kiefhaber et al.[18] in a larger uncontrolled series. They were successful in stopping variceal hemorrhage in 160 or 174 episodes of bleeding, but, because of a moderately high incidence of rebleeding, they recommended that sclerotherapy be performed early for more definitive treatment.

In summary, the Nd:YAG laser is effective in stopping active UGI bleeding and reduces the need for emergency surgery. The rebleeding from spurting arteries or new lesions can be managed successfully by repeated laser photocoagulation. Perforations have not been a problem. The argon laser, in randomized studies, has been shown to have no effect on the rate of rebleeding, necessity for operation, or mortality.[19,20]

Clinical Results in Other GI Bleeding Conditions

Colonic Hemorrhage Due to Benign Lesions

Colonic lesions can be treated with the Nd:YAG laser, bearing in mind the thinness of the distended colonic wall. Lesions such as bleeding diverticulae and arteriovenous malformations

TABLE 5.6. Belgium study of Nd:YAG in upper GI bleeding

Group	Type of bleeding	Total	Rebleed	Surgery	Died
1	*Spurting*				
	Laser	23	14	14	7
	Control		No Controls		
2	*Nonspurting*				
	Laser	38	2	1	6
	Control	32	12	4	5
3	*Stigmation – Recent Bleed*				
	Laser	14	3	2	2
	Control	22	7	5	3

may be coagulated by using 60- to 70-W power and an exposure time duration of 0.1 to 0.3 seconds, with noncontact and 8- to 12-W with exposure time of 2 to 3 seconds with the contact endoprobe and coaxial water. Coaxial water avoids distension and reduces the risk of perforation, and, by combining it with lower laser energy, it reduces thermal damage.

Nonbleeding Benign GI Lesions

The Osler–Weber–Rendu syndrome may exhibit as single or multiple, small or large vascular malformations. Following successful laser therapy, new lesions might appear in different sites. This requires "harvesting" of gastric and colonic lesions on a periodic basis to prevent further bleeding episodes. Other lesions that may bleed include benign polyps in the stomach, duodenum, or colon, which can be both photocoagulated and vaporized.

Malignant Lesions of the GI Tract

Laser therapy has been used to control bleeding in malignant lesions of the gastrointestinal tract, which either helps to prepare the patient for definitive surgery or obviates the need for further surgical intervention in an incurable situation.

Current Status

Lasers are readily available in the United States, Europe, and Japan. The Food and Drug Administration no longer classifies the laser as an experimental device for any gastrointestinal application. There are more controlled and uncontrolled data suggesting the safety and efficacy of the laser than are available for any other endoscopic method of treatment, whether by thermal means or not.

Previously, the laser had two inherent disadvantages. One was portability, and this problem is being addressed. The newer medium-powered Nd:YAG lasers require single-phase 208 to 220 V and are air cooled. This is opposed to three-phase electrical and special water hookups of the high-powered lasers. Mobility is now much less of a problem. The cost of lasers is approximately 5 to 20 times higher than that of other endoscopic hemostatic methods. This means that if a physician or hospital does not plan to use the laser for purposes other than the treatment of bleeding, it is unlikely to be cost-effective, unless the volume of cases to be treated is at least one per week. However, the Nd:YAG laser has other applications in GI, such as recanalization of obstructing carcinomas of the esophagus, stomach, and colon, as well as treatment of polyps and other tumors. In 1986, more than 500 medical centers worldwide, about 300 of which are in the United States, are using lasers to treat gastrointestinal disease.[14]

The various methods of endoscopic therapy of UGI bleeding in humans has been reviewed by Fleischer[14] (Table 5.7). The amount of information that exists from rigorously controlled scientific studies is small. Equally disturbing is the minimal information published on studies

TABLE 5.7. Evidence that endoscopic therapy is beneficial in upper GI bleeding

	Efficacy established							
	Bleeding from varices				Bleeding from ulcers			
Method	None	Anecdotal report	Uncontrolled series	Controlled trial	None	Anecdotal report	Uncontrolled series	Controlled trial
Topical	X			0		4		0
Injection			6	10			4	0
Mechanical	X			0			1	0
Thermal								
Monopolar	X		0	0			3	1
Bipolar	X		0	0			2	2
Heater probe	X		0	0			3	0
Laser			1	1			3	6

Number indicates number of published papers.
Adapted and updated from Fleischer D: Endoscopic therapy of upper gastrointestinal bleeding. Gastroenterology 90:22 234, 1986.

that compare the different modalities for treating the same lesion in humans. Some comparative information exists for animal models, which cannot always be translated into the clinical situation. Experimentally induced ulcers are pathologically, histologically, and hemodynamically different from those found in humans.

Contact Nd:YAG Laser Photocoagulation

Daikuzono and Joffe[15] recently developed a synthetic sapphire crystal attached to the end of the quartz fiber using a universal metal connector that allows contact Nd:YAG laser photocoagulation. The geometric shape of these synthetic sapphires provides the desired endoscopic effects of coagulation for bleeding and vaporization or excision of tumors. The power density (W/cm^2) is directly related to the distance of the probe from tissue. The contact probes prevent the backscattering of light, reduce the depth of tissue damage, and allow for much lower powers of laser energy to be used.

Several centers in Europe, Japan, and the United States[33] are currently evaluating the contact endoprobes in both upper and lower GI surgery.

Physical compression of the vessel walls allows a more effective form of closure with coagulation, known as coaptation. The noncontact Nd:YAG laser may be less effective than either of the other techniques, as pressure cannot be applied to tissue without burning and melting the fiber tip, making coaptation impossible. In order to stop bleeding from moderately large vessels, substantial amounts of energy must be applied to the tissue with the noncontact method, causing significant damage and occasionally even precipitating further bleeding. Moreover, the noncontact laser technique produces smoke that requires special evacuation, and the coaxial gas flow creates problems of patient distension, which increases risk of perforation and gas embolization.

The conventional noncontact method is typically used for endoscopic coagulation at powers in the 60- to 100-W range. Contact laser probes safely and efficiently seal vessels 1 to 3 mm in diameter, using powers below 10 W. Because of the low overall power and the reduction in scattered energy, there is virtually no smoke. Water irrigation applied coaxially at a low flow is adequate for cooling the fiber-to-probe junction. Contact laser probes can be applied directly to the tissue, which provides tactile feedback during YAG laser procedures, and allows tamponading of vessels for more effective hemostasis.

The *flat probe* is the instrument most often used for coagulation. The technique employed is similar to that used in the noncontact method of laser photocoagulation. Rosettes are formed around the periphery of the bleeding vessel to initiate edema. When bleeding visibly decreases, which may take up to 30–45 seconds, the probe can be used mechanically to coapt and seal the vessel with short pulses of energy.

To prevent heat dissipation of the absorbed Nd:YAG laser energy in a spurting blood vessel, and to create a sufficiently deep thrombosis, laser powers under 10 W, administered in 0.5- to 3-second pulses, are most effective. With the power off, the flat probe can be pressed directly onto the tissue. Firing the laser in pulses produces a high temperature change in the tissue (160–250°C), which, when applied to vessel walls, induces a glue-like adhesion, providing coaptation and coagulation of the vessel.

When properly employed, the contact laser endoprobe will not melt and can be reused. However, if the laser is activated for more than 2 seconds while a probe is not in contact with tissue—especially at higher powers—the probe may turn white and change shape. If this happens, the probe's optical and geometrical properties are irreversibly altered, and the probe must be replaced. The user should not deactivate the laser before removing the probe from the tissue or it may adhere. If sticking does occur, the probe should not be pulled off, but instead a short laser pulse should be given while gently withdrawing the probe from the tissue. Coaxial water irrigation further reduces the possibility of adhesion.

During the circumferential treatment of a bleeding site, one establishes a simple repetitive pattern. By setting the laser for 2- to 3-second intervals, the probe is placed on the tissue, the foot pedal pressed, the probe lifted off, and the foot pedal released. Alternatively, the laser is set in the continuous mode and the probe is "walked" around the bleeding site, touching the tissue for 0.5- to 2.0-second intervals at each spot. It is important when using contact endoprobes that the laser provide a stable output in a low power range, as sudden uncontrollable power bursts will not only damage the tissue being treated but will also cause irreversible damage to the probes.

Techniques may have to be altered, depending on the type of tissue, the lesion being treated, blood flow, and numerous other factors. The only true indication of coagulation is cessation of bleeding or blanching around the treatment site. Individual users with experience develop their own methods of treatment.

Each type of bleeding lesion must be identified and evaluated independently. Prior to endoscopy, if the patient is actively bleeding and/or there are blood clots in the stomach, the stomach must be emptied for adequate visualization of the bleeding site. This can be performed in one of several ways. The preferred technique is to pass a large-bore tube (Ewald) and irrigate the stomach with cold saline continuously until the effluent is minimally pink-stained and there are no further blood clots. If the endoscope is passed and blood clots are still found in the stomach, the procedures should be repeated. An alternative or supplementary method is to give intravenous injection of metoclopramide (Reglan) and a bolus of vasopressin (20 units over 10 minutes), provided that there are no contraindications. Endoscopy is performed in a standard manner under sedation. If the patient is actively bleeding and there is risk of aspiration, then endotracheal intubation should be performed.

At the end of the procedure, all lesions are gently washed off and observed for a minimum of 3 to 5 minutes to make sure that the bleeding has stopped completely. Fresh frozen plasma and blood are given as required. Clotting defects are corrected and antacids, H_2-receptor antagonists, and cytoprotective agents are prescribed. In the event of rebleeding, the procedure can be repeated.

Bleeding Gastric and Duodenal Ulcers with a Visible Vessel

The flat probe is applied circumferentially around the rim of the ulcer. Subsequently, the probe can be applied directly to the vessel for final coagulation and coaptation. If the probe sticks to the vessel, the laser power is set too high, producing vaporization of tissue. If adhesion occurs, the power should be adjusted down (under 10 W), and with the laser activated, the probe can be gently disengaged from the tissue.

When there is massive bleeding from a vessel, the flat probe can be pressed directly against the vessel and the laser activated at 8–10 W for 2 to 3 seconds. This will slow bleeding sufficiently to allow circumferential treatment.

Bleeding Erosions

Bleeding erosions have several punctate bleeding points from arteriolar and capillary vessels at the edges or in the base of the erosion. Using the flat probe, these can be directly photocoagulated. If there is a diffuse ooze, the Z-shooting technique is used. With laser power on, the probe is moved back and forth over the tissue surface in a zigzag fashion. This coagulates the vessels feeding into the bleeding area. The bleeding points within the triangular areas are then directly treated.

Bleeding Esophageal Varices

Bleeding is decreased using a vasopressin infusion and an inflated Sengstaken-Blakemore tube inserted 4 hours before the procedure. In a manner similar to the circumferential treatment, the flat probe is used to coagulate parallel lines on either side of the varix, either starting distally and working proximally or vice versa, but avoiding direct treatment of the varix. The procedure is repeated, working closer and closer to the varix until adequate vasoconstriction is obtained. Only when bleeding has decreased is the probe placed on the varix itself to coapt the vessel proximal to the bleeding site. If the varix is bleeding actively during the procedure, a gastric balloon is inflated and pulled up tightly to the cardioesophageal junction to decrease blood flow.

For a bleeding varix in the stomach, the feeding vessels around the bleeding site are coapted and waiting for 30–45 seconds to allow edema and coagulation of the feeding vessels to occur.

Bleeding Mallory–Weiss Tear

The flat probe is applied around the bleeding site, which coagulates the blood vessels supplying the bleeding point. Once bleeding has diminished, the bleeding point itself can be coagulated.

Lower GI Bleeding

Although there are many causes of lower GI bleeding, angiodysplasia is the condition for which the Nd:YAG laser, particularly when used in conjunction with contact probes, has demonstrated the clear advantages.

Contact photocoagulation with the flat probe is performed circumferentially around the angiodysplastic lesion in an attempt to seal off the feeding vessels. Immediately upon coagulation and coaptation of the feeding vessels, bleeding stops.

More recently we have been evaluating a *hollow cylindrical* contact probe at low power. The probe is used only with coaxial saline to prevent air embolization. The thermal effect simulates the noncontact high-powered laser, producing an effect on tissue at greater depth, but with the added advantage of coaptation. This endoprobe may be especially useful in the very actively bleeding visible vessel, such as arterial spurters.

The *frosted interstitial* probe provides interstitial irradiation with deep coagulation. Although primarily used in local hyperthermia and photodynamic therapy, it may have a place in GI bleeding. Pushed directly into the tissue up to its flange, adjacent to a bleeding site, either variceal or nonvariceal, it delivers a power density and thermal energy in a hemispherical volume up to a 2-cm radius. With powers of 5–7 W, it coagulates and can be moved circumferentially around the bleeding site. More clinical experience is required. A comparison of endoscopic hemostatic techniques, listing advantages and disadvantages, is given in Table 5.8, and features of contact and noncontact laser effects is given in Table 5.9.

Currently, the endoscopic method of contact laser photocoagulation has been used in over 200 patients with a success rate of over 90% in stopping bleeding without any complications or perforation. A randomized prospective study would help in its definitive evaluation, but this is most unlikely at present.

Conclusions

Endoscopic laser therapy for GI bleeding should be considered as one approach in the broad range of therapeutic possibilities. During emergency endoscopy for GI bleeding it is wise to anticipate that laser therapy may be required. If possible, the endoscopist should be prepared to deliver treatment, if appropriate, at the time he embarks on the diagnostic endoscopy. In

TABLE 5.8. Comparative endoscopic hemostatic techniques

Characteristic	Monopolar	Bipolar	Heat probe	Argon	Noncontact YAG	Contact YAG
Efficacy with major arterial bleeding	High	Sometimes	High	Low	Moderate	High
Tamponade during coagulation	Limited	Limited	Yes	No	No	Yes
Coagulation through desiccated tissue	No	Poor	Yes	Yes	Yes	Yes
Controlled coagulation depth	No	No	Yes	No	No	Yes
Tissue erosion potential	Yes	Yes	No	Yes	Yes	No
Risk of perforation	High	High	Low	Low	High	Low
Adjacent tissue damage	Yes	Yes	Yes	No	Yes	No
Coaxial irrigation possible	Yes	Sometimes	Yes	No	No	Yes
Gas insufflation required	No	No	No	Yes	Yes	Yes
Nonsticking probe	No	No	Yes	N/A	N/A	Yes
Large-channel endoscope needed	Yes	Sometimes	Yes	No	No	No
Interference with electronic equipment	Yes	Yes	No	No	No	No
Ability to cut and vaporize	No	No	No	No	Poor	No

TABLE 5.9. Contact versus noncontact Nd:YAG characteristics

Characteristic	Noncontact	Contact
Power levels		
Coagulation	60–100 W	10 W
Vaporization	70–100 W	8–15 W
Blood loss	High	Low
Smoke generation	High	Low
Width and depth of thermal damage	3–5 mm	0.2–1.0 mm
Energy lost to backscatter	30–40%	5%
Tamponading of bleeding vessels	No	Yes
Fiber maintenance requirement	Frequent	Infrequent
Tactile feedback	No	Yes
Pain to patient	Moderate	Low
Risk of perforation	High	Low

many instances, the treatment chosen will be dictated by the availability of therapeutic modality and the skill of the operator.

For variceal bleeding, only sclerotherapy and Nd:YAG laser treatment are options at present. For nonvariceal bleeding, injection therapy, electrocoagulation, laser photocoagulation, and the heater probe are reasonable considerations. The overwhelming evidence, however, points to the success of the Nd:YAG laser in this area.

Contact laser photocoagulation combines the coagulating properties of the Nd:YAG laser with the tactile feedback and coaptive features of the contact endoprobe. It provides safe, rapid, effective hemostasis. Accurately targeted low-power Nd:YAG laser energy causes less surface damage and lateral necrosis than other thermal techniques, yet offers a controlled penetrating thermal effect. Moreover, with a single versatile instrument, one has the ability not only to coagulate, but to cut and vaporize for other pathologic conditions.

The multidisciplinary applications of the Nd:YAG laser system make it a universal tool in the armamentarium of therapeutic endoscopy and open surgery. The incorporation of minimally invasive surgery, cost containment, and improved quality of patient care will expand its applications in the health care industry.

References

1. Fleischer D: Endoscopic laser therapy for gastrointestinal diseases. Arch Intern Med 144:1225–1230, 1984.
2. Joffe SN: The Nd:YAG laser—Past, present and future perspectives. Proceedings of the International Nd:YAG Laser Society, Tokyo, Japan, 1986.
3. Joffe SN, Muckerheide MC, Goldman L: Neodymium-YAG Laser in Medicine and Surgery. Elsevier, New York, 1983.
4. Goodale R, Okaka A, Gonzales R, et al: Rapid endoscopic control of bleeding gastric erosions by laser radiation. Arch Surg 101:211, 1970.
5. Nath G, Gorish W, Kiefhaber P: First laser endoscopy via a fiberoptic transmission system. Endoscopy 5:203, 1973.
6. Dwyer R, Havirback B, Bass M, Cherlow J: Laser-induced hemostasis in the canine stomach. JAMA 231:486, 1975.
7. Silverstein F, Auth D, Rubin C: Argon vs. Nd:YAG laser photocoagulation and experimental canine gastric ulcers. Gastroenterology 77:491, 1979.
8. Waitman AM, Grant DZ, Debeer R, Chryssanthou C: Endoscopic laser photocoagulation: Comparison of argon and Nd:YAG. Gastrointest Endosc 25:52, 1979.
9. Dixon JA, Berenson MM, McCloskey DW: Nd:YAG laser treatment of experimental canine gastric bleeding. Gastroenterology 77:647–652, 1979.
10. Johnston JH, Jensen DM, Mautner W: Comparison of endoscopic electrocoagulation and laser photocoagulation of bleeding canine gastric ulcers. Gastroenterology 82:904–910, 1982.
11. MacLeod IA, Bow DR, Joffe SN: A quantifiable bleeding gastric ulcer in dogs for assessing the neodymium YAG laser. Endoscopy 14:9–10, 1982.
12. Kelly DF, Bown SG, Calder BM, et al: Histological changes following Nd:YAG laser photocoagulation of canine gastric mucosa. Gut 24:916–920, 1983.

13. Joffe SN, Sanker MY, Brackett K: Effect of Intragastric Vagolysis on Acid Secretion. Elsevier, Optoelectronics, Munich, 1983.
14. Fleischer D: Endoscopic therapy of upper gastrointestinal bleeding. Gastroenterology 90:217–234, 1986.
15. Daikuzono N, Joffe SN: Artificial sapphire probe for contact photocoagulation and tissue vaporization with the Nd:YAG laser. Med Instrum 19:173–178, 1985.
16. Kiefhaber P: International experience with lasers for gastrointestinal bleeding. Proceedings of the International Laser Congress, Detroit, MI, 1979.
17. Kiefhaber P, Kiefhaber K, Huber F, Nath G: Endoscopic applications of neodymium YAG laser radiation in the gastrointestinal tract. In Joffe SN (ed): Neodymium-YAG Laser in Medicine and Surgery. Elsevier, New York, 1983, pp 6–14.
18. Kiefhaber P, Kiefhaber K, Huber F, Nath G: Endoscopic neodymium:YAG laser coagulation in gastrointestinal hemorrhage. Endoscopy 18(Suppl 2):46–51, 1986.
19. Vallon AG, Cotton PB, Laurence BH, et al: Randomized trial of endoscopic argon laser photocoagulation in bleeding peptic ulcers. Gut 22:228–233, 1981.
20. Swain CP, Storey DW, Northfield TC, et al: Controlled trial of argon laser photocoagulation in bleeding peptic ulcers. Lancet ii:1313–1316, 1981.
21. Jensen DM, Machicado GA, Tapia JF, et al: Endoscopic argon laser photocoagulation of patients with severe gastrointestinal bleeding. Gastrointest Endosc 28:151, 1982.
22. Rutgeerts P, VanTrappen G, Broekhaert L: Controlled trial of neodymium YAG laser treatment of upper digestive hemorrhage. Gastroenterology 83:410–416, 1982.
23. Ihre T, Johansson C, Seligsson U, et al: Endoscopic YAG laser treatment in massive UGI bleeding. Scand J Gastroenterol 16:633–640, 1981.
24. Escourrou J: Nd:YAG laser therapy for acute gastrointestinal hemorrhage. In Atsumi K , Nimsakul N (eds): Laser Tokyo 1981. Tokyo Intergroup Corp., 1981.
25. Swain C, Brown S, Salmon P, et al: Controlled trial of Nd:YAG laser photocoagulation in bleeding peptic ulcers. Lasers Surg Med 3:111, 1983.
26. MacLeod IA, Mills PR, MacKenzie JF, et al: Neodymium yttrium aluminium garnet laser photocoagulation for major haemorrhage from peptic ulcers and single vessels in a single blind controlled study. Br Med J 286:345–348, 1983.
27. Rohde H, Thon K, Fischer M, et al: Results of a defined therapeutic concept of endoscopic neodymium-YAG-laser therapy in patients with upper gastrointestinal bleeding. Br J Surg 67:360, 1980.
28. Krejs GJ, Little KH, Westergaard M, et al: Laser photocoagulation for the treatment of acute peptic ulcer bleeding: A randomized controlled clinical trial. NEJM 316, 1618–1621, 1987.
29. Trudeau W, Siepler JK, Ross K, et al: Endoscopic neodymium:YAG laser photocoagulation of bleeding ulcers with visible vessels. Gastrointest Endosc 31:138, 1985.
30. Fleischer D: Endoscopic Nd:YAG laser therapy for active esophageal variceal bleeding. A randomized controlled study. Gastrointest Endosc 31:4–9, 1985.
31. Fleischer D: Endoscopic laser therapy for upper gastrointestinal tract disease. Surv Dig Dis 1:42 53, 1983.
32. Swain CP, Kirkham JS, Salmon PR, et al: Controlled trial of Nd:YAG laser photocoagulation in bleeding peptic ulcers. Lancet i:1113–1116, 1986.
33. Joffe SN: Contact neodymium:YAG laser surgery in gastroenterology: A preliminary report. Lasers Surg Med 6:155–157, 1986.

6
Laser Treatment for Advanced or Recurrent Cancer of the Gastrointestinal Tract

Yoshiki Hiki, Tetsuhiko Yamao, and Hitoshi Shimao

In 1973, Nath et al.[1] were the first to publish the medical application of laser endoscopy. The trials for treating diseases of the digestive organs endoscopically began around 1975. Frühmorgen et al.,[2,3] Kiefhaber et al.,[4] Dwyer et al.,[5] and Waitman et al.[6] published the results of their experimental and clinical studies on the use of laser endoscopy in hemostatic therapy for digestive tract hemorrhage.

In Japan, reports on laser endoscopy appeared in 1979, and at the Congress of the International Laser Association held in Tokyo in 1981, the use of the laser for gastrointestinal tumors was discussed, in addition to its application for hemorrhage.

At present, digestive tract tumors are treated endoscopically by two procedures. One procedure is radical treatment with the high-energy Nd:YAG laser, which, by thermal action, coagulates, degenerates, and disperses the tumor. The other procedure is the photodynamic therapy of the low-energy argon-dye laser, which destroys the tumor photochemically in reaction with a hematoporphyrin derivative previously injected into the tumor.[7–10] In this chapter we will report our treatment of advanced and recurrent cancers of the digestive organs using the Nd:YAG laser with endoscope attachment.

Subjects

At Kitazato University, the Nd:YAG laser has been used in clinical applications since 1979. In our study, radiation therapy was administered 209 times to 108 patients. Among them, abdominal surgery was performed in 7 cases (7%), laparotomy was performed in 25 cases (23%), and gastrointestinal endoscopy was performed in 76 cases (70%) (Figure 6.1). In 64 patients, endoscopic Nd:YAG laser therapy was performed, first for hemostasis, followed by direct application to the tumor.

Benign tumors were treated in 25 patients: esophageal submucosal tumor, gastric polyp, gastric submucosal tumor, atypical cell tumor, rectal adenoma, and anal polyp. Malignant tumors were present in 39 patients, namely, 22 cases of early cancer (1 esophagus, 18 stomach, 3 rectum) and 17 cases of advanced and recurrent cancers (3 esophagus, 7 stomach, 7 colon) (Figure 6.2).

Method

In our study we used a laser-oscillation system, Molectron Model 8000 Nd:YAG laser and NIIC 130YZ. Intermittent radiation was performed under the following conditions of tip power output: noncontact type, 50–70 W of power for 0.5–1.0 second and contact type, 15–20 W of power for 0.5–2.0 second.

Efficacy-Evaluating Criteria for Laser Therapy of Advanced and Recurrent Cancer

In judging the therapeutic efficacy of cancer treatment, longevity must be the primary criterion in the case of radical surgery, while treatment of early cancer, with fewer clinical symp-

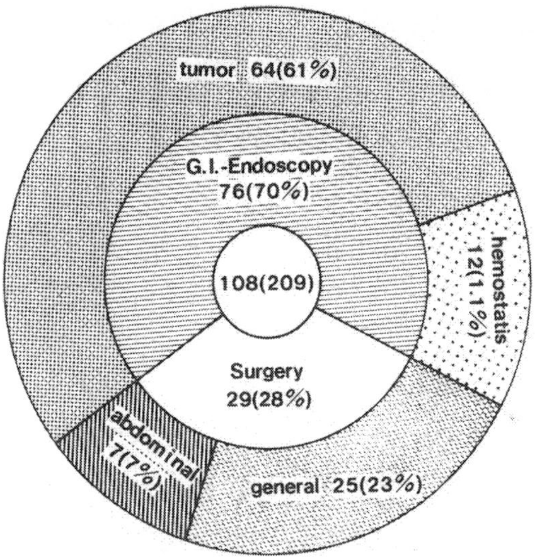

FIGURE 6.1. Nd:YAG laser treatment.

toms, may be judged by the result of histologic examination and the eradication of the tumor. In those cases of advanced and recurrent cancer that preclude surgical treatment, symptoms such as intermittent flare-ups, pain, hemorrhage, or exudation should be relieved conservatively. When longevity is the therapeutic goal, a standard for efficacy is needed. Therefore, we have established the criteria shown in Table 6.1.

Results

In 18 of the 22 patients treated with the Nd:YAG laser for early cancer, the tumor was eliminated and histologic examination was negative. Of the remaining 4 patients, 2 received radiotherapy during surgery, 1 required hemostasis, and 1 died from the disease. The tumors ranged from 0.5 to 4.0 cm, and radiation was administered from 1 to 5 times. Some cases were treated by repeated radiation for depressed lesions and larger tumors. No recurrent symptoms appeared for 56 months.

The efficacy of laser treatment was observed in 11 of 17 patients with advanced and recurrent cancers. Symptoms were mitigated in cases of gastrointestinal cancer aggravated by hemorrhage and in cases of rectal esophageal stenosis. Moreover, tumors were reduced in combined use with local immunotherapy, and longevity was seen in some cases. In one case of Borrmann type I stomach cancer, the tumor was eradicated after four doses of radiation and histologic examination was negative. There was no recurrence after 7 months. In another case of the same diagnosis, there was local recurrence after rectotomy (perineal-type rectal cancer). This patient suffered from exudation and hemorrhage; however, after 10 local laser treatments in 6

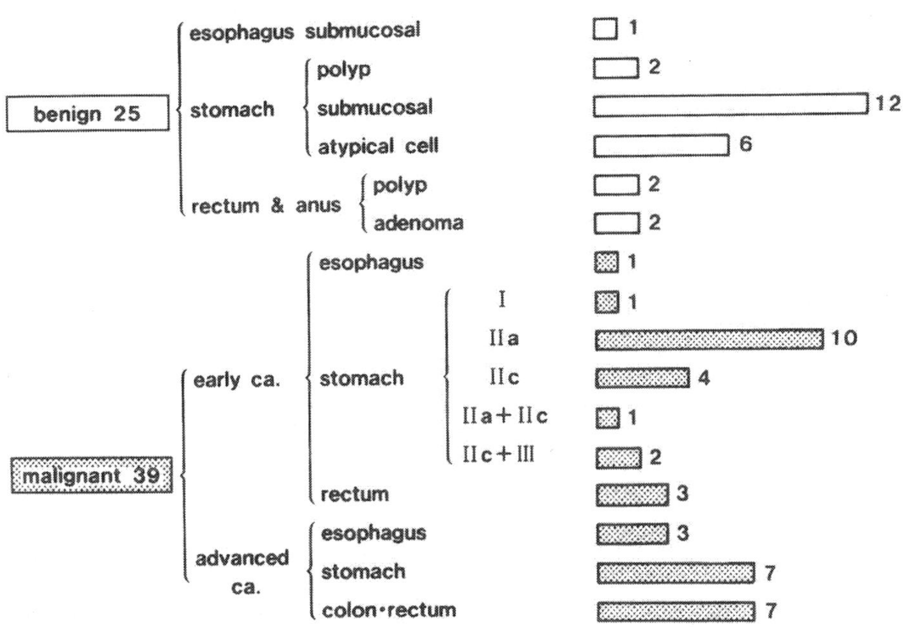

FIGURE 6.2. Endoscopic laser treatment for gastrointestinal tumor [n = 64 (157)].

TABLE 6.1. Criteria of laser effect

Tumor	Evaluation	Criterion
Malignant (palliative cases)	Excellent	Tumor is destroyed and pathohistologic examination is negative.
	Good	Tumor size is reduced over half and clinical courses are improved.
	No change	Tumor size is same as before and clinical courses are not improved.
	Worse	Tumor becomes big and clinical courses are getting worse.
Benign	Complete remission	Tumor is vanished.
	Partial remission	Tumor size is reduced as before.
	Stable	Tumor size is same as before.

months, the ninth biopsy was negative. Then the injury became a clear granular wound. No change was seen in 4 cases: in one case where there was no improvement of colonic cancer with longer stenosis; in two cases where there was tracheal infiltration of esophageal cancer; and in one case of stomach cancer where the hemorrhage was not controlled (Table 6.2).

Therapy for Cancer

At present, the basic therapy for cancer is resectional surgery. Systemic chemoimmunotherapy is mainly given for those cases impossible to excise or in those cases where surgery is contraindicated by being medically unfit, serious complications, or age. Today, laser therapy is indicated for these latter patients. However, the purpose and procedure may vary for early cancer and advanced or recurrent cancer.

Early Cancer

For early cancer, radical treatment is the goal, but, as cancer is a systemic disease, lymphatic metastasis is always a problem.

Lymphatic spread and depth of the cancer—"m" (mucosal) and "sm" (submucosal) was reviewed in those cases treated with surgery for early cancer. Simultaneously, cancer size was also surveyed. As a result, it was found that no lymphatic metastasis occurred when the cancer "m" depth was less than 2 cm. Therefore, a radical cure of early stomach cancer can be achieved by the laser alone, if it is an m-cancer

TABLE 6.2. Results—recurrent or advanced cancer (N = 17)

Organ	Case (times)	Type	Indication	Excellent	Good	No change
Esophagus	3 (5)	Stenosis	Obstruction 1		X	
		Tracheal invasion	Obstruction 1			X
		Stenosis	Obstruction 1		X	
Stomach	7 (23)	IIc + III-like	Tumor reduction 1			X
		IIa + IIc-like	Tumor reduction 1		X	
		Borrmann I	Tumor reduction 2	X	X	
		Borrmann II	Tumor reduction 1		X	
		Borrmann III	Bleeding 1		X	
		Post operative recurrence	Obstruction 1		X	
Colon-rectum	7 (42)	Post-LAR	Recurrence 3		X X	X
		Post-Miles	Recurrence 2	X	X	
		Borrmann III	Obstruction 2		X	X

smaller than 20 m without an ulcer. In this case, the premise is the exact identification of cancer depth with endoscopic diagnosis including the biopsy. These results should be considered when the choice of cancer therapy is the laser alone.

Advanced and Recurrent Cancer

Use of the laser for local radical cure is conservative therapy. However, the laser can increase longevity by palliating the symptoms of patients with advanced and recurrent cancer, who complain of bleeding, pain, or exudation. Of course, advanced cancer is not necessarily complicated by lymphatic metastasis, in which case the tumor may be disintegrated by repeated laser radiation. Also, the judgment of radical cure can be made by the results of this therapy over time.

Discussion

When laser radiation is indicated for digestive tract tumor, consideration should be given to the necessity of combined treatments, and to the selection of endoscopic devices for the lesion site, size, depth, and tissue type.

The laser can be used as direct therapy for raised, epithelial lesions such as adenomas, types I and IIa, whereas the larger masses, such as polyps, should first be reduced by high-frequency polypectomy, and then the laser can be applied. Polypectomy of type IIb (flat lesion) is performed by injecting physiologic saline solution into the submucosa, so-called strip biopsy, and applying laser radiation to the excised end.

In radical laser therapy for the depressed type of early cancer (IIc, IIc + III, III + IIc), it is essential to grasp the full range of the lesion. Irradiation should be executed from the peripheral site of the lesion. Radiation from the center may cause edema in the peripheral site, which would make the range of the lesion indistinct, resulting in insufficient radiation and, concomitantly, a residue of cancer at the peripheral site. Of course, a cancer residue may remain under the necrotic ulcer caused by the laser after radiation of deep sm-cancer. In such cases, repeated—but not excessive—radiation should be administered in order to minimize the danger of perforation that may occur in high-power one-time radiation treatment.

A radical cure may be effected by repeated radiation for the advanced cancer. However, in most cases, the laser is used for the relief of stenosis, relief of pain, or to obtain hemostasis. For the distinct lesion with residual cancer after radiation, including early cancer of the depressed type, local therapy in combination with OK-432 may induce better results. Frequent observations should be made over time with histologic examination following biopsy. For therapy with the endoscopic laser, especially the Nd:YAG laser, it is necessary to cut the lesion, therefore the exact range of the lesion must be in focus, as compared with the argon-dye laser's photodynamic therapy, for which it is important to keep the front of the lesion in view. The therapeutic approach must be fully understood to select appropriate laser equipment.

In comparison with the photodynamic therapy of the argon-dye laser, the Nd:YAG laser can be used simply and easily for retreatment of cancer residue after initial therapy, in a short treatment time. Also, it is useful for controlling the patients' symptoms or the side effects of hematoporphyrin derivative.

References

1. Nath G, et al: First laser endoscopy via a fiberoptic transmission system. Endoscopy 5:208, 1973.
2. Frühmorgen P, et al: Experimental examination on laser endoscopy. Endoscopy 6:116, 1974.
3. Frühmorgen P, et al: The first endoscopic laser coagulation in the human GI tract. Endoscopy 7:156, 1975.
4. Kiefhaber P, et al: Endoscopical control of massive gastrointestinal hemorrhage by irradiation with a high-power neodymium-Yag laser. Prog Surg 15:140, 1977.
5. Dwyer RM, et al: Laser-induced hemostasis in the canine stomach. JAMA 231:486, 1975.
6. Waitman AM, Grant DZ, Debeer R, Chryssanthou C: Endoscopic laser photocoagulation: comparison of argon and Nd:YAG. Gastroint Endoscopy 25:52, 1979.
7. Itoh K, et al: Endoscopic laser therapy for stomach tumor. Gastroenterol Endosc 23:1517, 1981.
8. Atsumi K: Challenge to the future medicine by laser. J Jpn Laser Med Assoc 3:1–4, 1982.
9. Kasugai T, et al: Laser-endoscopic therapy for early stomach cancer. J Jpn Nippon Rinsho (Japanese Clinic) 42:2282, 1984.
10. Hiki Y: Laser endoscopy. Jpn Text New Med Ser, yearly ed 84-A:51–60, 1984.

7 Videoendoscopy

David E. Fleischer

Fiberoptic endoscopy has revolutionized the management of gastrointestinal diseases. Since its advent, in the late 1950s, endoscopy has altered both the diagnosis and management of numerous medical problems. It provided the first nonsurgical option for examining the digestive tract in vivo and also provided the opportunity for biopsy with histopathologic evaluation and therapy. A wide variety of therapies can now be carried out endoscopically; for example, endoscopic laser therapy for bleeding lesions and gastrointestinal neoplasms is commonplace.

The key innovation in flexible endoscopy was the use of the fiberoptic bundle to transmit light for the visual image. In 1983, Sivak and Fleischer[1] reported the first use of the videoendoscope, using equipment developed by Welch-Allyn, Inc. The videoendoscope looks similar to the fiberoptic endoscope, but there are numerous differences (Figure 7.1). The physician looks at the video monitor rather than through an eyepiece. The image is transmitted electronically rather than through fiber bundles. This means that several observers can watch the procedure simultaneously (Figure 7.2). Electronic transmission opens up numerous options for both display and analysis.

The key to the development of the electronic endoscope was the charge-coupled device (CCD), invented in 1969 by Boyle and Smith. The CCD is generally referred to as a chip, and it was first incorporated into gastrointestinal endoscopes by Welch-Allyn, Inc. Sivak[2] has presented a detailed and lucid description of the CCD and its application with videoendoscopes.

Component Parts of the Videoendoscopic System

The component parts of the videoendoscopic system are the (1) videoendoscope, (2) videoprocessor, (3) display monitor, and (4) accessories (Figure 7.3).

A videoendoscope is somewhat similar in appearance to a fiberoptic endoscope, though it need not be. The control head is shown in Figure 7.4. No viewing eyepiece is required, since the physician looks at a television monitor. Suction and air/water buttons are shown in the figure. Cabled knobs control movement at the distal part of the tip. Intubation is performed through the mouth or the anus, as with routine fiberoptic endoscopy.

Information is then carried to a videoprocessor (Figure 7.5). The videoprocessor converts the information from the CCD which is an analogue device to discrete numerical values. Once the information is converted from an analogue system to a digital system, the data can be translated to a binary code that can feed into computers. Therefore, television images can be transmitted from one room of the hospital to another, from one medical area to another many miles away, or even, via a satellite communication system, over very far distances. Also, once the information exists in a binary language, the videoendoscopic system can be interfaced with computers and a wide variety of analytic functions can be carried out. In addition, the endoscopic images can be stored for retrieval at a later date.

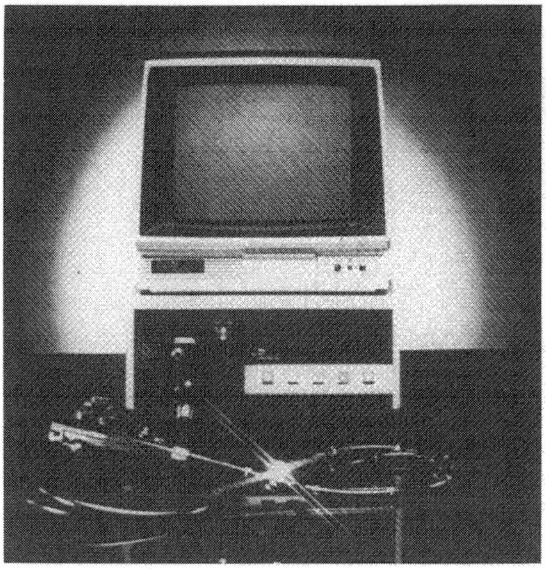

FIGURE 7.1. Videoendoscope (Welch-Allyn).

The display monitor can be a standard television or a computer monitor. In addition to the visual images, information about the patient and the procedure can be typed into the picture with a standard keyboard (Figure 7.6).

A wide variety of accessories can be matched to the videoendoscopic system. A videotape recorder can be used to record the proceedings to review at a later date. Photographic systems can be utilized that present an instant picture, a 35-mm slide, or a hard copy (Figure 7.7). A storage retrieval system, for example, using a laser disk, can be hooked up to the system for storage of a large number of video pictures. Additional monitors can be placed so that more persons in more sites can view the image. Finally, perhaps most importantly, a computer interface can be established so that the potential for analysis of the video image can be realized. This new and exciting area holds great promise for videoendoscopy and will be discussed in detail later in this chapter.

New Developments with Videoendoscopy

Videoendoscopy offers several opportunities that did not exist with standard fiberoptic endoscopy. Some of these that currently exist are (1) video advantages, (2) advantages for personnel and patients, (3) specific advantages distinct from fiberoptic instruments, and (4) documentation.

The first apparent video advantage is that high-quality images can be projected for multiple

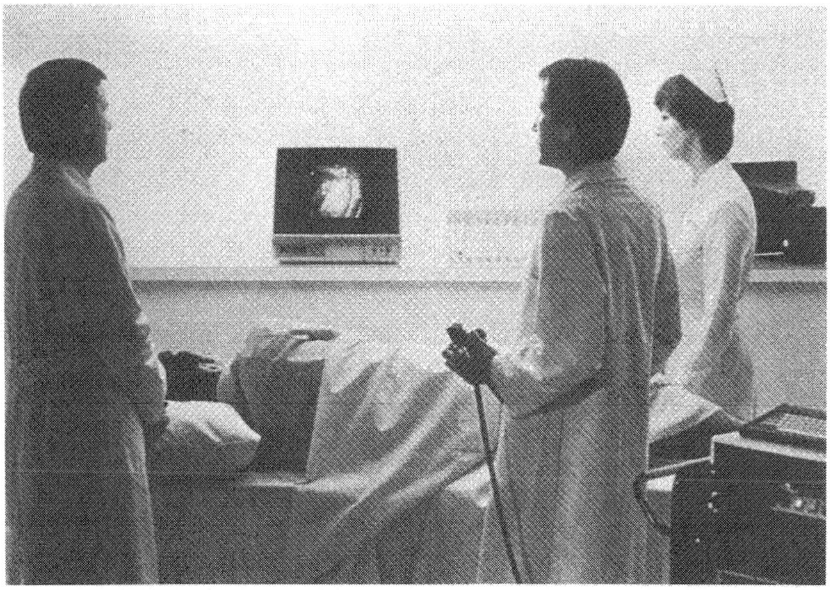

FIGURE 7.2. With videoendoscopy, the image is displayed on a monitor. Several observers can watch the procedure.

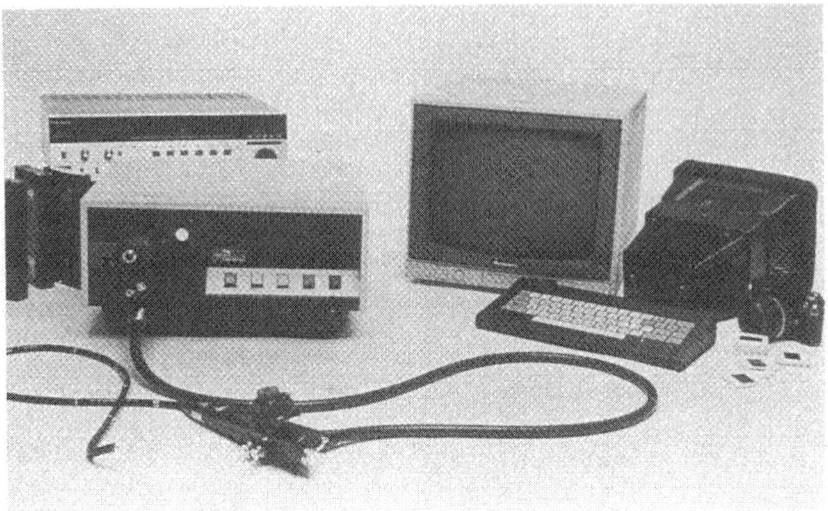

FIGURE 7.3. Component parts of the videoendoscopic system include the videoendoscope, videoprocessor, display monitor, and accessories.

viewers to observe in the same room. A teaching attachment is not required and verbal discussions can take place among multiple observers. If a record is to be made of the procedure, an additional television camera system is not required. The obvious video advantage of documentation will be discussed below.

There are certain advantages that are obvious to health personnel and patients. The endoscopist experiences less eyestrain when viewing the procedure through a monitor as opposed to through an eyepiece. It is also apparent that better coordination occurs between the endoscopist and the gastrointestinal assistant, since they are both observing the same procedure simultaneously. The gastrointestinal assistant finds the procedure more enjoyable because he can glance at the television monitor as well as at the patient. Since the assistant does not have to hold a lecture scope to his eye, his hands are now free to assist with the procedure or the patient. Coordination between the assistant and the physician is logically better if the assistant has better use of his hands. Initially, there was con-

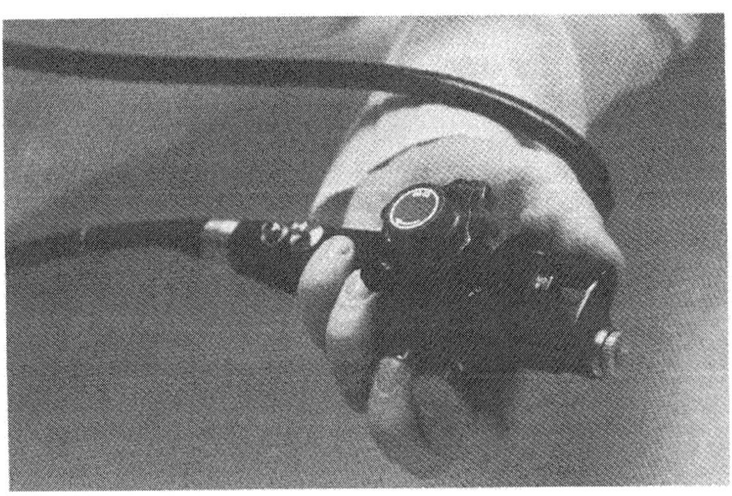

FIGURE 7.4. The control section of the videoendoscope is similar to the fiberoptic endoscope. Suction and air/water buttons are seen.

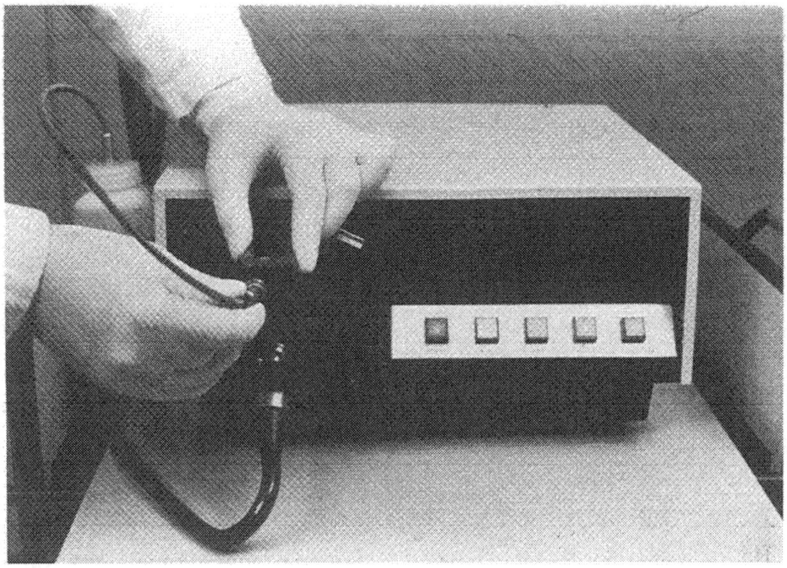

FIGURE 7.5. The videoprocessor serves as the light source, but also processes information received from the videoendoscope.

cern that it may be frightening for the patient to observe the procedure while it is being carried out, which is possible with the television monitor.However, most patients prefer to see the procedure, and those who choose not to look can "tune out" during the procedure. The physician naturally uses discretion as to when observation by the patient is appropriate. The ability to have a record that can be reviewed with the patient at a later date is often of much value.

The videoendoscope has numerous potential benefits, in contrast to fiberoptic instruments. Obviously, there will be no fiber breakage, since the electronic endoscope does not employ fibers. It is possible that the cost of both the instrument and the repair will be reduced when electronic endoscopes are used more extensively. Also, as

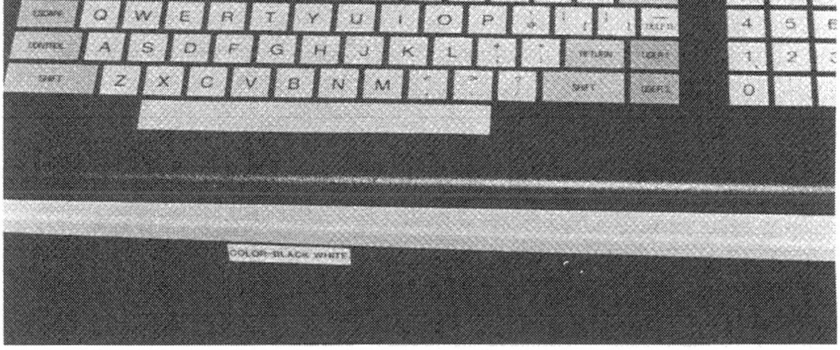

FIGURE 7.6. Keyboard (character generator) of the Welch-Allyn videoendoscopic system.

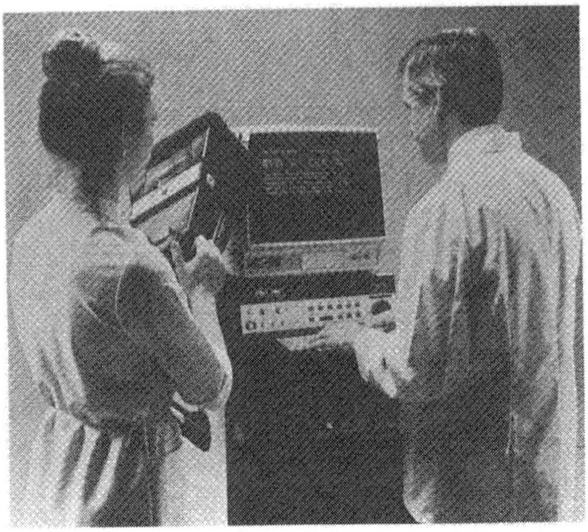

FIGURE 7.7. Photography from a videoendoscopic system can be instant, 35 mm, or hard copy.

the chips become smaller, the potential for smaller endoscopes and larger channels will exist.

Perhaps the most obvious immediate advantage of videoendoscopy is in the area of documentation. Here there are important opportunities for teaching. During the actual endoscopic procedure the teacher, the trainee, and other related observers can all view the activity simultaneously. It presents an opportunity for the trainee to review the procedure after it has been carried out and to glean some information about how the examination was performed. Since the videotape is potentially available immediately after the procedure, it can be used at conferences on the same day, as well as on other days.

The existence of a videotape means that the only record of an endoscopic procedure is no longer just a dictated description. Instead, the videotape can be reviewed by other physicians who will be seeing the patient—much like an x-ray film is reviewed. There is the opportunity for preoperative review by the surgeon. Long-distance live consultations could be carried out while the procedure is being performed or at a later date. This videotape record of the procedure permits comparisons with other endoscopies. Since the information can be stored and retrieved, records from a single patient can be compared much like x-ray records. The fact that the procedure is documented also lends potential for quality control and other means of accessing performance and management.

Limitations of Videoendoscopy

Technological advancement usually carries with it some tradeoffs. Currently, videoendoscopic systems are more expensive than routine fiberoptic endoscopic systems. Videoendoscopic systems have more component parts and they are larger; therefore operational space and storage of the equipment is of some concern. They are less portable than the current fiberoptic system, so that if an emergency procedure is required, for example, in an intensive care unit, transporting the system is awkward.

There is a learning period for physicians who are accustomed to the fiberoptic endoscope. When these physicians confront the videoendoscopic system for the first time, they need to observe and participate in five to ten procedures before they become comfortable with its use.

Currently, videoendoscopes exist for standard upper endoscopy and colonoscopy. There are few specialized instruments. Although some duodenoscopes do exist, these are not commonly employed at the present time.

Another concern about videoendoscopy is the rapidity with which the technology is changing. Therefore, there tends to be a real concern on the part of the purchaser that he may be purchasing a system that will be outdated in a few months or years.

None of these problems is insurmountable, but they indicate some of the limitations of videoendoscopy at the present time.

The Future of Videoendoscopy

The videoendoscopic system, as described, represents an important advancement. Several of the advantages have been cited. However, it is my opinion that if videoendoscopes are to replace fiberoptic systems (and I believe that they will), it will be new developments that allow them to do so. I think that the two areas that will determine the future of videoendoscopy are the computer interface and the analytic potential. Since it is the computer interface that is likely to enhance the analytic potential, the two areas actually are one. With computer interface, the electronic image can be evaluated in several fashions. Computerized image enhancement will be possible with edge enhancement evaluation.

Increased enhancement of the topography of the gastrointestinal tract can provide hitherto unavailable data useful for diagnostic interpretation (Figure 7.8). Magnification of electronic images is also possible, whereby an area can be enlarged and evaluated in greater detail. The potential for color evaluation and manipulation is reasonably straightforward. The gastrointestinal polyp that we see as a pink excrescence may contain multiple colors. It may be that normal cells are one color, and pathologic areas are another. By varying the color and manipulating it, distinctions that are not currently apparent may be highlighted. The videoendoscope is not limited to the light spectrum visible to the human eye, therefore, infrared and ultraviolet sensing may be possible. Endoscopic thermography may allow us to distinguish small differences in temperature, and this may have diagnostic benefits. At the present time thermography is used in the evaluation of normal and abnormal medical conditions. Of course, with a computer interface, the generation of an endoscopic report, even including pictures, is within easy reach.

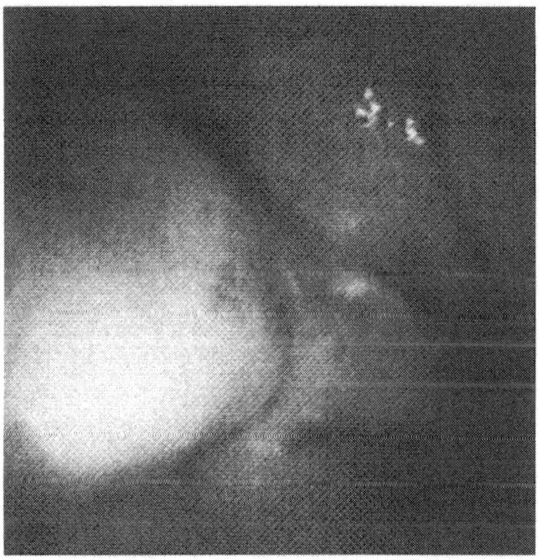

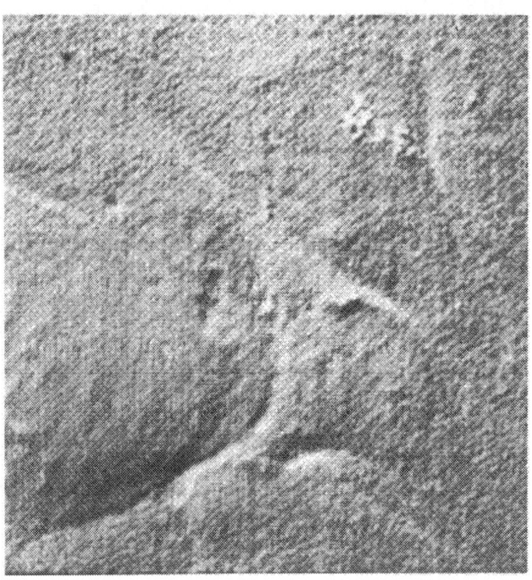

FIGURE 7.8. Small lesion in duodenum before image enhancement (*top*) and after (*bottom*).

The techniques described above greatly enhance the potential for analysis. It may be possible to determine blood flow with videoendoscopes. A more precise measurement of the size of the lesion—depth and height as well as length and breadth—can be obtained. Currently, ultrasonic endoscopy is used to determine the depth of lesions. The density of a lesion, as determined by computerized tomography, may be assessable with the videoendoscope, and this could give important information about the nature of the lesion. Ideally, the distinction between malignant and nonmalignant lesions might some day be made with a videoendoscope.

Application of the Videoendoscope for Use with Lasers

Some of the potential advances discussed above would be important for laser application. With regard to the management of gastrointestinal bleeding, if blood flow could be determined before and after laser therapy, one could get a better idea of both the hemodynamic nature of the lesion being treated and the efficacy of the therapy. One limitation of laser treatment of gastrointestinal neoplasms is in the pathologic evaluation of the lesion. In contrast to a snare polypectomy for the treatment of a gastrointestinal polyp, laser ablation does not allow for the delivery of the entire specimen to the pathologist. However, if videoendoscopy allowed for histologic interpretation, pathologic analysis would not be as critical. Also, the laser endoscopist often does not know how deep the laser therapy should be delivered, since he does not know the depth of the tumor in the gastrointes-

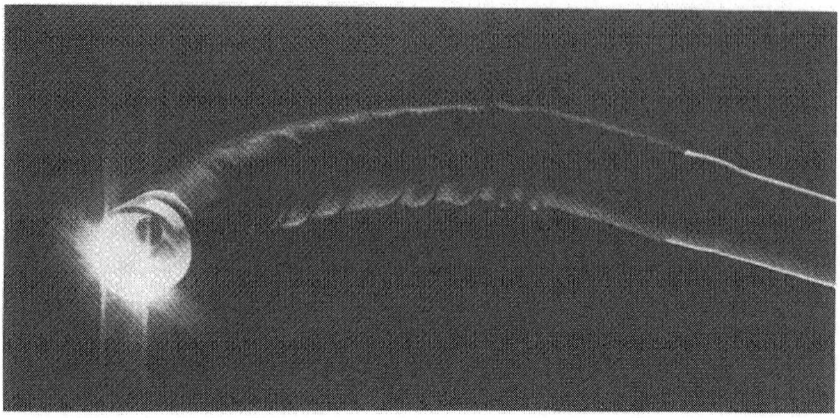

FIGURE 7.9. Welch-Allyn videoendoscope adapted for laser use. The white tip reflects the Nd:YAG beam. A filter at the tip protects (CCD) and reduces return from the aiming light, which could overwhelm the CCD and reduce the quality of the picture when the white aiming light is present.

tinal wall. If the depth of the lesion could be ascertained, a more precise delivery of the laser energy would be possible, and, in fact, the surgeon could determine whether or not curative therapy with the laser was possible. This would have an immediate application for the management of early gastric cancer and the possibility of the laser as a means of curative therapy.

Some modifications of endoscopes are necessary for use with lasers. The white aiming light from the laser fiber will overwhelm the CCD (chip) with its bright intense light. Therefore, the filter must be placed either into the laser or at the tip of the endoscope so that the video picture will not be wiped out. Additionally, this filter provides some protection for the chip. The videoendoscopic system by Welch-Allyn employs such a filter (Figure 7.9). The Welch-Allyn instrument also has a white tip on the endoscope, which is more apt to reflect than to absorb the beam from the most commonly employed Nd:YAG laser, which is the one most commonly employed. An enlarged biopsy channel also is important in endoscopic laser therapy because it permits the exhaust of gas from the laser fiber. It should be mentioned again that an added advantage of the videoendoscope when employed with lasers is that special protective eyeglasses are not required for the endoscopist or the other health personnel, since the laser beam is not observed directly through the eyepiece of the endoscope, but rather the endoscopy team watch the procedure on a television monitor.

Conclusion

Videoendoscopy represents a revolutionary advance in the evaluation and management of patients with gastrointestinal diseases. In its current form, it is an interesting and appealing alternative to fiberoptic endoscopy. However, the key to the future is in its analytic potential, and, when this is fully realized, videoendoscopes will completely replace fiberoptic instruments.

References

1. Sivak MV Jr, Fleischer DE: Colonoscopy with a videoendoscope: Preliminary experience. Gastrointest Endosc 30:1–5, 1984.
2. Sivak MV Jr: Videoendoscopy. Clin Gastroenterol 15:205–234, 1986.

8
Endoscopic Laser Therapy of Carcinoma of the Esophagus and Gastric Cardia

Richard C. Ranard and David E. Fleischer

In the United States, the largest experience with laser treatment of neoplasms of the gastrointestinal tract is with carcinoma of the esophagus. The great majority of these lesions are squamous cell carcinomas, although adenocarcinoma of the esophagus occurs in 3 to 7% of cases. The endoscopic laser therapy (ELT) of these lesions, as well as of adenocarcinomas of the gastric cardia, is effective in the palliation of these too-often incurable diseases.

The incidence of cancer of the esophagus is increased in blacks, males, and the socioeconomically disadvantaged. It is postulated that this is partly because the two major risk factors for carcinoma of the esophagus, cigarette smoking and alcohol ingestion, are more prevalent in these groups. The risk of esophageal carcinoma is increased geometrically when both of these factors are present. Washington, DC is one of the several areas in the United States where there is an increased incidence of esophageal carcinoma. This is where investigation of ELT of esophageal carcinoma was initiated.[1]

Patients most commonly present with symptoms of obstruction or bleeding. They have often experienced considerable weight loss as a reflection of their poor nutritional status. Dysphagia, the most common presenting symptom, almost always reflects advanced disease, where cure is seldom possible. The average time interval between onset of dysphagia symptoms and the diagnosis is over 3 months. The esophagus is distensible and surrounded by a rich lymphatic system. This permits extensive tumor growth before symptoms occur, allowing little possibility for cure. Median survival time from presentation with advanced squamous cell carcinoma of the esophagus in the United States is less than 6 months. Palliation, with minimization of morbidity and duration of hospitalization, is often the goal for patients with esophageal carcinoma who have limited survival.

In recent years, the medical community has witnessed the emergence of ELT for the palliation of cancers of the esophagus and gastric cardia. ELT, however, must be reviewed in the context of the available alternatives. Radiation therapy, surgery, chemotherapy, bougienage with or without prosthetic stent placement, and gastrostomy or pharyngostomy all are used in the palliation of cancer of the esophagus and/or gastric cardia, but each has specific limitations.

Radiation therapy, with a full course of 6000 rad or more delivered to the mediastinum, is the most common modality employed in the treatment of carcinoma of the esophagus. It is often employed in patients with locally advanced or widespread disease, and in those with other medical problems that lessen the chance for a good surgical outcome. Although short-term relief of symptoms is common, prolonged control of local disease is rare. Most patient have celiac axis node involvement or distal metastases at the time of autopsy. No controlled trials compare radiation therapy to surgery for squamous cell carcinoma of the esophagus, but survival rates are similarly poor. In a comprehensive review by Earlam and Cunha-Melo[2] of collective radiotherapy results on esophageal cancer, a 1-year survival of 18% and a 5-year survival of approximately 6% were reported. These rates are similar to that of surgically treated patients.

Compilation and evaluation of numerous surgical studies by Earlam and Cunha-Melo[3] determined that, of every 100 patients with cancer of the esophagus, 58 will be operative candidates and 42 will not be operative candidates. Of those 58, 39 will have the tumor resected and 19 will be unresectable. Of those 39 who come to operation, 13 will die in the hospital and 26 will leave the hospital with the tumor excised. Of these 26, 18 will live 1 year, 9 will live 2 years, and only 4 will live 5 years. Given these figures, the authors point out that an informed patient might ask about alternative treatment.

Both radiation therapy and surgery for cancer of the esophagus have limitations apart from poor survival. Radiation therapy may take several weeks to provide symptomatic relief. It cannot be administered for recurrences after the maximum dose has been reached. Its effect is not organ-specific. Nausea, malaise, pulmonary fibrosis, and spinal cord lesions leading to paraplegia, as well as radiation-induced esophageal strictures can occur.

Surgery is limited because the location of the lesion or the condition of the patient make most lesions unresectable at presentation. Many institutions consider surgery only with lesions of the distal third of the esophagus, reserving radiation therapy for proximal lesions. Surgical morbidity is high. Surgical mortality in patients considered operable is reported as high as 29%[3] although mortality in the range of 10% is more commonly reported.

Past results have generally been disappointing, but encouraging data are emerging on chemotherapeutic intervention in squamous cell carcinoma of the esophagus. Single-agent therapy has not been effective, with brief responses at rates usually in the range of only 15–20%.[4] More encouraging results have occurred with combination chemotherapy, often with *cis*-platinum-based regimens. Response rates up to 53% or more with prolongation of survival are reported.[5] Prospective randomized trials originating at the National Cancer Institute indicate that patients responding to preoperative and postoperative combination chemotherapy have longer disease-free and overall survival—more than 3 years. However, the failure to stratify nutritional factors may have affected these results.[6] These findings, and favorable results with short-term continuous infusion of 5-fluorouracil (5-FU) instead of the traditional bolus infusion, have led to the recent initiation of trials at Georgetown University Hospital, investigating chemotherapeutic intervention with continuous infusion 5-FU and intermittent *cis*-platinum preoperatively and postoperatively, with concurrent ELT for palliation of obstruction or bleeding as indicated. Despite some suggestions of increased response rates, incomplete responses and significant morbidity in patients with limited survival will continue to restrict the use of chemotherapy in the palliation of carcinoma of the esophagus.

Bougienage, with or without prosthetic stent placement, is relatively safe and efficacious, and provides symptomatic relief in many patients. Reported complication rates vary widely. Heit et al.[7] reported improvement in 24 of 26 patients, with only one perforation. Cassidy et al.[8] reported on 154 patients with malignant strictures undergoing more than 1300 individual dilatations, with only three serious complications—two perforations, and one massive hemorrhage—although 15% of the patients required peroral prosthesis placement to maintain a patent lumen. Mean survival after prosthesis insertion was 4.5 months. Graham et al.[9] reported one perforation and one fatal hemorrhage in 18 patients, 5 of whom were dilated prior to prosthetic stent placement for esophagorespiratory fistulas.

Bougienage may be unworkable if the stricture is too tight to allow clinically significant dilatations. Although successful initially, the procedure often becomes increasingly difficult and painful, and intervening periods of improved symptoms are of progressively shorter duration. While patients with stenosing tumors of the gastric cardia are often afforded temporary symptomatic benefit, dilatation is technically more difficult because the narrowed area often diverges at a sharp angle from the esophageal lumen.

Atkinson's group[10] reported satisfactory restoration of swallowing in 121 patients with endoscopic insertion of prosthetic tubes. There were 5 fatal and 10 nonfatal perforations, thirty-three of 121 patients survived for 6 months or more. Den Hartog Jager et al.[11] reported generally good palliation, with restoration of food passage, in 200 patients with esophagogastric malignancies after endoscopic placement of plastic prostheses. Complications included 16 perforations with 1 death, obstruction of the prosthesis in 35 patients, and tube migration in 44 patients. Seventeen percent of patients survived more than 6 months.

Restrictions on prosthetic stent placement are technical in some cases. Many investigators feel that stents are contraindicated for treatment of lesions in the proximal esophagus if the stent is adjacent to the cricopharyngeus, or for lesions in the distal esophagus if the prosthesis crosses the gastroesophageal junction. Occasionally, a malignant stricture cannot be dilated to accommodate stent placement, although in patients with malignant obstruction and fistulae, ELT has been reported to establish a lumen sufficient to allow prosthesis placement. Some patients have required general anesthesia. Besides the major complications of bleeding, perforation, obstruction, and severe gastroesophageal reflux, some reports have associated stent placement with premature mortality.[9]

Gastrostomy, jejunostomy, and pharyngostomy provide effective relief from obstructing esophagogastric malignancies. The patient's dignity, however, is too often compromised during his final days. The basic pleasure of eating is forfeited and the patient's self-esteem is hindered when it should be fostered. These procedures, as well as the other modalities for palliation of esophagogastric cancer, can each be beneficial in selected cases. Shortfalls and restrictions, however, have led to the description and critical evaluation of ELT as an effective adjunct in the palliation of these malignancies.

A study by Fleischer et al.[1] only 5 years ago, was the first to describe the safe and effective use of ELT for palliation of carcinoma of the esophagus. Their pilot study has formed the basis of a much larger experience, so that the Federal Food and Drug Administration no longer classifies ELT for obstructing carcinoma of the esophagus as an experimental procedure. Treatment is almost always initiated as palliation. Most commonly, symptoms are related to obstruction or bleeding. The majority of patients treated with ELT have undergone previous radiation therapy or surgery. In some cases, ELT is the only course left, short of feeding gastrostomy-jejunostomy. After appropriate instruction and experience, ELT is technically easy to perform. The endoscope gives direct visualization at the margin of the tumor. With the possible exception of lesions extending up to the cricopharyngeus, ELT is applicable to lesions anywhere in the esophagus. Surgery with general anesthesia and its attendant morbidity are avoided. Symptomatic relief is gained in a relatively short time with often dramatic improvements in quality of life. Most patients are able to leave the hospital.

In the evaluation of a patient for palliation with ELT, a CBC, coagulation parameters, multiple chemical analyses, chest x-ray, and barium swallow, as well as chest and abdominal computerized tomographic (CT) scans are obtained. Consensus can be sought from the surgeons, radiation oncologists, and medical oncologists that curative treatment is not possible. Many patients have had recurrence after prior radiation therapy or surgery. Others are unable to tolerate radiation therapy and a few are potentially curable, but nutritional or medical status precludes surgery. Once a course of ELT is chosen, the radiographic studies are reexamined. They will affect technical decisions and help gauge the number of treatments required. A CT scan, for example, can define the extent of disease. It may show if the wall at an anastomotic site is thick enough to allow ELT with a low risk of perforation. Alternatively, it may reveal lesions outside the esophagus.

The patient is fasted for 12 hours before each session. He is reminded that dysphagia may worsen before it improves, secondary to the local inflammation and swelling that follows ELT. These factors make the maintenance of an often impaired nutritional status problematic during long courses of ELT. Based on pretreatment nutritional status, initial lumen diameter, and tumor length, a judgment is made on the patient's ability to ingest oral feeding during therapy. If it is anticipated that ELT will take longer than 1 week, parenteral nutrition is sometimes initiated.

A screening examination with a small-diameter endoscope is generally done by the therapeutic endoscopist at an earlier session or just before the first endoscopic laser treatment. The point of maximum obstruction is discerned, with the smallest luminal diameter used as a reference point. It is determined where the tumor is, whether it is predominantly mucosal or submucosal, and if there is a large polypoidal component, better debulked by polypectomy snare than by ELT. It is important to know the course of the lumen just below the area being treated to help guide the laser beam appropriately.

ELT can be performed in a conventional endoscopy suite, although practical modifications optimize logistics. Optimally, one assistant attends the patient and assists with the equipment, and a second assistant records medical observations. Several commercially produced lasers are available. We use a Nd:YAG laser (Cooper LaserSonics or Lasers for Medicine) with a power output of 10–100 W. The Nd:YAG beam is preferred to the argon beam. Although the latter is more superficial, theoretically reducing the risk of perforation, it does not produce the deeper tissue effect and subsequent sloughing of the Nd:YAG laser, which enables an increased volume of tumor to be destroyed at each session.

Laser energy is preselected and conveyed by a quartz waveguide through the biopsy channel of a therapeutic endoscope. Fleischer usually uses 90–100 W in 2.0- to 2.5-second pulses. Lower powers (40–50 W) have been advocated by some physicians who believe that effective tissue damage can be accomplished at these powers and that there is less smoke and debris to interfere with vision. Coaxial gas flow serves to cool the fiber tip and clear it of debris. The coaxial gas can overdistend the stomach, causing patient discomfort and vasovagal responses, unless the gas can be exhausted. Therefore, rates (20 cc/second) are recommended.

The patient is prepared with topical anesthetic, and intravenous meperidine and midazolam sedation. Secretions may be controlled with an anticholinergic agent when completely obstructing lesions or extremely proximal lesions are present. The patient is placed in the standard left lateral decubitus position.

In the original technique described by Fleischer and Kessler,[12] the endoscope is advanced to the proximal tumor margin. The quartz waveguide carrying the laser beam is passed out and initially directed centrally, aiming at tumor closest to the lumen, then circumferentially around the luminal opening. The circle of treatment is widened concentrically toward, but never directly to, the esophageal wall. If there is a short submucosal segment, however, circumferential treatment is avoided, limiting treatment to a 180°–270° arc because of the increased risk of postlaser stricture and perforation. The laser beam is fired with the fiber at a 1.0-cm distance from the tumor. Tissue contact is avoided with noncontact probes, and it is often necessary to withdraw the fiber to clean the fiber tip.

Recently, newly developed sapphire tips that attach to the distal fiber allow the laser to be used as a contact device. Different tip shapes alter the effect so that coagulation, vaporization, and/or excision can be better achieved. With these contact fibers, the laser energy is concentrated at the point of interaction between the probe tip and the tissue. Since the energy density will be very concentrated at the tip, much lower energies can be applied to achieve coagulation (8–12 W). There are many appealing aspects to this technique. Its actual role in the endoscopic therapy of esophageal malignancies is not, as yet, fully defined.[13]

The first tissue reaction is a white circular burn where the beam hits tumor tissue. After initial treatment, the tissue will be coagulated and whitish-yellow. With continued treatment the tissue is vaporized and blackened. Cavitation occurs if the laser beam is continuously focused on the same site and if the fiber is close (<1.0 cm) to the tissue and the power is high (90–100 W). As it is not possible to control tissue temperatures with currently used endoscopic lasers, the endoscopist must use visual clues and his own experience to determine the tissue effect of the laser.

The treatment of tumors of the gastric cardia is similar to treatment of esophageal tumors, with some technical differences. The tumor is more likely to distort the anatomy, with the lumen more apt to diverge from the vertical axis of the esophagus at an acute angle, increasing the technical difficulty. Functional improvement is potentially lessened because food must pass through a rigid aperistaltic, horizontal segment without the advantage of gravity.

If the lumen of the malignant stricture of the esophagus or gastric cardia is markedly decreased, a biopsy forceps, ERCP cannula, or a laser-resistant guidewire can be passed to act as a probe to map out the luminal pathway. If the lumen is completely occluded, the treatment is more difficult, with increased risk of perforation. However, as long as tumor protrudes into lumen and lumen can be visualized distal to the treatment site, the margin of error is wide and the risk of complications lessened.

Usually, the first session is completed when the superior margin is treated with the cross-section of tumor vaporized. However, if the lumen is wide enough to pass a scope, treatment can be continued at various levels distally during the first session. Unfortunately, proximal edema with swelling at the superior margin often precludes this approach.

Alternatively, ELT may be initiated at the distal tumor margin. The advantage is that when edema from treatment ensues at the treatment site, the endoscope can be withdrawn proximally and treatment can be continued on a longer vertical segment of tumor. Unfortunately, the lumen can often accommodate only a single-channel endoscope with its limited capability to exhaust smoke and coaxial gas flow. Sometimes, when the luminal narrowing is marked, there is no option because even the smallest endoscope cannot traverse the tumor, even with the aid of a guiding device.

After the initial session, succeeding sessions are carried out at 48- to 72-hour intervals. This allows a convenience Monday – Wednesday – Friday schedule of treatments. This time frame seems to allow maximal tumor necrosis and is readily tolerated by patients. When the treated area is observed at 48 hours, it is whitish-yellow, soft, and necrotic. Serial treatment at less than 48-hour intervals does not allow for maximal sloughing of necrotic tissue, and longer intervals unnecessarily prolong the full course of therapy.

Before treatment is begun on underlying, previously untreated tumor, it is necessary to evacuate destroyed tumor from the prior treatment. Large biopsy forceps, polyp graspers, and polypectomy snares can be employed to remove necrotic tissue, but the softness of the tissue after laser therapy limits their utility. Sometimes, endoscopy cleaning brushes and Water Piks are helpful. Multiple retrievals can be anticipated when multiple levels of the tumor have been treated in one session. In this circumstance, and when the chunks of tissue are too large to be withdrawn through the biopsy channel, an overtube can be passed to facilitate removal and reduce trauma to the pharynx and cricopharyngeus. Often, no one method is entirely adequate, and, sometimes, it is quickest and most effective to just push treated tissue distally with the endoscope or a dilator.

After evacuation of necrotic tissue, subsequent treatment of tumor is performed. Laser treatment is continued until the lumen can permit passage of an 11-mm endoscope into the stomach, or until the patient can eat solid foods. Passage of an 11-mm endoscope usually correlates clinically with the ability to ingest many solid foods, although the correlation is poor in patients with cervical tumors. In his cumulative experience, Fleischer required a mean of 3.3 sessions per course of treatment for patients with esophagogastric cancer (unpublished data). Squamous cell carcinoma has required a mean of 3.6 treatments and adenocarcinoma, primarily arising in the gastric cardia, required 2.8 treatments on average.

Dilatation is performed when necessary 1 to 2 days after the last laser treatment. This may stretch the lumen still further and may aid in debridement. Tapered polyvinyl dilators are preferred. They are firmer than Maloney dilators, and may be safer and easier than Eder-Puestow dilators.[13] A barium swallow is helpful after a course of ELT to document improvement relative to baseline radiographs and to reveal any unsuspected perforation.

Pietrafitta and Dwyer[14] have reported success in obtaining a patent 13 – to 20-mm diameter esophageal lumen with a single-session treatment in five patients. After widening the lumen to 15 mm with Savary-Guillard dilators over a guidewire, they advance a 9.8-mm endoscope into the stomach. Then, retracting the endoscope, starting at the distal tumor margin, they apply ELT to the entire length of the tumor, using a Nd:YAG laser with a power setting of 85 W and a pulse duration of 0.5 seconds. Subsequently, vigorous debridement is performed with biopsy forceps. Four patients tolerated a regular diet after a single treatment. One patient required two subsequent treatments.

In the first full series on ELT of esophageal carcinoma by Fleischer and Kessler,[12] 14 patients for whom no curative therapy was possible were treated with the Nd:YAG laser. An arbitrary grading system to quantitate dysphagia, odynophagia, and chest pain was used to compare symptoms before and after ELT. All 14 patients had clinical, endoscopic, and radiographic improvement. All patients could eat solid food after treatment, while only four could do so before treatment. Mean survival was 14 weeks. Although survival compared favorably with other treatments, it must be noted that many patients treated with ELT had recurrence of tumor after surgery or radiation therapy or were not considered suitable for these modalities. For many, even dilatation was either no longer effective or was technically impossible.

In a similar group of patients, using historical controls, Mellow et al.[15] evaluated the effect of ELT on the survival of patients with carcinoma of the esophagus. They reported a longer duration of time free from dysphagia and prolonged survival when the laser-treated group was compared to similar patients treated with radiation therapy. They also documented the efficacy of re-treatment after tumor reocclusion, a mean of 10 weeks after the initial course of ELT was finished.

In a study by Fleischer and Sivak,[16] 15 patients with advanced adenocarcinoma of the gastric cardia were treated with endoscopic Nd:YAG laser therapy. Seven patients had been explored, but palliative surgery was not believed to be possible, and four patients had recurrence after prior surgery. All patients had clinical benefit in terms of increased food intake, and most could eat all foods. On one or two later occasions 3 of 15 patients received ELT for recurrent tumor reobstructing the lumen, and the response to therapy was similar to that of initial therapy. Mean survival was in excess of 5 months, and again similar to that of other treatments reported in the literature.

Certain parameters affect the initial outcome of ELT of esophagogastric cancer. Fleischer and Sivak[17] examined the affect on outcome of tumor histology and endoscopic appearance, clinical performance status, and tumor location. No difference in response was discerned between squamous cell carcinoma and adenocarcinoma of the esophagus. This is not surprising, as both are thermally destroyed. Outcome was better for treatment of mucosal tumors than of submucosal or extrinsic tumors, although the distinction is not always precise. The former tend to be exophytic and polypoid and, therefore, technically easier to treat. Luminal closure and scarring may occur more rapidly if the treated tumor is submucosal. Performance status conferred better prognosis for ambulatory patients in comparison with the bedridden and anorectic patients who fared worse.

Tumor location and length were important determinants of outcome. Outcome was better for tumors in straight segments of the mid-esophagus or distal esophagus, particularly if they were less than 5 cm in length. Tumors that recurred at the anastomotic site after a previous esophagogastrectomy were particularly easy to treat and afforded the most dramatic relief because the obstructed segment was short. If obstruction occurred in a sharply angulated, anatomically distorted site at an anastomosis or near the gastroesophageal junction, both the technical difficulty and the probability of perforation were increased. The outcome tended not to be as good. Such horizontal, aperistaltic segments would require food to cross without the aid of gravity, thereby increasing the likelihood of obstruction.

Tumors of the cervical esophagus had the poorest outcome. When the proximal tumor margin is within 3 to 4 cm of the cricopharyngeus, it can be difficult to know where to deliver treatment. The lumen may not be clearly defined and the maneuverability of the endoscope is lessened, making it difficult to aim the laser beam. Risk of aspiration is also greater with cervical tumors. Also, with cervical tumors, it is not unusual to have little or no improvement in swallowing after ELT, even though standard endoscopes readily pass through the laser-treated area.

This exemplifies the difference between technical and functional success, later examined by Mellow and Pinkas.[18] In their series, 30 consecutive patients with advanced carcinoma of the esophagus and gastroesophageal junction underwent palliative ELT. Functional success was not an implicit sequela for the 97% of patients for whom luminal patency was achieved. Functional success as they defined it—the ability to ingest all necessary calories and leave the hospital for home—was possible for 70% of patients. These figures mirror the experience of Fleischer and his cumulative series of 120 patients with esophagogastric cancer, where 95% had technical success, while 73% had functional success (unpublished data). This schism was greater for adenocarcinoma than for squamous cell carcinoma, probably reflecting the greater percentage of adenocarcinomas involving the gastroesophageal junction. In addition to location of tumor in the cervical esophagus or gastroesophageal junction, reasons for poor functional success are radiation-induced pharyngeal dysphagia, anorexia, painful tumor load, debility, and treatment complications.

Procedure-related death and perforation are the major complications of ELT of the esophagogastric lesions. Procedure-related death is rare and was not encountered in Fleischer's cumulative series. In that 120-patient series, there were 7 (6%) perforations. This is in line with data reported at the Washington Symposium on ELT in April 1985, where 13 investigators reported perforation rates of 0 to 4%, and 13 investigators reported rates of 5 to 10%.[19] Erosion of laser-treated necrotic tissue can cause mediastinal or abdominal perforation and tracheoesophageal fistula. It can occur days to months after ELT. It is often difficult to solely implicate ELT in the etiology of perforations, given that a previous course of radiation therapy or dilatation can also be responsible and that they also can occur spontaneously without any treatment. The potential for perforation is higher when the laser damages the luminal wall, as can be expected with endoscopists inexperienced in ELT, or when technical difficulty is great, as when treating the cervical esophagus. Such perforation can be avoided by focusing the beam on the central luminal area, and avoiding, as much as possible, treatment of tumor adjacent to esophageal wall. Conservative treatment with fasting, parenteral nutrition, and antibiotics often suffices. Tracheoesophageal fistulas require prosthetic stent placement.

Occasionally, perforation is suspected clinically, as when free intraperitoneal air is seen on routine postlaser x-rays, but no perforation is found at surgical exploration. This benign pneumoperitoneum may be due to the passage of coaxial gas through necrotic laser-treated tumor tissue. Therefore, a barium swallow is recommended to confirm suspected perforations.

Minor complications that are not uncommon include low-grade temperature elevations and milk leukocytosis. In most patients, both resolve without treatment in less than 24 hours. Blood cultures and chest x-rays typically reveal no evidence of bacteremia or aspiration pneumonia, suggesting that tissue inflammation and necrosis are the etiologies for these findings.

While severe pain during ELT is unusual, pain can infrequently make patients uncomfortable enough to temporarily halt treatment. Pain is much more common in patients with submucosal disease in whom it is necessary to burn through normal mucosa than in patients with mucosal tumor. Additional intravenous meperidine invariably relieves the pain, but some patients may benefit from pretreatment with 2% xylocaine delivered through a sclerotherapy needle. Mild pain after the procedure is handled with a mild analgesic. Infrequently, more severe pain may last for up to 1 week before resolving spontaneously.

Minor bleeding can be expected with the destruction of friable, malignant tissue during ELT. It occurs in approximately 50% of patients, but is easily managed and usually stops spontaneously. If not, laser coagulation at a lower power setting is usually satisfactory. Uncontrolled bleeding secondary to ELT was not observed in the 120 patients in Fleischer's cumulative series.

Gastric overdistension before opening the esophageal lumen may cause discomfort, vasovagal response with bradycardia, or respiratory distress in approximately 12% of patients.[17] Frequent evacuation of air and turning down the coaxial gas flow can quickly reverse this complication. Aspiration was unusual and was suspected in only 5 of 120 patients in Fleischer's series.

Summary

Cure of obstructing tumors of the esophagus and gastric cardia is rare. After the possibility of cure is ruled out, palliation is the primary goal. ELT provides effective palliation with minimization of morbidity and mortality. With proper training, the technique is easily learned by experienced endoscopists. The place of ELT versus modalities for palliative therapy is not as yet fully defined. The focus of further investigation should be on how these modalities can interface in a complementary manner and in what situations one treatment is truly preferable to another.

References

1. Fleischer D, Kessler F, Haye O: Endoscopic Nd:YAG laser therapy for carcinoma of the esophagus: A new palliative approach. Am J Surg 143:280, 1982.
2. Earlam R, Cunha-Melo JR: Oesophageal squamous cell carcinoma: II. A critical review of radiotherapy. Br J Surg 67:457, 1980.
3. Earlam R, Cunha-Melo JR: Oesophageal squamous cell carcinoma: I. A critical review of surgery. Br J Surg 67:381, 1980.
4. Kelsen D: Chemotherapy of esophageal cancer. Semin Oncol 11:159, 1984.
5. Kelsen D, Coonley C, Hilaris B, et al: Cisplatin, vindesine, and bleomycin combination chemotherapy of local, regional, and advanced esophageal carcinoma. Am J Med 75:639, 1983.
6. Roth J: Personal communication, M.D. Anderson Hospital, Houston, TX. (1986)
7. Heit HA, Johnson LF, Siegel SR, Boyce HW: Palliative dilatation for dysphagia in esophageal carcinoma. Ann Intern Med 89:629, 1978.
8. Cassidy DE, Nord HJ, Boyce HW: Management of malignant esophagus strictures. [Abstract]. Am J Gastroenterol 76:173, 1981.
9. Graham DY, Dobbs SM, Zubler N: What is the role of prosthesis insertion in esophageal carcinoma? Gastrointest Endosc 29:1, 1983.
10. Ogilvie AL, Dronfield MW, Ferguson R, Atkinson M: Palliative intubation of oesophagogastric neoplasms at fiberoptic fibreoptic endoscopy. Gut 23:1060, 1982.
11. den Hartog Jagar FCA, Bartelsman JFWM, Tytgat GNH: Palliative treatment of obstructing esophagogastric malignancy by endoscopic positioning of a plastic prosthesis. Gastroenterology 77:1078, 1979.
12. Fleischer D, Kessler F: Endoscopic Nd:YAG laser therapy for carcinoma of the esophagus: A new form of palliative treatment. Gastroenterology 85:600, 1983.
13. Joffe SN: Preliminary clinical applications of the contact surgical rod and endoscopic microprobes with one Nd:YAG laser. Gastrointest Endosc 31:155, 1985.
14. Pietrafitta J, Dwyer R: Endoscopic laser therapy of malignant esophageal obstruction. Arch Surg 121:395, 1986.
15. Mellow MH, et al: Endoscopic therapy for esophageal carcinoma with Nd:YAG laser: Perspective evaluation of efficacy, complications, and survival. Gastrointest Endosc 29:165, 1983.
16. Fleischer D, Sivak MV: Endoscopic Nd:YAG laser therapy as palliative treatment for advanced adenocarcinoma of the gastric cardia. Gastroenterology 87:815, 1984.
17. Fleischer D, Sivak MV: Endoscopic Nd:YAG laser therapy as palliation for esophagogastric cancer: Parameters affecting initial outcome. Gastroenterology 89:827, 1985.
18. Mellow MH, Pinkas H: Endoscopic laser therapy for malignancies affecting the esophagus and gastroesophageal junction: Analysis of technical and functional efficacy. Arch Intern Med 145:1443, 1985.
19. Fleischer D: The Washington Symposium on Endoscopic Laser Therapy. April 18–19, 1985. Gastrointest Endosc 31:397, 1985.

9
Endoscopic Laser Treatment of Gastrointestinal Tract Cancer in Japan: Update

Yanao Oguro and Hisao Tajiri

Owing to the recent advances in gastroenterologic endoscopy, it has become possible to treat radically some types of early gastric cancer by endoscopic procedures. In 1973, we were the first in Japan to treat an elevated type of early gastric cancer by endoscopic polypectomy. Since then, 12 cases of such lesions have been treated by this method, without surgery, in our hospital. Of these patients, 11 have been alive for more than 5 years, and one died from renal cancer, independent of the gastric malignancy treated 6 years ago.[1]

In 1978, we began to study laser endoscopy in the radical treatment of early gastric cancer and the recanalization of obstructions of the gastrointestinal tract. Endoscopic laser treatment for these malignancies has now been performed in many hospitals and medical institutes in Japan.

In April 1981, the Laser Endoscopy Committee of the Japan Society for Gastroenterological Endoscopy (Chairman: Yanao Oguro) began a study of the current status of laser endoscopy, especially for the treatment of gastrointestinal cancers, throughout Japan.[2] Subsequent studies were performed in November 1982,[3] in June 1984, and in November 1985. The results of the last study is reported here, comparing it to former studies.

Method of the Studies

Questionnaires were mailed to 133 hospitals and institutes, where endoscopic laser systems were available and endoscopic laser treatment was being performed, especially for gastrointestinal cancers. The addresses were obtained from former studies, from papers presented in selected symposia, and from laser companies in Japan. Answers were collected from 75 institutions in November 1985. The response rate was 56.4%. Of these 75 institutions, endoscopic laser equipment for use in gastroenterology was available in 66 hospitals.

Results of the Studies

Endoscopic Laser Equipment Available for Gastroenterology

In November 1985 there were 82 endoscopic lasers in use for gastroenterology in Japan, of which 63 were Nd:YAG lasers (Table 9.1). Compared with the June 1984 study, there was an increase of 20 lasers: 19 Nd:YAG and one N_2-dye. The number of argon and/or argon-dye lasers, remained the same 15 in both studies.

Endoscopic Laser Treatment for Gastrointestinal Cancers

As of November 1985, 1558 cases of gastrointestinal cancer had been treated by laser endoscopy in Japan, an increase of 569 cases since the June 1984 study. Radical treatment was performed in 1076 cases (an increase of 311 cases), of which, 963 cases were gastric cancer. Symptomatic and/or palliative treatment was administered in 482 cases (an increase of 228), and, of

TABLE 9.1. Laser apparatus in digestive endoscopy

Type of laser	Manufacturer	No. of Units
Nd:YAG	MBB	30
	Molectron	25
	Olympus	3
	Aloka	3
	Pentax	1
	Fujinon	1
	subtotal	63
Argon or Argon dye	Spectra Physics	6
	Lexel	3
	Coherent Radiation	4
	Cooper Medical	2
	subtotal	15
Krypton	Spectra Physics	2
N_2-dye	Molectron	1
	Cooper Medical	1
Total		82

November 1985, Japan.

TABLE 9.2. Laser treatment for gastrointestinal cancer

Treatment	Site	No. of cases
Radical (Curative) purpose	Esophagus	54
	Stomach	963
	Colon	52
	Others	7
	Subtotal	1076
Palliative, symptomatic	Bleeding	102
	Stenosis	327
	Others	53
	Subtotal	482
Total		1558

November 1985, Japan.

these, recanalization was performed in 327 cases (Table 9.2).

Radical Treatment with Laser Endoscopy for Early Gastric Cancer and Its Lymph Node Metastasis

Endoscopic laser treatment for early gastrointestinal cancers may be indicated for the following two conditions: (1) absence of lymph node or distant metastasis, and (2) complete vaporization of the cancerous lesion by laser irradiation. As shown in Table 9.3, we studied the frequency of lymph node metastasis in early gastric cancer cases after radical laser irradiation, in which there was no residual carcinoma in the surgically removed stomach. Of 68 patients who had been surgically treated for early gastric cancer, there were 3 cases (4.4%) with lymph node metastasis, all being the type IIc early gastric cancer. These three cases give a 7.7% incidence for the group of 39 cases of IIc having lymph node involvement. According to these results, the frequency of lymph node metastasis is higher in IIc with an ulcer or ulcerous scar (U1), than a IIc without ulceration. Therefore, the indication for radical laser endoscopy treatment for IIc type with U1 should be determined carefully.

According to our pathologic study on the surgically operated cases with early gastric cancer,[1] there was no lymph node metastasis nor distant metastasis in the following four types:

1. Pedunculated polypoid type (type I) of early gastric cancer, restricted to the mucosal layer only

TABLE 9.3. No residual carcinoma in surgically removed organs, after radical irradiation with laser endoscopy

Site	Type of carcinoma	No. of cases	Lymph node metastasis (+)	Lymph node metastasis (−)	Percentage of (+) lymph node metastasis
Esophagus	Superficial	2		2	0
Stomach	I	4		4	
	IIa	19		19	
	IIa + IIc	2		2	
	IIc	39	3	36	3/39 = 7.7%
	IIc + III	4		4	
Total		68		65	3/68 = 4.4%
Colon	I	2		2	0

November 1985, Japan.

TABLE 9.4. Radical endoscopic lasar treatment of early gastric cancer

	No. of patients in each group			
Laser	Group A*	Group B**	Group C†	Total patients
Nd:YAG	325	88	349	762
Argon	9	2	0	11
Argon + HpD	1	0	4	5
Argon-dye + HpD	28	2	50	80
Others	1	3	5	9
Total	364	95	408	867
Percent	42.0	11.0	47.0	100.0

November 1985, Japan.
HpD = hematoporphyrin derivative.
*Negative biopsy more than 1 year after treatment.
**Positive biopsy 1 year after treatment.
†Evaluation pending—less than 1 year follow-up.

2. IIa type of early gastric cancer, less than 3 cm in diameter
3. Gastritis-like early gastric cancer, less than 2 cm in diameter
4. Focal cancer

The first lesion in the list would be managed more effectively by endoscopic polypectomy than by laser irradiation. However, radical laser irradiation is indicated for the remaining three types of early gastric cancer. Laser irradiation with endoscopy can be performed as radical therapy for almost any type of early gastric cancer, in those patients with other serious diseases, those whose advanced age prohibits surgery, and those who simply refuse surgery.

Results of Endoscopic Laser Treatment for Early Gastric Cancer, for the Purpose of Radical Therapy Without Surgery

As shown in the Table 9.4, 867 patients with early gastric cancer were treated with radical laser irradiation without surgery. Among them, 762 cases were treated by Nd:YAG laser, 80 cases by argon-dye laser, 5 cases by argon laser, and 9 cases by the other lasers. More than 1 year posttreatment, 364 patients (42.0%) had negative biopsy (Group A in Table 9.4). In the same series, 95 patients (11.0%) showed positive biopsy after 1 year (Group B in Table 9.4). Evaluation was pending at the time of this writing in another 408 cases (47.0%) because follow-up was less

TABLE 9.5. Symptomatic endoscopic laser treatment for gastrointestinal cancers

Symptom	Effective	Noneffective	Total	Effectiveness (%)
Bleeding	76	26	102	74.5
Stenosis				64.6
Esophagus	41	28	69	
Cardia	55	19	74	
Pylorus	35	36	71	
Stoma	44	8	52	
Others	42	28	70	
Subtotal	217	119	326	
Tumor reduction, etc.	33	11	44	75.0
Total	326	156	472	69.1

November 1985, Japan.

TABLE 9.6. Complications resulting from accidents, endoscopic laser irradiation gastrointestinal cancers

Type of treatment for accident	Bleeding	Perforation	Pyloric stenosis	Death by laser	Total no. of accidents
Laser hemostasis	4				4
Nonsurgical	19				19
Surgery	6	1	1		8
Ethanol injection	2				2
Others	1		1		2
Total	32	1	2	0	35
Total treated cases					1558
Percent	2.0	0.1	0.1	0	2.2

November 1985, Japan.

than 1 year (Group C in Table 9.4). The high percentage of pending results attests to the recency of laser treatment for early gastric cancer.

Result of Symptomatic Treatment with Laser Endoscopy for Gastrointestinal Cancers

As shown in Table 9.5, laser photocoagulation was performed in 102 cases of cancer-related gastrointestinal bleeding with 74.5% success. Laser endoscopy for obstruction caused by cancer of the esophagus, cardia, pylorus, stoma, and other sites was performed in 326 cases, with 64.6% success overall. Laser endoscopic irradiation for the purpose of tumor reduction, and so on, was performed in 44 cases, with 75.0% success.

Complications of Endoscopic Laser Irradiation for Gastrointestinal Cancers

In our series of 1588 patients with gastrointestinal cancer treated by endoscopic laser irradiation we experienced 35 complications. The most frequent complication was bleeding encountered in 32 cases (2.0%). There were two cases of pyloric stenosis and one perforation. Most of the complications were treated nonsurgically; a few required surgery, laser hemostasis, ethanol injection, or other methods (Table 9.6). There were no deaths as a result of a complication.

References

1. Oguro Y, et al: Endoscopic treatment of early gastric cancer:polypectomy and laser treatment. Jpn J Clin Oncol 14(2):271–282, 1984.
2. Oguro Y, et al: Collective studies on gastroenterological laser endoscopy in Japan. Prog Dig Endosc 19:62–64, 1981.
3. Oguro Y, et al: Present status of laser medicine and laser endoscopic treatment for cancers of gastrointestinal tract in Japan. Prog Dig Endosc 26:152–157, 1985.

10
New Modalities of Contact Nd:YAG Laser Endoscopy for General Application in the Gastrointestinal Tract

Sohtaro Suzuki, Jun Aoki, and Takeshi Miwa

It is generally recognized that fiberoptic endoscopy has both diagnostic and therapeutic uses and is one of the most common procedures in clinical gastroenterology. In the last decade, several endoscopic modalities for the treatment of gastrointestinal hemorrhage and neoplasms have been applied clinically. They include laser irradiation,[1–5] electrocoagulation,[6] topical injection, sclerotherapy, thermoprobes,[7] and intubation of prosthesis.[8] All of these procedures naturally have both advantages and disadvantages. Laser endoscopy is an unique procedure. Since the middle 1970s, Nd:YAG lasers have been applied using the noncontact method with the optical quartz fiber.[1–5,8,9] There are distinct disadvantages of noncontact irradiation, such as the difficulty in keeping a constant distance from the tip of the quartz fiber to the lesion, allowing reliable tissue changes to occur related to the applied power. Furthermore, the quartz tip will be damaged when it comes into contact with tissue or blood. To overcome these disadvantages, the SLT contact method® with SLT endoprobes® directly connected to the quartz fiber was developed following reports of experimental research with the surgical probe, which was made of new ceramic materials.[10–12] We initiated experimental and clinical studies of endoscopic Nd:YAG laser therapy, comparing the new SLT contact ceramic endoprobes with the single noncontact quartz fiber endoprobes, in order to evaluate the histologic effects and safety of each method. In this chapter, we discuss the possibilities of the clinical application of SLT contact endoprobes as a new endoscopic modality in the gastrointestinal tract.[13–16]

Contact Irradiation with SLT (Surgical Laser Technologies Inc) Endoprobes®

Properties of Endoprobes

Newly developed SLT contact endoprobes are made of a ceramic obtained from Al_2O_3 powder (Surgical Laser Technologies Melvel, PA and Japan Co. Ltd.). Many of the physical characteristics of aluminum oxide are advantageous for medical equipment: high melting point, low thermal conductivity, high mechanical strength, hardness, and good transmission of the Nd:YAG laser beam compared to that of the quartz fiber. It is easy to produce several different probe shapes to get a number of divergent angles and power densities with this transparent new ceramic material (Figure 10.1). These endoprobes can be screwed into a metal universal connector attached to the tip of a quartz fiber. The outer diameter of the tip is 2.2 mm, and so is able to pass through the biopsy channel of a standard upper gastrointestinal fiberscope (Figure 10.2).

Histologic Findings with Contact Endoprobes

One to two weeks after Nd:YAG laser exposure, the canine stomach was removed and fixed in 10% formalin. Each irradiated lesion was sectioned into 5-mm slices to select the central area of deepest injury for histologic examination. The histologic findings were studied by hematoxylin-eosin staining and Elastica-van Gieson staining[13] (Figure 10.3).

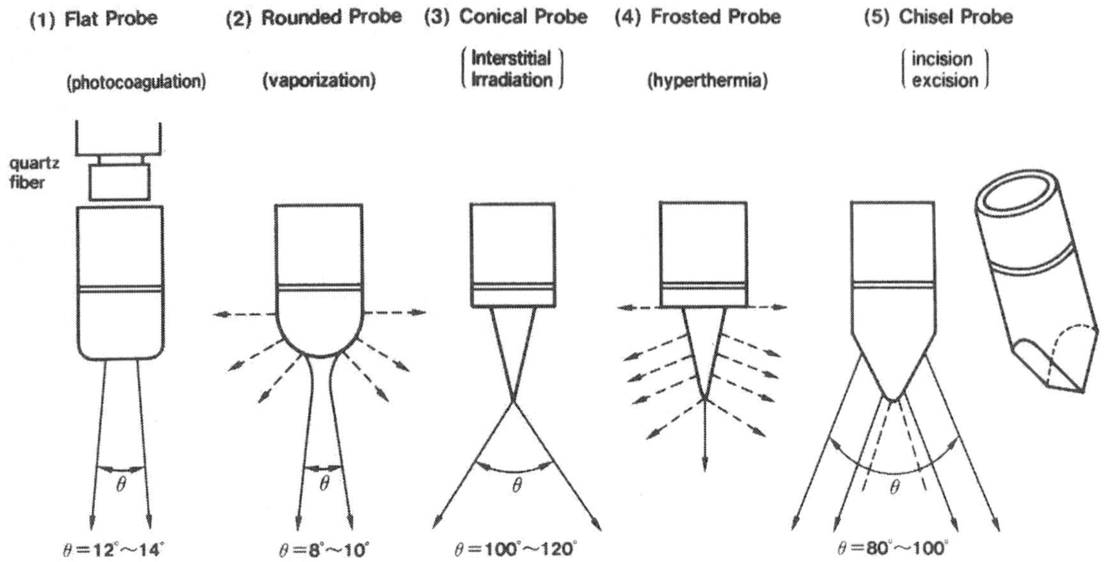

FIGURE 10.1. Contact method of laser endoscopy: type and beam divergence of endoprobes.

Effects with the SLT Flat Probe® and the SLT Rounded Probe®

The histologic examination of the canine gastric wall showed that photocoagulation and vaporization through the mucosal layer to the submucosal layer occurred from contact irradiation with the flat probe and the rounded probe, with less than 20 W power and a short pulse (1.0 to 2.0 seconds) duration. We reported earlier[13] that high-power contact irradiation—>30 W—with continuous pulse (>3.0 seconds) duration produced transmural damages and might lead to excessive penetration and perforation of the gastric wall.

Effects with the SLT Chisel Probe®

Irradiation with the chisel probe at a power of 20 W and a duration of 1.0 to 2.0 seconds can incise the mucosal surface with less hemorrhage. This procedure may be applied for the recanalization of benign or tumorous strictures, and mucosal incision or excision for complete biopsy

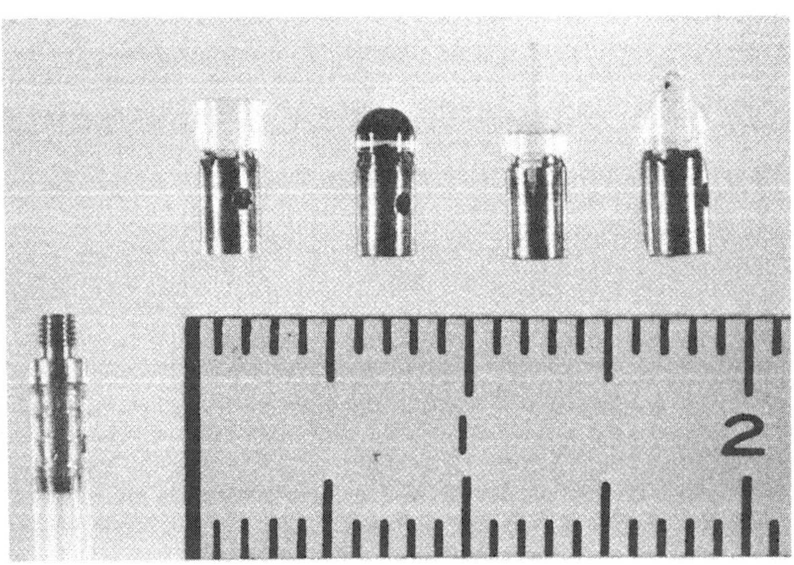

FIGURE 10.2. Contact endoprobes.

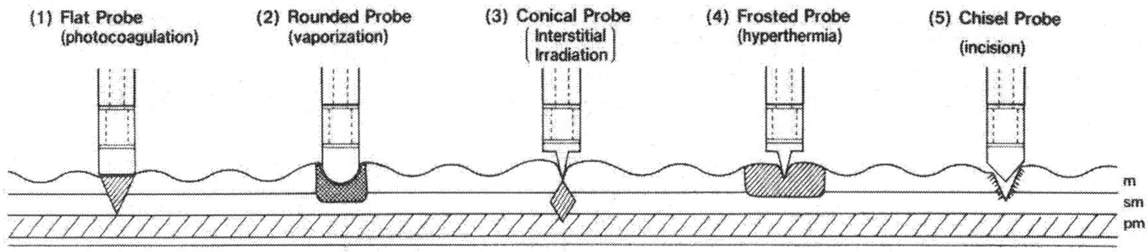

FIGURE 10.3. Histologic effects on canine gastric wall with contact method of Nd:YAG laser. m, mucosa; sm, submucosa; pm, proprial muscle.

of submucosal tumor in the gastrointestinal tract.

Effects with the SLT Frosted Probe®

Interstitial irradiation with the frosted probe[14] effectively stops bleeding and reduces local hyperthermia (laserthermia) with lower power (<5 W) and longer continuous duration (5 to 20 minutes). Among the remarkable histologic changes after low-power interstitial irradiation were intravascular coagulation and thrombosis in the submucosal layer, mucosal edema and hyperemia (Figures 10.4 and 10.5).

Clinical Application

Photocoagulation with the flat probe is easier and safer to use than the noncontact endoprobes for controlling the irradiation depth and area in relation to the exposed power and duration. Therefore, the flat probe may be indicated for all types of gastrointestinal diseases, such as

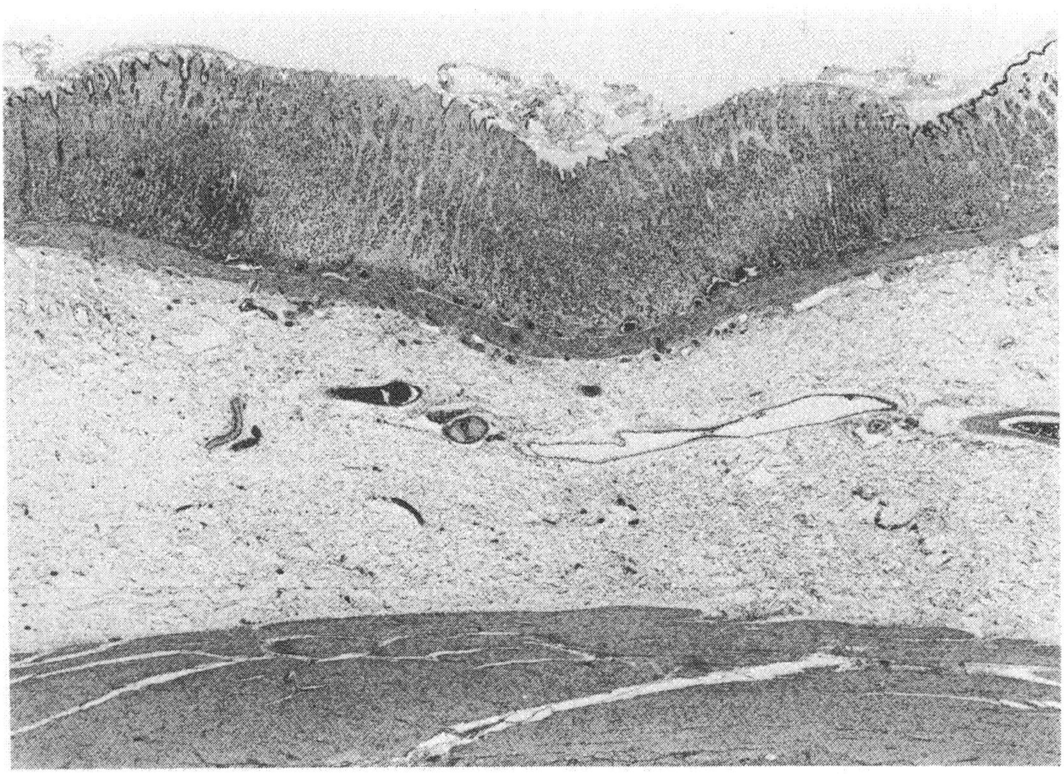

FIGURE 10.4. Soon after laserthermia for 5 minutes, mucosal edema and hyperemia were apparent. (Hematoxylin and eosin, ×20).

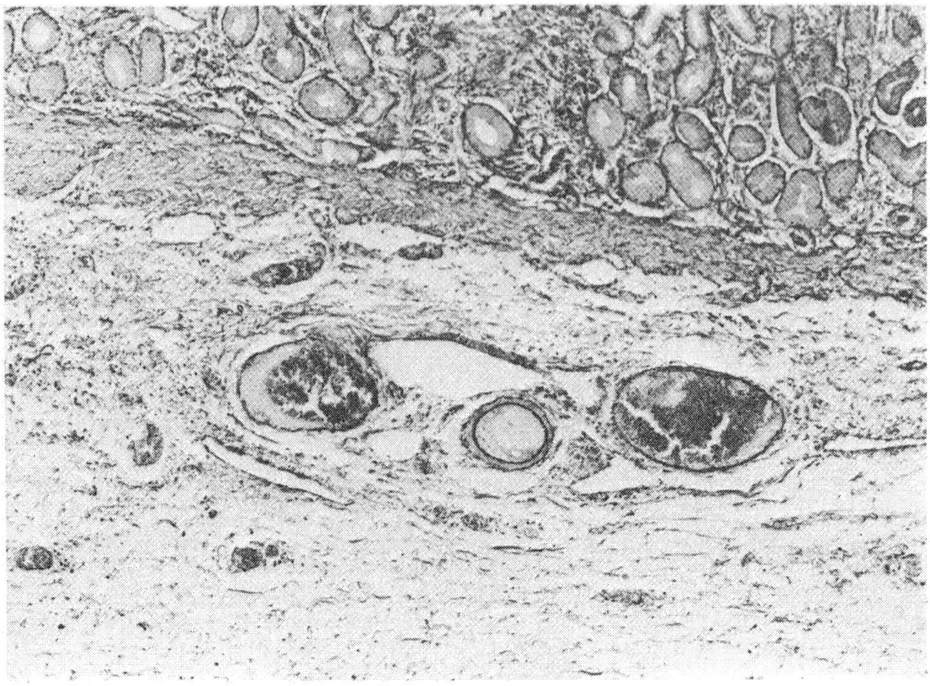

FIGURE 10.5. Soon after laserthermia, intravascular coagulation in the submucosal layer without ulceration was seen. (EVG, ×112).

depressed or protruded lesions. Vaporization with the rounded probe can reduce the tumor mass. From August 1980 to June 1986, we treated 50 patients—63 lesions—with the Nd:YAG endoscopic laser as initial therapy. These patients had contraindications for surgery because of associated diseases. Noncontact irradiation was administered to 30 of the lesions: 2 esophageal superficial cancers, 10 adenomas, and 9 early gastric cancers. In this group, 21 lesions (70.0%) were effectively cured. In another group of 19 lesions—1 superficial esphageal cancer, 15 adenomas, and 3 early gastric cancers—irradiated with contact endoprobes, 16 lesions (84.2%) were cured. The local curative rate by the contact endoprobe method was 14.2% higher than the curative rate by the conventional noncontact method.

Other clinical benefits of this new modality of the contact method are as follows: One case of pyloric stricture due to a peptic ulcer and four cases of a submucosal tumor in the middle esophagus were treated and diagnosed by excisional procedures with the chisel probe, and interstitial irradiation with the frosted probe in a case of gastric ulcer hemorrhage caused by stress.

Endoscopic Laserthermia®

According to S.G. Bown,[17] Nd:YAG laser hyperthermia can be induced by placing a bare quartz fiber into the tumor tissue. We have been studying Nd:YAG laser hyperthermia (Laserthermia®) with the SLT contact endoprobe, which has a conical shape and diffused laser beam on its surface, at a low-power density of about 0.05 W/cm^2 for 1 W of total irradiated energy.

Computer-Controlled Laserthermia System®

We developed the computer-controlled endoscopic contact Nd:YAG laser systems for local interstitial hyperhermia.[14] This system is shown in Figures 10.6 and 10.7. The measuring of the tissue temperature with the thermo-

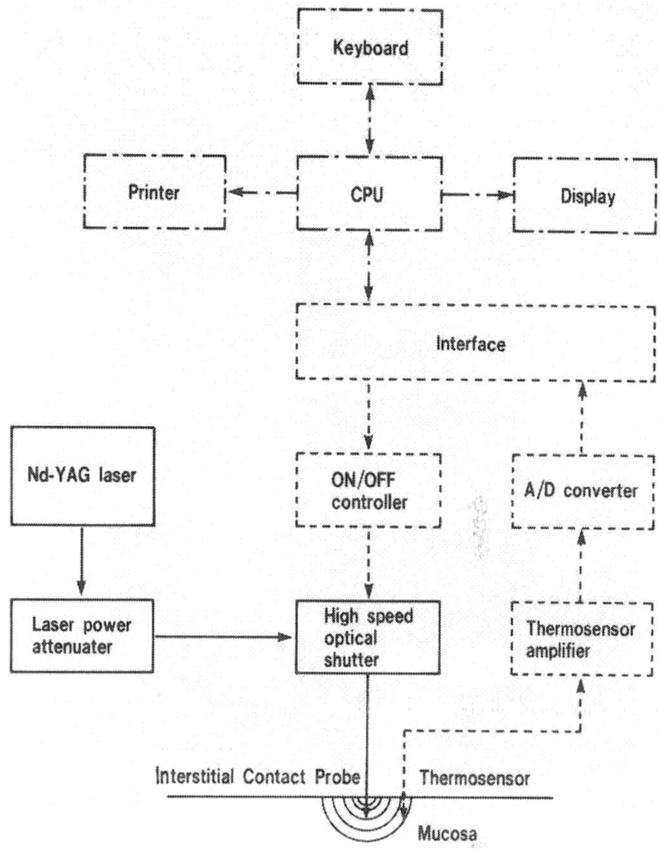

FIGURE 10.6. Computer-controlled Nd:YAG laserthermia system. (—) Nd:YAG laser system; (---) control and monitor system. (—-—-—) computer system.

couple was confirmed by comparative studies of simultaneous measurements from the thermocouple and the thermogram showed no interference during the low-power Nd:YAG laser irradiation.

The control mode for temperature with laser delivery is shown in Figure 10.8. For the first stage of irradiation by laserthermia, laser energy was delivered continuously from the basal temperature of the subject until the "lower control temperature" of 42.0 or 43.0°C was reached. When the tissue temperature reached the "upper control temperature" of 43.5°C, it stopped delivering laser energy. During the laserthermia treatment, this control pattern was carried out in the operating mode.

Histologic Findings

For 5 to 10 minutes after laserthermia, wide superficial mucosal edema and hyperemia (Figure 10.4) developed, and intravascular coagulation appeared in the submucosal layer. Two weeks after the procedure the mucosal surface was covered with thin regenerating epithelium, and fibrosis and thrombosis was seen in the submucosal layer around the irradiated area, about 1.0 cm in width (Figure 10.9).

Application to an Experimental Gastric Tumor

The computerized laserthermia system was applied to an ENNG-induced gastric tumor in Beagle dogs. Thermal control of this system was stable and safe with a power of 3 W for a duration of 20 minutes (Figure 10.10). Laserthermia was repeated at 2-week intervals. Each session was performed for 20 minutes at temperatures between 43.0 and 43.5°C with a laser power of 3 W and 0.5-second pulse duration. The size of the tumor reduced during these procedures, eradicating the largest tumor which was 3.0 cm in diameter after four sessions.

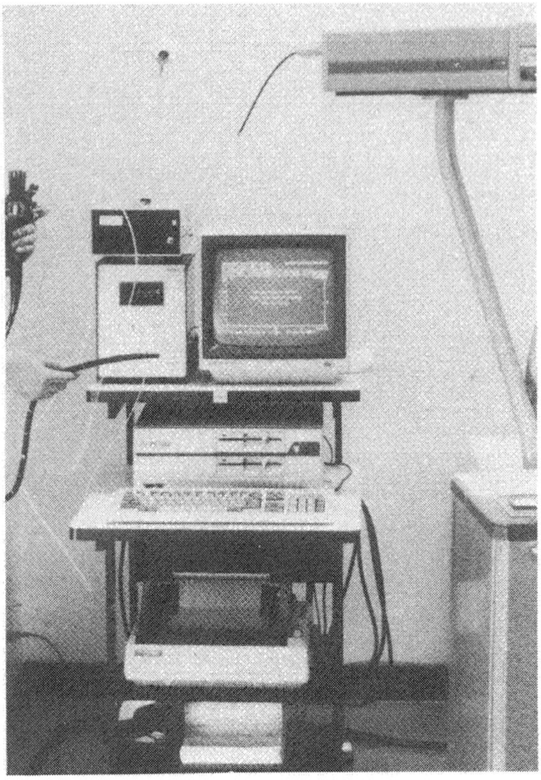

FIGURE 10.7. Computer system with Nd:YAG endoscopy.

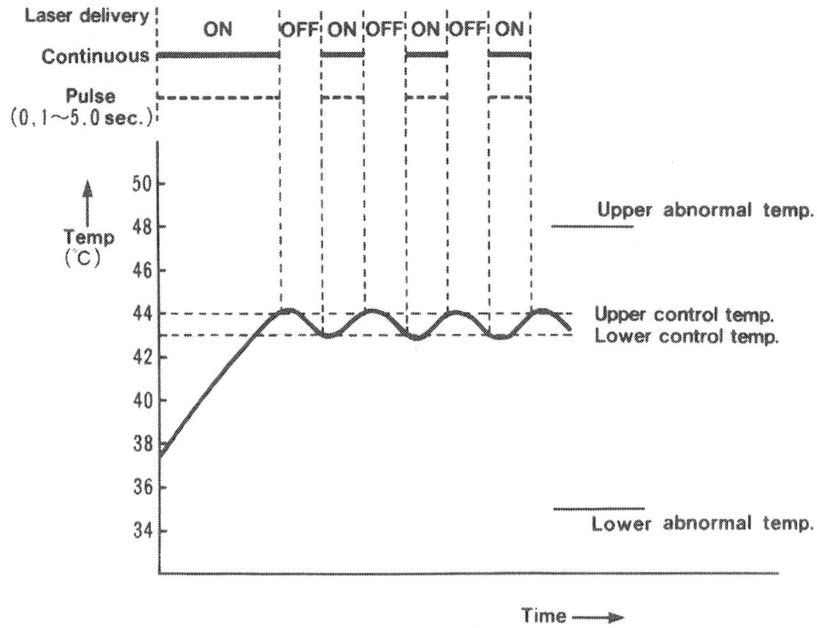

FIGURE 10.8. Control method for temperature with laser delivery.

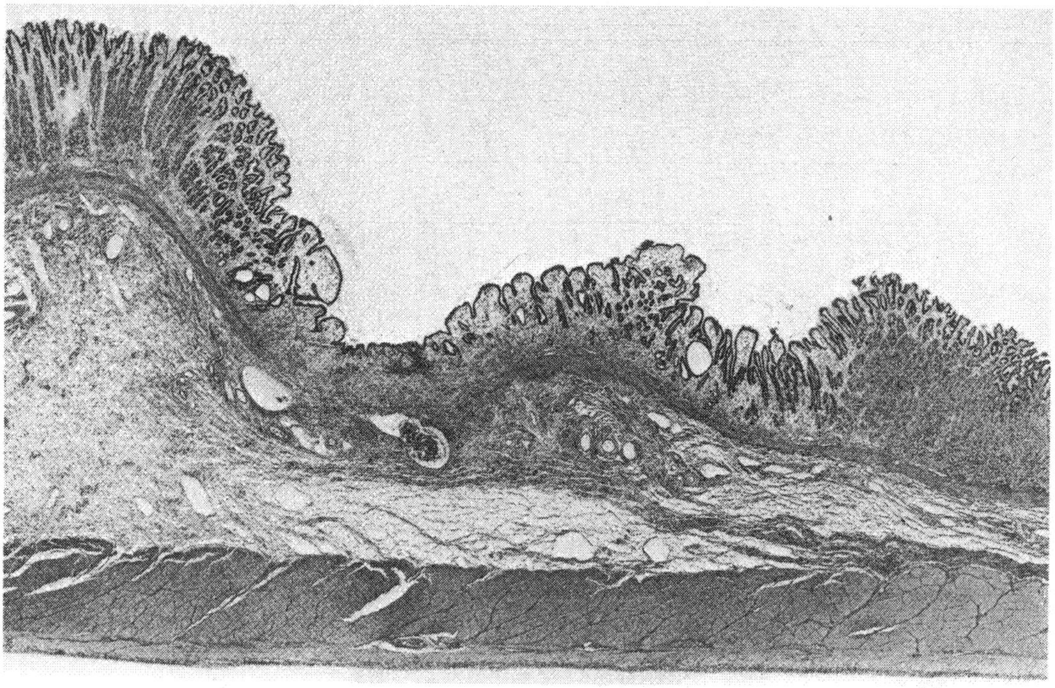

FIGURE 10.9. After 2 weeks, laserthermal irradiation for 5 minutes, *42.0 ± 1.0°C,* showed thin regenerating epithelium and submucosal fibrosis. (Hematoxylin and eosin, ×12).

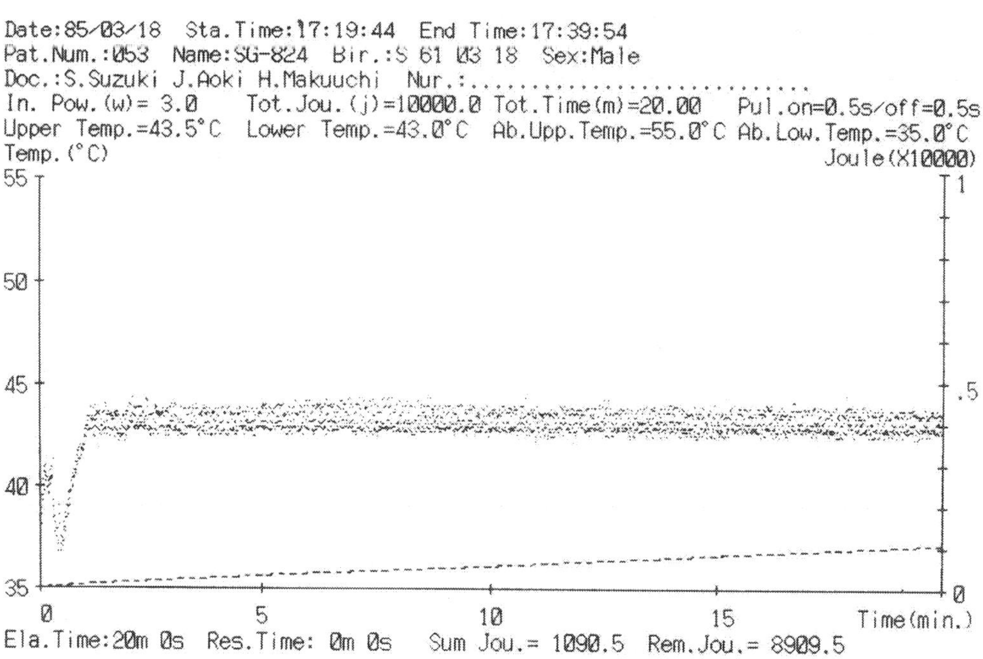

FIGURE 10.10. Computer-controlled Nd:YAG laserthermia of an experimental gastic tumor.

Discussion

Since the middle of the 1970s, the noncontact Nd:YAG laser method with a single quartz fiber has been applied to clinical endoscopy. Although the Nd:YAG laser for therapy of acute upper gastrointestinal bleeding was effectively hemostatic, it was technically more difficult to use and potentially could cause complications.[1–5] Only 70 to 80% of the patients studied were hemostatically controlled. This was discussed in detail at the symposium "Problems of Hemostatic Procedures" at the 25th annual meeting of the Japan Society of Gastroenterological Endoscopy (JSGE) in May 1983. There were no differences reported in the clinical results of the various hemostatic procedures for upper gastrointestinal hemorrhage, whether H_2-recepter antagonists, secretin, laser irradiation, electrocoagulation, topical injection of absolute ethanol or epinephrine, and sprays of thrombin or fibrinogen were used. Several reasons that no increased benefits were reported from laser therapy, compared to other endoscopic modalities, may be that the noncontact method requires the quartz tip to be at least 1.0 cm from the lesion. About half of the applied energy is lost by the noncontact irradiation by backscattering. Therefore, a large amount of energy is required for endoscopic noncontact Nd:YAG laser therapy. In addition, the tip of the quartz fiber can be damaged upon contact with tissue, blood or fluid during laser exposure.

It was demonstrated in our studies that the SLT contact endoprobes® made of synthetic sapphire, in reference to their various physical properties, including beam divergence and thermal conductivity, have been more effective than the conventional noncontact method with a quartz fiber. Deeper histologic effects by low-power Nd:YAG laser irradiation may be produced by concentrating the power density and decreasing the backscatter.[11–13]

Although clinical results of endoscopic contact laser therapy with SLT contact endoprobes® has improved, there are still some residual areas of tumor tissue after irradiation. It is still difficult to treat certain local lesions curatively even if contact irradiation is superior to the effects of the noncontact method. This has now led to endoscopic local hyperthermia (Laserthermia®) with the SLT contact frosted endoprobe® as a local curative treatment.

It is suggested that wider areas of histologic damage from the mucosal layer to the middle layer of the gastric wall by Nd:YAG laserthermia with the computer control system will be better able to treat mucosal malignant tumors in the gastrointestinal tract. As for new modalities of endoscopic laser therapy, the SLT contact method with the various endoprobes makes it possible for applying interstitial irradiation mucosal incision or excision, and local laserthermia either alone or in combination. In accordance with the advance of modern technology, the contact method with endoprobes will not only make progress in endoscopic modalities but will also encourage the reduction of price of the laser equipment leading to even greater utilization.

References

1. Dwyer RM, Haverback BJ, Bass M, Cherlow J: Laser-induced hemostasis in the canine stomach. JAMA 231:486–489, 1975.
2. Kiefhaber P, Nath G, Moritz K: Endoscopical control of massive gastrointestinal hemorrhage by irradiation with a high-power neodymium-Yag laser. Prog Surg 15:140–155, 1977.
3. Silverstein FE, Protell RL, Gilbert DA, et al: Argon vs. neodymium YAG laser photocoagulation of experimental canine gastric ulcers. Gastroenterology 77:491–496, 1979.
4. Rutgeerts P, Vantrappen G, Broeckaert L, et al: A new and effective technique of Yag laser photocoagulation for sever upper gastrointestinal bleeding. Endoscopy 16:115–117, 1984.
5. Fleischer D: Endoscopic laser therapy for upper gastrointestinal tract disease. Surv Dig Dis 1:42–53, 1983.
6. Sugawa C, Shier M, Lucas CE, Walt AJ: Electrocoagulation of bleeding in the upper part of the gastrointestinal tract. Arch Surg 110:975–979, 1975.
7. Bate CM, Aziz LA: Electrohydrothermoprobe—A simple alternative to laser therapy in the management of acute gastrointestinal hemorrhage. Gut 26:477–480, 1985.
8. Ogilvie AL, Dronfield MW, Ferguson R, Atkinson M: Palliative intubation of oesophagogastric neoplasms at fiberoptic endoscopy. Gut 23:1060–1067, 1982.
9. Fleischer D, Silvak MV: Endoscopic Nd:YAG

laser therapy as palliative treatment for advanced adenocarcinoma of the gastric cardia. Gastroenterology 87:815–820, 1984.
10. Joffe SN: Contact Neodymium:YAG laser surgery in gastroenterology: A preliminary report. Laser Surg Med 6:155–157, 1986.
11. Suzuki S, Shiina Y, Miura T, et al: Effects of Nd-YAG laser radiation on the gastrointestinal mucosa. 6th report: Experimental studies with a new contact type of the YAG laser rod. Gastroenterol Endosc (in Japanese) 26:705–710, 1985.
12. Daikuzono N, Joffe SN: Artificial sapphire probe for contact photocoagulation and tissue vaporization with the Nd:YAG laser. Med Instrum 19:173–178, 1985.
13. Suzuki S, Aoki J, Shiina Y, et al: New ceramic endoprobes for endoscopic contact irradiation with Nd:YAG laser: Experimental studies and clinical applications. Gastrointest Endosc 33:282–286, 1986.
14. Suzuki S, Aoki J, Shiina Y, et al: Endoscopic local hyperthermia with Nd-YAG laser—Experimental study and development of computed thermosystem. J Soc Laser Med (in Japanese) 6:347–350, 1986.
15. Symposium: Problems of hemostatic procedures Gastroenterol Endosc (in Japanese) 25:1593–1629, 1983.
16. Halldorsson TH, Rother W, Langerholc J, Frank F: Theoretical and experimental investigations prove Nd:YAG-laser treatment to be safe. Int Med Laser Symp, 29:3–31, 1979.
17. Bown SG: Tumor therapy with the Nd-YAG laser. In Joffe SN, Muckerheide M, Goldman L (eds): Neodymium-YAG Laser in Medicine and Surgery. Elsevier, New York, pp 59–70, 1983.

11

Contact Nd:YAG Laser Treatment of Gastrointestinal Tract Cancer

Hisao Tajiri and Yanao Oguro

Although general surgery is probably still the usual modality for most clinicians in the management of gastrointestinal cancer, recent refinements in endoscopy have stimulated support for this tool. Laser endoscopy, in particular, has become widely used, with excellent results. This usage has sharpened an awareness of its indications and problems.[1]

Since 1980, when laser endoscopy was clinically adopted at our hospital, the number of patients selected for this therapeutic course for gastrointestinal cancer has been increasing yearly. As laser endoscopy is still in the stage of early development, progressive features appear from time to time, and just recently we adopted the new synthetic sapphire contact endoprobe.[2,3] This chapter reports our study of the relative advantages of the contact endoprobe (contact method), in contrast to the traditional noncontact method.

Patients and Methods

From 1980 to April 1986 at our National Cancer Center Hospital (Tokyo), 81 patients with gastrointestinal cancer have undergone treatment with the use of the endoscopic laser. The types of cancer we encountered were as follows: 8 patients with superficial esophageal cancer, 55 patients with early gastric cancer (23 type IIa and 32 type IIc), 15 patients with advanced gastric cancer, and 2 patients with colon cancer. We used the Nd:YAG laser (Medilas, MBB) in 59 cases, the HpD + argon-dye laser (Lexel Model 504) (photodynamic therapy) in 15 cases, and a combination of both lasers in 7 cases. The contact endoprobe (provided by Surgical Laser Technologies Japan Co., Ltd.) was therapeutically administered to 31 patients. The clinical details are given in Tables 11.1 to 11.3.

The treatment performance of the Nd:YAG laser with contact endoprobe required a power output of 10 to 30 W, with a duration of 1 to 2 seconds. The types of endoprobes used for case studies 1 to 27, except case 7, were the SLT Rounded Probe (most frequently used), Flat Probe, or Hollow Probe. The frequency of radiation ranged from 100 to 600 times, depending on the size of the lesion. Case 7 received photodynamic therapy with the Frosted Probe for coagulation and interstitial irradiation. In this case, hematoporphyrin derivative (HpD) in a dose of 2.5 mg/kg was given intravenously 72 hours before the therapy. The argon-dye laser, 300 mW, was radiated at six points on and around the lesion, 7 minutes each, for a total of 42 minutes. We attempted to treat three cases of stenosis of postsurgical anastomosis with the contact endoprobe after operations on esophageal cancers. We also attempted histologic diagnoses of submucosal tumors.

Results

We used the SLT contact Nd:YAG laser system to treat 26 of 27 cases of early gastric cancer. Photodynamic therapy was administered to one case in this group (Case 7). All 27 patients had macroscopic cancers: 18 cases of type IIc and 9 cases of type IIa. The cancers were small—less than 2 cm in diameter (Figure 11.1). Most of these patients were elderly, 78% were 65 or

TABLE 11.1. Clinical details of patients with early gastric cancer treated by the contact method: Resected cases and follow-up cases after more than one year

Case no.	Age (years)	Sex	Macroscopic type	Location	Size (cm)	Period following therapy (prognosis)*
1	84	M	IIa	Corpus post.	1.0	Operation (L)
2**	65	M	IIc	Remnant stomach	4.0	Operation (L)
3**	73	M	IIa	Antrum post.	2.0	16 m (died of heart failure)
4	57	F	IIc	Angle less.	1.5	20 (L)
5	77	F	IIc	Antrum less.	1.0–2.0	19 (L)
6	83	F	IIc	Angle less.	4.0	18 (L)
7†	85	M	IIc	Antrum great.	1.5	16 (L)
8	56	M	IIc	Angle less.	1.0	13 (L)
9	65	M	IIa	Corpus less.	1.5	12 (L)
10	72	M	IIa	Angle ant.	2.0	12 (L)
11	88	F	IIa	Antrum post.	1.5	12 (L)
12**	65	M	IIc	Antrum great.	1.0–2.0	12 (L)

May, 1986, National Cancer Center Hospital, Tokyo.
*L, living.
**Both the contact and the noncontact methods were used.
†Photodynamic therapy was used with the Frosted Probe.

older, with various coexisting complications, such as heart disease and liver disease, which made them unfit to undergo surgical treatment.

Two patients were subsequently treated by surgery after the laser treatment, and the resected specimens were examined histopathologically. For Case 1, no cancer residue was apparent. However, residual cancer in the submucosa was detected in Case 2. The remaining 25 cases were followed up as outpatients with endoscopy and multiple biopsies. More than 1 year had passed since the initial laser treatment for 10 of the 25 patients (Cases 3 to 12). With the exception of Case 3, there was no recurrent

TABLE 11.2. Clinical details of patients with early gastric cancer treated by the contact method: Follow-up cases for less than one year

Case no.	Age (years)	Sex	Macroscopic type	Location	Size (cm)	Months following therapy (prognosis)*
13	77	F	IIc	Antrum less.	0.5	10 (L)
14	84	F	IIc	Angle post.	2.0	9 (L)
15	74	M	IIa	Corpus great.	1.5	8 (L)
16	74	M	IIc	Corpus ant.	2.0	7 (L)
17	81	M	IIa	Corpus post.	1.5	6 (L)
18	65	M	IIc	Antrum post.	4.0	5 (L)
19**	69	M	IIc	Remnant stomach	2.0	4 (L)
20	76	M	IIa	Antrum less.	1.0	4 (L)
21	57	M	IIc	Antrum less.	1.0	3 (L)
22	52	M	IIc	Angle ant.	1.0	3 (L)
23	75	M	IIc	Antrum less.	1.0	3 (L)
24	63	M	IIa	Corpus great.	1.5	2 (L)
25**	60	M	IIc	Corpus post.	1.5	2 (L)
26**	79	F	IIc	Corpus post.	4.0	1 (L)
27**	69	M	IIc	Corpus post.	4.0	1 (L)

May, 1986, National Cancer Center Hospital, Tokyo.
*L, living.
**Both the contact and the noncontact methods were used.

TABLE 11.3. Clinical details of patients administered palliative therapy with the contact Nd:YAG laser method.

Case no.	Age (years)	Sex	Macroscopic type	Location	Purpose of therapy	Condition (power × second × pulse)	Result
1	72	F	Borrmann 3	Cardia	Alleviation of stenosis	15–20 W × 1.5 s × 324	Effective
2	61	M	Borrmann 3	Cardia	Alleviation of stenosis	30 W × 1.5 s × 400	Effective
3	77	F	Borrmann 2	Cardia	Alleviation of stenosis	30 W × 1–1.5 s × 353	Effective
4	74	M	Borrmann 3	Cardia	Alleviation of stenosis	20–25 W × 1–1.5 s × 420	Effective
5	88	M	After operation of esophageal cancer	Middle esophagus	Alleviation of stenosis	10–15 W × 1 s × 40	Effective
6	71	M	After operation of esophageal cancer	Middle esophagus	Alleviation of stenosis	10–15 W × 1 s × 83	Ineffective
7	40	M	After operation of esophageal cancer	Middle esophagus	Alleviation of stenosis	10–15 W × 1 s × 67	Ineffective → operation
8	40	M	Submucosal tumor	Antrum post.	Histologic diagnosis	15 W × 2 s × 5	Confirmed (glomus tumor)

May, 1986, National Cancer Center Hospital, Tokyo.

cancer. For 5 of the remaining 15 cases, less than 1 year—after the initial laser treatment, residual or recurrent cancer persisted, and the treatment was followed up more than twice. All of these were the depressed type of cancer.

The results of palliative treatments, using the contact Nd:YAG laser method, are shown in Table 11.3. Cases 1 to 4 underwent treatment in order to alleviate the stenosis that extended from the lower part of the esophagus to the cardia due to the advanced gastric cancer (Figure 11.2). Total obstruction was imminent. At least one month following the treatment, these 4 patients were freed from intravenous hyperalimentation (IVH) and were eating normally. Case 1 was even released from the hospital and thus became an outpatient. The Rounded Probe was used for vaporization of this lesion. The treatment was successful and excessive tissue damage and other adversities were avoided. In Case 8, 1.0 cm of the mucosa around the submucosal tumor was cut for histopathologiac diagnosis, and a biopsy of the submucosal tumore was done. This diagnosis, and a biopsy of the submucosal tumor was done. This was the first attempt using this method, and for confirmation of the histopathologic diagnosis, a local excision was performed. The tumor was confirmed to be a glomus tumor, 3 × 3 × 2 cm.

The Chisel Probe and Frosted Probe were used to treat the stenosis of the anastomosed portion that resulted from the treatment of esophageal cancer in Cases 5 to 7 in Table 11.3. The recovery of case 5 from the stenosis symptoms after the treatment was excellent and it was not necessary to see him at the hospital for 3 months.

Cases 6 and 7 also underwent incision for treating the stenosis. However, in these cases the stenosis recurred 2 to 4 weeks after therapy. In Case 6 the stenotic portion was resected, and he is still healthy. Case 7 died of metastatic carcinoma after 3 months of this therapy.

When we first used these probes, sometimes we observed mechanical problems between the probe and its metal sleeve. However, owing to the recent improvements in this instrument, no more damage has occurred, regardless of the number of times it is used.

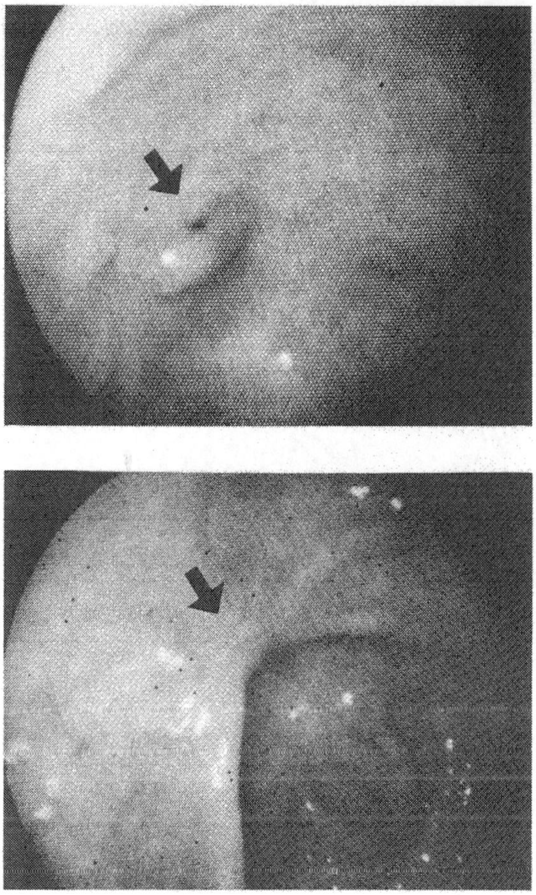

FIGURE 11.1. Type IIa of early gastric cancer (Case 20 in Table 11.2). (*Top*) Before Nd:YAG therapy. (*Bottom*) After 4 months of therapy.

Discussion

The laser generator was introduced in Japan for use with laser endoscopy in 1978, and from that time on, much research has been conducted, especially on its use for the treatment of gastrointestinal and bronchial cancers. At our hospital, many patients have recovered from superficial esophageal cancers and early gastric cancers by laser endoscopy. For some of these patients, 5 years have passed without the recurrence of cancer.

However, in regard to the endoscopic laser treatment, there still remain problems concerning the instrumentation itself, the technique, and the selection of materials that will achieve the best results. Earlier, we reported on the types of cancers that can be treated most effectively, focusing mainly on gastric cancers.[1,] Technically, since we have clinically adopted a new material, a synthetic sapphire for the contact endoprobe, it is possible to state that we have approached a new stage of progress.[4,5] A comparison of the contact and the noncontact treatment methods will demonstrate the superior advantages of the former: (1) reproducible radiation on the lesion was possible, (2) damage to the blood or mucous membrane by the tip of the fiber was avoidable, (3) the time period needed for treatment was shortened, (4) the thermal efficiency was high due to less backscattering of the beam and low thermal conductivity, thereby reducing the need for high power, and (5) pain and abdominal distension was reduced by the use of water delivery instead of gas.

In order to maintain the low power output necessary for laser endoscopy, inexpensive and stable laser generators are now available, for example, the SLT Contact Laser. In the treatment of early gastric cancers, those portions that were especially difficult to irradiate with the traditional noncontact method—for example, the antrum and the upper part of the corpus or the cardia, which were radiated in a U-turn technique—can now be treated with ease.

Another important accessory is the power attenuator, which controls the instability of the laser and assures the low power, less than 10 W from the Nd:YAG laser, needed for endoscopic laser therapy.

According to a nationwide investigation by the Laser Endoscopic Committee for the Japanese Society for Gastroenterological Endoscopy, of the 66 Japanese institutions that treat gastric cancers, 25 have already adopted the contact method as routine, and it has proved to be very effective.[6]

In conclusion, the contact method has many advantages over the noncontact method. For this reason, it should be more widely used for laser endoscopic treatment. However, there still remains a need for further improvements concerning (1) the problems of adhesion of the tissue to the contact laser Tip (or Rod) during the treatment and (2) the most appropriate conditions, such as the precise power and duration, for this technique. Furthermore, we are now in the process of seeking a highly effective and safe

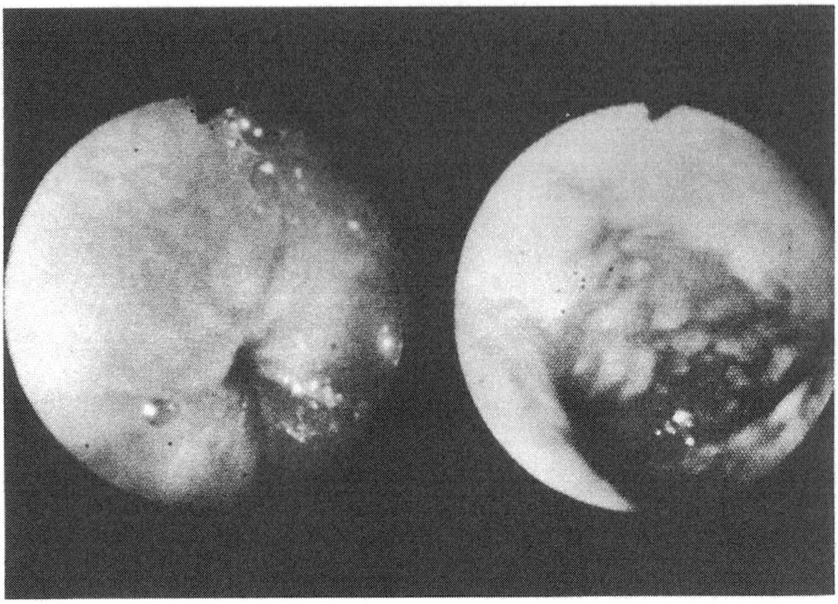

FIGURE 11.2. Palliative therapy for advanced gastric cancer of the cardia (Case 2 in Table 11.3). (*Left*) Before therapy. (*Right*) After 1 week of therapy.

method for radiation into the tissue and of its clinical adoption, such as local laser hyperthermia using a low-power Nd:YAG laser.[7]

References

1. Oguro Y, Tajiri H, Hirashima T: Endoscopic treatment for gastric cancer. Stomach Intest 19:855–863, 1984.
2. Daikuzono N, Joffe SN: Artificial sapphire for contact photocoagulation and tissue vaporization with the Nd:YAG laser. Med Instrum 19:173–178, 1985.
3. Suzuki S, Shiina Y, Miura T, et al: Effects of Nd-YAG laser radiation on the gastrointestinal mucosa, the sixth report: Experimental studies with a new contact type of the YAG laser rod. Gastroenterol Endos. 26:705–710, 1984.
4. Tajiri H, Oguro Y, Hirota T, et al: Present status and problems of photoradiation therapy for gastrointestinal cancer. Jpn Soc Laser Med 5:119–124, 1985.
5. Tajiri H, Oguro Y, Shiotani H, et al: Laser endoscopic treatment of gastrointestinal cancer—A new approach to treatment by using contact probe. J Jpn Soc Laser Med 6:549–522, 1986.
6. Oguro Y, Tajiri H, Takemoto T: Present status of laser medicine and laser endoscopic treatment for cancers of gastrointestinal tract in Japan. Laser Optoelectronics in Medicine. p.323–327, 1985. Springer-Verlag (Berlin, West Germany)
7. Tajiri H, Saito D, Ohkura H, Oguro Y: A study on local interstitial hyperthermia using low power Nd:YAG laser. Oncologia 17:161–163, 1986.

12 Use of Lasers in Nonbleeding Gastrointestinal Lesions: A European Experience

J.M. Brunetaud, V. Maunoury, J.P. Ancelin, D.Cochelard, A.Cortot, and J.C. Paris

Lasers were developed in gastrointestinal (GI) endoscopy for their hemostatic properties. They are now used increasingly for tumor destruction.[1,2] From December 1979 to April 1986, we treated 409 patients with a GI tumor at the Lille Laser Center. The lasers were used (1) for palliation of esophagogastric (esophagus or gastroesophageal junction) or rectosigmoid cancers in nonsurgical patients, (2) for a curative effect in selected patients with a rectosigmoid villous adenoma, and (3) for the destruction of small sessile polyps in patients with a familial polyposis after total colectomy and ileorectal anastomosis. Finally, for a few nonsurgical patients with a small esophagogastric or rectosigmoid cancer, the purpose of the laser treatment was to completely destroy the lesion and to obtain negative biopsies. Small lesions were defined as a tumor less than 3 cm in length, with a circumferential extension of the base less than one-third of the circumference, without signs of infiltration, and primarily exophytic without ulceration.

Patients and Methods

Methods of Treatment

Patient Preparation

Patients were treated on an outpatient basis, without anesthesia or sedation. Patients with a low GI tumor were prepared with a small enema at the Laser Center and no special diet was required before the treatment. Treatment was administered once or twice a week until there was functional improvement (esophagogastric or rectosigmoid cancer) or until the lesions (rectosigmoid villous tumor or rectal polyposis) were completely destroyed. Then patients with cancer were re-treated every month, and patients with benign lesions were followed up and re-treated if new lesions appeared or if there was a recurrence of lesions.

Laser Treatment Modalities

Two types of laser were used for GI endoscopic treatment: an argon laser and a Nd:YAG laser. The argon laser was a 770 Lasersonics (Santa Clara, California) with a 10-W maximum power output. The argon wavelength is well absorbed by the tissue; it was used for vaporization of superficial tumoral zones (until a flat surface was obtained, as delayed necrosis is negligible) at a power of 8 W, a spot size of 1 mm (power density: 1000 W/cm^2) with a continuous beam. The Nd:YAG lasers were the YM 100 and 101 CILAS (Marcoussis, France) with an 80-W maximum power output. The Nd:YAG wavelength is less absorbed by the tissue than the argon wavelength. The volume of delayed necrosis occurring after noncontact Nd:YAG vaporization can be difficult to predict from the macroscopic aspect of the tissue during the treatment.[3] Therefore the Nd:YAG laser was used only for coagulation (blanching) of the tumor and an interval of 3 days to 1 week between two treatments allowed the coagulated parts of the tumor to slough off. Reproducible effects without unexpected necrosis were obtained at 70 W, 2-mm spot size (2000 W/cm^2), and 0.7-second exposure time.

Only the exophytic parts of the tumor were

treated by laser. In case of obstructing lesion, the treatment was preferentially performed from the distal part to the proximal part. For esophagogastric tumors, when the endoscope was unable to pass through the stenosis, dilatation was performed the day before the laser treatment. In the rectosigmoid, a snare resection was used to debulk the most exophytic parts of the tumor before laser treatment.

The Laser Fibers

A 200-μm core optic fiber was used for argon laser transmission and a 400 μm (YM 100) or a 600 μm (YM 101) were used for Nd:YAG. In both cases the fiber was protected by a Teflon catheter; the external diameter of the laser probe was 1.6 mm for upper GI endoscopy and 2.2 mm for lower GI endoscopy. Nitrogen gas was injected at a flow rate of 2 liters/minute to protect the fiber tip. For upper GI endoscopy, coaxial gas escaped through the 2.2-mm biopsy channel of the endoscope, which was maintained open. For lower GI endoscopy a cannula was introduced in the rectum along the endoscope. In a few cases where the conventional fiber reached an esophageal lesion tangentially and was difficult to use, a special contact probe with a synthetic sapphire (Surgical Laser Technologies, (Melvern, PA, USA) was used with the Nd:YAG laser at 15 W.

Patient Population

Seventy-Nine Patients with an Esophagogastric Cancer

The average age was 71 years (range 46 to 95 years). Sixty-eight patients had an advanced lesion (60 with dysphagia, 8 without), and 11 had a small lesion without dysphagia. Table 12.1 gives the localization of the lesions, and Table 12.2 gives the circumferential extension of the tumor bases. C1 indicates less than one-third of the circumference, C2 between one-third and two-thirds, and C3 more than two-thirds.

121 Patients with a Rectosigmoid Cancer

The average age was 79 years (range 51 to 93 years). An advanced tumor was treated in 106 patients. Reasons for treatment, localization, and circumferential extension are given in Tables 12.3, 12.4, and 12.5. The main symptom at the beginning of the treatment was abnormal rectal discharge in 88 patients and obstructive symptoms in 18. A small lesion was found in 15 patients. The reason for treatment and localization are given in Tables 12.3 and 12.4.

192 Patients with a Rectosigmoid Villous Adenoma

The average age was 74 years (range 40 to 93 years). The indications for laser treatment were nonsurgical patients (74), a small tumor requiring major surgery (57), recurrent tumor after a previous nonlaser treatment (56), and patient's refusal of surgery (5). Localization and circumferential extension of the tumor base are given in Table 12.6.

Seventeen Patients with a Rectal Polyposis

The average age was 29 years (range 11 to 48 years). Twelve patients had a familial polyposis and 5 had Gardner syndrome. All patients underwent colectomy with an ileorectal anastomosis before rectal treatment.

TABLE 12.1. Localization of the esophagogastric lesions

	Advanced lesions		
Localization	With dysphagia	Without dysphagia	Small lesions
Upper third	11	0	5
Middle third	6	5	3
Lower third	16	3	1
Cardia	27	0	2

TABLE 12.2. Circumferential extension of the esophagogastic lesions

	Advanced lesions		
Circumferential extension	With dysphagia	Without dysphagia	Small lesions
C1 ($<\frac{1}{3}$)	3	3	11
C2 ($\frac{1}{3}$–$\frac{2}{3}$)	11	3	0
C3 ($>\frac{2}{3}$)	46	2	0

TABLE 12.3. Reasons for treatment in patients with advanced and small rectosigmoid cancers

Reasons for treatment	Advanced lesions	Small lesions
Nonsurgical without metastasis	65	11
Nonsurgical with metastasis	15	1
Colostomy and abnormal discharge	16	0
Recurrence after surgery	7	1
Refusal of surgery	3	2

Results

Results in Esophagogastric Cancers

Of the 60 patients with dysphagia, 47 (78%) were improved. The average duration of the initial treatment was 13 days. In 43 of the 47 improved patients the treatment was ended and the average duration of improvement (ADI) after the initial treatment to recurrence of obstructions could be recorded. The ADI was 110 days (range 10 to 886) in these 43 patients. The ADI was 141 days (range 13 to 886) in the 26 patients with an adenocarcinoma, and 63 days (range 10 to 253) in the 17 patients with a squamous cancer. The ADI was 48 days for upper third lesions, 44 days for middle third, 95 days for lower third and 149 days for lesions of the cardia. The ADI was 156 days for a C2 tumor and 94 days for a C3. Thirteen patients (22%) presenting with dysphagia were not improved. In 12 patients the lack of success was related to a very advanced stage of the lesion. In the last patient acute gastric dilatation occurred during the first treatment, which required a gastrostomy.

In the 8 patients with an advanced lesion without dysphagia, 4 died without dysphagia after an average of 3 months, 3 were lost to follow-up, and 1 required a gastrostomy after 1 year.

Eight of the 11 patients with a small carcinomas had negative biopsies after the treatment. However, one tumor recurred 6 months later. In 2 patients negative biopsies could not be obtained with treatment, and they were treated by radiation therapy. The last patient with a small lesion is still under laser treatment.

Complications occurred only in the group of patients with dysphagia. This included 2 fistula, 1 fatal hemorrhage, and 1 acute gastric dilatation.

TABLE 12.4. Localization of advanced and small rectosigmoid cancers

Localization	Advanced lesions	Small lesions
Rectum	71	11
Rectosigmoid junction	21	1
Sigmoid	14	3

Results in Rectosigmoid Cancers

Of the patients with an advanced lesion, 89% were improved after an average duration of 18 days for the initial treatment. Treatment was completed in 65 patients and the ADI was 9.4 months (0.1 to 38.2). Using life table analysis 39% of the patients are alive at 1 year, with 82% of them remaining improved. The improvement rate was higher in surviving patients with initial abnormal rectal discharges (95% at 6 months) than in those with obstructive symptoms (60%).

TABLE 12.5. Circumferential extension of the advanced rectosigmoid cancers

Circumferential extension	Advanced lesion
C1 (<⅓)	15
C2(⅓–⅔)	40
C3 (>⅔)	51

TABLE 12.6. Localization and circumferential extension of the 192 villous tumors

Localization	Villous tumor	Circumferential extension
Lower rectum	51	C1 (<⅓) : 87
Middle rectum	71	C2 (⅓–⅔) : 80
Rectosigmoid junction	38	C3 (>⅔) : 25
Sigmoid	32	

Patients with a C1 tumor did much better than the other groups. The 11% failure rate depended on the circumferential extension of the tumor: no failure in the 15 C1 patients, 1 failure in the 40 C2 patients, and 11 (22%) in the 51 C3 patients.

Two of the 15 patients with a small rectosigmoid cancer are still under treatment. Negative biopsies were obtained in all the 13 others after an average treatment duration of 3.7 months. However, 1 patient who had metastasis before the treatment died 8 months later. The average follow-up of the 12 patients with negative biopsies is 18.2 months (8–43.3).

Three complications occurred in the group of patients with advanced rectosigmoid carcinoma. This includes perforation at the rectosigmoid junction which proved fatal, 1 perirectal abscess, and 1 rectovaginal fistula.

Results in Rectosigmoid Villous Adenomas

Treatment was incomplete in 52 patients, 8 patients were lost to follow-up, 14 died from another etiology during the treatment and 30 are still under treatment. The treatment was successful for 131 patients, with an average of 22.6 months follow-up (0.2 to 61.6). Among them, 12 had a recurrence after an average period of 7.9 months, which was easily re-treated, and 7 had a stenosis. However, only 2 stenoses were symptomatic and required dilatations. No perforation or massive hemorrhage occurred. The circumferential extension was the main factor that influenced the duration of treatment and the frequency of recurrence and stenosis (Table 12.7).

In 8 of the 192 patients with a villous adenoma, treatment was discontinued because of a positive

TABLE 12.7. Influence of the circumferential extension of the tumor base on the treatment duration and on the percentages of recurrences and stenosis in patients with rectosigmoid villous adenomas

Extension	Treatment duration (months)	Recurrences (%)	Stenosis (5)
C1	3.1	8.6	2.9
C2	5.3	6.3	4.2
C3	9.2	23.1	23.1

biopsy for carcinoma. However, only 6 had a true adenocarcinoma. One patient could not be successfully treated. He had a circumferential lesion previously treated by electrocoagulation, which resulted in a very tight stenosis. Only a diverting colostomy could be performed.

Results in Rectal Polyposis

No rectal carcinoma was observed in the 12 patients with familial polyposis. Eleven were regularly treated at the Laser Center with an average follow-up of 8.5 years (range 1 to 15 years) after the colectomy. One patient was lost to follow-up 10 years after the colectomy. Among the 5 patients with Gardner's syndrome, 2 were lost to follow-up 1 and 1.5 years after colectomy, 2 have been regularly followed for 2 years, and the last patient required a proctectomy 5 years after the colectomy for an adenocarcinoma. No complication occurred in this group of patients.

Discussion

Our technique of using both argon and Nd:Yag lasers is rather unique. The use of the argon laser in GI endoscopy is not common, probably because the purchase of a second laser is found too expensive by most of the gastroenterologists. The multidisciplinary use of lasers[4] is a solution in sharing the expenses with other specialties, and to have the appropriate laser wavelength for each particular lesion. In fact, those who have access to an argon laser[5] appreciate the absence of delayed effects, risk of perforation, and thermal stenosis.

The method of using the noncontact Nd:YAG laser is also controversial. Some vaporize the tissue with a very high-power density (over 10,000 W/cm^2).[6] We prefer to coagulate with a lower power density (between 1500 and 2000 W/cm^2) and wait until the coagulated areas slough off. Others[7,8] have an intermediate position; they coagulate the small lesions with the Nd:YAG and vaporize the larger ones.

Our ambulatory treatment without special diet or medications is well adapted to our population of elderly patients. Among the 409 patients of this study, only 16 (4%) were lost to follow-up during the treatment. Our treatment technique (association of argon and Nd:YAG lasers, and limitation of the Nd:YAG laser effects to coagulation is also safe. Major complications occurred in only 9 of our 409 patients (2.2%). They consisted of 5 perforations (3 fistulas, 1 perirectal abscess, and 1 free perforation), 1 hemorrhage, 2 stenoses, and one complication from the gas insufflation (acute gastric dilatation). Two complications (0.5% of the patients) were fatal due to a free perforation and hemorrhage. The major complications occurred only in advanced cancers or large villous adenomas. The complication rate was 6% for esophagogastric cancers, 3% for the rectosigmoid cancers, and 1% for the rectosigmoid villous adenomas. The complication rate for esophagogastric treatment is similar to that of Fleischer and Sivak[9] or to a European survey of 326 patients.[10] The complication rate for rectosigmoid cancers or villous adenomas is smaller than the 10% reported by Mathus-Vliegen and Tytgat.[7,8]

The 78% immediate success rate in palliation of obstructive esophagogastric cancer is similar to that of Fleischer and Sivak's study.[9] The average duration of improvement is short (110 days), but it parallels the patients' survival, and gastrostomy could be avoided for most patients. Radiation therapy was combined with the laser treatment of squamous cancers whenever it was possible. However, in contrast to Fleischer's experience, our results are better in adenocarcinomas (ADI: 141 days) than in squamous cancers (ADI: 63 days).

The 89% immediate success rate in palliation of advanced rectosigmoid cancers was not significantly dependent on the initial symptomatology. However, at 6 months, 95% of surviving patients with previous abnormal rectal discharge and 60% of those with obstructive symptoms remained improved. Mathus-Vliegen and Tytgat[7] and Escourou and co-workers[10,11] have, respectively, an immediate success rate of 93% and 100% in hematochesia and 83% and 67% in obstructive symptoms. The laser treatment appears to be somewhat more effective for patients with predominant hematochesia than for those with obstructive symptoms.

A complete local destruction with negative biopsies of small esophagogastric os rectosigmoid cancers can be achieved by endoscopic laser treatment. This result was obtained by in 7 of 9 upper gastrointestinal lesions and in all the 13 lower gastrointestinal lesions. Similar results were reported by others.[11-14] However, possible local or regional spread of these tumors cannot be detected, and their endoscopic treatment is limited to nonsurgical patients.

A large proportion of patients with a villous adenoma were difficult cases with 55% having a large lesion (C2 and C3) and 30% had a recurrence after previous nonlaser treatment. However, all patients (except one) with a successfully completed treatment were cured by the laser treatment. These results are slightly better than those from Mathus-Vliegen and Tytgat,[5] who have only a 40% cure rate in almost the same type of lesion. Six malignancies (3%) occurred in our series. Mathus-Vliegen had also the same problem with a higher rate of 20% of malignant degeneration. Therefore it is important to get adequate histology before tumor treatment, using a large snare biopsy or resections. We also select our patients and we limit the indications as mentioned above in the patients' population paragraph.

The management of patients with a previous resection and ileorectal anastomosis for familial polyposis is more difficult. The risk of malignancy, even in patients regularly treated, is not negligible. One patient developed a carcinoma 5 years after colectomy. Laser treatment has the same limitations as electrocoagulation in this type of condition. Its main advantage over electrocoagulation is the excellent quality of healing without scarring, as demonstrated by Mathus-Vliegen and Tytgat.[8]

Conclusions

Endoscopic laser treatment is a safe and effective technique for the treatment of sessile GI tumors. The main disadvantage of the lasers remains their higher price, which can be lowered by a multidisciplinary use. In the future, newer techniques like the large multipolar probe[15] may be available for tumor destruction. However, endoscopic laser therapy is the most feasible technique for treatment. Its safety and efficacy having been proven in many studies including our own results in 409 patients.

References

1. Jensen DM: Lasers in the GI cancer war and other fronts. Gastroenterology 87:974–976, 1984.

2. Fleischer D: Lasers and colon polyps. Technology and pathology: The courtship continues. Gastroenterology, 90:2024–2025, 1986.
3. Brunetaud JM, Mosquet L, Houcke M, et al: Villous adenomas of the rectum: Results of endoscopic treatment with argon and Nd:Yag lasers. Gastroenterology 89:832–837, 1985.
4. Brunetaud JM, Mosquet L, Bourez J, et al: Organization of a multidisciplinary laser center. In Fleisher D, Jensen D, Bright-Asare P (eds): Therapeutic laser endoscopy in gastrointestinal disease. Martinus Nijhoff, Boston, 1983, pp 167–172.
5. Dixon JA, Burt RW, Roetering RH, McCloskey DW: Endoscopic argon laser photocoagulation of sessile polyps. Gastrointest Endosc 28:162–165, 1982.
6. Naveau S, Poitrine A, Poynard T, et al: Traitement palliatif des cancers de l'oesophage et du cardia par le laser YAG néodyme (essai préliminaire non contrôlé) Gastroenterol Clin Biol 8:545–550, 1984.
7. Mathus-Vliegen EM, Tytgat GN: Nd:YAG laser photocoagulation in gastroenterology: Its role in palliation of colorectal cancer. Laser Med Sci 1:75–80, 1986.
8. Mathus-Vliegen EM, Tytgat GN: Nd:YAG laser photocoagulation in colorectal adenoma. Evaluation of its safety, usefulness, and efficacy. Gastroenterology 90:1865–1873, 1986.
9. Fleischer D, Sivak M: Endoscopic ND:YAG laser therapy as palliation for oesophagogastric cancer. Gastroenterology 89:827–831, 1985.
10. Delvaux M, Escourou J: Complications observées au cours du traitement par laser des tumeurs du tractus digestif supérieur Acta Endosc 15:13–17, 1985.
11. Escourou J, Delvaux M, Frexinos J, et al: Traitement du cancer du rectum par le laser neodyme YAG. Gastroenterol Clin Biol 10:152–157, 1986.
12. Patrice T, Jutel P, Le Bodic L: Traitement par laser des cancers intra-muqueux de l'oesophage chez des patients inopérables. Gastroenterol Clin Biol 4:374, 1985.
13. Oguro Y, Hiroshima T, Tagiri, et al: Endoscopic treatment of early gastric cancer, polypectomy and laser treatment. Jpn J Clin Oncol 14:815–820, 1985.
14. Lambert R, Sabben G: Photodestruction par laser des tumeurs colorectales: résultats précoces. (Abstract). Gastroenterol Clin Biol 7:59A, 1983.
15. Johnston J, Quint R, Petruzzi C, Namihira Y: Development and experimental testing of a large probe for palliative treatment of obstructing esophageal and rectal malignancy. (Abstract). Gastrointest Endosc 32:9, 1986.

13
YAG Laser Therapy for Intractable Gastric Ulcer

Kazumichi Harada and Masayoshi Namiki

At present a number of excellent therapeutic agents including H_2-blocker antagonists have been developed for peptic ulcers. As a result, so-called intractable gastric ulcers have come to be encountered less frequently, though there are still some cases of gastric ulcer with repeated relapse and recrudescence that follow an intractable clinical course. We have been applying endoscopic local injection therapy for the treatment of intractable gastric ulcers for 20 years. Using this therapy, which consists of an injection of steroid solution and 0.5% Alantoine solution into the ulcer edge area and base, we have obtained favorable results. In the present study we used YAG laser irradiation in lieu of the injection of steroid solution for the treatment of intractable gastric ulcer and observed healing in all cases. In the following, our procedures are described, with a presentation of the cases.

Subjects

In this study, gastric ulcers not showing scarring after more than 3 months of pharmaceutical treatment irrespective of an in- or out-patient status were handled as cases of intractable gastric ulcer. The study subjects comprised 30 individuals, 23 males and 7 females. Twenty-seven patients showed relapsed ulcer, whereas 3 had had no previous history of ulcer. The patients ranged from 48 to 70 years of age with a mean of 55 years. As to the site of gastric ulcer, the lesion was found in the angulus area in 15 patients, lower corpus area in 6 patients, middle corpus area in 3 patients, and upper corpus area in 6 patients.

Methods

For irradiation of the laser, the YAG laser Model 8000 (produced by former Molectron Co., now incorporated into Cooper Co., USA) was used.

The laser was initially irradiated at a power of 50 W, which was recently increased to 30 W, for 1 second to several sites (3 to 5 sites) of the ulcer edge from a distance of 1 to 2 cm (Figure 13.1). In addition, using an apparatus by which the laser can be irradiated in contact with the

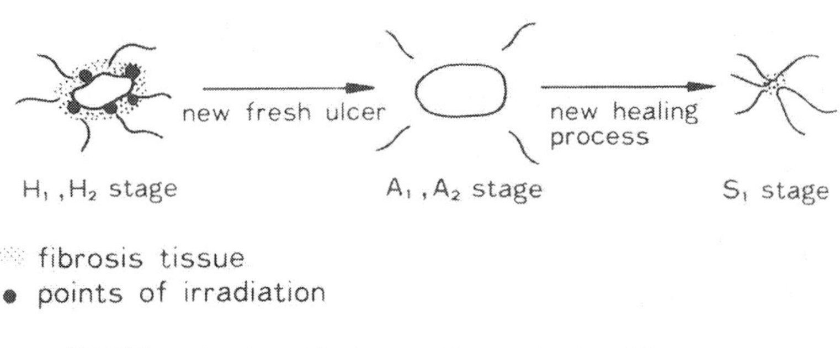

FIGURE 13.1. Scheme of YAG laser treatment for intractable gastric ulcer. No contact method: 30 W, 1 second per site at 1-2 cm distance. Contact method (by microrod): 10 W, 1 second per site.

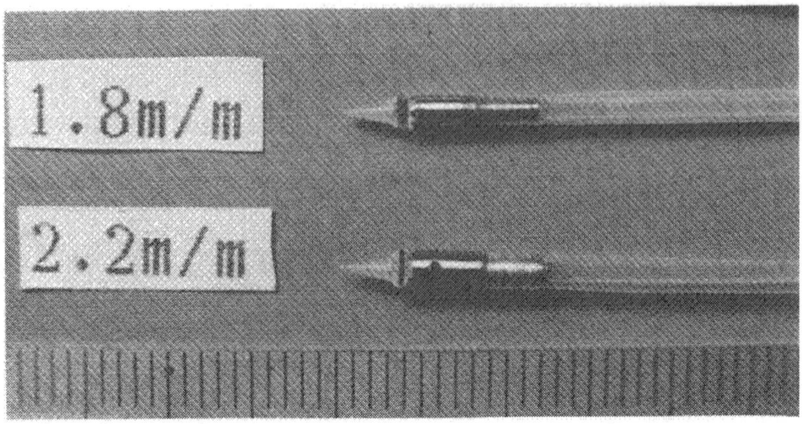

FIGURE 13.2. (*Top*) SMRP-3. (*Bottom*) MRP-3. (SLT, Japan).

mucosa, a microrod (Figure 13.2, SLT, Japan) laser was irradiated at 10 W for 1 second to several sites of the ulcer edge. Use of this microrod has made it possible to apply irradiation to the specific site more precisely.

In most cases, favorable results were obtained with only 1 day's treatment with the laser. In only 2 cases was it required to give laser therapy twice.

With respect to antiulcer drugs, the same drug as a rule was used before and after laser therapy.

Results

In all 30 cases of intractable gastric ulcer which could not achieve ulcer healing despite endoscopic local injection therapy or administration of the H_2-blocker antagonist, scarring of the ulcer was obtained in a mean period of 2.6 months after our laser therapy.

In 2 cases the ulcer relapsed, indicating that recurrence of the ulcer cannot be prevented even with laser treatment. It is considered important to take psychological precautions in addition to local therapy in order to prevent a relapse. In none of the cases were any complications that may be associated with local therapy including laser irradiation therapy observed.

Case 1

The left portion of Figure 13.3 shows the case of a 65-year-old male who had an intractable ulcer with a marked rand wall in the posterior wall of the upper gastric body. The right portion is

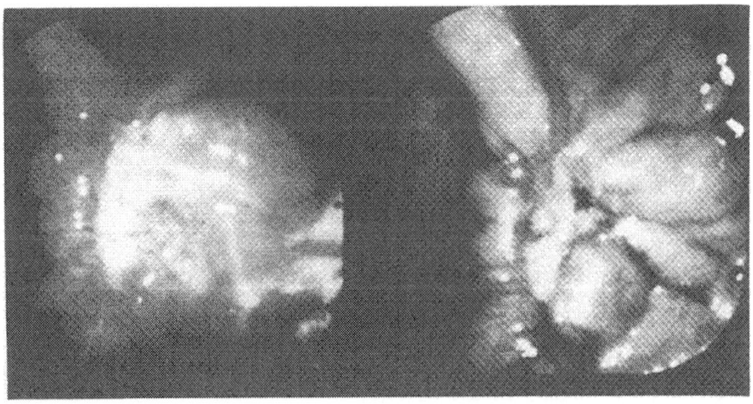

FIGURE 13.3. Endoscopic findings of the intractable gastric ulcer. (*Left*) Before injection of dye. (*Right*) After injection of dye.

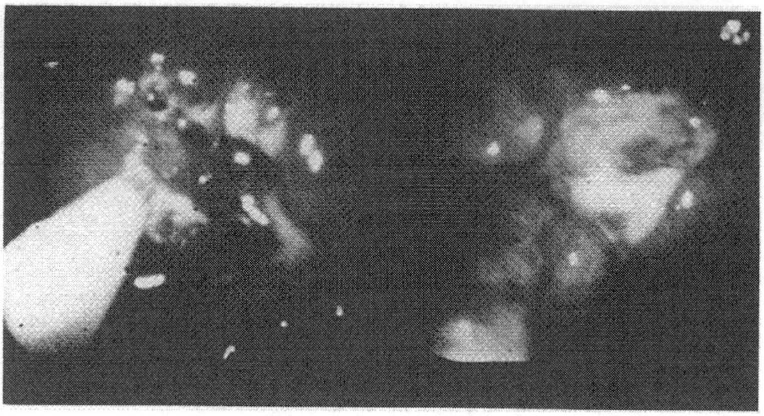

FIGURE 13.4. Endoscopic findings of the intractable gastric ulcer. (*Left*) During laser treatment. (*Right*) Four days after treatment.

a view using the dye contract method which makes the rand wall more apparent.

The left portion of Figure 13.4 shows an endoscopic view of laser irradiation with 50 W/second on 3 sites of the edge of the ulcers. The right portion shows an endoscopic view 4 days after irradiation in which the elevated ulcer edge became lower but the ulcer became larger in the active stage.

The upper left portion of Figure 13.5 shows an endoscopic view 6 weeks after irradiation and the upper right portion is of 8 weeks after irradiation. The lower portion of Figure 13.4 shows a view 10 weeks after irradiation in which cicatrization of the ulcer developed. This case took the longest time in our study but still the patient recuperated within 3 months.

Case 2

Figure 13.6 shows the case of a 43-year-old male who had an intractable ulcer in the lesser curvature at the gastric angle. He had no particular subjective symptoms. The upper left portion of Figure 13.7 shows the ulcer after laser irradiation on 4 sites of the ulcer edge with 50 W/second/site in which the irradiated sites discolored to white. The right upper portion of Figure 13.7 shows an endoscopic view 4 days after irradiation in which the ulcer became larger and shifted to the active stage. The left lower portion of Figure 13.7 was taken 5 weeks after irradiation in which the ulcer is markedly healed. Eight weeks after irradiation, cicatrization of the ulcer developed as shown in the right lower portion of Figure 13.7.

The upper portion of Figure 13.8 shows the histology of a biopsied specimen of the previous case which was obtained from the edge of the ulcer before laser irradiation. This manifested extensive inflammation accompanying fibrosis and regeneration of the epithelium. The lower portion of Figure 13.8 shows the histology of a biopsied specimen which was obtained from the same site 4 days after laser irradiation in which the mucosa manifested marked edematous alterations. This allows the inference that a new healing process might have been initiated for the mucosa around the ulcer.

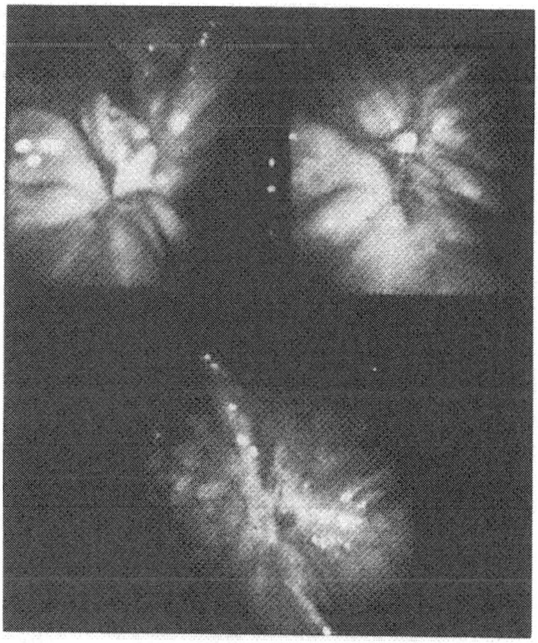

FIGURE 13.5. Endoscopic findings of the intractable gastric ulcer. (*Top left*) Six weeks after treatment. (*Top right*) Eight weeks after treatment. (*Bottom*) Ten weeks after treatment.

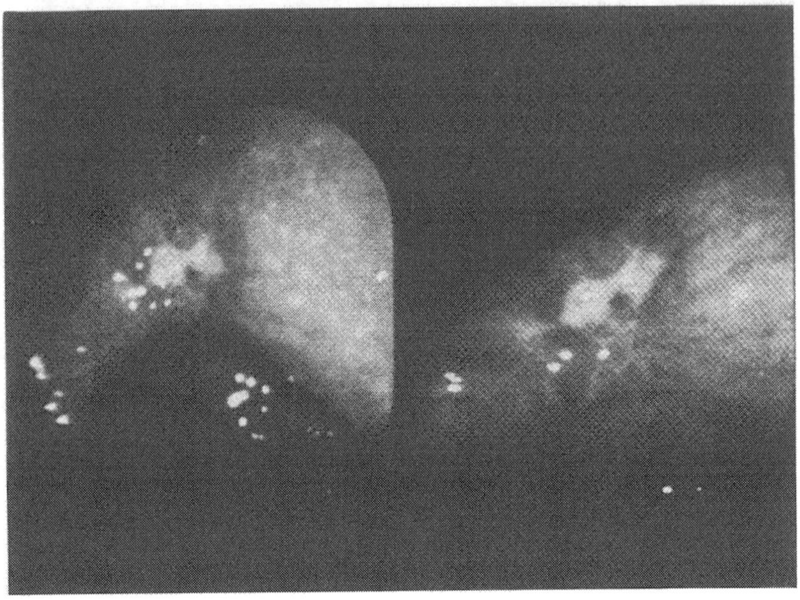

Figure 13.6. Endoscopic findings of the intractable gastric ulcer Small ulcer is seen in the angle.

Case 3

The upper left corner of Figure 13.9 shows the case of a 50-year-old man who had an intractable ulcer in the lesser curvature at the gastric angle. The upper right corner was taken after laser irradiation on 4 sites of the ulcer edge with 10 W/second per site by using microrod. The lower left corner of Figure 13.9 is the view 1 week after irradiation in which the ulcer became larger in the active stage. The lower right corner shows the ulcer 11 weeks after treatment in which a scar developed.

Discussion

As a treatment for chronic intractable ulcers, we have employed endoscopic local injection

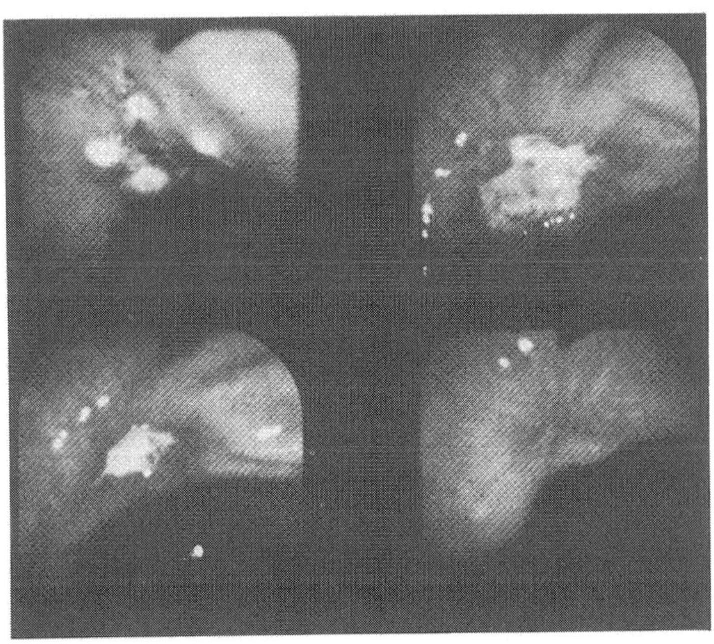

Figure 13.7. Endoscopic findings of the intractable gastric ulcer. (*Top left*) Immediately after laser treatment. (*Top right*) Four days after treatment. (*Bottom left*) Five weeks after treatment. (*Bottom right*) Eight weeks after treatment.

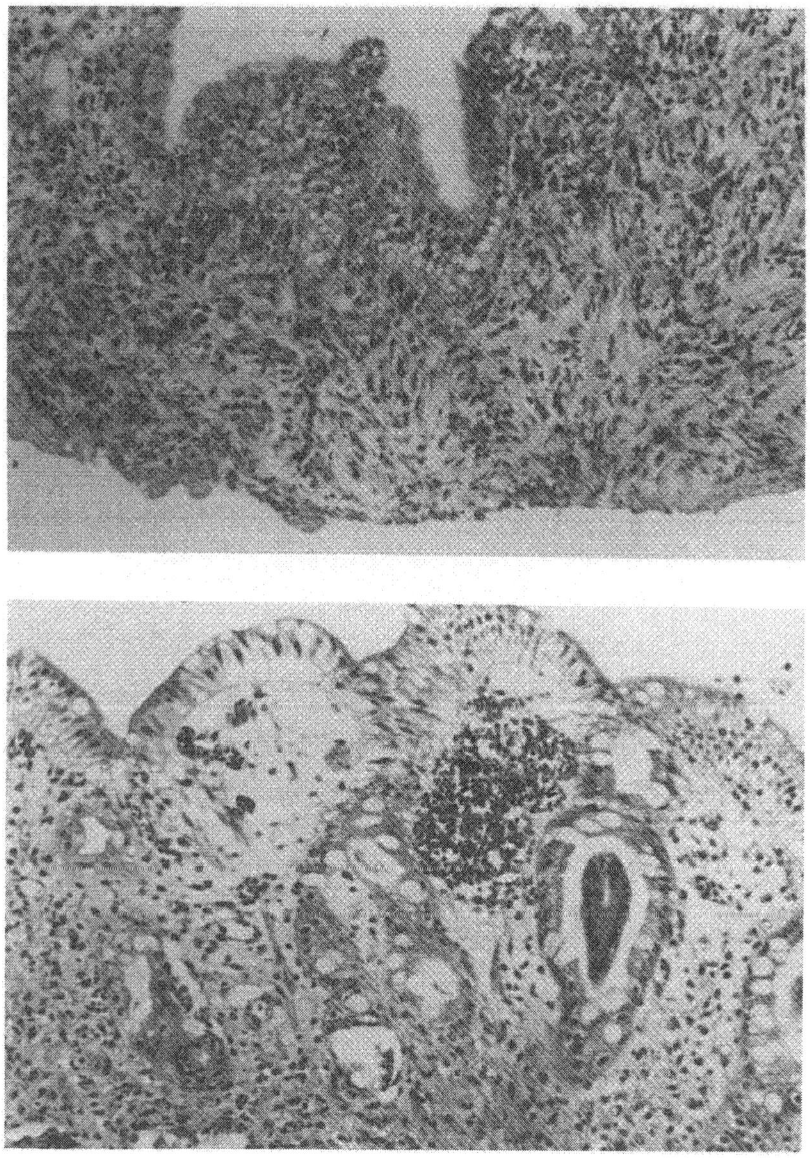

FIGURE 13.8. Histological findings of the biopsy specimen. (*Top*) Before laser treatment. (*Bottom*) Four days after laser treatment.

therapy for 20 years. Two factors are thought to contribute to the intractability of these ulcers, i.e., general factors including psychosomatic and local factors. In treating ulcers, it is necessary to deal pertinently with these two factors. Endoscopic local injection therapy is one means of treating the local factors.

In chronic intractable gastric ulcers, the healing process appears to be hindered by extensive fibrinoid tissue around the edge and extending to the base. We thought that we could expect favorable healing by removing these hard fibrinoid tissues. This means that a chronic ulcer is turned into a fresh new ulcer for which a new healing process can be expected. For this purpose, we injected a steroid hormone to lessen the hardness of the fibrinoid tissue and also injected 0.5% alantoine to facilitate favorable granulation formation.

After clinical application of the laser began[1,2], we had the idea to utilize the laser instead of steroids although we have had satisfactory results from the local injection therapy. We expected to facilitate the healing process following the formation of a fresh new ulcer by laser irradiation. Generally speaking, ulcers engen-

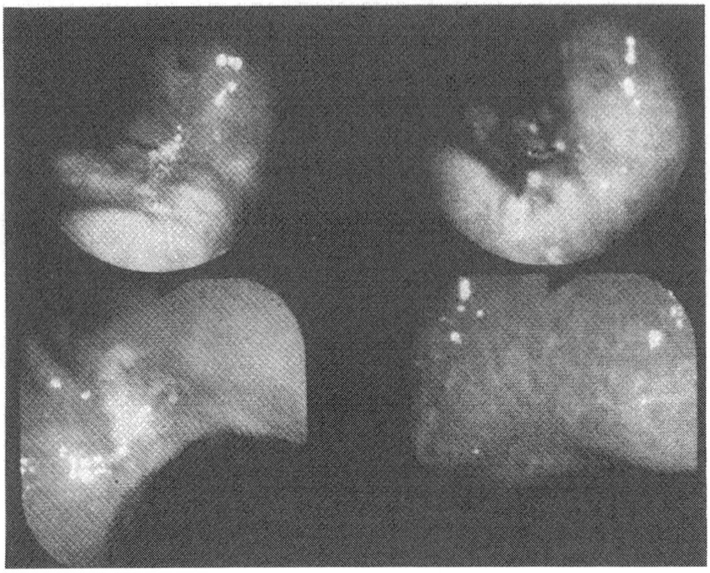

FIGURE 13.9. Endoscopic findings of the intractable gastric ulcer. (*Top left*) Before treatment. (*Top right*) Immediately after laser treatment using microrod. (*Bottom left*) One week after treatment. (*Bottom right*) Eleven weeks after treatment.

dered by laser irradiation heal within a short period, so our speculation seemed to be rational.

In most of the cases of intractable peptic ulcer the lesion is relatively small in size (about 5 to 10 mm) and at the healing stage (H_1, H_2). Therefore, endoscopic observation at 1 week after laser therapy on our cases revealed that the ulcer became a fresh one of a little larger diameter and at the active stage (A_1, A_2) following treatment with a mere irradiation by laser to several marginal sites of the ulcer. These findings indicate that the laser irradiation may play a role in the debridement of the old ulcer which has hardened with fibrosis. As one of the causes to prevent healing of the peptic ulcer, a decrease in gastric mucosal blood flow has been enumerated. When the gastric mucosal blood flow at the edge of an intractable gastric ulcer was determined by the H_2-gas clearance method before and after laser therapy, it was found that the blood flow at 1 week after laser irradiation was increased as compared to the pretreatment value. This circumstance is also considered advantageous for the healing process of peptic ulcers.

We have described laser treatment for chronic intractable gastric ulcers for which the healing process was hindered by local factors. The reason why we restricted the area of irradiation to the edges of the ulcer was that the edge is the site of epithelial regeneration.

Studies describing the efficacy of some types of acupuncture laser therapy at low power for cutaneous ulcer and oral aphta have increasingly been published. It is assumed that YAG laser also plays a role as a stimulator in addition to the role of providing energy. We are going to investigate further the power of the laser, time, site of irradiation, etc.

Summary

A total of 30 cases of intractable gastric ulcer were treated with YAG laser at a relatively low power, scarring the ulcer in a mean period of 2.6 months after irradiation in all cases. We believe our method is valuable as a new clinical application of the endoscopic YAG laser.

References

1. Harada K et al.: YAG laser treatment for intractable gastric ulcers. Gastroenterol Endosc 23:1752–1758, 1981.
2. Mizushima K et al.: Laser endoscopy and its clinical application. Asian Med J 25:575–595, 1982.

14
Use of the Nd:YAG Laser in Cholangioscopic Surgery

Teruo Kouzu and Yoshikazu Yamazaki

In recent years cholangioscopy has become a widely used technique. By the introduction of the Nd:YAG laser this procedure has come to be used not only in endoscopy but has been aggressively applied in the treatment of biliary tract diseases. In this chapter we focus on the treatment of biliary tract calculi, using the Nd:YAG laser. In the treatment of hepatolithiasis, the most important point to be observed is that with whatever method of treatment used, bile duct calculi should leave no residual. As a means for attaining this goal various methods are reported: (1) lithotomy using a wire under fluoroscope[1]; (2) treatment by various tools used in lithotomy[2]; (3) lithotomy by Dormia catheter[3]; and (4) lithotomy by steel catheter.[4] There are also many reports on lithotomy under direct observation endoscopy.[5–7] In endoscopic lithotomy, the goal is to crush impacted calculi and calculi larger than the diameter of the fistula from which they are to be extracted and to extract these stones without any trauma. Since 1980 we have used the Nd:YAG laser as a means for lithotripsy in cholangioscopic lithotomy and previously reported on its value and safety.[8] This chapter discusses recent progress in use of this method.

Method

Cholangioscopy is performed while perfusing with a saline solution or distilled water. In postoperative cases, the route for inserting the cholangioscope into the bile duct is through the T-tube tract. In a preoperative case or a case of recurrence we use the percutaneous transhepatic choledoco drainage (PTCD) fistulous tract. We insert the cholangioscope after having dilated the PTCD fistula to the size of 18 French. We proceed to extract small stones that can be seen under the endoscope using the conventional Fogarty catheter, basket forceps, and alligator forceps. However, in cases where large stones and stones are impacted within the bile duct which absolutely refuse to yield and cannot be removed even though graspable by the basket forceps, lasers are used in the performance of the lithotripsy. The Medilas YAG laser was used in our study. The method of lithotripsy is to first make a fistula through the surface of the calculus by applying the laser. If and when the direction of the stone can be altered we proceed to produce multiple holes from a number of angles. In a case where we cannot move the stone and can only open a single hole on facet, the laser beam is used to gradually enlarge the defect that has already been made. Then, having enlarged the hole sufficiently and grasping firmly with the alligator forceps, the stone that was so hard it could not be crushed previous to the laser irradiation can now easily be broken into small fragments. We proceed to extract fragments as in the conventional manner. With fragments too large to be removed, we once again apply added laser irradiation to the surface and extract the now smaller fragments in the same manner.

There are at the present time two laser irradiation methods: Noncontact irradiation and contact irradiation. In the noncontact irradiation method, allowing for a space of 3 to 5 mm between the fiber tip and the surface of the calculus, we perform high-power irradiation. In this method we previously constructed a quartz fiber-tip device, but at present we use a digestive tract fiber tip from which the metal nozzle has been removed. In the noncontact irradiation method, a 70 W, 0.5-second repeated irradiation for calcium bilirubinate stone and a 70 to 80 W, 2-second repeated irradiation for cholesterol stone are the laser settings used for irradiation. Contact irradiation is a method in which a synthetic SLT contact probe is fitted directly to the quartz fiber tip, when placed in contact with the surface of the calculus, it directly irradiates it.

As to the shape of the contact probe (Surgical Laser Technologies, Japan), we learned through an initial study that the bullet-shaped type is most suitable for lithotripsy (Figure 14.1). Furthermore, the shape and size of the probes can be easily changed. When this contact probe is used we can produce a sufficient opening leading to a hole in cholesterol stones with irradiation of as little as 15 W at pulsed intervals of 1 second. This probe's endurance is relatively good, but with long use it degenerates. When this occurs, this probe is simply changed and a new one inserted. The SLT laser now used is very stable at low power outputs, and we believe it will lead to greater use in the field of research and clinical application in gallstone lithotomy and lithotripsy.

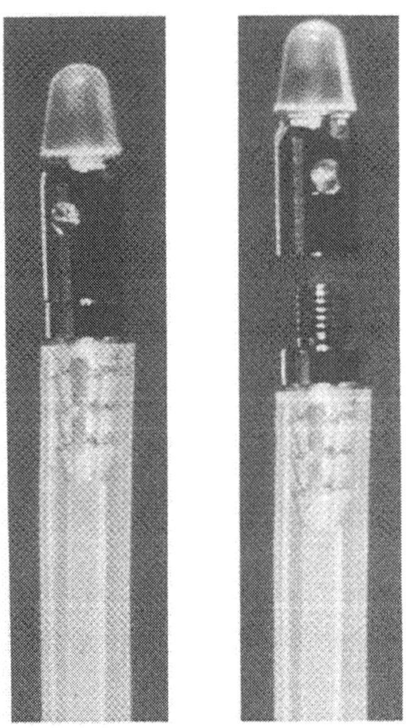

FIGURE 14.1. The contact rod made from ceramics for lithotripsy.

Results

From 1974 to April 1986 cholangioscopic lithotomy was performed in 106 cases. Of these, there were 27 cases of lithotripsy by laser, 13 cases of hepatolithiasis postoperative residual calculi, 5 cases of hepatolithiasis with nonsurgical history, 5 cases of retained stones in the common bile duct, and 4 cases of gallbladder lithotomy.

The cholangioscope is inserted through the T-tube tract. In many cases however, we used the PTCD route through the dilated tracts. The success rate of complete cholangioscopic lithotomy using the Nd:YAG laser was 91.5% (54 of 59 cases). Using one of the forceps techniques, the success rate for complete lithotomy was only 66% (31 of 47 cases). This indicates that laser gallstone lithotripsy is a much more successful technique in our institution when both methods were being evaluated simultaneously.

Case 1

The patient was a 39-year-old man (Figure 14.2). Upon being diagnosed 4 years ago as a case of hepatolithiasis, the patient underwent a cholecystectomy, a cholodochotomy, and an intraoperative lithotomy. After the operation, the T-tube inadvertently slipped out. He was observed as an outpatient, postponing the planned cholangioscopic lithotomy. Recently, hospitalized with pyrexia and abdominal pain, a PTCD tube was inserted into the right and left hepatic ducts. In the left duct, several stones were identified. In addition there was cystic duct dilation and a large stone in a right hepatic ductule. Dilation of the right and left PTCD fistulas was performed for reaching the right and left hepatic duct. Laser lithotripsy of the large calculus allowed a complete removal of all stones by cholangioscopy over a total of 22 procedures. After the lithotomy, the right hepatic duct dilation returned to a normal size over time. Insertion of the cholangioscope into the common duct was easy. Also, the area thought to be a severe stenosis before lithotomy, has returned to normal after lithotomy.

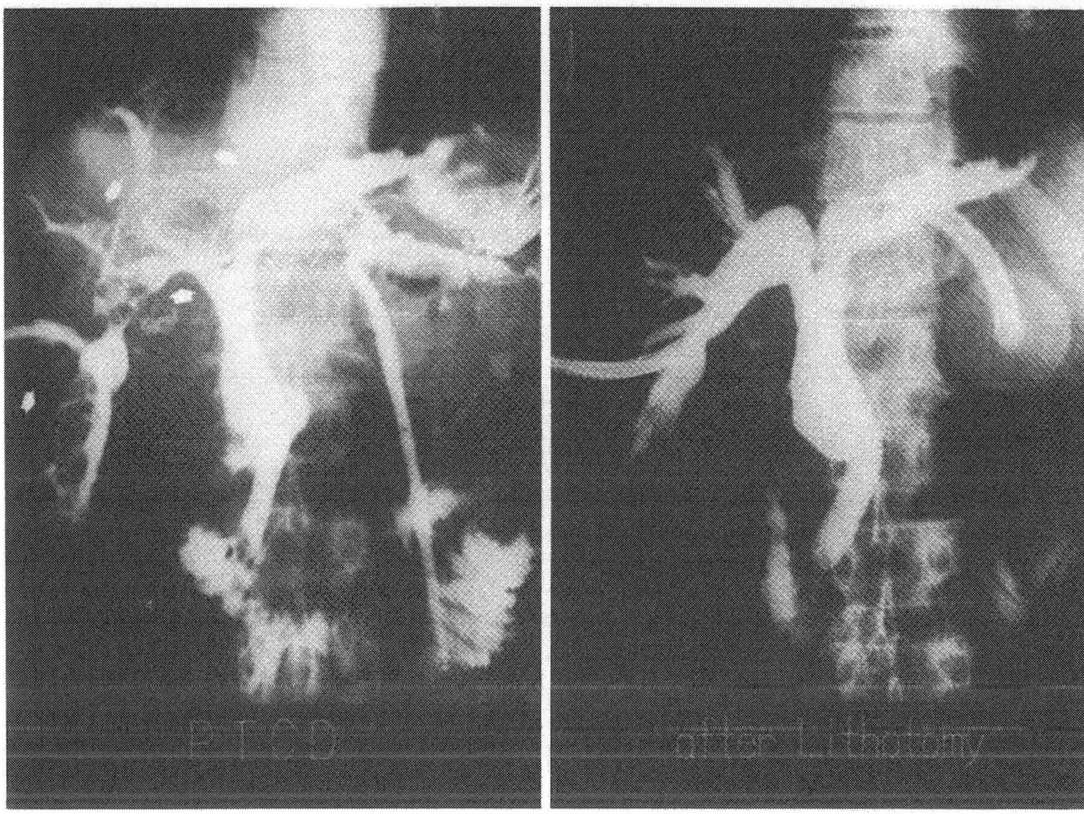

FIGURE 14.2. (*Left*) *Arrows* indicate stones in right and left lobe of liver before treatment. PTCD – percutaneous transhepatic choledoco drainage. (*Right*) After stone extraction by endoscopic lithotomy by Nd:YAG laser irradiation.

Case 2

The patient was a 59-year-old woman (Figure 14.3). Complaining of pain in the hypochondrillum, she was hospitalized with a diagnosis of cholelithiasis. Past history included an appendectomy at the age of 20 years, an exploratory laporotomy at 30 years, a reexploration at 37, an excision of a uterine myoma at 50, an operation for intestinal obstruction at 54 years, and a mastectomy for breast cancer at the age of 57 years. With the previous five abdominal operations, and severe myocardial ischemia it was decided to perform cholangioscopic surgery. Under ultrasound-guided cholecystography a larger stone was seen occupying half the gallbladder lumen. Dilating the percutaneous transhepatic cholecyst drainage tract the cholangioscope was inserted. The stone was a white, 3 cm diameter, cholesterol stone. Using the Nd:YAG laser the calculus was fragmented and extracted from the gallbladder. During lithotomy, part of the fragments passed into the common duct and accumulated in the distal end failing to pass into the duodenum and an endoscopic papillotomy was added to the procedure. With a total of nine cholangioscopic lithotomies and one endoscopic papillotomy removal of the stone and its fragments was achieved.

Case 3

The patient was a 73-year-old man. He was hospitalized with complaints of pyrexia and pain in the right hypochondrium. With a PTCD from the right hepatic duct stones were recognized in the common duct and the right and left hepatic ducts and a stricture identified in the right duct with small stones in its periphery. The left hepatic duct and common duct stones were easily

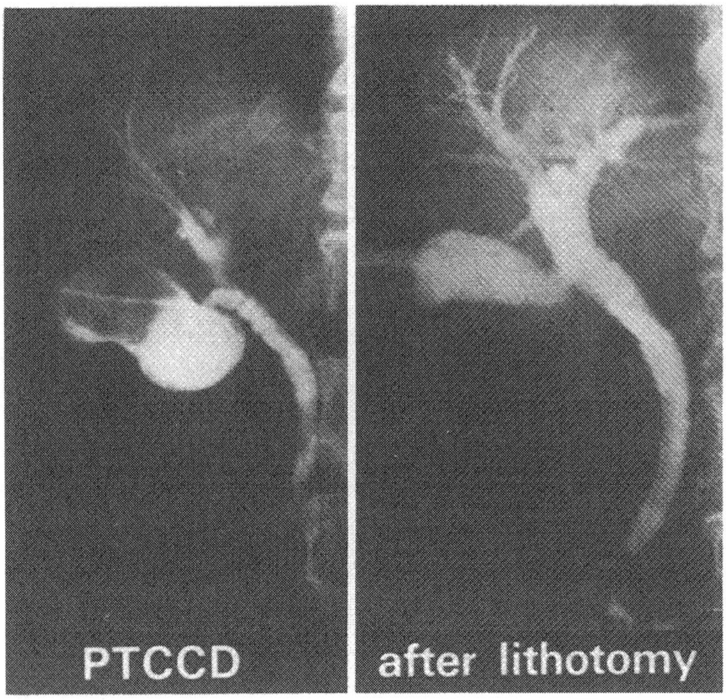

FIGURE 14.3. (*Left*) Cholesterol stone in the gallbladder. PTCCD, percutaneous transhepatic cholecyst drainage. (*Right*) After lithotripsy using the YAG laser through the PTCCD fistula and added endoscopic papillotomy.

removed by use of a laser. The right duct stricture was dilated using the SLT contact probe with 20 W for a 1-second repeated irradiation. After dilation insertion of a 5 mm diameter cholangioscope was possible, and all the stones in the distal ducts were removed.

Discussion

Recently, bile tract endoscopy has become an increasingly popular mode of therapy. The Nd:YAG laser is the instrument of choice in this treatment. In the near future the endoscope is also likely to be commonly used for the curative treatment of early bile duct carcinoma, while cholangioscopic surgery with the use of laser in relieving stenosis and in bile tract calculi lithotomy is already quite popular.

Hepatolithiasis requires that there be no residue and the stenotic bile duct must be unobstructed. Cholangioscopic lithotomy offers a new treatment and an alternative to a formal hepatectomy. Following removal of intrahepatic stones, the dilated ducts return to normal and strictures often disappear. We believe in the future, assessment of each case will lead to a natural approach distinguishing those requiring major operative surgery compared to cholangioscopic lithotripsy. Also, in using the Nd:YAG laser in lithotrity, progress has been made from the noncontact irradiation method to the SLT contact method.

At present both modes are being used. For example, in a situation where the length of the rigid part of a contact rod interferes with the irradiation of the calculi surface, we adopt a noncontact mode by using the quartz fiber of the tip from which the metal nozzle has been removed. Although the irradiation is performed under water, a spark is visible, but there is no danger of duct damage in the area of the calculi.[8] During irradiation, the point of greatest concern is performing the irradiation within a good and confident field of vision while simultaneously confirming the depth of the opening made on the surface of the calculus.

When calculi are found in the periphery of a stenotic duct into which a choledochoscope cannot be inserted, it may be well to insert a percutaneous transhepatic drainage tube into the periferial ductule. From a pathologic study of these stenoses however, it is considered a simple

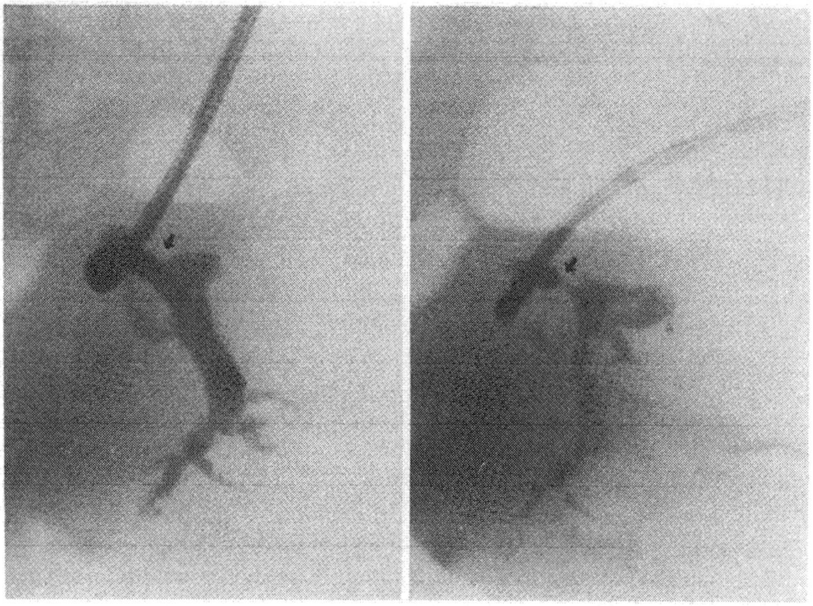

FIGURE 14.4. (*Left*) The stricture of the right hepatic duct and stones in the periphery of the duct. (*Right*) After dilatation with the use a contact rod.

procedure to dilate it sufficiently to pass a fiberscope through.[9] The trick in dilating the stenosis with a laser is not to create carbonization on the irradiated area but rather to stop the procedure when tissue becomes pale. Some two days later, insert the choledochoscope and perform the lithotripsy becomes possible when passing a Fogarty catheter through. At this point, laser irradiation can be performed on all calculi.

In the early stages of this study, it was thought that calcium bilirubinate stones were the only ones suited for laser lithotripsy. However, with the development of contact probes, cholesterol stones, which comprises the majority of gallbladder calculi, are easily fragmented and removed. Bile duct calculi extraction, with duct dilation, is now an established technique.

In the future, photodynamic therapy using photosensitizers and Nd:YAG laser treatment may be expected to advance to include even bile duct carcinomas using cholangioscopy.

Summary

In this study we have reported our experience with cholangioscopic surgery using the Nd:YAG laser. This includes bile duct calculi lithotripsy and dilation of duct stenosis. The laser irradiation method has evolved from the noncontact mode to the contact mode. The numbers of patients requiring this treatment are increasing. It is hoped that in the future this method will be adopted for bile duct carcinoma.

References

1. Mahorner H, Bean WJ: Removal of a residual stone from the common bile duct without surgery. Ann Surg 173:857–860, 1971.
2. Mazzariello RM: A fourteen-year experience with nonoperative instrument extraction of retained bile duct stones. World J Surg 2:447–455, 1978.
3. Magarey CJ: Non-surgical removal of retained biliary calculi. Lancet 1:1044–1046, 1971.
4. Burhenne HJ: Nonoperative instrument extraction of retained bile duct stones. World J Surg 2:439–445, 1978.
5. Warshaw AL, Barlett MK: Technique for finding and removing stones from intrahepatic bile duct. Am J Surg 127:353–354, 1974.
6. Yamakawa T, Komaki F, Shikata J: Experience with routine postoperative choledocoscpy via T-tube sinus tract. World J Surg 2:379–385, 1978.
7. Hwang MH, Yang JC, Lee SA: Choledocofiberscopy in the postoperative management of intrahepatic stones. Am J Surg 139:860–864, 1980.
8. Kouzu T, Sato H: Endoscopic laser treatment of intrahepatic stones. In Intrahepatic Calculi. Alan R. Liss, New York, 1984, pp. 321–332.
9. Yamazaki Y: Basic and clinical investigation of cholangioscopic lithotomy. Gastroenterol Endosc 27:27–43, 1985.

15
Nd:YAG Laser Treatment of Bladder Tumors

A.G. Hofstetter

Since 1976 we have treated more than 1000 patients with urinary bladder tumors of stages pT_A–pT_4 with the Nd:YAG laser.[1,3]

The advantages of this technique are: (a) contact-free tumor destruction in excellent visual conditions, since there are no or only unimportant hemorrhages during the operation; (b) blocking tumor supplying blood and lymphatic vessels; (c) general anesthesia is not required in the most cases, only adapted sedation; (d) dispensing with a postoperative catheter treatment, so that nosocomial infections can be largely avoided; and (e) replacing of electrolyte-free flushing solutions by sterile water, leading to saving in costs.[1]

Apart from these advantages, the question as to the degree of efficacy of the Nd:YAG laser as compared to conventional transurethral resection techniques has to be checked. Therefore we performed a prospective, randomized study.

Techniques

Endoscopic destruction of bladder tumors is carried out in three steps if the tumors are bulky. In these cases, the exophytic portion is first resected with the electric snare deep into the bladder wall after prior coagulation of the margins of the tumor. The base and edges of the tumor are then postcoagulated with the Nd:YAG laser. Smaller tumors are primarily destroyed with the Nd:YAG laser. Here, we first irradiate until blanching of the tissue surrounding the tumor occurs to a breadth of about 0.5 to 1 cm, in order to seal off the afferent blood vessels and lymphatics. Subsequently, the tumor is necrotized linearly.

Immediately after irradiation, the tumor is removed with biopsy forceps. This tissue removed immediately after the Nd:YAG irradiation can be subject to histological workup to confirm the diagnosis and to classify the tumor.

Before the operation, biopsies are taken from the base of the tumor and the tissue immediately surrounding the tumor for a distance of 1 cm at 3, 6, 9, and 12 o'clock. This procedure is supplemented by "quadrant biopsy." Since no, or only very insignificant, hemorrhage occurs under Nd:YAG laser irradiation, a transurethral catheter can as a rule be dispensed with after the operation. This is important to avoid nosocomial infections.

The patient should be kept under observation for 1 day after the operation, in order to detect a possible intestinal perforation in good time, in particular when large areas are irradiated at the posterior wall of the bladder. With a radiation dose of up to 45 W, using water as a flushing fluid, we have yet to observe such a complication, although we have treated several thousands tumors. Within 8 years only in three cases did small intestinal perforations occur after faulty irradiation at too high a power (about 80 W). Clinically, these perforations manifested as signs of acute abdomen with 12 h after the irradiation.

Clinical Results

As mentioned above, we have compared the efficacy of the Nd:YAG laser with the results obtained with TUR, using the rate of recurrence as a criterion. Patients with stage pT_A–pT_2, N_o, M_o urothelial carcinomas (n = 66; 39 men, 27

TABLE 15.1. Primary Tumors (pT_A–pT_2, N_0, M_0)

Number:	40 (M = 23, F = 17)	
Age:	Males	45–81 years, $\bar{x}_M$ = 66.5 years
	Females	54–84 years, $\bar{x}_F$ = 69.1 years

TABLE 15.2. Relapse Tumors (pT_A–pT_2, N_0, M_0)

Number:	26 (M = 16, F = 10)	
Age:	Males	40–79 years, $\bar{x}_M$ = 62.1 years
	Females	53–83 years, $\bar{x}_F$ = 72.1 years

TABLE 15.3. Classification and Incidence distribution of transitional cell carcinoms (PT) in 24 (M = 15/F = 9) Patients of Laser Group and 16 (M= 11/F = 5) of TUR Group

	Laser Group				TUR Group			
pT/G	1	2	3	*N*	1	2	3	*N*
A	7	4	1	12	6	4	0	10
1	4	4	1	9	1	0	2	3
2	0	1	2	3	0	2	1	3

TABLE 15.4. Classification and Incidence distribution of transitional cell carcinom (RT) in 20 (M = 12/F = 8) Patients of Laser Group and 6 (M = 4/F = 2) Patients of TUR Group

	Laser Group				TUR Group			
pT/G	1	2	3	*N*	1	2	3	*N*
A	3	3	0	6	1	3	0	4
1	5	6	3	14	1	1	0	2
2	0	0	0	0	0	0	0	0

women; average age 68 years) were included in the study. Laser or TUR treatment was carried out in accordance with a randomization scheme. In addition, adjuvant chemotherapy with mitomycin C (20 mg/14 days) was administered 8 days after the operation. The control group received no chemoprophylaxis. The study was commenced on September 1, 1981. The patients were divided into a group with primary tumors (Table 15.1) and a group with relapse tumors (Table 15.2). The classification of primary tumors is shown in Table 15.3 and the classification of relapse tumors in Table 15.4.

The therapeutic results obtained in primary tumors are shown in Table 15.5 It can be seen that laser application with and without chemotherapy is superior to TUR with and without chemotherapy, as indicated by the relapse rate ($p < 0.0001$ four fields test). The superiority of laser application was also seen in relapse tumors (Table 15.6). In addition, a particularly important observation is, we believe, that after laser application hardly any local relapses occurred in contrast to the results obtained with TUR (1 to 40%). Otherwise it is interesting to note that there was never any change from localized to multiple tumor growth after laser irradiation, unlike TUR. Our experience has been confirmed in general by Meier et al.[2]

Summary

Our 10-year clinical experience with the Nd:YAG laser permits us to state that the conventional TUR method for treatment of bladder

TABLE 15.5. Therapeutic results after Nd:YAG laser coagulation V.C. TUR (PT) (N = 40)

	Laser + MC (N = 15)	Laser (N = 9)	TUR + MC (N = 13)	TUR (N = 3)
Number of patients with recurrence	1	1	6	3
Recurrence rate[a]	0.17	0.27	1.32	7.89
Mean follow-up (months)	38.00	41.00	25.00	13.00
Deaths	1[b]	0	1[b]	0
Total months of follow-up	581.0	372.0	329.0	38.0

[a]Recurrence rate $= \dfrac{\text{No. recurrences}}{\text{Month follow up}} \times 100.$

[b]Not due to cancer.

TABLE 15.6. Therapeutic results after Nd:YAG Laser Coagulation VZ. TUR (RT) ($N = 26$)

	Laser + MC ($N = 15$)	Laser ($N = 5$)	TUR + MC ($N = 2$)	TUR ($N = 4$)
Number of patients with recurrence	2	3	2	4
Recurrence rate[a]	0.4	2.2	7.14	11.1
Mean follow-up (months)	27.4	27.2	14.0	9.0
Deaths	0	0	0	0
Total months of follow-up	411.0	136.2	28.0	36.0

[a]Recurrence rate $= \frac{\text{No. recurrences}}{\text{Month follow up}} \times 100.$

tumors should be reconsidered. Randomized, prospective studies comparing the efficacy of TUR and laser treatment indicate the superiority of Nd:YAG application.

References

1. Hofstetter A, Frank F: The Nd:YAG Laser in Urology. Editiones Roche, Basel, 1979.
2. Meier U, Hofstetter A, Pflüger H: Effects of intravesical instillation of mitomycin after endoscopic treatment with TUR or laser on recurrence rate of bladder tumors. XXth Congress of the International Society for Urology, Vienna, 1985.
3. Staehler G, Hofstetter A, Schmiedt E, Keiditsch E: Endoskopische Laser-Bestrahlung von Blasentumoren des Menschen. Fortschr Med 95:3, 1977.

16
Contact Laser Treatment for Bladder Cancer

Hiroto Washida

The word laser, an acronym for Light Amplification by Stimulated Emission of Radiation, was coined by Maiman,[1] who succeeded in the amplification of electromagnetic waves in the region of visible light, using a ruby crystal. As laser equipment must fulfill many requirements for use in the medical field, the following laser systems have become available only today: (1) the ruby laser, (2) the argon laser, (3) the Nd:YAG laser, and (4) the CO_2 laser. Among these lasers, the Nd:YAG laser developed in 1962 by Johnson and colleagues[2] and described in 1966 by Snitzer[3] has been increasingly accepted because of its possibility to transmit the Nd:YAG laser beam by means of a flexible quartz fiber, as well as a highly efficient coagulation and penetration capability.[4] However, such distinct disadvantages as damage to the tip of the laser light guide, instability, and uncertainty, have been pointed out for endoscopic surgery due to the noncontact method for delivering laser energy.[5,6] We devised and prepared a new probe called an endorod, which can transmit laser light interstitially.[7] This chapter discusses the features of contact laser irradiation using the endorod for the treatment of bladder cancer, namely, transurethral laser destruction of bladder cancer (TULD).

The Endorod (SLT Contact Endoprobe®)

The endoprobe is made out of new ceramic which is a fusion product of aluminum oxide (Al_2O_3). The probe has been shaped into a fine needle forming a conical trapezoid of 2.0 mm in diameter at the part of incidence connected with a quartz fiber, 5.0 mm in length and 0.1 mm in diameter at the tip (Figures 16.1 and 16.2).

Method of Operation

The surgeon and his staff wear protective eyeglasses during the operation. The patient is placed in the lithotomy position as for any transurethral intervention. Prior to laser treatment, specimens for histologic examination were taken from the apex and base of the tumor. The laser is set for a continuous period and is controlled by the surgeon with an on and off foot switch similar to using electrocautery. The power is around 15 W/second. A modified 27 French size sheath and telescope with Albarran element (Olympus Co.) are inserted transurethrally. The SLT endoprobe connected to a quartz fiber is passed into the bladder and passed into the cancer under direct vision. It is possible to drive the endorod freely into any area by moving the Albarran element and/or the scope itself. The irradiation effect can be distinguished by a whitish discoloration of the cancer. The bladder is filled and irrigated continuously with 10% Urigal solution (Nikken Chemical Co., Japan) during the surgery. The progress of the cancer destruction can be observed. The operation is further carefully conducted until the cancer disappears.

Subjects and Results

The subjects were 25 patients with bladder cancer hospitalized at the Department of Urology of Anjo Kosei Hospital from February to Oc-

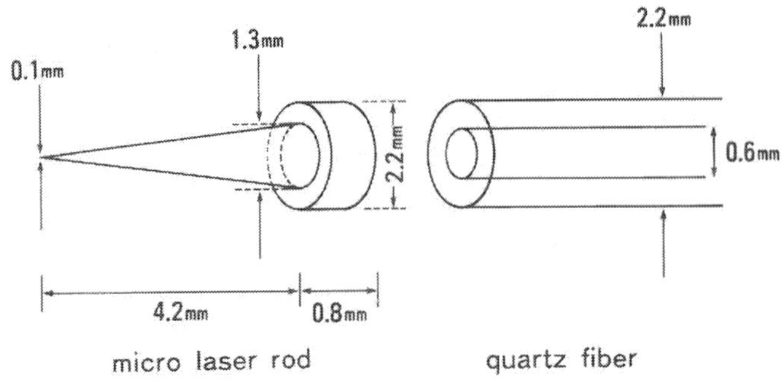

FIGURE 16.1. Scheme of the endorod. Diagramatical representation of the SLT contact endoprobe.

tober 1984. The cancers were classified by the Japanese Association of Urology for bladder cancer care. There were 19 cases of single tumors, six cases of large tumors. Histologically, there were 24 cases of transitional epithelial cancer, one being a mixed type with squamous epithelial cancer, and 1 case of adenocarcinoma. The malignancy was of Grade I in eight cases, Grade II in eight cases, Grade III in six cases, one case being mixed with squamous epithelial cancer. Further, one case of a single large Grade III tumor was diagnosed as cancer of the ureter infiltrating into the bladder by subsequent examinations. To completely treat a bladder cancer of such a background with TULD alone, 16 treatments were required. With TUR-Bt 6 treatments were required and TULD combined with laparotomy (cases in which the total cystectomy was judged desirable from the histologic type) was applied in three cases, including one case of cancer of the ureter, as mentioned before (Table 16.1). In six cases, where the treatment could not be completed with TULD alone, bleeding was marked, and TUR-Bt was required, but these were all cases in the early period when TULD was started, resulting from lack of experience with the laser apparatus, techniques, and so on.

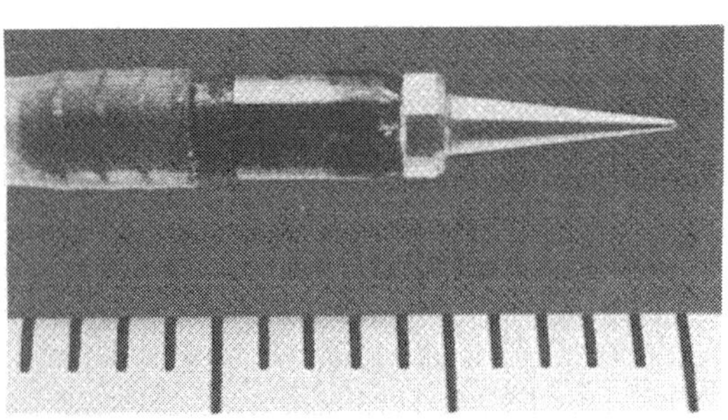

FIGURE 16.2. An endoprobe connected to the quartz fiber. (SLT contact endoprobe.)

A tumor in the vicinity of the ureteral orifice was seen in five cases, but in none of them was the ureter affected in the bladder wall or the ureteral orifice, and no abnormality was noted in the upper urinary tract using the indigocarmine excretion test and excretory urogram immediately after operation.

Case 1: A 56-Year-Old Man

The patient was examined with a chief complaint of hematuria. The cystoscopy revealed a papillary tumor with a stalk, about 1 cm large, on the left lateral wall (Figure 16.3A). TULD was performed after biopsy of the tumor. The SLT contact endoprobe was placed superficially into the neck of tumor and laser irradiation started

TABLE 16.1. Summary of clinical cases of bladder tumors treated by SLT contact laser surgery

Treatment	TULD	TULD + TUR-Bt	Open surgery after TULD
Number			
Single	11	5	3
Multiple	5	1	0
Size			
Small	3	0	0
Medium	8	2	0
Large	5	4	3
Grade			
I	8	0	0
II	6	5	0
III	1	2 + SCC 1	3
AC	1	0	0

TULD = transurethral laser destruction (of bladder cancer).
TUR-Bt = transurethral surgery for bladder tumor.

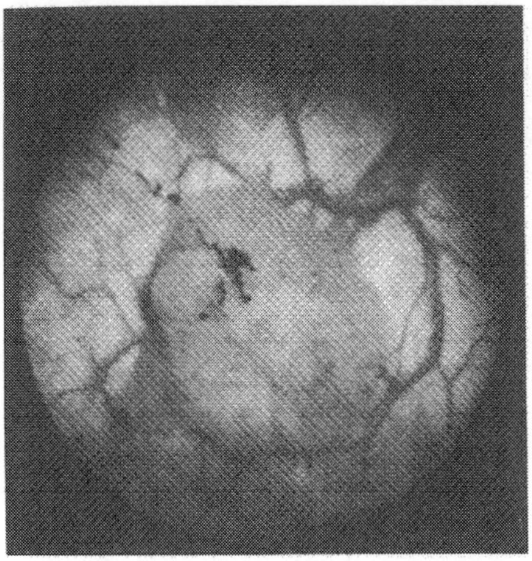

A

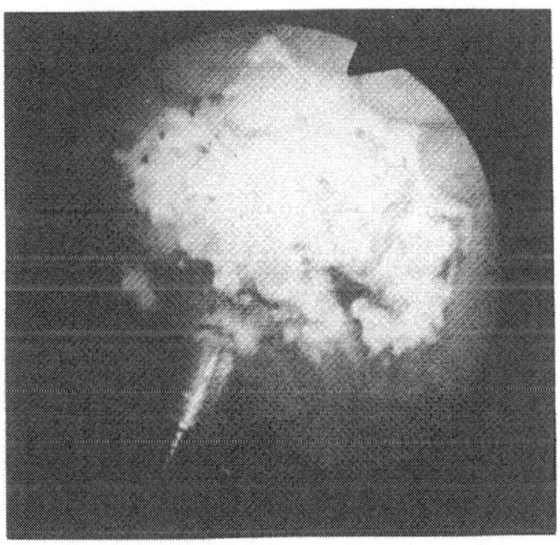

B

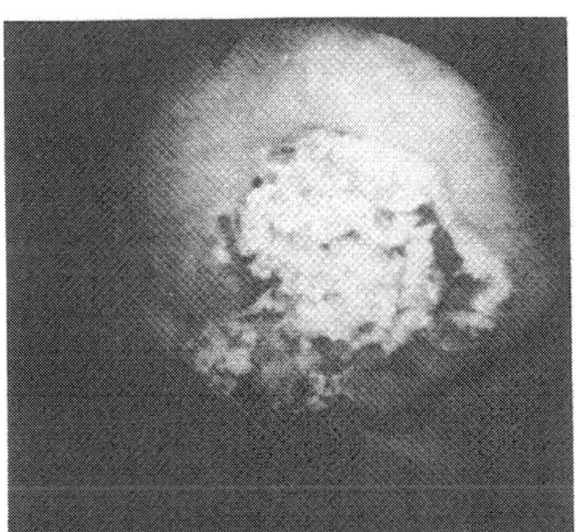

C

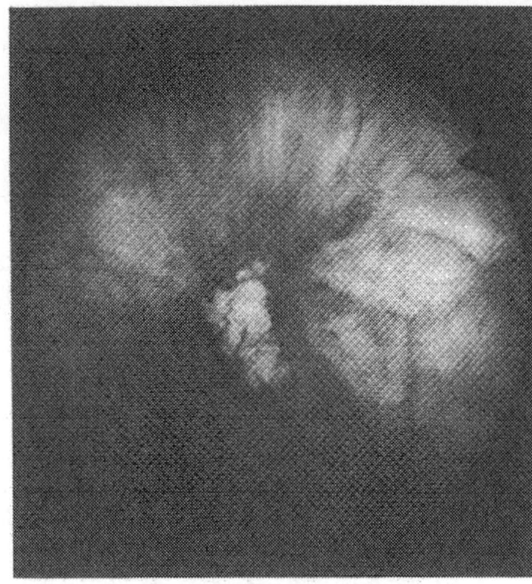

D

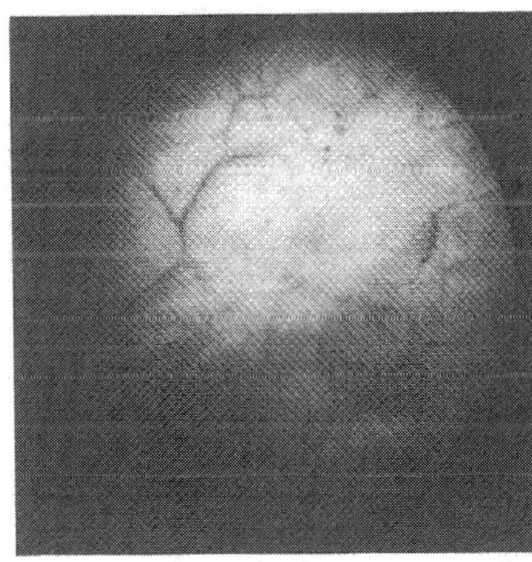

E

FIGURE 16.3. (*A*) A papillary tumor about 1 cm large on the left lateral wall of the bladder. (*B*) During the TULD. Showing an SLT contact endoprobe in the tumor (*arrow*). (*C*) Tumor site immediately after laser treatment. (*D*) Treatment site at 4 weeks. (*E*) Treatment site at 8 months showing a healed mucoser with no evidence of recurrence on biopsy.

with a 15-W power output. The tumor was destroyed instantaneously and this action was repeated to complete the operation using a total of 2800 J (Figure 16.3B,C). It had taken about 2 months for the wound to heal (Figure 16.3D,E). The histologic changes of the cancer are shown in Figure 16.4.

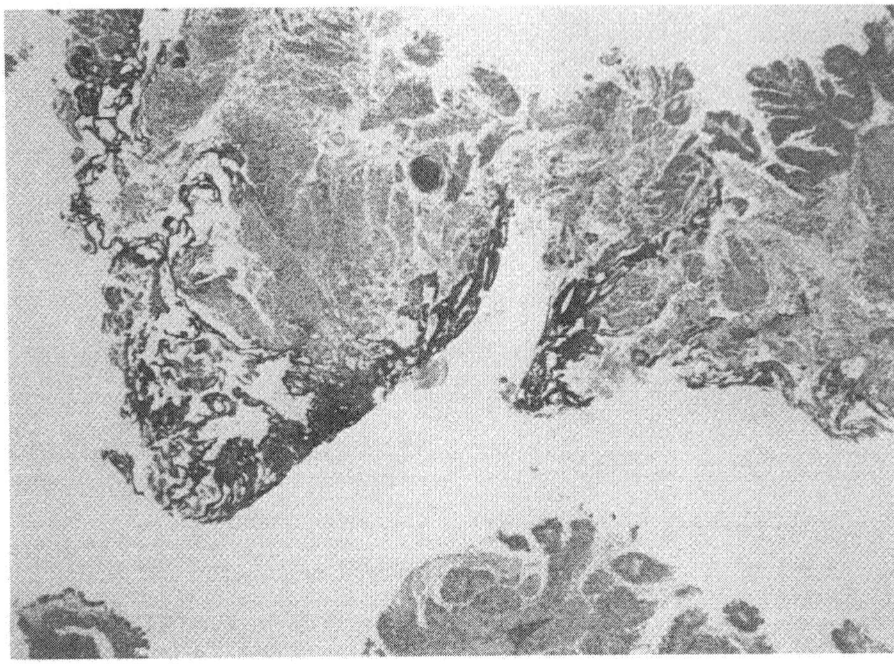

FIGURE 16.4. Histologic changes of a bladder tumor after transurethal contact laser surgery.

Discussion

Since it became possible to use a flexible fiber in the conduction of light,[8] the laser has come into use for endoscopic operations. The Nd:YAG laser, in particular, has shown an excellent capacity for coagulation and hemostasis, and has been applied to excise tumors of the digestive tract or bladder and others.

The treatment of bladder tumors with the Nd:YAG laser was started by Staehler and colleagues.[9] They reported excellent results and stated such advantages as absence of bleeding, short period of hospitalization and less risk of perforation, as compared with TUR-Bt. In Japan, in 1980, Murase and colleagues[10] published a pessimistic report on laser treatment using Nd:YAG laser irradiation in the rabbit bladder, while others[11] recognized its significance as a new treatment method for bladder tumors from basic and clinical studies.

We started the treatment of bladder cancer with the Nd:YAG laser beam in 1983. Due to laser instability and uncertainty of tissue damage, we studied the laser conduction path of the SLT contact endoprobes for transurethral endoscopic operations.[12] Daikuzono and Joffe[7] had previously developed the laser surgical scalpel, and we clinically applied it from February 1984 after completing basic studies on the transurethral laser destruction of bladder cancers.

At about the time when this technique was started, we were not sufficiently experienced using lasers and method for manipulation of the SLT contact laser system and thus a TUR-Bt was initially needed. Since it was found that an output of about 15 W at a time was the most suitable, the purpose of the treatment has been sufficiently achieved.

Based on this present experience, the following aspects of the laser apparatus need to be considered or improved. Concerning the laser apparatus, a high output (around 100 W) was necessary for the noncontact laser treatment. If the endorod is used, the output needs to be stable at a low setting (less than 20 W). For instance, the MediLas YAG (MBB, GFR), is frequently used in Japan and is suitable for a high output only. When compared to Cooper 8000 (Cooper, USA), the output of the MBB laser is unstable at low powers (< 20 W). Further, it takes several seconds for the laser energy to become stabilized. (Immediately after switching on the MBB laser, the output at the fiber tip is very different from the output displayed, often by a several-fold difference at low power. This leads to difficulty in safely and effectively carry out contact laser surgery.

When using the contact laser system, destruction of the tumor is excessively rapid at a power output of 30 W, with potentiation of bleeding and TUR-Bt is needed. However the SLT laser and the Cooper 8000 have a stable output of 10–15 W. The transurethral endoscopes for laser operations available at present are unsatisfactory. It will be necessary to develop endoscopes suitable for these operations.

The treatment of bladder cancer using the SLT contact laser system is in the early stages and there are still some problems to overcome. The technique, however, is simple to apply in practice, bleeding is hardly seen, there is less damage to surrounding tissue. All these factors suggesting the possibility that interstitial laser irradiation is superior to TUR-Bt. Work is currently in progress to evaluate a larger number of patients with a longer follow-up period.

References

1. Maiman TH: Stimulated optical radiation in ruby. Nature, 187:493, 1960.
2. Johnson LF, Boyd GD, Nassau K, Soden RR: Continuous operation of a solid-state optical laser. Phys Rev 126:1406, 1962.
3. Snitzer E: Glass lasers. Appl Opt 5:1487, 1966.
4. Hofstetter A, Frank F: The neodymium-YAG laser in urology. Roche F (ed): Hoffmann-La Roche, Basle, 1980, pp 17–30.
5. Suzuki S, Shiina Y, Miura T, et al: Effects of Nd-YAG laser radiation o the gastrointestinal mucosa the sixth report: Experimental studies with a new contact type of the YAG laser rod. Gastroenterol Endosc 26:705, 1984.
6. Washida H, Tsugaya M, Hirao N, et al: Interstitial laser irradiation for bladder cancer using laser micro rod. Jpn J Urol 76:1524, 1985.
7. Daikuzono N, Joffe SN: Med Instrum 19, 173, 1985.
8. Nath G, Gorisch W, Kiefhaber P: First laser endoscopy via a fiberoptic transmission system. Endoscopy 5:208, 1973.
9. Staehler G, Hofstetter A, Schmiedt E, et al: Endoskopisch Laserbestrahlung von Blasentumoren des Menschen. Fortshr Med 95:3, 1977.
10. Murase T, Matsumoto K, Nishisaka T: Histological change of the rabbit bladder by irradiation of the Nd-YAG laser. Nishinihon J Urol 42.1147, 1980.
11. Amagi T: Experimental and clinical studies for laser application to the treatment of bladder tumor. Nichidai Ishi 40:985, 1981.
12. Washida H, Tsugaya M, Hirao N, et al: Fundamental and clinical study of micro laser rod for endoscopic laser surgery. Jpn J Laser Med 5:521–524, 1985.

17 Endoscopic Nd:YAG Laser Treatment in Airway Lesions

Kenkichi Oho and Ryuta Amemiya

A CO_2 laser was first employed in the treatment of respiratory diseases by Strong et al.,[1] who treated a papilloma of the airway. However, the CO_2 laser has been used only with the rigid bronchoscope because it cannot be transmitted by a quartz fiber as its wavelength is long (10,600 nm). Hence the CO_2 laser has been used primarily for lesions located in the larynx to the main bronchus that can be seen by the rigid bronchoscope. As a result, the CO_2 laser has been used mainly in the field of ENT.

With the advent of the neodymium:yttrium-aluminum-garnet laser (Nd:YAG laser) which has a short wavelength (1064 nm) that can be transmitted by quartz fibers, high-energy laser treatment of airway lesions with the fiberoptic bronchoscope became possible. In 1979 Godard et al.[2] first reported treatment of a bronchial tumor using the Nd:YAG laser.

On the other hand, photodynamic therapy (PDT), a method which involves intravenous injection of the photosensitizer, hematoporphyrin derivative, followed by application of an argon-dye laser as an activator of the photosensitizer, has been widely performed in lung cancer cases by Hayata et al.[3] since 1979. Its application for the diagnosis of lung cancer was reported by Doiron et al.[4]

We have performed basic research on the applications of the Nd:YAG and argon lasers in dogs, beginning in 1978.[5,6] On the basis of those results, in 1980 we began to use this modality in clinical cases of airway stenosis as far distal as the segmental bronchi; tracheal tumors; lung cancer; and tumors metastatic to the airway in addition to cases of cicatricial lesions due to tuberculosis and granuloma.[7,8]

In this chapter, the present status and points at issue concerning endoscopic Nd:YAG laser treatment in airway lesions are discussed based on the experience of the authors.

Materials and Methods

Between 1980 and 1985 we have treated a total of 136 cases consisting of 64 lung cancer, 9 primary tracheal cancer, 33 benign lesions, and 30 metastatic airway lesions. In 107 cases (79%) effective results were obtained.

All procedures were performed under local anesthesia except in an 11-year-old boy with a mucoepidermoid carcinoma in the left main bronchus. The standard method of topical anesthesia using a 4% Xylocaine spray is performed, followed by the insertion of the fiberoptic bronchoscope with the patient in a supine position. After the target site has been brought under observation the transmission fiber is inserted through the instrumentation channel and is projected about 5 mm from the distal tip of the endoscope. The fiber is maintained at a distance of about 5–10 mm from the target. Air is flushed continuously and coaxially through the Teflon sleeve of the laser fiber in order to prevent fragments of carbonized material from adhering to the tip. A red helium–neon laser beam is employed as a pilot beam. In cases of severe ventilatory disturbance with PaO_2 below 60 torr, 15–30 mg pentazocine and 10 mg diazepam are administered to temporarily reduce the level of consciousness in order to facilitate the performance of the laser procedure.

We used an Olympus model MYL-1 continuous wave laser with a power output of 1 to 100 W. The time interval of irradiation is set at 0.2 to 2.0 seconds.[9]

Results

Our standard of "therapeutic effectiveness" means only that the desired result was obtained and is not related to long-term survival. Many of the cases were treated for emergency relief of stenosis and obstruction, not for cure of the underlying disease. When detected, the majority of central-type lung cancer cases have already invaded extensively along the longitudinal axis of the bronchus, or show stenosis due to submucosal invasion connected with many metastatic lymph nodes, or else show invasion continuing to the periphery from the tumor in the main bronchus. Considering the developmental behavior of the lung cancer, it is natural that the effectiveness of endoscopic Nd:YAG laser treatment be limited. The purposes for the performance of endoscopic Nd:YAG laser treatment differ significantly according to each individual case. Cases in which the procedure is indicated can include malignant and also benign diseases. The purposes of the procedure are hemostasis in some cases and palliative widening of the airway in other cases. Consequently, it is difficult to establish uniform criteria to evaluate the effectiveness of this procedure. Many cases have been treated and represent a wide and varying range of advanced malignant diseases and clinical symptoms. Furthermore, since this procedure is intended to produce only a local effect, it would not be tenable to attempt to evaluate its effectiveness in terms of length of survival. For the meantime therefore, it is unavoidable that a certain amount of subjectivity be involved in the evaluation of effectiveness.

This procedure has been performed in a total of 136 cases up to February 1986, using an Nd:YAG laser. These cases consisted of 47 cases of tracheal lesions, 15 cases of tracheal and bronchial lesions, and 74 cases of bronchial lesions. Out of the 52 emergency cases in which the procedure was performed to widen the airway, effective results were obtained in 49. It was also effective in 47 of 66 cases in which the procedure was performed for palliative (staged) widening of the airway. In 11 of 18 cases in which the procedure was performed for curative vaporization of tumor and 1 of 3 cases in which the procedure was performed for hemostasis, successful results were obtained. Effective results were obtained in 46 of 64 cases (70%) of lung cancer. Results were effective in all 9 cases of primary tracheal cancer. Effective results were obtained in 27 of 33 cases (82%) of benign airway lesion cases. Effective results were obtained in 25 of 30 cases (71%) of metastatic airway lesions (Table 17.1).

ABLE 17.1. Cases treated by endoscopic Nd:YAG laser treatment.

Lesion	Cases	Effective cases	Effective: Emergency widening of airway	Effective: Palliative widening of airway	Effective: Curative vaporization of tumor	Effective: Hemostasis	Noneffective cases
rimary lung cancer bronchial lesions	51	34 (66.7%)	3/3 (100%)	25/37 (65.5%)	6/10 (60.0%)	0/1 (0%)	17
racheal and bronchial lesions	13	12 (92.3%)	10/11 (90.9%)	1/1 (100%)	1/1 (100%)		1
rimary tracheal cancer	9	9 (100%)	8/8 (100%)		1/1 (100%)		0
enign airway lesions	33	27 (81.8%)	6/6 (100%)	20/26 (76.9%)		1/1 (100%)	6
letastatic airway lesions	30	25 (71.4%)	22/24 (91.7%)	1/2 (50.0%)	3/3 (100%)	0/1 (0%)	5
otal	136	107 (78.7%)	49/52 (94.2%)	47/66 (71.2%)	11/15 (73.3%)	1/3 (33.3%)	29

ebruary 1986.

Indications

There is a tendency to consider a wide range of conditions as indications for endoscopic Nd:YAG laser treatment, because this procedure can vaporize and remove tissue easily.[10] However, great caution is necessary in deciding the indications of this procedure in advanced cases of lung cancer. We consider that the indications are limited to an extremely small number of cases. At present we judge the indications of this procedure as follows:

1. Pathologic changes of the trachea causing ventilatory disturbances or bleeding, regardless of the histologic diagnosis and requiring immediate treatment (Figure 17.1). Moreover, there is no other therapeutic option for these cases at present apart from this procedure. However, in cases of malignant disease it is frequently impossible to totally vaporize the entire lesion, even if most of the lesion can be eliminated. In advanced cases this method is high-energy vaporization of tissue and must be halted before damaging normal tissue.
2. Pathologic changes located from the trachea to segmental bronchi limited to within the cartilage. We have experienced 12 cases of this type of lesion (Figure 17.2). This procedure may be a possible alternative method to conventional surgery, to curatively treat certain malignant lesions limited to within the bronchial cartilage as far as the vicinity of the orifices of segmental bronchi. However, it would not be indicated in lesions located in the right upper lobe segmental bronchi and left B^{1+2} and B^3, and both right and left B^6, due to the difficulty of maneuvering the quartz fiber.
3. Maintenance of airway, regardless of depth of lesions, and cases in which improvement can be expected by widening the airway. In such cases this procedure is performed as a noncurative treatment. In cases in this category it is necessary that the peripheral airway and the parenchyma distal to the stenosis or obstruction be viable in terms of ventilation and circulation.
4. Benign tumors originating from the trachea to segmental bronchi are good indications (Figure 17.3). This procedure is often the treatment of choice for a benign tumor. Lesions of cicatricial stenosis are indications for this therapeutic modality. However, lesions extending 1 cm or more longitudinally in length and cases in which tuberculous granulomatous tissue are ob-

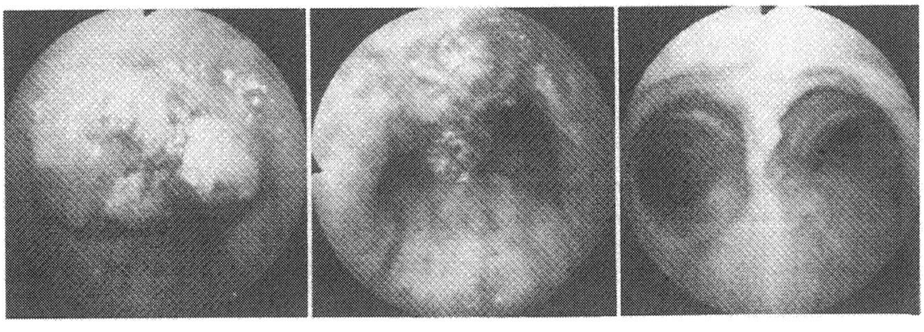

FIGURE 17.1. *(Left)* A 75-year-old man with squamous cell carcinoma was admitted with orthopnea even receiving oxygen (PaO_2 on admission: 58 torr). Chest x-ray revealed no tumor, atelectasis, or obstructive pneumonia in either lung field. Endoscopic Nd:YAG laser treatment was performed as emergency treatment in an attempt to render him a candidate for radiotherapy and chemotherapy. *(Center)* One week after the first session a part of the necrosis-covered tumor was observed to move on respiration and when a small aperture was made at the site with the laser a flood of pent-up secretions appeared. Following aspiration of the secretions opening of the left main bronchus was recognized. The PaO_2 increased to 78 torr breathing room air, and he was subsequently able to receive radiotherapy and chemotherapy. *(Right)* Ten months after completion of a 60 GY course of Linac radiotherapy good regeneration of the mucosa and sharpening of the bifurcation was recognized. Local and general conditions improved remarkably. The laser treatment consisted of 24.345 J over two sessions, at a power level of 60 to 80 W. Treatment was considered successful because most of the lesion was exposed in the airway lesion and endoscopic laser treatment was the first step in a multimodality therapeutic approach, rather than being treatment for relapse.

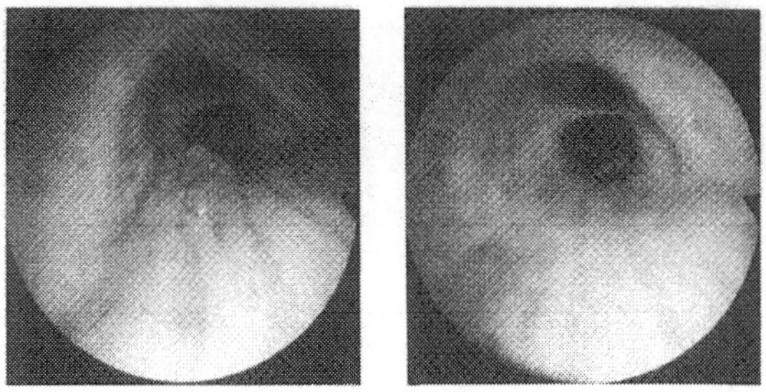

FIGURE 17.2. (*Left*) A 59-year-old nonsmoker had undergone left lower lobectomy for a squamous cell carcinoma in the left basal bronchus. Following the appearance of bloody sputum 17 months later a second squamous cell was discovered in the truncus intermedius. Deep bite biopsy specimens revealed that the extent of invasion was limited to within the extramuscular layer and the peripheral margin of the tumor was endoscopically visible. Since the poor lung function of this patient contraindicated operation, endoscopic Nd:YAG vaporization was performed as a curative procedure. The Nd:YAG laser treatment was spread over 3 sessions during a during a period of 3 weeks. The power intensity was 20 to 50 W delivered in 0.1 to 2.0-second shots, with a total of 823 J. No other method of treatment was employed. (*Right*) The findings 3 weeks after completion of the third vaporization procedure show that the tumor has disappeared and that there is good regeneration of the mucosa at the site where it was located, although the longitudinal folds are interrupted. Follow-up bronchoscopy and sputum cytology are being performed at 3-month intervals and he is apparently disease-free 8 months after the first vaporization session.

tained from the lesion should be excluded from the indications for this treatment.

Discussion

Endoscopic Nd:YAG laser treatment has recently gained popularity. The main airway disease in which this procedure is employed in these institutions is advanced lung cancer.[11,12] Therefore, we should keep in mind that the primaratory disturbance due to obstruction or marked stenosis by a tumor growing as a polypoid in a large airway. Only in such cases in which the peripheral airway can be maintained and in which the parenchyma distal to the stenosis or obstruction is viable in terms of ventilation and circulation, can laser vaporization be considered. Therefore, indications are limited to a relatively small number of cases. Considering the reasons for the noneffectiveness in 19 of 64 lung cancer cases in this series, these included 2 procedures for emergency widening, 12 procedures for palliative widening of the airway, 4 for curative vaporization of a tumor, and 1 for hemostasis. An underestimation of the extent of cancer invasion was recognized as the single most important factor in these noneffective cases. In 14 cases, of which 2 cases were performed for emergency widening and 12 cases for palliative widening of airway, the reasons for failure was that cancer invasion continued to the periphery. There is no completely reliable diagnostic method to obtain information concerning the peripheral airway and the parenchyma distal to the stenosis or obstruction, although Pearlberg et al.[13] reported that chest CT provides useful information and also Joyner et al.[14] reported the effectiveness of instillation of contrast medium distal to the sites of airway stenosis or obstruction.

In 4 cases residual carcinoma or carcinoma in situ were found in resected specimens following an attempt at curative laser vaporization. At present the major indications for curative endoscopic Nd:YAG laser treatment in squamous cell carcinoma of the airway are as follows: (1) The deepest portion of cancer invasion is limited to the extramuscular layer of the bronchus. (2) The tumor invasion is localized to the site of possible laser irradiation. (3) The peripheral margin of the cancer invasion is seen via the endoscope. For these lesions laser treatment is performed at a power of 40 to 50 W at 1 second or less for areas of apparent cancer invasion and 20 to 40 W, for 0.2 to 0.5 seconds for surrounding areas. These power conditions are advisable to prevent perforation of the bronchial wall and to minimize the damage of normal bronchial architecture and to obtain early and good reepithelialization.

For the treatment of airway diseases, especially for tracheal, tracheobronchial, and bronchial malignant tumors, there are two types of endoscopic laser treatments. One is using endoscopic hematoporphyrin derivative (Hpd) and photodynamic therapy (PDT) and the other is endoscopic Nd:YAG laser treatment. Cases presenting with respiratory insufficiency due to

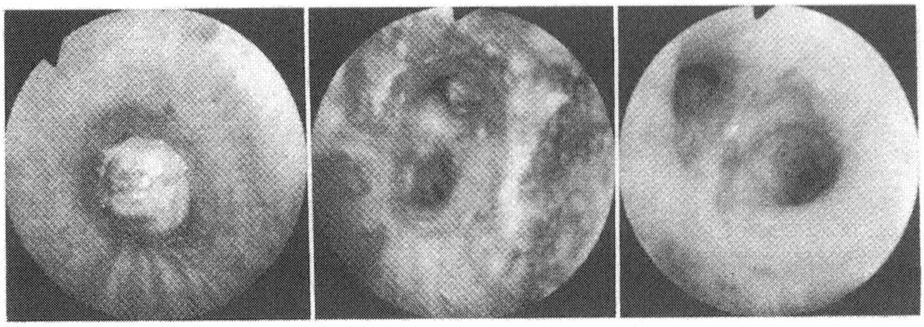

FIGURE 17.3. (*Left*) A 41-year-old female presented with episodes of frequent cough, sputum, and slight dyspnea during the past year. Endoscopically, a polypoid tumor can be seen in the left main bronchus. No tumor invasion can be recognized in the surrounding bronchial wall. The tumor appears to obstruct the main bronchus. (*Center*) Findings before the second session. The tumor originated in B^4 and polypoid proliferation to the left main bronchus was recognized in the left upper lobe bronchus. (*Right*) Findings of the treated portion 2 months after endoscopic Nd:YAG laser treatment. The left upper is the upper division bronchus and the lower right is the lingular bronchus in which tumor originated after treatment by Nd:YAG laser. No edema or scar can be recognized. Reepithelialization also appears to be completed in this area. Glomus tumor was diagnosed by biopsied specimen. We can say that endoscopic Nd:YAG laser treatment for such benign tumors in the airway is a most appropriate therapeutic modality, which not only can be performed with the least damage to bronchial architecture and the least complications but is also a single therapeutic modality to replace thoracotomy.

obstruction or stenosis by tumors in the trachea, the carina or main bronchi are good indications for endoscopic Nd:YAG laser treatment. Tumors occupying the airway lumen are vaporized, leading to a rapid improvement of the condition. Such cases are not indications for PDT. However, in cases not presenting with ventilatory insufficiency even if there is obstruction or stenosis due to a tumor in main bronchi or lobar bronchi, both PDT and Nd:YAG laser treatment can be employed. In order to prevent perforation of the airway wall in cases of tumor invasion extending beyond the bronchial wall, YAG laser treatment should be stopped, even if the widening of the airway is incomplete. With PDT, delayed complications should be kept in mind, such as bronchial fistula, bronchoesophageal fistula, and massive bleeding.[15] In tumors limited to within the bronchial wall originating in bronchi larger than lobar bronchi, both types of endoscopic laser treatments can be used. However, lesions such as those limited to within the bronchial wall extending to segmental bronchi differ according to each individual case. As mentioned above, it is imperative that the peripheral margin of cancer invasion be recognized within the extent of the visual field of the endoscope. Even if the invasion is limited to within the bronchial wall, if the lesions extend to the subsegmental bronchi the case should not be considered for either type of endoscopic laser treatment because it is difficult to treat such lesions safely and effectively. PDT needs great care to ensure that the PDT beam reaches only the lesion in order to prevent possible destruction of the architecture of the surrounding normal bronchial wall in segmental or subsegmental bronchi. If this is not done, in cases of lesions located in segmental bronchi, bronchial stenosis or obstruction and delayed reepithelialization will occur. In the case of Nd:YAG laser, care must always be exercised concerning the depth of irradiation in order to prevent perforation of the airway wall.

Preoperative laser treatment to widen the range of indications for surgery and to reduce the extent of resection has come to be performed in a few institutions.[16] However we consider that the indications of preoperative laser treatment are limited to a small number of cases because exact evaluation of the actual extent of submucosal invasion and lymphatic involvement is extremely difficult. Cases of adenocarcinoma should in general be excluded because of the tendency toward submucosal extension of this histologic type.

The limitations of this procedure are as follows:

1. The procedure requires skill in the manipulation of the endoscope, skill in laser irradiation, and strict analysis of endoscopic findings. Simultaneously, as the Nd:YAG laser beam is a high-energy laser, perforation of the bronchial wall and massive bleeding will follow mistaken irradiation. Therefore a detailed anatomic knowledge concerning the branching of bronchi and pulmonary vessels is required. In addition, the level of endoscopic expertise largely influences the therapeutic results.
2. Pulmonary function limitations of this procedure are PaO_2 below 50 torr, or $PaCO_2$ above 50 torr due to the danger of postprocedural acute respiratory insufficiency and cardiac decompensation.
3. In cases of lesions in the trachea or main bronchi, destruction by a tumor involving 2 or more cartilaginous rings can result in an airway collapse following treatment, even if a temporary opening is achieved by this procedure. Therefore most lesions such as those with compressive stenosis are generally not indications for this procedure.
4. Finally, less extensive lesions along the longitudinal axis of the airway causing stenosis and obstruction can be vaporized more safely and quickly. In general, vaporization of tumors less than 3 cm in length can be performed safely and easily.

References

1. Strong MS, Vaughan CW, Polanyi T, Wallace R: Bronchoscopic carbon dioxide laser surgery. Ann Otol 83:769, 1974.
2. Godard P, Draussin M, Lopez FM, et al: Utilization du rayonnement laser en bronchologie. Resection de deux tumeurs trachebronchique. Pulmon 35:147, 1979.
3. Hayata Y, Kato H, Konaka C, et al: Hematoporphyrin derivative and laser photoradiation in the treatment of lung cancer. Chest 81:269, 1982.
4. Doiron DR, Profio E, Vincent RG, Dougherty TJ: Fluorescence bronchoscopy for detection of lung cancer. Chest 76:27, 1979.
5. Amemiya R, Oho K, Ohtani T, et al: Laser photoradiation via the fiberoptic bronchoscope: Effects on the bronchial wall. In Bronchology. Martinus Nijhoff, The Hague, Boston, and London, 1980, p 540.
6. Hayakawa H, Oho K, Amemiya R, et al: Photodynamic effect of laser surgery on the trachea and bronchi of mongrel dogs. In Bronchology. Maltinus Nijhoff, The Hague, Boston, and London, 1980, p 543.
7. Oho K, Ohtani T, Amemiya R, et al: Laser surgery in the trachea and bronchus via the fiberoptic bronchoscope. 4th Congress of the International Society for Laser Surgery. Laser Tokyo '81 14, 1981.
8. Oho K, Ogawa I, Amemiya R, et al: Indications for endoscopic Nd-YAG laser surgery in the trachea and bronchus. Endoscopy 15:302, 1983.
9. Oho K, Amemiya R: Practical Fiberoptic Bronchoscopy, 2nd ed. Igaku-Shoin, Tokyo and New York, 1984, p 174.
10. Dumon JF, Reboud E, Garbe L, et al: Treatment of tracheobronchial lesions by laser photoresection, Chest 81:278, 1982.
11. Hetzel MR, Millard FJC, Ayesh R, et al: Laser treatment for carcinoma of the bronchus. Br Med J 286:12, 1983.
12. Dumon JF, Shapshay S, Bourcereau J, et al: Principles for safety in application of Neodymium-YAG laser in bronchology. Chest 86:163, 1984.
13. Pearlberg JL, Sandler MA, Kvale P, et al: Computed-tomographic and conventional linear-tomographic evaluation of tracheobronchial lesion for laser photoresection. Radiology 154:759, 1985.
14. Joyner LR, Maren AG, Sarama R, Yakaboshi A: Neodymium-YAG laser treatment of intrabronchial lesions, a new mapping technique via the flexible fiberoptic bronchoscope. Chest 87:418, 1985.
15. Cortese DA, Kinsey JH: Hematoporphyrin derivative phototherapy in the treatment of bronchogenic carcinoma. Chest 86:8, 1984.
16. Kato H, Konaka C, Ono J, et al: Preoperative laser photodynamic therapy in combination with operation in lung cancer. J Thorac Cardiovasc Surg 90:420, 1985.

18
Developments in Bronchoscopic Nd:YAG Laser Resection

J-F. Dumon and B. Meric

Medical lasers have not been available for very long. The Nd:YAG laser was not marketed for medical use until the late 1970s. Thus it is not an exaggeration to say that the laser is currently one of the frontiers of medical science. This notion of newness in laser medicine is important because it explains that techniques and equipment are still emerging and evolving. Bronchology is one of the first fields in which the laser was used "internally," and the basic principles are now well-defined. Today laser resection is one of the newest and most effective palliative modalities in medicine's arsenal against lung cancer. It has no aftereffects and requires no particular follow-up. In case of recurrence, it can be repeated as needed. It can be associated with any other form of treatment (e.g., radiotherapy or chemotherapy). The purpose of this chapter is to discuss the current status of laser technology in lung medicine with respect to laser systems, instrumentation, and methodology. We also wish to take this opportunity to repeat the principles of our laser resection technique and to update our results.

Laser Systems

Not all laser systems are suitable for endoscopic use. At the present time the three main biomedical lasers are the CO_2, the argon, and the Nd:YAG. The CO_2 laser, which is a very precise cutting instrument, is not well adapted to endoscopy. Although it may soon be available, there is no optical fiber that can transport the CO_2 laser beam. Delivery of CO_2 energy is achieved by means of a cumbersome mirror arm delivery system, and, although the last mirror can be positioned at the entrance of the bronchosope, no other instrumentation, including the viewing lens, can be used during firing. Obviously under these conditions aiming is problematic and accuracy difficult. For this reason, up to now the CO_2 laser has been extensively used by ENT specialists and surgeons, but rarely by bronchoscopists.

Argon laser beams can be delivered through an optical fiber, but, because the power output of these lasers is low, they do not penetrate the tissue and consequently are not very useful in endoscopy. One notable exception to this is an endoscopic technique called hematoporphyrin phototherapy in which small, very local, inoperable lesions are destroyed by activation of hematoporphyrin retained in malignant tissues by a dye laser-pumped argon laser. On the other hand, argon lasers have been used advantageously in ophthalmology and dermatology.

As far as precision resection is concerned, it is the Nd:YAG laser that is, at the present time, the most valuable laser system for endoscopic use. With this system 20 to 100 W of power can be delivered to the tip of an air-cooled optical fiber measuring only 2.6 mm in diameter. Standard fibers are 4 m in length. The effects of the Nd:YAG laser on living tissue range from vaporization to coagulation and depend on power setting, firing range, pulse duration, and tissue color. On dark tissue vaporization is quickly achieved at high power and close range. Hemostasis is accomplished at medium power and range. In fact, coagulation is not a direct effect of the Nd:YAG laser. Rather, it is an indirect result of tissue shrinkage, which cuts off the flow of blood. A major danger with the Nd:YAG laser is that it is difficult to control the depth of penetration of the beam, especially when working on pale tissue. It behooves every physician using the Nd:YAG laser to be aware of the dreaded "popcorn effect." As described by Fisher, this phenomenon occurs as the temperature in underlying tissue rises and steam builds up in a pocket below the surface. Given these unseen effects, great care must be taken in the tracheobronchial tree to avoid inadvertently creating a fistula, especially on the backside of the trachea, which is not reinforced by cartilage, or damaging the cartilaginous rings themselves. In extreme cases the steam pocket may ultimately explode, causing extensive damage. It is ill-advised to use the laser in the continuous mode at any time and any power setting. Properly controlled, however, the ability of the Nd:YAG laser to penetrate into tissue can be used to stop a hemorrhage, to coagulate tissue before mechanical resection, and probably to kill viral infection (such as in the case of papillomas).

To conclude this discussion on biomedical lasers, it should be said that research and development will certainly lead to the design of other laser systems that can be used for biomedical purposes. One exciting innovation that should be ready in the very near future is the copper-vapor laser. The particularity of this laser is that its beam is made up of several different wavelengths—green, yellow, and red—which it is technically possible to filter and use separately. The green beam has the same characteristics as the argon laser, the yellow is a new wavelength never used in medicine, and the red is a tunable dye laser beam that may lead to the development of new photochemical modalities like the hematoporphyrin technique. We will soon begin an experimental program with such a laser in our unit in Marseille and will report our findings.

Instrumentation

The dangers of laser resection are now well known. They may be classified into two categories, namely, the irreversible ones that can and must be prevented by limiting the amount of laser exposure and the controllable ones. The complications in the first category, including perforation, pneumothorax, and fire, are catastrophic, and, once they have occurred, little can be done to prevent a fatal outcome. Those in the second category, hypoxia and hemorrhage, may, if left unattended, become life-threatening, but, if the endoscopic team is properly trained and equipped, it should respond quickly. In the area of instrumentation specifically suited to laser resection, some very interesting develpments have recently taken place.

Only very small lesions can be safely resected with a flexible fiberscope. Fiberscopic resection accounted for only 20% of our procedures. In our experience flexible instrumentation using optical fibers carried some major liabilities. The fiberscope is a solid tube measuring 5 to 6 mm in diameter; when it is introduced into the airway, it results in a considerable reduction of the tracheal lumen. In cases involving high-grade tumoral occlusion or intubated patients, 50% or more of the lumen is blocked. The fiberscope is inflammable and has reportedly ignited during laser resection. Though fiberscopic lenses now provide excellent definition, their location at the tip of the instrument exposes them to constant soiling by secretions. The most serious drawback of the fiberscope for laser resection, however, is that its working channel is, at the most, only 2.6 mm in diameter. This is too small to allow passage and simultaneous use of both the laser fiber and a suction tube.

In view of these problems, most endoscopists practicing laser surgery have learned how to use a rigid bronchoscope for laser resection. Indeed, the rigid open tube offers many advantages over the fiberscope for laser resection. Depending on the manufacturer and model, the working channel is 8 to 9 mm in diameter, which is large enough to allow simultaneous viewing, lasing, and suctioning. In cases of high-grade occlusion, the rigid scope can be used to prop open the airway, thereby restoring patency. Vision through a telescope is much better than through a fiberscope, and the lens is better protected against soiling. In addition to these advantages the tip of the rigid tube can be used to palp the lesion, thus providing "tactile" feedback that is crucial in deciding what and how much to resect.

Many of the bronchoscopes now being sold have in fact been designed specifically for therapeutic purposes and especially laser resection.

In collaboration with J. Harrell of the University of California in San Diego, we at Salvator Hospital have developed a third-generation universal bronchoscope especially suitable for lasing in the tracheobronchial tree. It comes with a set of interchangeable barrels, ranging in size from 3.5 to 9 mm in diameter, which can be used for children as well as adults. A second set of short barrels with no lateral ventilation ports is also available for the treatment of tracheal stenosis. The fact that barrels are interchangeable is a great advantage for tracheal stenosis, since progressively larger barrels must be used to dilate and gauge the trachea as tissue is resected. In addition to the main entrance through which the telescope and/or other instrumentation is introduced, the head of the bronchoscope has a side port that is designed to accommodate the laser fiber and one suction tube, and to allow removal of resected fragments. All openings can be sealed with Silastic caps so that closed-circuit ventilation is possible. With regard to ventilation, it should also be noted that the T-tube adaptor is mounted on a swivel so that it is not necessary to interrupt lasing under closed-circuit conditions. The Dumon–Harrel bronchoscope is thus a truly all-purpose instrument that can be used on adults or children under closed- or open-circuit conditions, with or without jet or high-frequency ventilation.

Experience has shown that suction tubes are a key component of the equipment setup for tracheobronchial laser surgery. The presence of at least one suction catheter in the airway is an absolute requirement for most procedures, and, should hemorrhage occur, a second catheter is sometimes needed. These tubes are used not only to keep the operative field and airways clean by constant suctioning of blood and secretions, but also to palp the lesion and to seize and pull out resected fragments. The design and quality of the suction tube is very important. It must be made of rigid and ignition-resistant plastic. Catheters meeting these standards are now available from several manufacturers, and they should be used by any team that practices endoscopic laser resection.

Hypoxia during a laser procedure can result from the following: the presence of instrumentation in the airway, oversedation, tumoral occlusion, treatment-related complications (e.g., hemorrhage and secretion accumulation), or from any combination of these factors. Depending on the patient's cardiovascular status, hypoxia can very quickly lead to more serious problems, including bradycardia and cardiac arrest. In order to be able to respond to hypoxia promptly, blood oxygenation should be monitored. The Ohmeda Biox 3700 Pulse Oximeter is very well suited for noninvasive monitoring of arterial oxygen saturation. Light generated in a finger probe is passed through the tissue and is converted into an electronic signal by a photodetector. This signal is relayed back to the oximeter where it is amplified and processed. Patient data and status information, including SaO_2, pulse rate plethysmographic waveform, trend data, status messages, and alarm messages, are presented on two liquid crystal displays. At the first sign of a consistently negative trend, lasing should be interrupted long enough to oxygenate the patient and perform tracheobronchial toilet. An oximeter is also a great asset in the recovery room, where the risks of hypoxia are the same as in the endoscopy room.

Another useful accessory that is now available for Nd:YAG and argon lasers is the artificial sapphire laser tip designed to be attached to the end of the optical fiber for contact photocoagulation and tissue vaporization. Until now, laser energy has been delivered by noncontact irradiation. Contact irradiation has several advantages, including greater precision in aiming, lower power requirements for equivalent effects, greater control over depth of penetration, and protection of the laser fiber from soiling and deterioration. These advantages are particularly important for the application of laser energy in closed tubes like the esophagus, but the laser tip also opens up new possibilities in bronchology.

Methodology

Six years of experience has given us a good idea of the applications for laser resection. The best indications are inoperable tumors located in the trachea or main stem bronchi and causing dyspnea, regardless of the degree of malignancy. Patients with these lesions are often in acute respiratory distress, and palliative laser resection literally saves them from death. Another strong advantage of the laser is that it can be used repeatedly at each recurrence, thus greatly extending survival time. Inoperable malignant tumors in peripheral regions of the tracheobronchial tree can also be treated, but because of their inaccessibility, they are not very good indications. Although extrinsic compression is an absolute contraindication for laser resection, treatment of the endoluminal portion of inoperable extrabronchial tumors (tip of the iceberg) is possible. Finally, for benign tumors without extrabronchial involvement, laser treatment may be the treatment of choice. In this regard, it is interesting to note that papilloma recurrence after laser resection is lower than with other therapies.

With regard to nontumoral tracheal pathology, there are a few minor applications for laser resection, such as destroying granulomas on suture threads, cutting suture threads, controlling local bleeding, and removing impacted foreign bodies, but the most significant nontumoral indication for bronchoscopic laser therapy is tracheal stenosis. At our institution the laser has completely changed our approach to this type of pathology, which had previously been treated exclusively by sleeve resection—contraindicated for older patients or patients in poor condition. Presently, endoscopic laser resection is the initial treatment for most patients with tracheal stenosis. With a concentric web or a solitary tracheal granuloma, laser resection is usually curative in only one or two sessions. In order to maximize the effect of each treatment, resection should be complemented by forceful dilatation with various-sized open tubes. For more extensive lesions involving inflammation and chondromalacia, recurrence after laser resection is systematic. In these cases we either recommend the patient for sleeve resection, or, if his condition or age makes surgery unfeasible, we insert a Montgomery T-tube after the first laser session and then wait for the inflammatory process to subside before deciding on further treatment (laser or surgical). With respect to the T-tube, it should be stated that significant improvements have been made, and this device is now very reliable and easy to use. The greatest improvement is the presence of a lock ring on the perpendicular segment to prevent migration.

Certain other factors, such as the patient's general condition, the degree of obstruction, hemorrhagic potential (e.g., carcinoid tumors), and the age of the lesion, greatly influence the degree of risk. Probably the most important factor of all—even more than pathology—is location. All tracheal and main stem bronchial lesions are dangerous because the risk of hypoxia is high. Especially dangerous are lesions located on the posterior wall of the trachea and left main stem bronchus because of the added danger of esophagotracheal perforation. Also demanding great caution are lesions on the anterior wall of the lower third of the trachea due to the proximity of the aorta and in the left upper lobe due to the difficulty of access. However, the most dangerous lesions of all are recurrences after pneumonectomy.

In the previous section it was said that most laser procedures were carried out through a rigid open tube, but there are some for which the fiberscope can be used safely. Fiberscopic procedures can be carried out with no premedication other than atropine. The patient should lie on the pathologic side. This "safety position," first proposed by our team in 1980, prevents flooding of the healthy bronchus in the event of a hemorrhage. With regard to the choice of rigid and flexible bronchoscopy, it should be added that the endoscopist must have sound experience with both systems. After each laser resection, a fiberscopic inspection of the whole tracheobronchial tree is necessary to ensure that all secretions and/or debris have been removed. Along with careful coagulation of the resected zone, this inspection is the key to a complication-free recovery period.

A variety of general anesthesia techniques for rigid bronchoscopy is used by the different teams practicing laser resection. Because many drugs of proven reliability in Europe are unavailable in the United States, it is useless to give a detailed description of our protocol. Suffice it to say that we still recommend use of a "light" anesthesia, leaving the patient breathing spontaneously and allowing rapid awakening. We are against jet high-frequency ventilation, which, in our opinion, unnecessarily complicates the procedure and increases the risk for the patient. Gas anesthesia with a noninflammable agent like nitrogen pentoxide can be practiced but requires closed circuit conditions at all times. The Dumon-Harrel bronchoscope with its Silastic seals on all ports is compatible with gas anesthesia. Prior to general anesthesia, each patient must have a chest x-ray, an electrocardiogram, and laboratory tests, including an ionogram and a coagulation test. Other tests, such as measurement of blood gas levels, may also be performed.

Our experience has taught us that, in practice, cooperation between the endoscopist and the anesthetist is more important than the anesthesic technique itself. The main risks during laser resection are hypoxia and hemorrhage, which can lead to irreversible cardiovascular complications. To keep this from happening, it is necessary to monitor vital signs continuously. At the least sign of hypoxia, the endoscopist must interrupt lasing and allow the anesthesist time to seal off the bronchoscope for mechanical ventilation, if the procedure is not already being carried out under closed circuit conditions. A tracheobronchial toilet should also be performed. The exact response to hypoxia or hemorrhage depends on the location of the lesions. For tracheal lesions, the bronchoscope is distal to the main stem bronchi; thus, in order to have access to the lungs, it must be passed forcibly through the stenosed area. For lesions in one main stem bronchus, the bronchoscope must be withdrawn from the pathologic bronchus and positioned at the entrance to the healthy one. Once hypoxia has been reversed, or the hemorrhage is under control, lasing can be resumed.

The postoperative period is crucial to the success of a laser procedure. A recovery room in close proximity to the endoscopy room is therefore a very important facility in a unit practicing endoscopic laser surgery. The risk of hypoxia from secondary bleeding or secretion accumulation remains high. In the recovery room, the patient should be watched and monitored by a specially trained team until he or she awakes (another reason why "light" general anesthesia with a short recovery time is important).

TABLE 18.1. Indications for laser resection and methodology

Indication	No. of patients	No. of treatments
Tumors	463	807
Tracheal stenosis	136	333
Miscellaneous	152	227
Total	751	1367

Results

Our series now comprises 1367 resections on 751 patients. The vast majority (80%) of these procedures were carried out under general anesthesia with a rigid open tube. Table 18.1 summarizes indications and methodology. Tracheobronchial tumors were the most common indication for laser resection in our experience. Malignant tumors alone (463 cases) accounted for over half our indications (61%). The most frequent malignant entity was squamous cell carcinoma (Figure 18.1). Immediate results are easily assessed and depended mainly on location (Figure 18.2). Because they are the most accessible, tumors in the trachea or main stem bronchi are the best indications.

Assessment of long-term results is more difficult, if not impossible, since these patients were referred to us from all over the world and underwent a wide variety of complementary treatments. We did, however, record long survival times in several "last chance" cases with extensive tracheobronchial involvement. Laser resection should be considered as an emergency measure destined to reestablish airway patency. Resection can be also done to prepare a patient for radiotherapy or chemotherapy under optimal conditions. We also performed laser surgery on tumors with uncertain prognosis (Figure 18.3). Given the likelihood of extrabronchial involvement, carcinoid tumors are best treated surgically, even if they require a delicate procedure such as resection-reimplantation. For carcinoid patients beyond the reach of surgery, the laser can be called on as a palliative alternative. The endoscopist must, however, keep in mind that carcinoid tumors are highly hemorrhagic. Massive bleeding occurred in 2 of the 13 cases of carcinoid tumor that we treated. Adenoid cystic carcinoma is also a surgical entity, but recurrences are frequent. Furthermore, as these tumors almost always become refractory to radiotherapy, the laser is often the only treatment available to patients that are inoperable or present recurrences after surgery. One or two resections a year usually provide excellent palliation in cases of adenoid cystic carcinoma. One

FIGURE 18.1. Histology of malignant tumors.

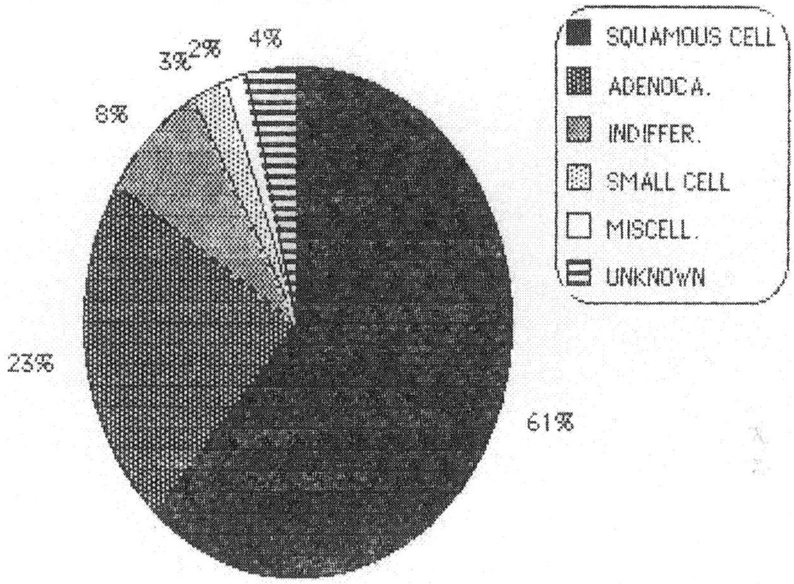

of our patients, who was referred to us with subtotal obstruction of the trachea and the left main stem bronchus, has been undergoing regular resections for 5 years. Though they are excellent indications for laser surgery, purely endobronchial benign tracheobronchial tumors are rare (only 44 cases in our series: Table 18.2).

After cancer, nontumoral tracheal stenosis is the second most frequent indication for laser resection (18% of our procedures). Stenosis caused by a solitary tracheal granuloma or a granuloma at the rim of a tracheostomy catheter can be easily resected endoscopically with the Nd:YAG laser. By contrast, genuine tracheal

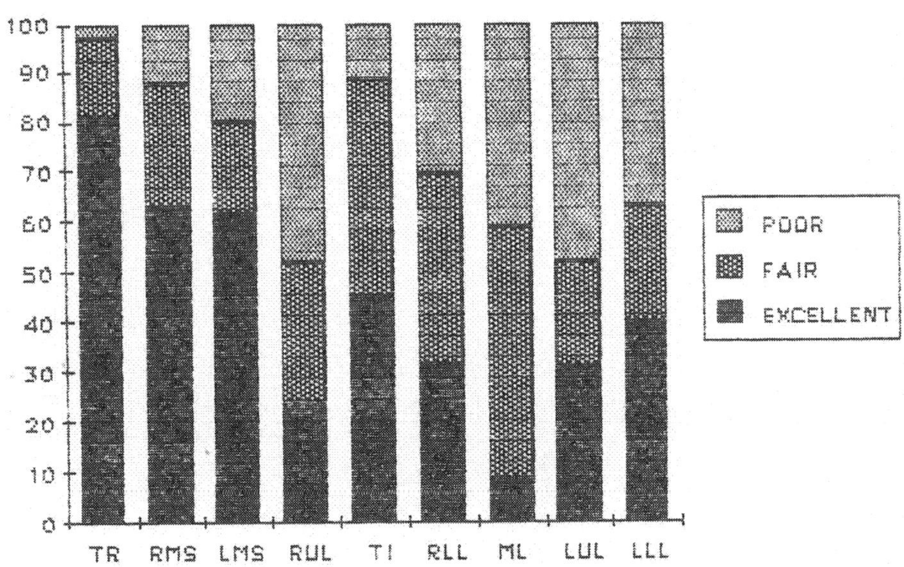

FIGURE 18.2. Immediate results of laser resection of tracheobronchial tumors in various locations. TR, trachea; RMS, right main stem bronchus; LMS, left main stem bronchus; RUL, right upper lung; TI, ; RLL, right lower lung; ML, middle lung; LUL, left upper lung; LLL, left lower lung.

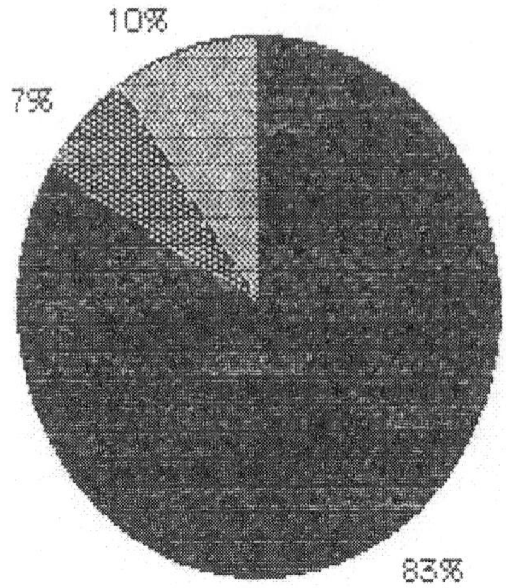

FIGURE 18.3. Prognosis of tumors treated with laser surgery.

TABLE 18.2. Forty-four benign tumors

Amyloidosis	5	Angioma	4
Botryoid tumor	2	Bronchoosteoblastoma	1
Chondroma	3	Fibroid leiomyoma	2
Fibroma	1	Hamartoma	7
Hemangioma	1	Lipoma	1
Lymphoma	3	Myoblastoma	2
Neurofibroma	1	Papilloma	7
Tuberculosis	4		

stenosis, that is, inflammatory stenosis following intubation or tracheotomy, are very difficult to manage due to the risk of recurrence. Treatment of these lesions must be undertaken in an institutional environment. Regardless of their type or location, our approach to these lesions is to examine the lesions endoscopically and then attempt to reestablish normal tracheal gauge by laser resection through a rigid bronchoscope under general anesthesia. A week after this initial session, the patient is reexamined fiberscopically, and, based d on the findings and the patient's condition, a decision about further treatment is made. There are four options: continued endoscopic observation, further laser resection, placement of a Montgomery T-tube, or sleeve resection. The therapeutic strategy may be modified in the light of future developments. In our series we treated 93 cases of genuine tracheal stenosis. In 70 cases the results were good and the patients have been in stable condition for over a year. In 13 cases, follow-up is too short to judge results. Six patients treated in intensive care were lost from view, and the remaining four are dead. One death occurred after surgery and one after removal of a T-tube (Figure 18.4). Miscellaneous indications include removal of suture threads, granulomas on suture threads, management of local bleeding, treatment of bronchial stenosis, and dislodgement of an impacted foreign body. These procedures can

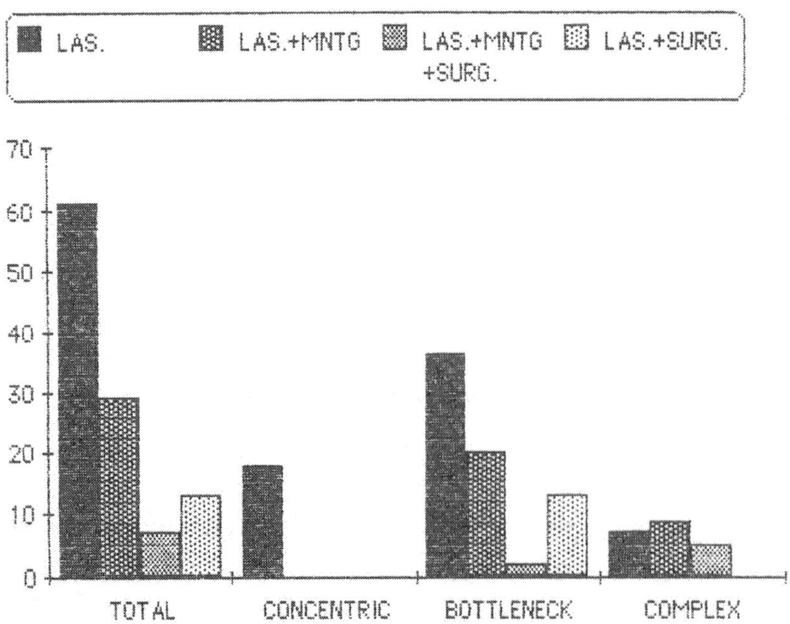

FIGURE 18.4. Therapeutic strategy for trachael stenosis.

usually be carried out with a flexible fiberscope under local anesthesia.

Serious complications have been rare and were always due to anoxia. We do not attempt to distinguish between anesthesia-related and resection-related complications, rather, we consider all problems to result from the technique as a whole. The most frequent incident was hemorrhage, which was always stopped; no death by exsanguination was recorded. We experienced 13 cases of bleeding in excess of 200 cc and 4 in excess of 700 cc. Hypoxemia-related cardiovascular complications also occurred intraoperatively, including 1 cardiac arrest, 3 severe bradycardias, and 1 bronchospasm. All were reversed. The postoperative period is especially dangerous. We recorded 2 deaths during this period: one from cardiac arrest after severe bradycardia two days after laser resection of a tumor in the right main stem bonchus of a patient with mediastinal and pericardial tumor, and one from respiratory arrest in an 82-year-old woman one day after removal of a Montgomery T-tube. We also recorded 2 cases of mediastinal emphysema and 2 cases of transient pneumothorax.

Conclusion

After 6+ years of use, the indications and protocol for endoscopic Nd:YAG laser resection are now well-defined. Considering the very serious condition of most of the patients treated, complications are rare and results often spectacular. This new modality constitutes an important advance in the field of pneumology.

19
Neurosurgical Applications of Laser Technology

William D. Tobler and John M. Tew, Jr.

It has now been a decade since lasers for neurosurgical applications have been widely available. Since then, the carbon dioxide and Nd:YAG lasers have gained a firm position in clinical neurosurgery. The carbon dioxide laser is more widely employed than the Nd:YAG laser and is used primarily as an ablative instrument for benign extraaxial tumors, usually at the base of the brain, or in the spinal canal. The Nd:YAG laser functions primarily as a coagulative instrument, to shrink and coagulate vascular tumors and vascular malformations. At the University of Cincinnati Medical Center our combined laser experience approaches 700 cases, beginning with the carbon dioxide laser first used in late 1981.

The development of the quantum theory paved the way for Einstein's landmark paper in 1917 entitled "Zur Quantum Theorie der Strahlung," which detailed the principles for stimulated emission of photons.[1] Bascow and Prokehnov further contributed to an understanding of stimulated emission. The first molecular oscillator or maser (microwave amplification by the stimulated emission of radiation) was produced by Gordon in 1954.[2] The 1958 paper by Schawlow and Townes, "Infrared and Optical Masers," described the structure and function of a laser, but it was Theodore Maiman who was credited with producing the first laser light in July of 1960 from a ruby crystal.

Early Neurosurgical Applications of Lasers

Most early efforts of pioneering neurosurgeons were directed toward describing the ablative effects of laser radiation.[3,4] The ruby laser, applied in a pulsed mode to experimental animals, produced cerebral contusions, subdural hemorrhage, and often death. Direct radiation of cortical surfaces of cats with ruby lasers showed various degrees of tissue destruction and in-depth reports of the histologic detail were provided.[5–8]

Stellar and colleagues[9] demonstrated the precise cutting and vaporization effects of the laser in 1968. In experimental tumors in mice, the carbon dioxide laser was shown to coagulate and vaporize entire masses of tumor. Histologic evaluation of experimental lesions consistently showed three zones of injury: (1) an inner charred layer; (2) a middle zone of desiccation, and (3) an outer layer of edema (Figure 19.1). In 1970, Stellar and collegues[9] reported the first human neurosurgical application of the carbon dioxide laser to partially vaporize a glioblastoma.

Development of the Carbon Dioxide Laser

The present era of laser neurosurgery began in 1976. The development of portable laser units that could easily be transported into the operating room enabled surgeons to develop and apply laser technology to clinical practice. Ascher[10–12] first used the laser in Austria to remove a brain tumor in 1976, and since then has accumulated an experience of greater than 1000 cases. Simultaneous reports of precise tissue effects and histologic studies of laser effects began to appear.

Shortly thereafter, neurosurgeons began to use the carbon dioxide laser in the United States. With improving technology and the recognition of significant benefits of laser application, the

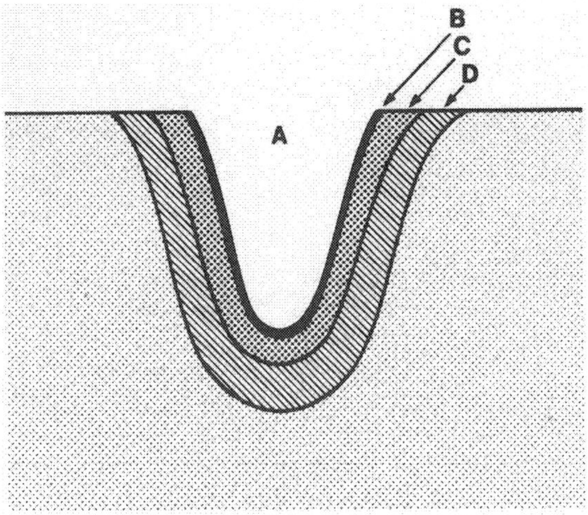

FIGURE 19.1. *A:* Morphology of layers of tissue injury after exposure to a pulse of carbon dioxide laser energy; *B:* char, 20–50 μm; *C:* middle layer desiccation, 100 μm; *D:* outer edema, 100 μm.

use of carbon dioxide lasers has become widespread in the United States. Training programs to familiarize the surgeon with the features and advantages as well as the safety aspects of laser surgery have become requisite.[13]

Encouraging reports of the efficacy of carbon dioxide laser techniques of vaporizing meningiomas, acoustic neuromas, and other tumors have appeared.[14–24] The carbon dioxide laser has become a standard part of the armamentarium of the neurosurgeon of the 1980s. It is used primarily as an ablative tool and, adapted to the microscope, becomes a precision microsurgical instrument. The area of greatest impact in laser microsurgery is the removal of basal, intraventricular, and spinal tumors.

Development of the Nd:YAG Laser

Development of the Nd:YAG laser for biomedical applications began in the late 1960s. The first clinical neurosurgical application was reported by Beck in 1976.[25] The deeper tissue scatter effect and its preferential pigment absorption provided neurosurgeons with a potent coagulation laser.[26] Initial clinical reports have shown the Nd:YAG laser to be effective for vascularized tumors such as meningiomas, hemangioblastomas, and chordomas.[27,28] More recently, attention has turned toward the application of the Nd:YAG laser for shrinking and coagulating arteriovenous malformations. Reports by Fasano and co-workers[29,30] Wharen and Sundt,[31] and recently by Tew and Tobler[32,33] indicate its usefulness, but there is not total consensus about its applicability to vascular malformations. Recent approval by the Food and Drug Administration now enables any trained neurosurgeon to use the Nd:YAG laser in the United States for coagulation of tumors and vascular malformations.

The Argon Laser

The argon laser has a minor but interesting role in neurosurgery. Edwards and his group[34,35] Powers and his associates[36] have reported the only significant neurosurgical experience with the argon laser to date. It has not gained widespread use because of the relatively low powers, making it inefficient as an ablative instrument. The production of dorsal root entry zone (DREZ) lesions has been reported with argon as well as with carbon dioxide laser.[36–38] Unless a more powerful argon system is developed, widespread use of this laser in neurosurgery is not likely.

Clinical Applications of Lasers

A consensus continues to evolve about the relative indications of laser for brain and spinal cord tumors. The following summary indicates our current opinions. We believe that the laser is absolutely indicated in basal tumors, including meningiomas, acoustic neuromas, chordomas, and para- and suprasellar tumors. The carbon dioxide laser is uniquely suited to remove very firm tumors that would require significant manipulation for removal by other techniques. Densely calcified meningiomas most commonly present this type of challenge. The laser is also useful in the removal of previously radiated, fibrotic pituitary tumors. The carbon dioxide laser, because of its precision, is indicated in the removal of all spinal cord tumors, especially intramedullary, intradural, and foramen magnum region tumors. The Nd:YAG laser is indicated for the removal of vascular tumors, such as glomus tumors, hemangioblastomas, and angioblastic meningiomas.

Relative indications for the carbon dioxide and the Nd:YAG laser are pituitary tumors. Hemostasis by coagulation of the dura by both lasers can be accomplished, but more easily with the Nd:YAG laser. In many cases, the laser facilitates intrasellar tumor removal, but a high level of concern for potential injury to surrounding arteries and nerves is critical. In any patient where blood loss is a factor because of medical condition or religious beliefs, the laser may be of significant benefit. There is no indication for the use of the laser in the excision of superficial, nonvascular tumors. However, the inexperienced surgeon may first develop his laser skills with these less critical cases.

The following case summaries represent categories where we find the laser to be indispensable. The discussions further emphasize the salient features of laser application.

Clinical Applications of the Carbon Dioxide Laser

A 60-year-old surgeon was found to have a large, densely calcified, left sphenoid wing meningioma (Figure 19.2). The surface of the tumor was easily exposed but very firm. Without any tugging or pulling, the tumor was vaporized in a noncontact technique. The central portion of this tumor was rock-hard and the lesion could not have been removed safely by mechanical force. The powerful carbon dioxide laser gently vaporized this tumor and its origin along the medial sphenoid wing and cavernous sinus. Postoperative computed tomography (CT) demonstrates complete removal of the lesion (Figure 19.2). The patient was neurologically intact postoperatively, and there is no evidence of recurrence four years later.

A 32-year-old woman with headaches was found to have a posterior fossa meningioma arising from and attached to the critical left transverse sinus (Figure 19.3). The dural attachment of the tumor at the juncture of the vein of Labbe and transverse sinus could not be removed, but the carbon dioxide laser enabled vaporization of the tumor origin at this critical vascular juncture.

A 69-year-old woman presented with numbness of the right hand, mistakenly diagnosed as carpal tunnel syndrome, was found to have an intraspinal mass at C1 placed anteriorly, causing posterior displacement of the spinal cord (Figure 19.4). This inaccessible lesion was exposed posteriorly and vaporized with a focused carbon dioxide laser beam. The noncontact, no-instru-

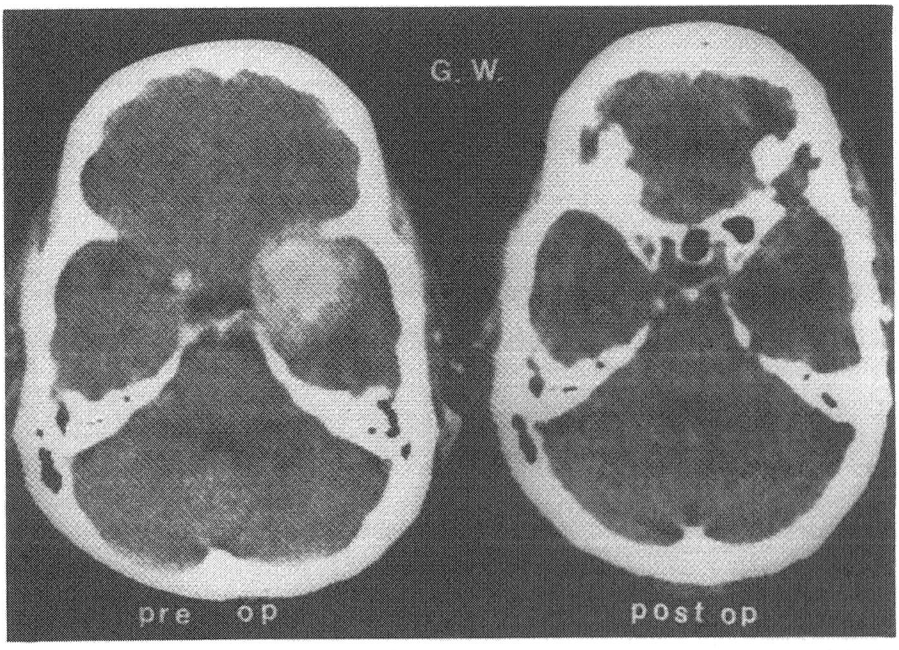

FIGURE 19.2. Heavily calcified left sphenoid wing meningioma. Tumor excision was facilitated with the carbon dioxide laser.

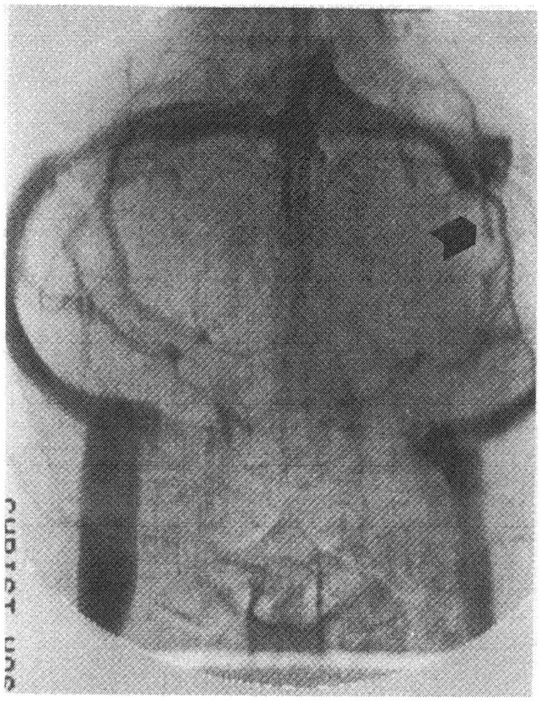

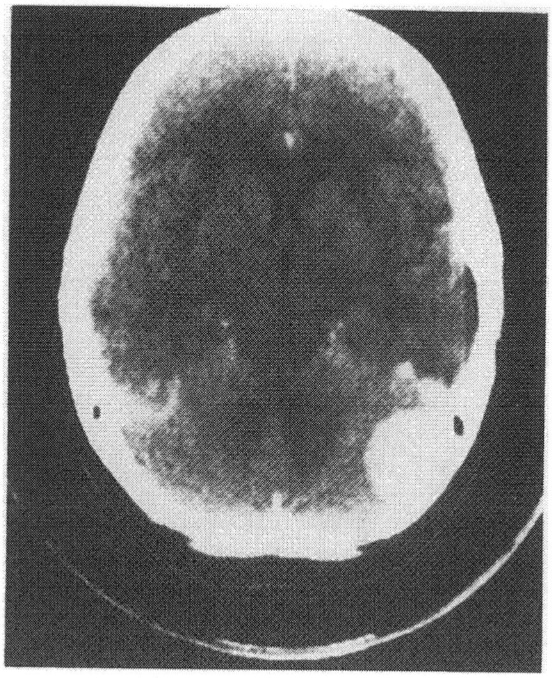

FIGURE 19.3. Posterior fossa meningioma attached to and obliterating a segment of the transverse sinus (*arrow*).

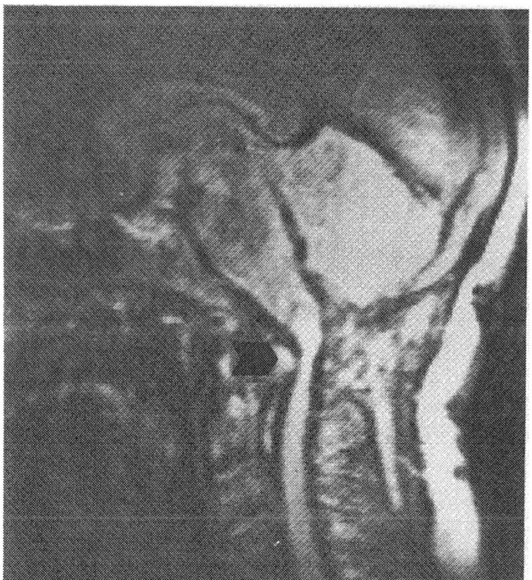

FIGURE 19.4. Magnetic resonance imaging (MRI) scan shows discrete lesion (chordoma) anterior to and displacing the spinal cord at C1.

mentation technique of laser technology permitted total removal of this chordoma through an exposure of less than 5 mm, with neurologic function spared.

Surgical removal of acoustic neuromas is one of the major applications of laser technology. Rapid debulking can be achieved without traction or transmission of heat to surrounding nerves, arteries, or the brainstem. Electrical interference with evoked potential monitoring is eliminated and delicate dissection of the tumor capsule from critical structures can be achieved with ease. Many of our acoustic patients have been operated on because the referring surgeon was unable to totally remove the residual capsule from the brainstem.

This 29-year-old man with von Recklinghausen's disease has had two subtotal resections of a right-sided acoustic neuroma with rapid recurrence (Figure 19.5). He also had a smaller left acoustic neuroma. Total excision of the tumor, especially the adherent portion attached to the brainstem, was achieved (Figure 19.5). Careful nontraumatic dissection and vaporization can be accomplished with the carbon dioxide laser. Routine monitoring of brainstem

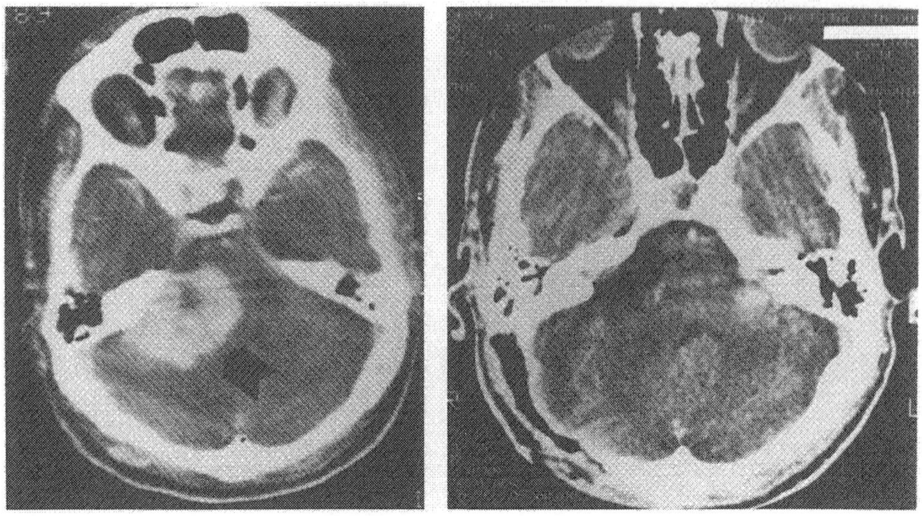

FIGURE 19.5. Pre- and postoperative scans of a patient with bilateral acoustic neuromas. The right-sided lesion was removed (*arrow*).

evoked potentials and facial nerve function has remarkably aided our ability to preserve neurologic integrity.

In 30 patients, we used a transcallosal approach to gain access to intraventricular tumors and vascular malformations. The laser is effective for incising the corpus callosum and improving access deep in the third ventricle because of the elimination of instrumentation. We are able to limit the opening of the corpus cal-

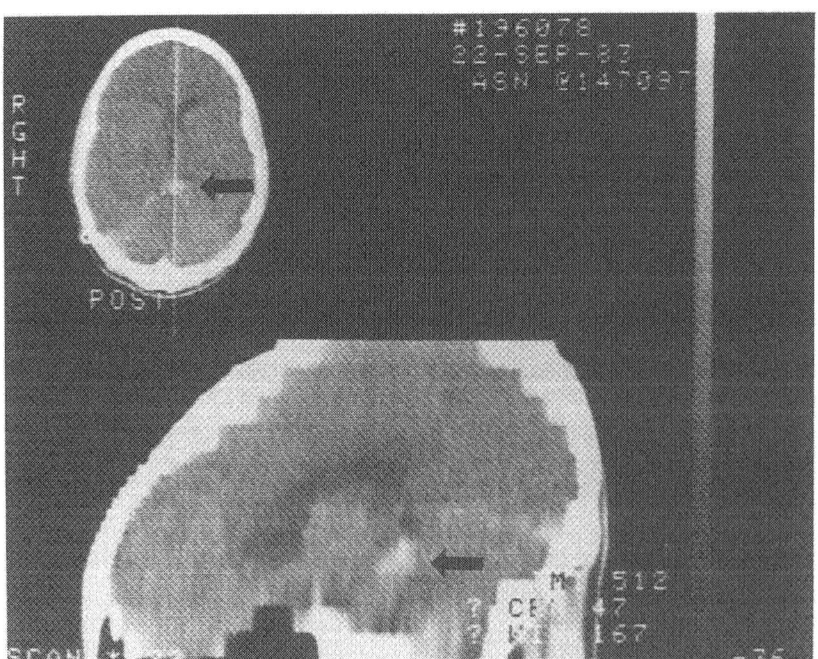

FIGURE 19.6. Hamartoma of the posterior thalamus pulvinar region excised by means of a transcallosal approach and carbon dioxide laser vaporization.

losum to no more than 2.0 cm to avoid disconnection symptoms.[39,40] Both the Nd:YAG and the carbon dioxide lasers are useful for removing these deeply placed lesions.

A 25-year-old male with headaches and hemisensory deficit was found to have an enhancing tumor in the left pulvinar region of the thalamus (Figure 19.6). At surgery this tumor was effectively and completely vaporized through a posterior transcallosal approach. The patient exhibited a temporary, partial visual disconnection syndrome, and improvement in his preoperative symptoms.

Clinical Applications of the Nd:YAG Laser

At our institution we began to use the Nd:YAG laser for clinical applications in late 1984. To date, we have treated 25 cases: 8 tumors and 17 arteriovenous malformations. Understandably, the range of applicability for the Nd:YAG laser is not as great as for the carbon dioxide laser in neurologic surgery. General availability of the Nd:YAG laser will permit the accumulation and evaluation of a larger experience in brain tumor and arteriovenous malformation surgery.

Brain Tumors Treated with Nd:YAG Laser

Although the Nd:YAG laser is not used as frequently as the carbon dioxide laser, it is an instrument of unique capabilities for a neurosurgeon. Specifically, its potent coagulative capabilities permit the removal of highly vascularized tumors, minimizing blood loss.

Hemangioblastomas are highly vascularized tumors associated with a very high operative mortality because of their vascularity. The chances of safe removal of this, fortunately, rare tumor can be increased with the Nd:YAG laser. Such a tumor was found in a 57-year-old woman with headaches and ataxia. A solid hemangio-

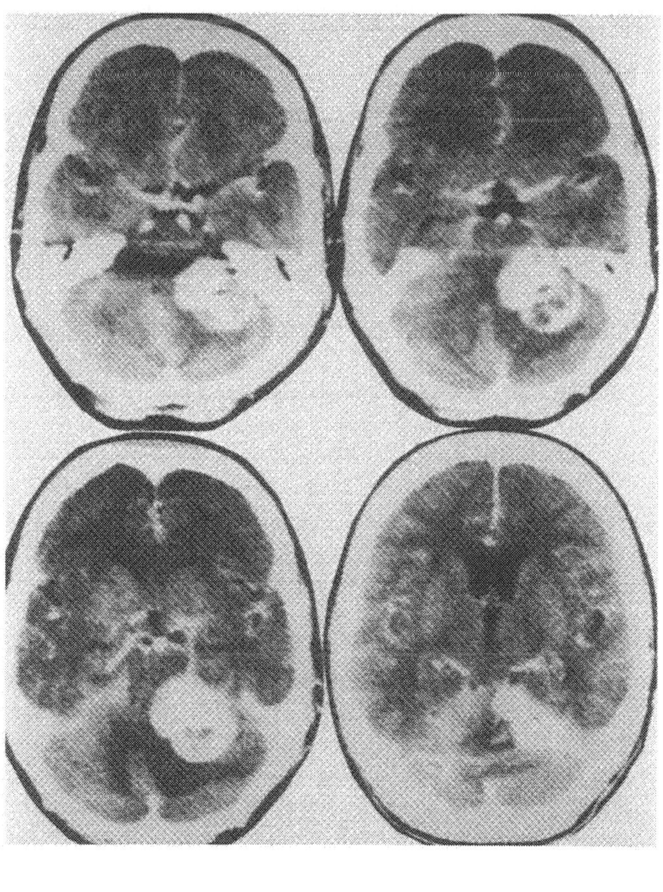

FIGURE 19.7. Densely enhancing solid hemangioblastoma of the posterior fossa removed with the Nd:YAG laser.

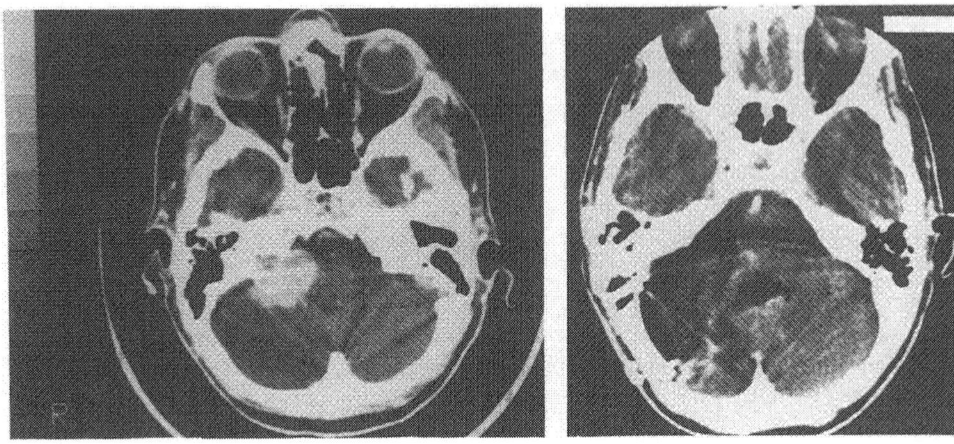

FIGURE 19.8. Glomus jugulare tumor growing through the base of the brain into the posterior fossa, coagulated with the Nd:YAG laser. Postoperative view on the right.

blastoma was found in the left cerebellar hemisphere (Figure 19.7). At surgery, this tumor was beefy-red and bled profusely when palpated with a dissector. The tumor was coagulated with the Nd:YAG laser, then vaporized with the carbon dioxide laser in alternating fashion until complete removal was obtained. The hemostasis provided by the Nd:YAG laser was excellent and enabled vaporization to be carried out rapidly, in a dry field. This case also demonstrates the limitation of the carbon dioxide laser as a coagulative instrument.

The addition of the Nd:YAG laser to the neurosurgeon's armamentarium will likely lead to dramatic improvements in the morbidity and mortality of this classification of tumor.

Glomus jugulare tumors are highly vascular and infiltrate the skull base. This tumor is ideally suited for the Nd:YAG laser. Like the hemangioblastoma, this is a rarely encountered lesion.

A 57-year-old woman underwent a posterior fossa craniectomy and biopsy of a glomus tumor in 1959, but surgical excision was not attempted. In January 1984, she presented with progressive headaches and loss of facial sensation. Computed tomography (CT) disclosed a large cerebellopontine angle tumor (Figure 19.8). Preoperatively, the patient underwent particulate embolization of the tumor, which significantly decreased blood flow to the tumor. At surgery, the Nd:YAG laser coagulated the tumor, and in a nearly dry field it was vaporized with the carbon dioxide laser for total excision.

Arteriovenous Malformations Treated with the Nd:YAG Laser

Reports concerning the clinical effectiveness of the Nd:YAG laser for coagulation and induction of hemostasis associated with vascular tumors,[41,42] aneurysms,[43] and arteriovenous malformations (AVMs)[43–45] have varied from enthusiastic to disappointing. Blood selectively absorbs the energy emitted by this laser wavelength, and obliteration of vessels can be effectively induced without imparting substantive damage to adjacent brain tissue. Because the operative removal of AVMs of the brain, and particularly those arising from the central core, remains one of neurosurgery's major unresolved technical challenges, we have directed our efforts toward technical developments of the Nd:YAG laser as a mode of therapy. We agree with Wharen and colleagues[45] that refinements are necessary. However, our experience in a substantial number of cases of complex AVMs confirms the safety of the device and indicates that it can be of inestimable benefit in the surgical extirpation of some malformations.

The Nd:YAG laser was first used at our institution in February 1984, and we have treated a total of 17 AVMs with this laser. The following summaries represent our more challenging cases.

A 27-year-old woman with headaches and temporal lobe seizures had a large temporal-Sylvian arteriovenous malformation. The nidus

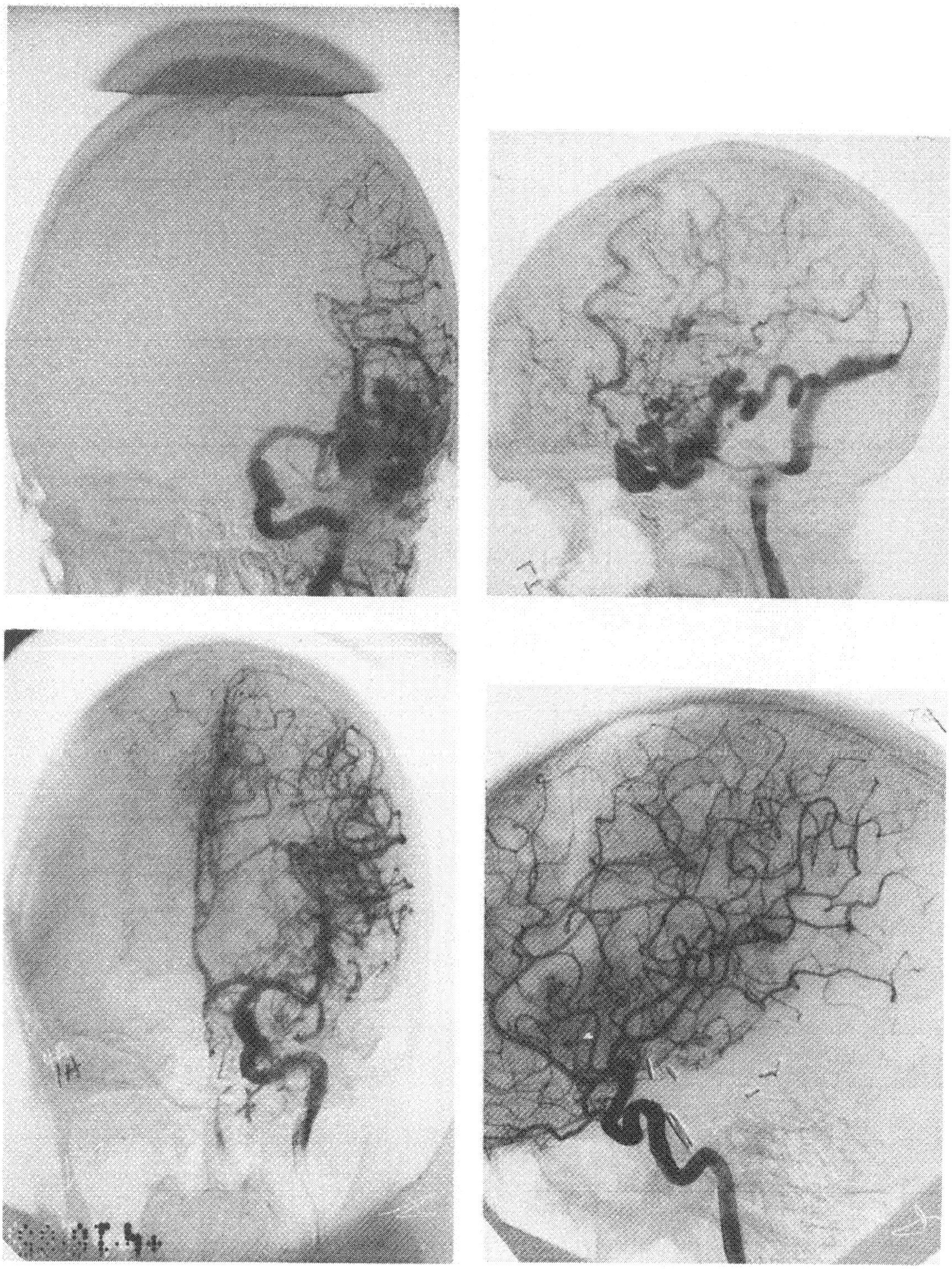

FIGURE 19.9. Dominant temporal lobe arteriovenous malformation vaporized with the Nd:YAG laser. (*Top*) Preoperative views. (*Bottom*) Postoperative views.

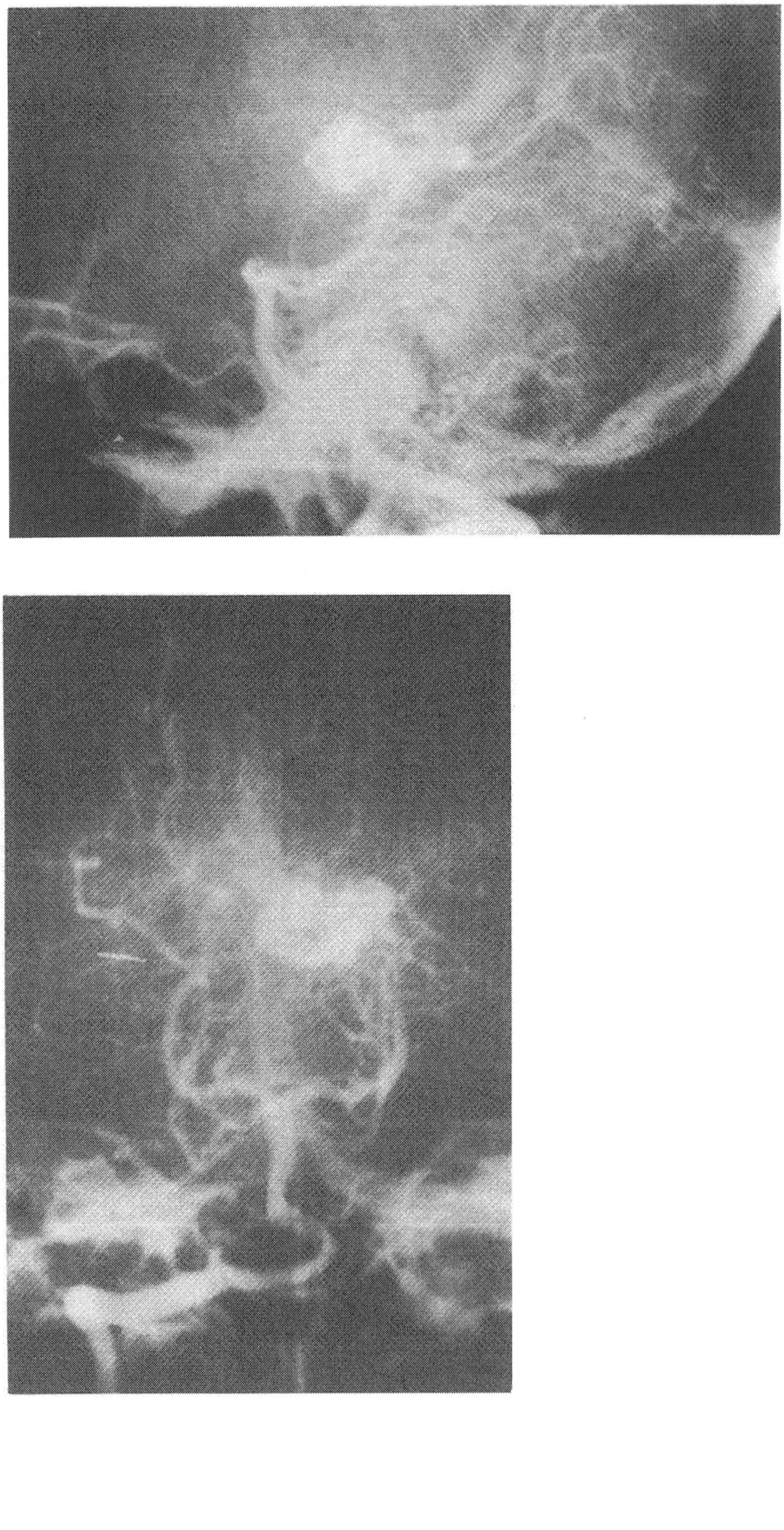

FIGURE 19.10. Left thalamic arteriovenous malformation fed by deep thalamoperforate and posterior cerebral artery branches.

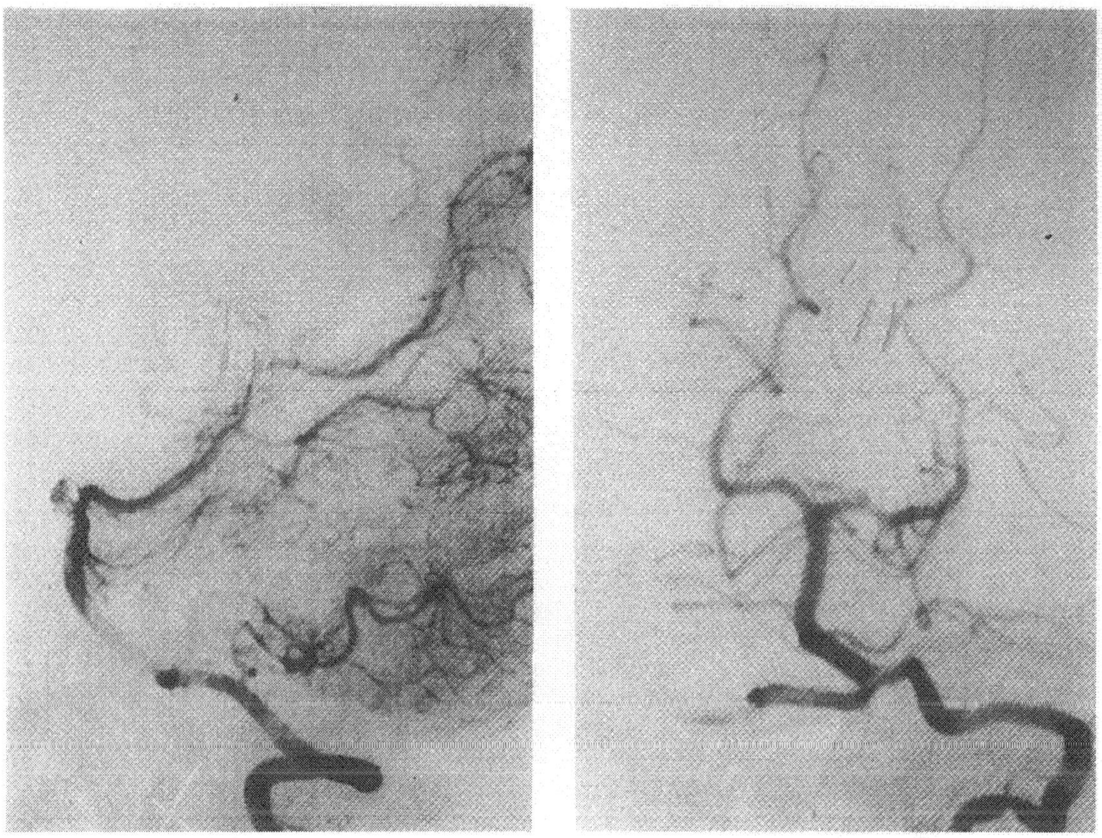

FIGURE 19.10. (*continued*) Postoperative angiogram.

of the malformation was treated with the Nd:YAG laser to reduce its bulk. Complete dissection and excision of the AVM was accomplished with a combination of bipolar and Nd:YAG energy (Figure 19.9). The patient made an excellent recovery with no detectable speech deficit. This experience demonstrated the capacity of the laser to effectively coagulate dural vessels and radically reduce the flow in a large malformation located adjacent to eloquent brain.

A 33-year-old female presented with sudden onset of a severe headache and a left intracerebral hematoma. Angiography confirmed a left thalamic AVM whose primary feeding branches were the thalamoperforate and posterior choroidal branches of the left posterior cerebral artery (Figure 19.10). Neurologic examination was normal except for athetoid movements of the right upper extremity.

The patient underwent a left parietal craniotomy and transcallosal approach to the left lateral ventricle. The left thalamus was entered, and the hematoma cavity was evacuated. The arteriovenous malformation was identified, and its vessels were coagulated with Nd:YAG laser energy. Some large feeders required bipolar coagulation and application of a surgical clip. A second-stage procedure was necessary to totally excise a few residual vessels of the AVM. The patient had no residual motor dysfunction, but did have short-term memory loss, which was temporary.

The last case chosen for illustration is a 48-year-old man who presented with intracerebral hemorrhage. His arteriovenous malformation was in the right posterior thalamus (Figure 19.11). At surgery, the nidus was coagulated with the Nd:YAG laser, and total excision was achieved (Figure 19.11). The patient's hemiparesis gradually resolved.

The Nd:YAG laser is helpful for dissecting the plane between nidus and normal brain, and also for achieving hemostasis in the bed of re-

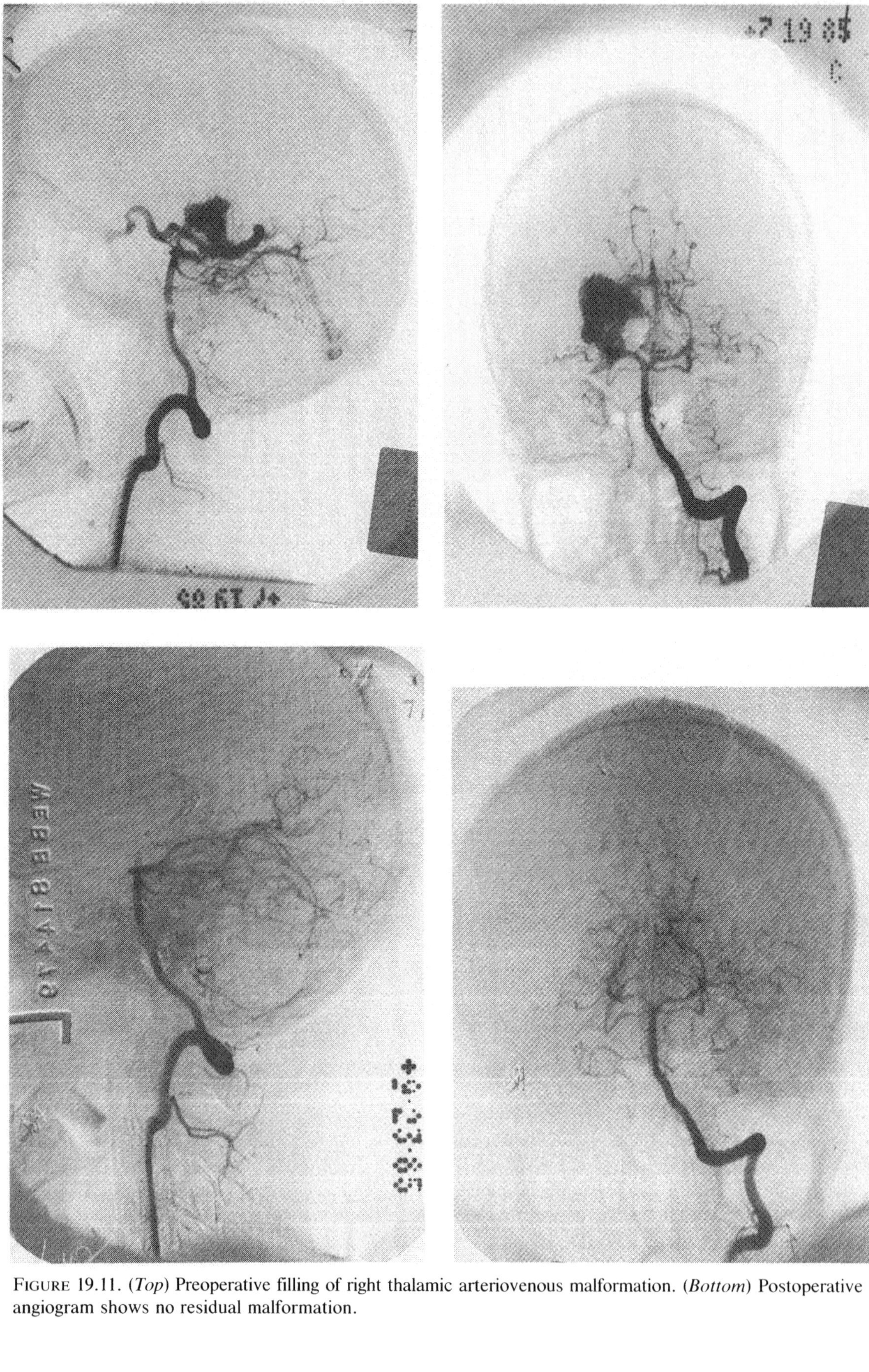

FIGURE 19.11. (*Top*) Preoperative filling of right thalamic arteriovenous malformation. (*Bottom*) Postoperative angiogram shows no residual malformation.

section. More importantly, direct radiation of the AVM nidus causes shrinkage of the AVM and reduces the blood flow through it. Heating of the radiated vessels causes contraction of the collagen fibers and results in narrowing of the vessel lumen. Often, however, high flow through a vessel reduces the heating effect on the vessel lumen, and results in failure to achieve shrinkage or thrombosis of the vessel. Therefore, it may not be possible to coagulate and occlude the end of a bleeding vessel with the Nd:YAG laser. High flow prevents the Nd:YAG laser from shrinking and totally occluding most AVMs with a noncontact technique. Bipolar cautery is still an important instrument for achieving control of high-flow vessels.

The development of a precise micromanipulator for the surgical microscope has greatly facilitated the precision of application. The spot size can be accurately controlled and the laser beam precisely directed under direct vision without the interposition of vision-obstructing handpieces. The application of microlaser techniques has improved results in deep-seated malformations of the ventricles, thalamus, and brainstem where direct approach with standard techniques is unusually difficult.

We are encouraged by our experiences with the technique of coagulation occlusion of arteriovenous malformations. Study of the histologic and physiologic consequences of Nd:YAG energy in neurosurgical applications continues. Development of new micromanipulators for combined CO_2 and Nd:YAG fibers is needed, and endoscopic techniques for Nd:YAG applications hold promise for future development in neurosurgery.

Great caution must be exercised in the use of the Nd:YAG laser, especially at the base of the brain in close proximity to critical vascular and neurologic structures, particularly the brainstem and cranial nerves. The scatter effect of this laser can cause irreversible injury to the nearby structures by heat transmission. In contrast, the CO_2 laser energy is virtually entirely absorbed on the surface.

We concur with the reports of others that the unique features of the Nd:YAG laser will ensure its future use in the treatment of brain tumors. These two lasers, the Nd:YAG and carbon dioxide, have become important tools for the neurosurgeon.

References

1. Einstein A: Zur Quantum Theorie der Strahlung. Phys Z 18:121–128, 1917.
2. Hecht J, Teresi D: Laser, Super Tool of the 1980s. Ticknor & Fields, New York, 1982.
3. Lambert PW, Fox JL, Earle KM: Cerebral edema after laser radiation. An electron microscopic study. J Neuropathol Exp Neurol 25:531–541, 1966.
4. Rosomoff HL, Carroll F: Reaction of neoplasm and brain to laser. Arch Neurol 14(2):143–148, 1966.
5. Fox JL: The use of laser radiation as a surgical "light-knife." J Surg Res 9:199–205, 1969.
6. Fox JL, Hayes JR, Stein MN, et al: Experimental cranial and vascular studies of the effects of pulsed and continuous wave laser radiation. J Neurosurg 27:126–137, 1967.
7. Fox JL, et al: Lasers and their neurosurgical application. Milit Med 131:493–498, 1966.
8. Liss L, Roppel R: Histopathology of laser-produced lesions in cat brains. Neurology 16:783–790, 1966.
9. Stellar S, Polanyi TG, Bredemeier HC: Experimental studies with the carbon dioxide laser as a neurosurgical instrument. Med Biol Eng 8:549–558, 1970.
10. Ascher PW, Heppner F: CO_2-laser in neurosurgery. Neurosurg Rev 7:123–133, 1984.
11. Ascher PW: The CO_2 laser in neurosurgery. Fortschr Med 98:253–254, 1980.
12. Ascher PW: Newest ultrastructural findings after the use of a CO_2 laser on CNS tissue. Acta Neurochir Suppl (Wien) 28:572–581, 1979.
13. Brown JT, Cerullo LJ: Laser workshops in neurological surgery. Lasers Surg Med 4:241–246, 1984.
14. Bartal AD, Heilbronn VD, Avram J, et al: Carbon dioxide laser surgery of basal meningiomas. Surg Neurol 17:90–95, 1982.
15. Gong-bai C: Laser vaporization on intracranial tumors. Lasers Surg Med 1:235–240, 1981.
16. Hara M, et al: Evaluation of laser surgery against brain tumor (Japan). No Shinkei Geka 8:363–369, 1980.
17. Hudgins R, Moody J, Sanders M, et al: Microsurgical laser vaporization of inaccessible tumors of the central nervous system. Dallas Med J 76:245–250, 1981.
18. James HE, Williams J, Brock W, et al: Radical removal of lipomas of the conus and cauda equina with laser microsurgery. Neurosurgery 15(3):340–343, 1984.
19. Mattos Pimenta LH, Mattos Pimenta A, Martins JL: The use of the CO_2 laser for the removal of

awkwardly situated meningiomas. Neurosurg Rev 4:53–55, 1981.
20. Robertson JH, Clark WC, Robertson JT, et al: Use of the carbon dioxide laser for acoustic tumor surgery. Neurosurgery 12:286–290, 1983.
21. Sawaya R, Hawley DK, Tobler WD, et al: Pineal and third ventricle tumors. In Youmans J (ed): Neurological Surgery, 3rd ed.
22. Takizawa T: The carbon dioxide laser surgical unit as an instrument for surgery of brain tumours—Its advantages and disadvantages. Neurosurg Rev 7:135–144, 1984.
23. Tew JM Jr, Tobler WD: The laser: History, biophysics, and neurosurgical applications. Clinical Neurosurg 31:506–549, 1984.
24. Tobler WD, Sawaya R, Tew JM Jr: Successful laser-assisted excision of a metastatic midbrain tumor. Neurosurgery 18(6):795–797, 1986.
25. Beck OJ: Use of the Nd:YAG laser in neurosurgery. Neurosurg Rev 7:151–158, 1984.
26. Beck OJ, Wilske J, Schoenberger J: Tissue changes following application of lasers to the rabbit brain. Neurosurg Rev 1:31–36, 1979.
27. Beck OJ: The use of the Nd:YAG and CO_2 laser in neurosurgery. Neurosurg Rev 3:261–266, 1980.
28. Handa H, Takeuchi J, Tamagami T: Nd:YAG laser as a surgical tool. Neurosurg Rev 7:159–163, 1984.
29. Fasano VA, Urciuoli R, Ponzio M: Photocoagulation of cerebral arteriovenous malformations and arterial aneurysms with the neodymium: yttrium-aluminum-garnet or argon laser: Preliminary results in twelve patients. Neurosurgery 11:754–760, 1982.
30. Fasano VA: The treatment of vascular malformation of the brain with laser source. Lasers Surg Med 1:347–356, 1981.
31. Wharen RE, Anderson RE, Sundt TM: The Nd:YAG laser in neurosurgery. Part 2: Clinical studies: An adjunctive measure hemostasis in resection of arteriovenous malformations. J Neurosurg 60:540–547, 1984.
32. Tew JM Jr, Tobler WD: Present status of lasers in neurosurgery. Adv Tech Stand Neurosurg Vol. 13, pp 1–36, 1986.
33. Tew JM Jr, Tobler WD, Zuccarello M: The treatment of arteriovenous malformations of the brain with the neodymium:YAG laser. Adv Tech Stand Neurosurg Vol. 14 (in press) 1988
34. Edwards MSB, Boggan JE: Argon laser surgery of pediatric neural neoplasms. Child Brain 11:171–175, 1984.
35. Edwards MSB, Boggan JE, Fuller TA: The laser in neurological surgery. J Neurosurg 59:555–566, 1983.
36. Powers SK, Adams JE, et al: Pain relief from dorsal root entry zone lesions made with argon and carbon dioxide microsurgical lasers. J Neurosurg 61:841–847, 1984.
37. Levy WJ, Gallo C, Watts C: Comparison of laser and radiofrequency dorsal root entry zone lesions in cats. Neurosurgery 16(3):327–330, 1985.
38. Levy WJ, Nutkiewicz A, Ditmore QM, et al: Laser-induced dorsal root entry zone lesions for pain control. Report of three cases. J Neurosurg 59:884–886, 1983.
39. Apuzzo MLJ: Transcallosal interfornical exposure of lesions of the third ventricle. In Schmidek HH, Sweet WH (eds): Operative Neurosurgical Techniques. Grune & Stratton, New York, 1982, pp 585–594.
40. Winston KR, Cavazzuti V, Arkins T: Absence of neurological and behavioral abnormalities after anterior transcallosal operation for third ventricular lesions. Neurosurgery 4:386–393, 1979.
41. Fasano VA: Observations on the use of three laser sources in sequence (CO_2-argon-Nd:YAG) in neurosurgery. Lasers Surg Med 2:199–203, 1983.
42. Takeuchi J, Handa H, Taki W, Yamagami T: The Nd:YAG laser in neurological surgery. Surg Neurol 18(2):140–142, 1982.
43. Fasano VA, Urciuoli R, Ponzio RM: Photocoagulation of cerebral arteriovenous malformations and arterial aneurysms with the neodymium: yttrium-aluminum-garnet or argon laser: Preliminary results in twelve patients. Neurosurgery 11(6):754–760, 1982.
44. Fasano VA: The treatment of vascular malformation of the brain with laser sources. Lasers Surg Med 1:347–356, 1981.
45. Wharen RE Jr, Anderson RE, Sundt TM Jr: The Nd:YAG laser in neurosurgery. Part 2. Clinical studies: An adjunctive measure for hemostasis in resection of arteriovenous malformations. J Neurosurg 60:540–547, 1984.

20
The Use of Contact Lasers (Nd:YAG and Argon) in Neurosurgery: Clinical and Experimental Data

Victor Aldo Fasano

Recent technical improvements have resulted in the introduction of laser contact-delivery systems. These combine the main features of the laser source with the tactile feedback. A new contact laser technique has thus taken its place beside conventional noncontact lasers. The ideal material for contact irradiation should prevent tissue adhesion and combine several properties: physiologic neutrality, hardness, mechanical strength, and low thermal conductivity. The standard surgical laser light transmitter, that is, the single quartz crystal fiber, has proved to have several drawbacks, as far as beam irradiation and damage to the quartz tip are concerned, when used in contact with tissues or blood. Several natural and artificial substances have therefore been investigated.

Daikuzono and Joffe[1] have shown that a single Al_2O_3 artificial sapphire crystal is a good transmitter of the Nd:YAG laser and combines the coagulating properties of the source with cutting capabilities previously offered by the CO_2 laser only. This preliminary work has shown that noncontact irradiation from a noncontact quartz fiber entails backscattering, accounting for 30–40% of the total irradiated power, whereas with a contact probe there is no sideward irradiation and all the power is delivered at the distal end.[1] Because of this feature the sapphire crystal provides the substantial reduction in laser energy required. Even when on low power, the thermal energy is always enough for sharp incision by means of rapid vaporization of tissue. In addition, the beam from a contact probe has greater divergence and provides a concentric circular pattern due to interference attributable to laser light coherence and the conical shape of the probe. This accounts for a more uniform distribution of energy on the target and less extent of the lesion in depth.

In this chapter, the advantages and limits of contact delivery systems in neurosurgery are discussed in the light of personal clinical and experimental results.

Subjects and Methods

All experiments were obtained using a synthetic SLT sapphire contact probe (manufactured by Surgical Laser Technologies Inc., Malvern, PA) attached to a handpiece and connected by a universal metal adapter to the conventional fiberoptic delivery system of commercially available lasers (a Teflon-coated quartz fiber light guide with 0.6 mm diameter).

Experimental Studies

In a first series of experiments the distribution of brain tissue temperature was studied at time of surgery after Nd:YAG laser impact. Power settings were 10 to 30 W (noncontact) and 5 to 20 W (contact). The exposure time was 5 seconds. Iron-constantan thermocouples were placed at variable distances and depths from the target (0.1 to 10 mm). The recording system used for thermal measurements was a Honeywell E 195 LAB/TEST recorder. Successively, the angular distribution of Nd:YAG laser light in a noncontact system (bare fiber) and a contact surgical scalpel (0.6 mm Tip) has been measured.

The dependence of the probe/temperature and corresponding thermal radiated power on the radiated laser power has been studied in order to discriminate the responsibility of a direct thermal diffusion from the probe in the expression of the biologic damage. For the experimentation we used:

1. Thermopile Scientech model 360203 with a maximal resolution of 10 μW and 10 μJ, constant spectral answer in the wavelength range 0.25 to 35 μm.
2. Optics of collection in NaCl.
3. Calibrated filters for the selection in the infrared range. The effects of heating and thermal radiation from the Tip and the bare fiber have been evaluated by a germanium filter, which is able to absorb the Nd:YAG radiation with high transparency for the thermal radiations at the temperature of interest (less than 2000°C).

In a second series, the modifications occurring in perilesional areas, after contact laser radiation with a contact probe, were studied by electron microscopy. The experimentation was performed during neurosurgical procedures on gliomas (10 cases), on meningiomas (7 cases), and on normal brain whenever the surgical approach to the lesion made it necessary to remove peritumoral tissue (8 cases). Irradiation was delivered at a power output of 3–5 W with argon and 15 to 20 W with Nd:YAG for 5 seconds. Thin sections were observed in a Siemens Elmiskop 1A electron microscope.[2]

Series of Cases

Since 1985 we have treated 147 cases: 104 intra-axial lesions (60 subcortical cerebral gliomas, 13 cortical metastases, 7 cerebral abscesses, 1 lymphoma, 1 radionecrosis, 3 ependymomas of the fourth ventricle, 15 cerebellar spongioblastomas, 1 cerebellar hemangioblastoma), and 40 intracranial extracerebral tumors (15 dural endotheliomas, 14 parasagittal meningiomas, 6 sphenoid wing meningiomas, 5 meningiomas in the cerebellar region).

Depending on tissue consistency, powers ranging from 12 to 20 W with Nd:YAG and 2 to 5 W with argon were used. Exposure time was 5 seconds with 2-seconds interval after each pulse; to avoid melting of the tip, probes had to be replaced after three sequential pulses. SLT Contact Laser Probes were used for

1. hemostasis, either on the surface or in cavities (SLT Flat Probe®);
2. cutting poorly vascularized tissues, mainly white matter, using a 0.1-mm SLT Probe® designed for microsurgery (a 0.05-mm diameter probe will be available in the near future); and
3. cutting highly vascularized tissues with a the SLT Frosted Probe®. The beam is emitted both at the probes distal end and along the lateral aspect of the crystal to improve the hemostasis.

Results

Physical Data

From the mathematical evaluation of 75 thermal measurements the thermal increase seems to be governed by the following law:

$$\Delta T = T_0 e - ar,$$

where T_0 and a are two parameters whose values can be deduced by best fitting: we found T_0 = 269°C and a = 0.21 mm-$_1$. The analysis suggests, moreover, that, because of the loss of heat by vaporization, only 37% of the power used produces thermal effects. The law enables us to calculate the radius of the hemisphere in which the tissue temperature after laser impact is a certain value T.

$$r = \ln \frac{[Pt_0/P_0(T - T_1)]}{a},$$

where T_0 and a are known, P_0 is a reference power value: 28 W for noncontact irradiation and 36 W for contact irradiation, P is the power used, and T_1 is the tissue temperature on the surface or in depth.

Figure 20.1 indicates the radius of the hemisphere in millimeters, in which the temperatures of 42°C (threshold of cellular damage), 60°C (tissue coagulation), and 100°C (tissue carbonization) are reached on the assumption that only 37% of the power used produces thermal effects. A comparison of the contact and noncontact delivery systems has demonstrated the following characteristics.

In Nd:YAG laser light transmitted through bare quartz fiber, 80% of the laser power is emitted in a cone-shaped beam of about 12° (Figure 20.2). The power density at the end of the fiber is about 400 W/cm^2 for a laser power

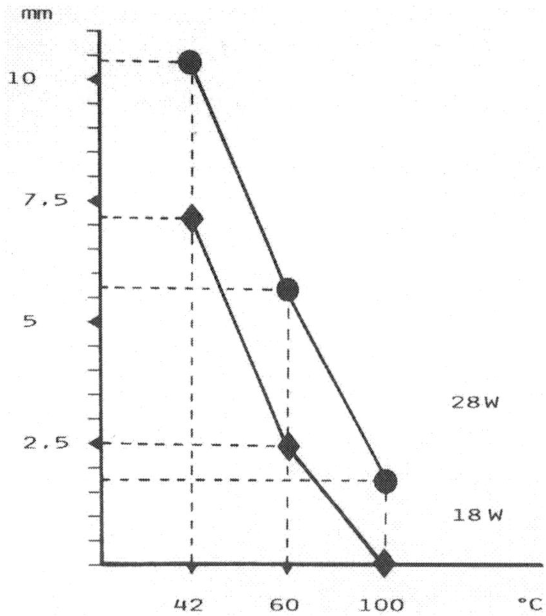

FIGURE 20.1. Thermal diffusion in cerebral tissue. The graph shows the values of the radius in millimeters, in which temperatures of 42, 60, and 100°C are reached, at corresponding powers of 18 and 20 W. ♦, contact Nd:YAG laser; •, noncontact Nd:YAG laser.

of about 13 W. The thermal radiation is not appreciable (less than 1/10,000 of the total laser power).

In Nd:YAG contact delivery systems 80% of the laser power is emitted in a cone-shaped beam of about 90°; the angular distribution shows a peak in the axis and two symmetrical lateral lobes (Figure 20.3). The power density at the Tip is about 2.5 kW/cm^2 for a laser power of about 6.5 W. At a distance of 2 mm from the probe the power density is reduced to 50 W/cm^2, while for the quartz bare fiber at the same distance the power density is unchanged. The thermal radiation power is in the range of 1/1000 of the total laser power. Table 20.1 shows the temperature of the Probe for various levels of the laser power. Values of 1800 K are reached for a laser power of 23.5 W and a 10-second irradiation time.

Histologic Data

The following data apply only to the periphery of the lesion (approximately 1.5 to 3.0 mm away from the center of the lesion). Significant tissue or microvascular lesions were not observed after contact argon irradiation; slight modifications in morphology of the blood-brain barrier and nervous tissue constituents (slight swelling of astrocyte pedicles, small vesicles in the basement

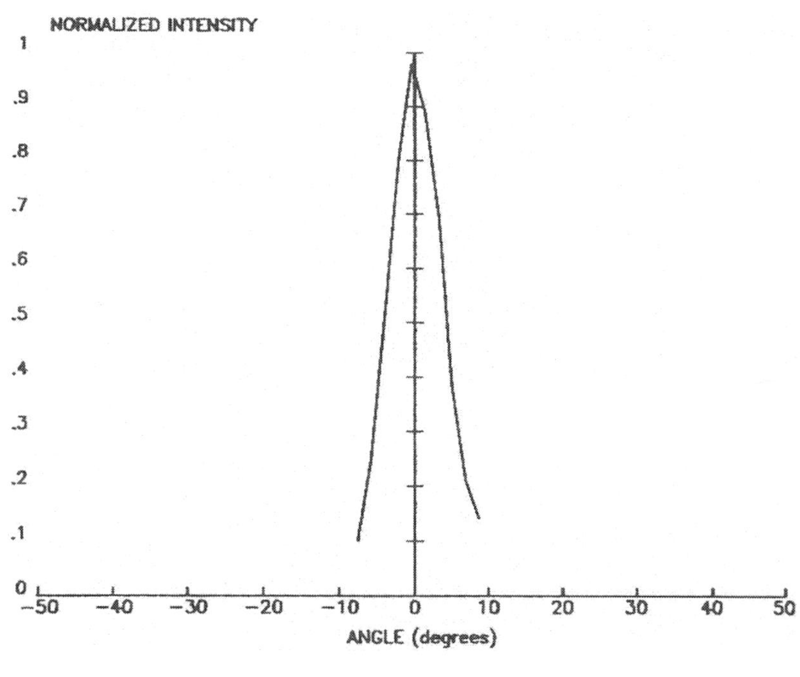

FIGURE 20.2. Angular distribution of Nd:YAG laser light. Noncontact surgical system (bare fiber).

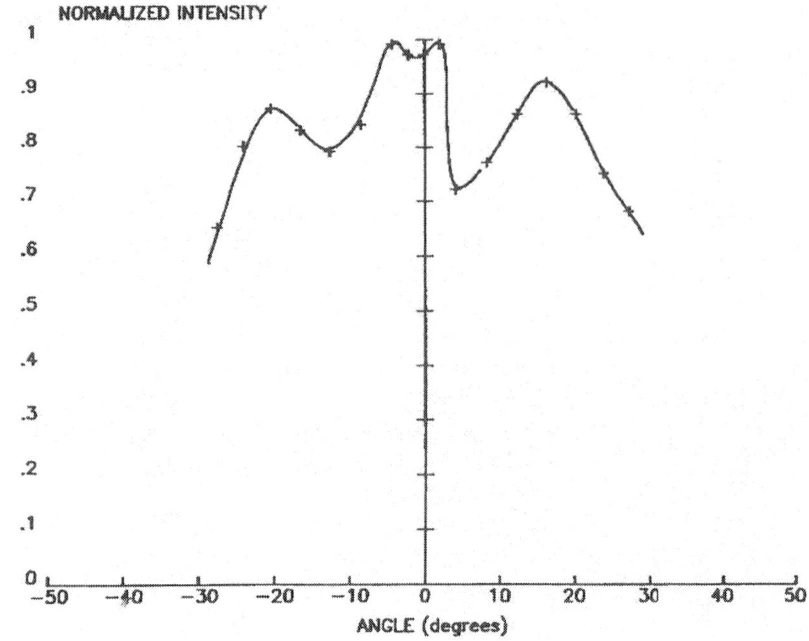

FIGURE 20.3. Angular distribution of Nd:YAG laser light. Contact surgical system (0.6-mm Tip).

membrane) with complete preservation of capillary patency and tissue architecture were detected (Figure 20.4).

Lesions were more severe with the contact Nd:YAG laser. At the blood-brain barrier level, erythrocytes were aggregated, the astrocytes and the endothelial cells were vacuolized and swollen. The structure of the basement membrane was well retained and capillary patency preserved. Neurons and myelin sheaths retained their structure sufficiently well to be fully recognizable (Figure 20.5).

TABLE 20.1. Direct thermal radiation in a Nd:YAG contact surgical system

P-laser (W)	P-thermal (mW)*	Temperature (K)
23.5	21	1800
16.5	15	1650
11	9	1450
8.5	7	1350

Dependence of the tip temperature and corresponding thermal radiated power (P-thermal) on the radiated laser power (P-laser)

Irradiation time: 10 seconds.

*P-thermal is normalized to the same angular aperture of the outcoming laser radiation.

Surgical Results

The procedures used to approach intraaxial lesions (incision of cortex and subcortical layers) and to separate residual infiltrating tumors from surrounding fibrous, neurovascular, and parenchymal deep structures were effective and rapid in all cases, even in the presence of blood or liquids. In the extraaxial tumors the dissection of the arachnoid was performed with conventional instruments, and then the tumor was dissociated from the surrounding healthy structures with a contact laser with good results in all cases treated. In tumors adjoining nerves or important vessels, the neurovascular structures involved were always preserved. The base of tumor implant on falx, tentorium, and durk is easily resected.

Maneuvers were difficult in hard, heavily calcified tissues (separation of thick abscessed capsula from marked perilesional gliosis; incision of calcified meningiomatous capsulae) and in procedures on grey matter because of the diffuse bleeding; this maneuver, however, has been highly improved by the use of the SLT Frosted Probe. Cutting the arachnoid is ineffective. Hemostasis has been often insufficient in tumors fed by arteries larger than 1 mm and in the presence of bleeding vessels. Another disadvantage is the frequent rupture of the contact probe,

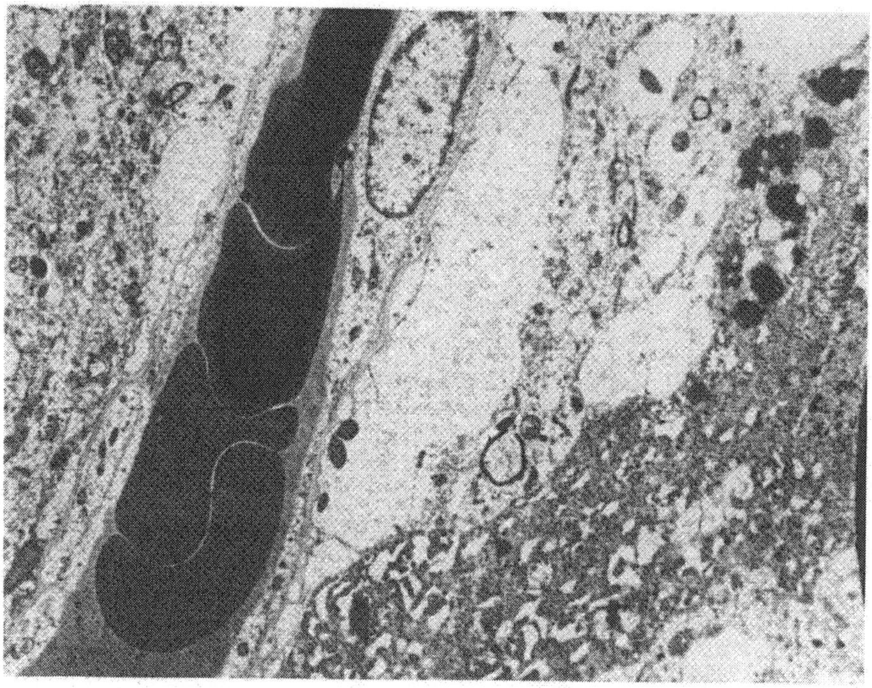

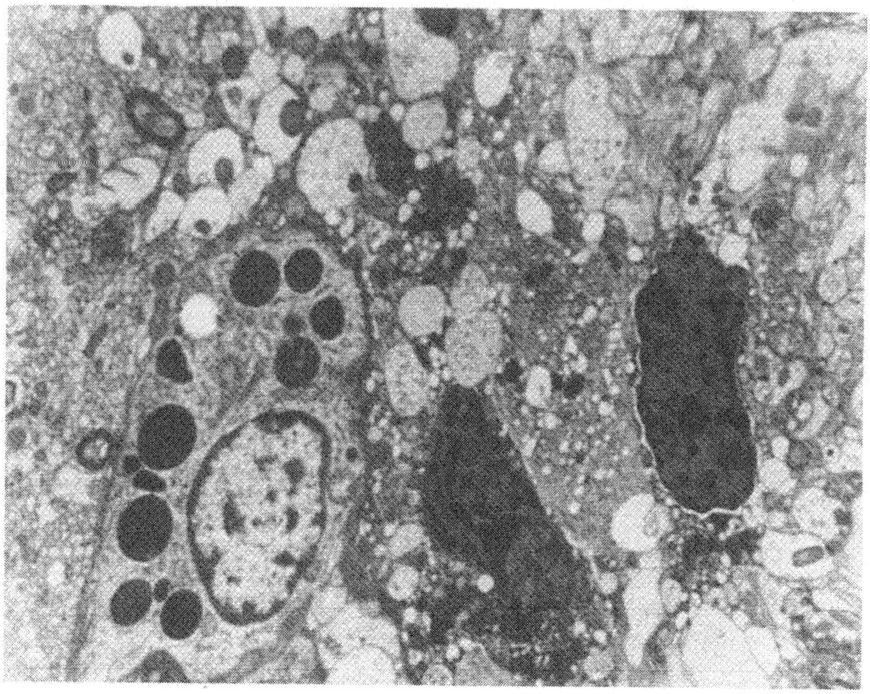

FIGURE 20.4. (*Top*) Cerebral capillary after contact irradiation with argon laser. Slight swelling of astrocyte pedicles; vesicles into the basement membrane. (*Bottom*) Cerebral tissue after contact irradiation with argon laser. No important morphologic changes.

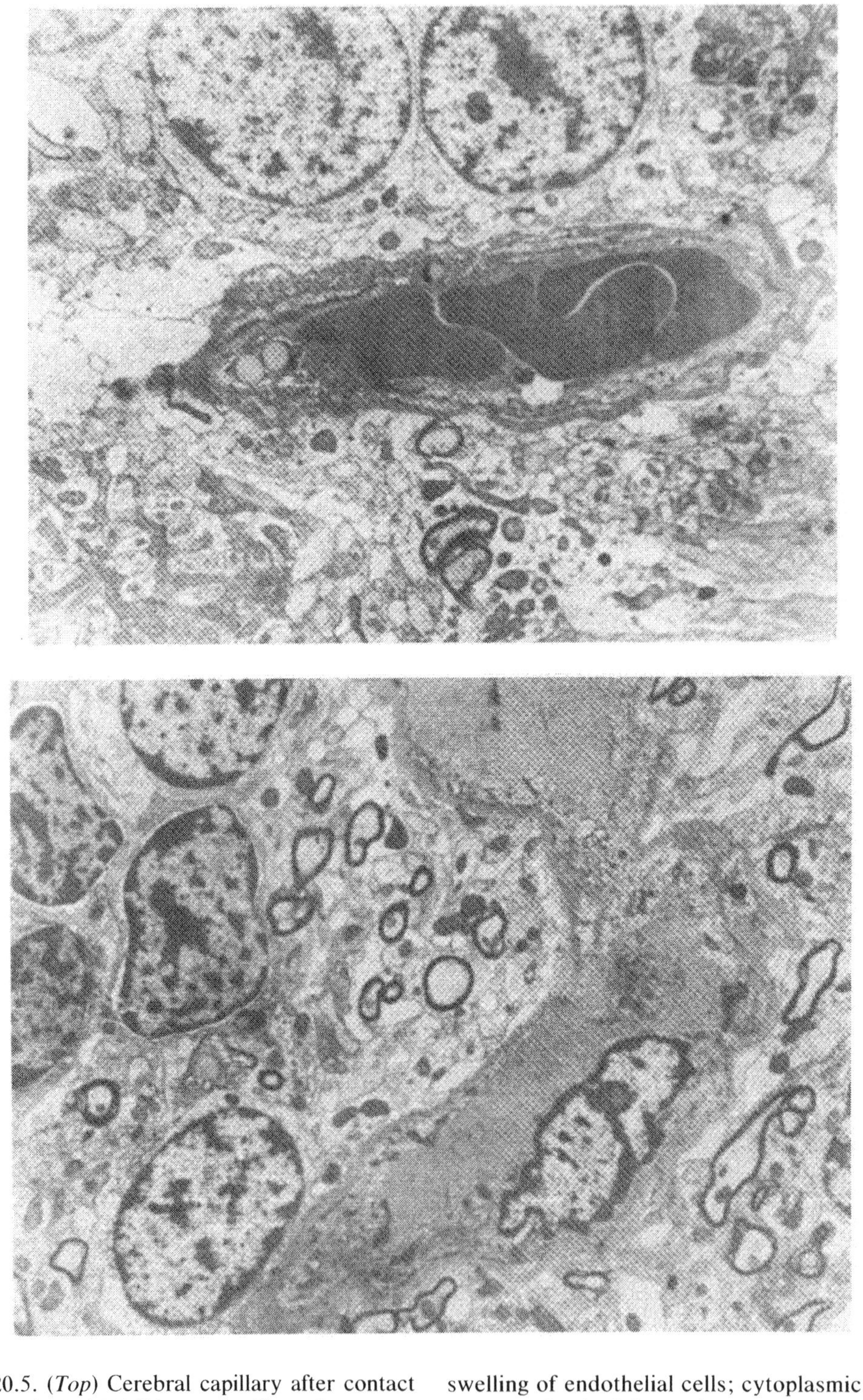

FIGURE 20.5. (*Top*) Cerebral capillary after contact irradiation with Nd:YAG laser. Swelling of astrocyte pedicles, shrinkage of basement membrane and swelling of endothelial cells; cytoplasmic vesicles. (*Bottom*) Cerebral tissue after contact irradiation with Nd:YAG laser. No important morphologic changes.

which depends on the fluctuations in energy delivery, because of the instability of the power range in high-power laser systems.

Discussion

The literature indicates that the most important difference in morphology between contact and noncontact radiation is related to the depth and volume of necrotic tissue found at the target site. The standard noncontact technique resulted in a lesion depth of 1.0 to 4.4 mm, the mean values increasing with the amount of energy delivered. The contact technique resulted in a lesion depth of only 0.1 to 0.2 mm, with no significant changes related to alterations in the power range.[3] Data on the morphology of perilesional tissues after laser impact are limited to our histologic observations on the effects of noncontact CO_2 and Nd:YAG irradiation.[4] The damage appeared to be related to the duration of radiation, rather than to the power of the source. Accordingly, only minimal damage of the astrocyte-capillary junctions were observed after CO_2 and Nd:YAG exposure at 20–40 W for 2–3 seconds; tissue changes (more severe after Nd:YAG) consisted of swelling of astrocyte pedicles and endothelial cell cytoplasm, while the basement membrane was unaffected.[4] Similar findings have now been observed with argon and Nd:YAG contact irradiation. Conversely, after noncontact CO_2 and Nd:YAG exposure at 20 to 40 W for 5 to 10 seconds, prominent lesions up to complete destruction of the tissue and occlusion of capillaries were observed; with Nd:YAG, perivascular hemorrhages occurred in highly vascularized brain tumors.[4,5] Such lesions were never observed in the present study after contact irradiation. The similarity between effects produced by short noncontact irradiation and contact irradiation can thus be attributed to the reduced thermal diffusion of the latter technique. The greater extension of damage after noncontact irradiation explains why this technique is indicated for vaporization of small deep-seated lesions or tumor remnants in the cavity.[6] Experimental results also support indication of the contact laser technique for dissection and cutting.[7–9]

The SLT laser scalpel shows many advantages over traditional and noncontact laser techniques. Cutting with bipolar forceps is irregular and coagulation of diffuse superficial bleeding can extend the tissue damage; moreover, the dissection of tumors adjoining neurovascular structures is more traumatic with this technique.

Poorer control of the maneuver means that separation of irregular-shaped lesions from surrounding structures is difficult with noncontact CO_2 irradiation. The main risk being damage to nerves or important vessels by accidental deviation of the beam. Moreover, hemostasis is limited to vessels up to 0.1 to 0.2 mm.

With contact irradiation the incision is sharp, the cut is thinner than that produced by noncontact irradiation, there is no smoke, and carbonization of the edges is avoided; moreover, the control of subadjacent planes is continuous, and the hemostasis is complete for veins and arteries up to 1 mm. Less laser energy is required and thermal diffusion is reduced.

Due to the shape and the small diameter of the probe there is less interference with the field of vision, even under the operating microscope. The feeling and appreciation of the texture of tissues increases the safety and rapidity of the maneuver. To assure maximal precision in deep lesions, expecially in proximity of neurovascular structures, direct constant visual control is required by sufficient exposition of all sectioned planes. Due to its very limited side effects the argon laser scalpel has distinct indications for procedures near important vessels or nerves. Contrary to noncontact Nd:YAG exposure, the decreased thermal spreading allows the Nd:YAG laser scalpel to be used safely even in critical areas; uncontrolled deepening of the irradiation and postoperative hemorrhages from residual infiltrating tumors, in fact, were never observed in our series.

The two laser techniques can occasionally be associated, such as in preliminary vaporization of a small lesion and subsequent separation of remnants from surrounding structures. In highly vascularized tissues, laser scalpel incision can be preceded by noncontact irradiation with defocused Nd:YAG laser or contact coagulation so as to improve hemostasis.

In conclusion, contact laser systems are suitable for progressive dissection and cutting in depth, while noncontact lasers seem to be useful mostly for the vaporization and tissue ablation in surface. In the future, surgical procedures will be deeply conditioned by the proper selection between the two techniques.

References

1. Daikuzono N, Joffe SN: Sapphire probe for contact photocoagulation and tissue vaporization with the Nd:YAG laser. Med Instrum 4:173–178, 1985.
2. Karnowsky MJ: A formaldehyde-glutaraldehyde fixative of high osmolarity for use in electron microscopy. J Cell Biol 27:137A–138A, 1965.
3. Diaz FG, Dujovny M, King PK, et al: Use of the contact Nd:YAG laser scalpel in neurosurgery. Proceedings of the 4th General and Scientific Meeting of the LANSI (Laser Association of Neurological Surgeons International), Venice, pp. 30 1986.
4. Fasano VA, Peirone SM, Ponzio RM, et al: Effects at the periphery of the laser lesion in human brain and its tumors after CO_2, Nd:YAG and CO_2 high peak pulsed radiation. Lasers Surg Med 6:308–317, 1986.
5. Yain KK: Complications of the use of the Nd:YAG laser in neurosurgery. Neurosurgery 16:759–762, 1985.
6. Fasano VA: Advanced Intraoperative Technologies in Neurosurgery. Springer-Verlag, Wien and New York, 1986.
7. Fasano VA, Ponzio RM, Bolognese P: Preliminary experiences with contact Nd:YAG and argon laser in neurosurgery. Clinical data. Proceedings of the 4th General and Scientific Meeting of the LANSI (Laser Association of Neurological Surgeons International), Venice, pp 13–14 1986.
8. Fasano VA, Peirone SM, Fiscella B, et al: Preliminary experiences with contact Nd:YAG and argon laser in neurosurgery. Experimental data. Proceedings of the 4th General and Scientific Meeting of the LANSI (Laser Association of Neurological Surgeons International), Venice, pp. 32–33 1986.
9. Fasano VA, Ponzio RM, Lanotte M, Gawlik J: Preliminary Experiences with Argon and Nd:YAG Scalpel Laser in Neurosurgery. Proceedings of the 7th International Congress of Laser/Optoelectronics in Medicine with 2nd International Nd:YAG Laser Conference. pp 424–427 Springer Verlag, 1986.

21 Fiberoptic Laser Endoscopy in Neurosurgery

P.W. Ascher

Flexible fiberoptic endoscopy and stereotaxic procedures are of interest to neurosurgeons. Stereotactic psychosurgery is now rarely performed, due to the availability of specific drugs, and is used only in certain chronic pain syndromes and extrapyramidal movement disorders. Stereotactic procedures are invaluable for the biopsy of deep and often inaccessible tumors and abscesses. These procedures also allow the interstitial laser therapy of benign tumors, such as astrocytomas grades 1 and 2. Following topographic localization, these tumors are biopsied, examined bylight microscopy, and, finally, implanted with radioactive seeds.

Neurosurgical fiberoptic endoscopy was initially used for diagnosis. Following a spinal puncture, the cerebellopontine angle and the spinal cord can be inspected, and, with a ventricular puncture, the ventricles can be viewed. Today, flexible fiberoptic endoscopy, used with the Nd:YAG laser, will permit minimally invasive neurosurgical procedures.

Development of Nd:YAG Laser Endoscopy

The combination of the Nd:YAG laser with an endoscope was first used clinically in urology and gastroenterology. This led neurosurgeons in Graz to use the laser initially with a flexible bronchoscope (Figure 21.1). In Munich in 1982 O. Beck, using the rigid pediatric cystoscope, punctured a ventricular cyst, aspirated its contents, and coagulated the cyst wall. Coagulation of the ventricular choroid plexus was then tried in animals, as a potential treatment of hydrocephalus.

Between 1982 and 1983 L.M. Auer developed a rigid encephaloscope for the evacuation of acute cerebral hematomas. The biopsy channel would be used for suction, irrigation, and insertion of the laser fiber. The original device was then modified to produce a neuroendoscope with a 6.0-mm diameter shaft. These endoscopes were used to puncture and evacuate cystic tumors. For all other procedures a pediatric 5.5-mm cystoscope with wide-angle optics is used (Figure 21.2). Still, some technical improvements are needed, for example, the shaft of the endoscope should be longer.

Indications

Nd:YAG laser endoscopy is currently used in three main areas: (1) intraventricular and periventricular tumors, especially meningiomas and ependymomas, (2) acute intracranial hematomas, and (3) cystic tumors.

Meningiomas and ependymomas in the lateral and third ventricles are extremely responsive to laser irradiation. These tumors shrink following photocoagulation of the vasculature. After this procedure, as shown in our study of four patients, open surgical removal of the tumor, whether in toto or piecemeal, is technically easier and less traumatic to the patient.

Two patients with inoperable tumors of the thalamus were treated with the Nd:YAG laser via a pediatric cystoscope. The tumor disappeared, as confirmed by computed tomography. Neither patient had any neurologic deficit at a

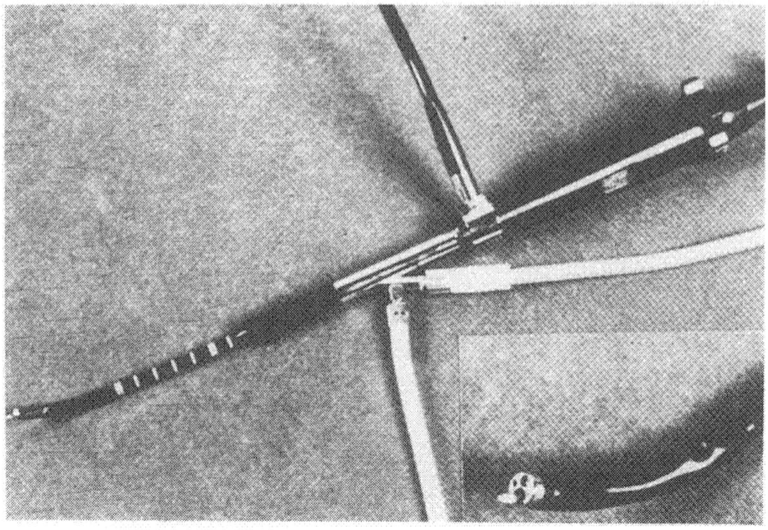

FIGURE 21.1. Flexible bronchoscope used in neurosurgery.

2-year follow-up. Since 1983, L.M. Auer has evacuated over 150 intracranial hematomas, using the neuroendoscope in combination with the Nd:YAG laser for photocoagulation. Following aspiration, the cystic tumors were evacuated. Tissue samples were obtained for light microscopy, and the stroma or cavity of the tumor was lasered on the internal surface, leading to tumor shrinkage in all cases. One week later, a less complicated surgical operation was performed.

Future Indications

The Nd:YAG laser is currently being evaluated in three main areas: in the treatment of intervertebral disk disease; as a method of performing a thoracic sympathectomy, and in the management of occlusive carotid artery disease.

Daniel Choy (New York) suggested introducing a laser probe through a needle puncture directly into the intervertebral disk, which would

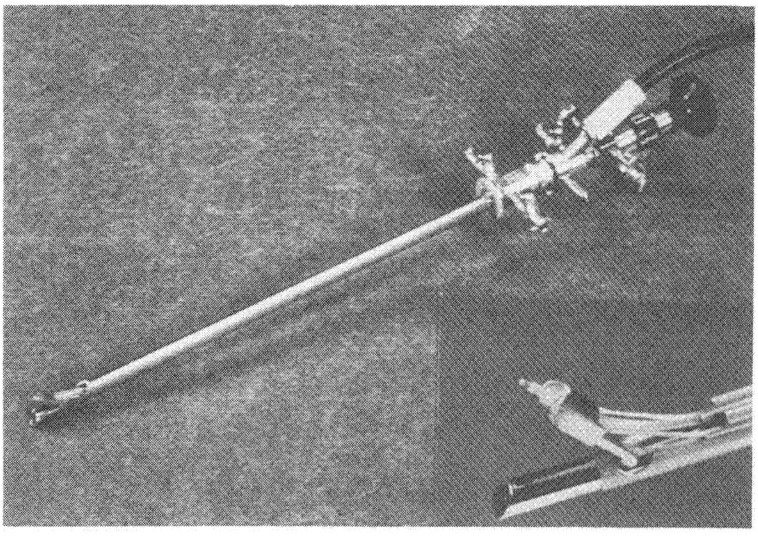

FIGURE 21.2. Rigid pediatric cystoscope used in encephaloscopy.

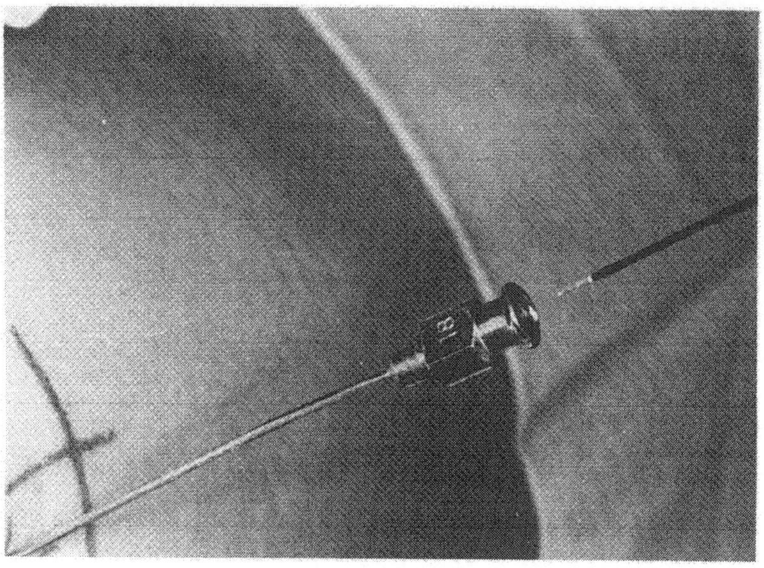

FIGURE 21.3. Lumbar puncture needle inserted into L4–L5 disk space for vaporization of nucleus pulposus.

cause the disk to collapse, thereby relieving the symptoms. Theoretically, the CO_2 laser would be suitable for vaporizing the nucleus pulposus because of its high water content. As suitable CO_2 fibers are not yet available, the Nd:YAG laser, coupled to either a 400 or 600 μm diameter quartz fiber, is being used (Figure 21.3). To minimize the Nd:YAG laser light absorption in water, the nucleus pulposus is first stained by injecting methylene blue. In the first 12 patients we treated with the Nd:YAG laser, 20 to 35 pulses at a total energy output of 350 to 500 J reduced the intervertebral disk sufficiently to alleviate the symptoms in all patients with a 4-month follow-up to date. A larger number of patients now need to be treated and carefully evaluated. The current technique used with the future the CO_2 laser fiber, or the Nd:YAG at a 1.32-μm wavelength, may allow between 10 and 15% of patients currently undergoing conventional surgery to be treated by laser vaporization of the nucleus pulposus.

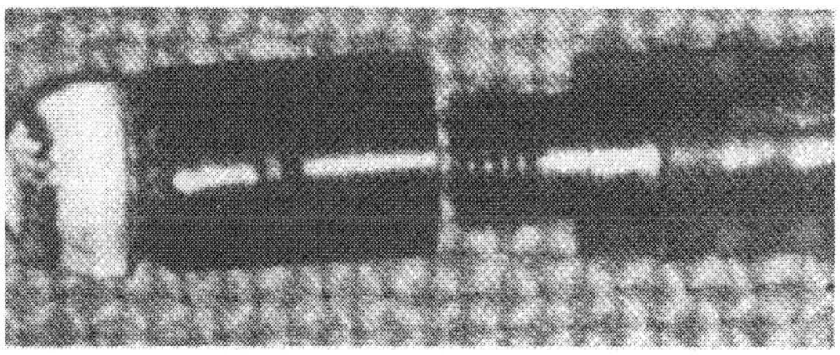

FIGURE 21.4. Contact synthetic sapphire used with the Nd:YAG laser for therapeutic fiberoptic and rigid neurosurgical procedures.

Thoracic sympathectomy used in the treatment of upper limb hyperhydrosis and various pain syndromes has been made easier by using the Nd:YAG laser endoscopically. Experience and follow-up is too short at present. The sympathetic cord is vaporized for three segments beneath the stellate ganglion, but laser photocoagulation may be an adequate form of treatment without total excision (Figure 21.4).

Carotid laser angioplasty was initially performed with the argon laser by using the percutaneous transfemoral approach. Although feasible, it was technically very complicated. The Nd:YAG laser (1.06 μm wavelength) with the contact synthetic sapphire point has provided excellent results in a limited number of patients. Other wavelengths (1.32 μm) and new lasers (excimer) need to be evaluated. Current experimental and clinical studies will lead to greater applicability of this technique. Vascular endoscopes that permit direct visualization with the contact probes are also being evaluated.

Conclusions

New and exciting applications of the Nd:YAG continue to increase since the advent of YAG laser endoscopy in neurosurgery. Endoscopic procedures previously performed for diagnosis are now routinely being used in treatment.

In the near future, based on the present experience with benign ventricular astrocytomas, stereotactic laser probes will be used with magnetic resonance imaging. Newer optic systems, including the contact sapphire probe, which prevents overheating of the quartz fiber, reduce tissue damage and allow selective and uniform heating of tumor tissue. This will increase the applications of the Nd:YAG laser in neurosurgery.

Coagulation of the choroid plexus may treat certain types of hydrocephalus. The use of selective tumor dyes (hematoporphyrin derivatives) and corresponding laser wavelength will treat tumors, and may prevent tumor recurrence following excision. The era of lasers in neurosurgery is just beginning.

22 The Contact Nd:YAG Laser in Neurosurgery

Hirotsugu Samejima, Satoshi Iwabuchi, and Nobuo Yoshii

It took 10 years to recognize the laser for its neurosurgical application since Rosomoff[1] tried to use a ruby laser for surgery on a brain tumor. Today three lasers, CO_2, argon and Nd:YAG, are widely used for neurosurgery. Among these lasers, the Nd:YAG has been evaluated to be inappropriate for neurosurgery, in spite of its excellent hemostatic capability, because of an unsatisfactory cutting-off effect. At the same time, this ability to achieve hemostasis has been highly successful in endoscopic procedures.

We have found a way to resolve this problem for neurosurgery. We can now obtain a satisfactory cutting-off effect, in addition to good hemostasis, by using a contact laser scalpel, with a rod made of artificial sapphire, attached to a Nd:YAG laser. The experimental and clinical results of our study are discussed in this chapter.

Equipment

The Medilas Type 2 Nd:YAG laser (Messerschmitt Bolkow Blohm, Munich, Germany) was used and its laser beam was conducted by an optic conduit of the 600-μm core quartz fiber-optic delivery system. The handpiece with focusing lens was used for the noncontact laser scalpel and the artificial sapphire rod was used for the contact laser. The contact laser has also been used with a quartz fiber inside a Burnett handpiece developed for neurosurgery.

The laser rod is structured as a single artificial sapphire crystal of aluminum oxide (Al_2O_3). Its melting point is 2030–2050°C and the thermal conductivity is 0.0016–0.0034 W/cm^2 /second at 40°C and it transmits more than 90% of the Nd:YAG laser beam.[2,3] Compared to the quartz scalpel, which was developed as a contact optic delivery conduit, the laser rod has a higher thermal resistance and a lower thermal conductivity, which concentrates energy more effectively by a sharp increase of local temperature at the distal end. This may be the most distinctive characteristic of the equipment. The laser beam shows a markedly wide degree of divergence—more than 100° at the distal end of the laser rod, in contrast to 7–8° at the end of the optical quartz fiber. It shows a remarkable attenuation of power density at a distance in a straight line to high energy concentration at the distal end. Moreover, the laser rod is said to rarely cause backscattering on the surface of the tissue, while the quartz fiber causes a fair amount.[2]

Confirmation of Safety

In Vitro Effects

We studied the effect of a noncontact laser and a contact laser, fixed vertically on the surface of a pig liver, on the depth of the liver tissue irradiated for 6, 4, and 2 seconds at 50 W. The noncontact laser vaporized the target tissue to a depth of 2.5 mm for 6 seconds, 1.8 mm for 4 seconds, and 1.1 mm for 2 seconds, while the depth of vaporization produced by the contact laser was 1.8 mm for 6 seconds, 1.4 mm for 4 seconds, and 1.1 mm for 2 seconds. The depth of edema in the heat-affected pale zone that ensued from the noncontact laser application was 2.1 mm for 6 seconds, 2 mm for 4 seconds, and

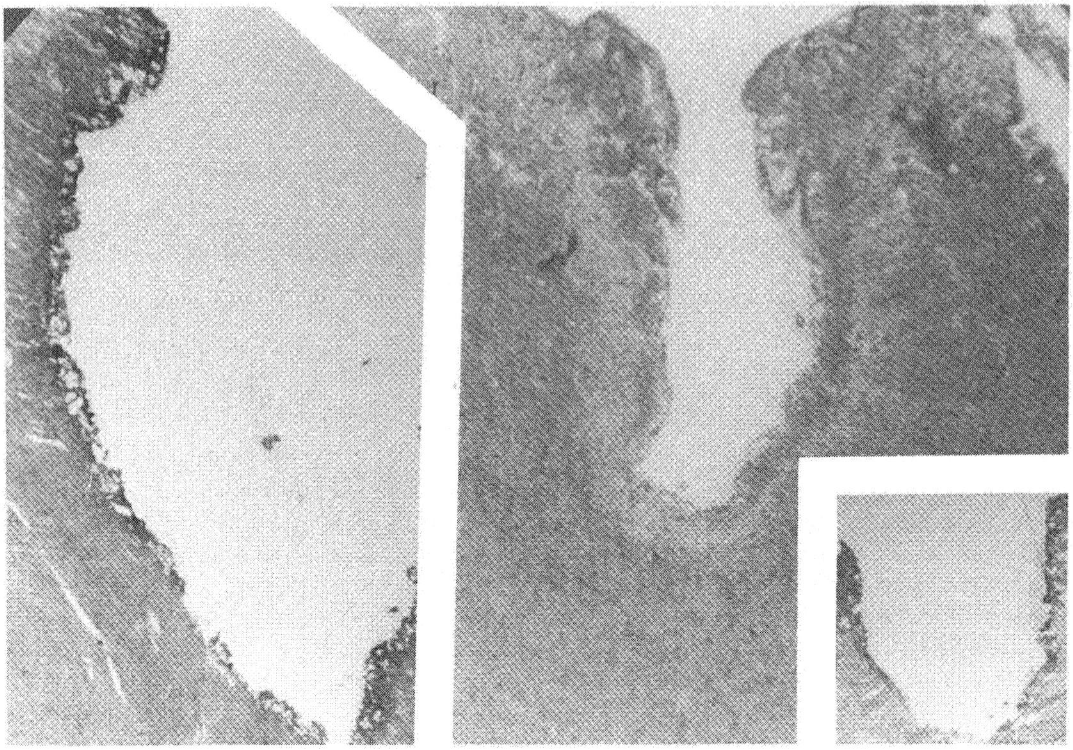

FIGURE 22.1. Light micrograph of tumor tissue vaporized by the laser rod immediately after extirpation at an output of 70 W. Duration of the current was 6 seconds (*left*); 4 seconds (*right*); 2 seconds (*inset*). H & E, × 20.

0.9 mm for 2 seconds, and from the contact laser the edema was 0.7 mm for 6 seconds, 0.5 mm for 4 seconds, and 0.4 mm for 2 seconds. Compared to the quartz fiber directly, the effect on the tissue was decreased by 30% in vaporized depth and 70% in the pale zone at the distal end of the laser rod point.

To observe a direct effect of the laser rod on tumor tissue immediately after the extirpation, the surface of a meningioma was irradiated for 2, 4, and 6 seconds at 30, 50, and 70 W. Even with the irradiation at 70 W, the maximum output, the extent of thermocoagulation beyond the vaporized zone was 410 μm, and it was only 700 μm including the peripheral edema zone. Effects on tissue deeper than that observed in the pig liver, were not found in meningioma, perhaps because of the solidity of this tumor. The extent of irradiation, that is, the depth of the honeycomblike area seen in the pale zone, was generally invariable in the hematoxylin-eosyn stain (Figure 22.1).

In Vivo Effects

In the frontal region craniotomy of a white rabbit under intravenous anesthesia the frontal lobe was irradiated by the contact laser rod. Thirty minutes after the irradiation, for 5 seconds at 25 W, demention of the vaporized crater did not exceed 2 mm. There was no clear boundary line between the coagulation zone and the edema zone,[4] and a microcystic honeycomblike zone was found in the outer stratum. An engorgement was caused by intravascular thrombi and an accumulation of erythrocytes in and partial transudation occurred, but no obvious hemorrhagic lesion was found. Brain tissue directly under the pale zone, that resulted from the thermal effect, showed a normal structure. With irradiation for 5 seconds at 40 W, which caused a comparatively greater depth of edema than at 25 W, the extent of the thermocoagulation zone was nearly the same and no hemorrhagic lesion was observed. One week after irradiation for 5 seconds at 25 W, the boundary between the microcystic

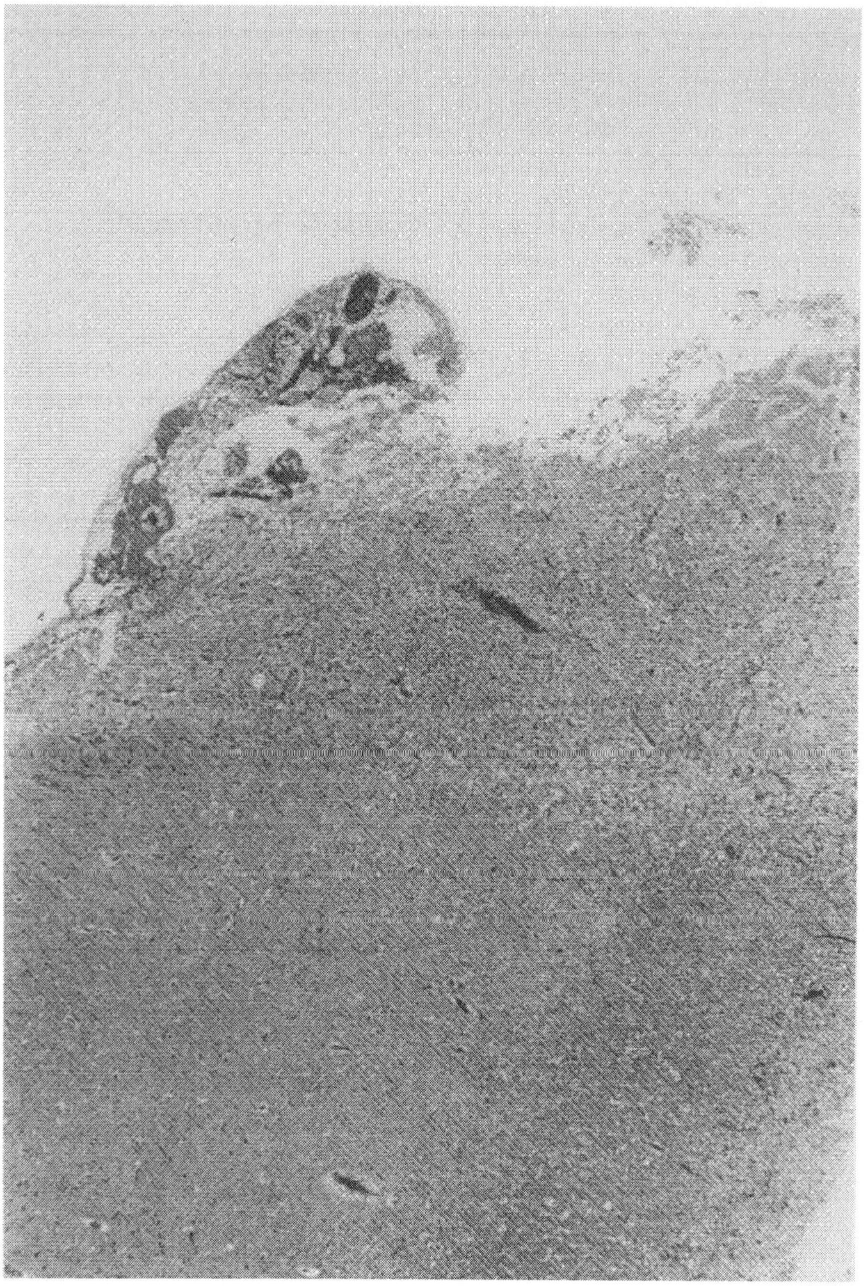

FIGURE 22.2. Light micrograph of rabbit brain section one week after the laser rod irradiation at 25 W for 5 seconds. Microcysts were observed in the edematous zone. H & E, × 20.

tissue and normal tissue became clearer than in its acute stage, the edema zone contained many macrophages, fibroblasts, and glial cells, and the number of nerve cells decreased. Vessels were shrunken and there were no signs of hemorrhagic lesions (Figure 22.2).

Discussion

There have been many reports on the medical applications of the laser, and its safety has been rather firmly established.[5–8] However, some clinicians are still apprehensive of the safety of the

Nd:YAG laser, owing to its optical characteristics.[9,10] Edwards[9] explained it in terms of absorption coefficiency and extinction length, showing that the depth in the tissue laser beam is derived from photobiology. The Nd:YAG laser, which is a scattering-dominated instrument, as opposed to the absorption-dominated CO_2 laser, has an extinction value of 60 mm in length to water, but 2.3 mm to the stomach wall and 3.5 mm to the human brain.[11] Even if the extinction length to water is 80 mm, such depth in tissue will not be affected due to the scattering effect.[7] In in vitro transmission, the ratio of the Nd:YAG absorption of blood to brain was 100:1, and the in vivo change in tissue by the thermal effect was only 2 mm at the acute stage and 3 mm at the chronic lesion by irradiation for 8 seconds at 10 W and 2.5 mm and 4 mm by 8 seconds at 40 W irradiation. This was because the Nd:YAG laser was preferentially absorbed by hemoglobin in blood.[8] In acute and chronic experiments on the rat brain, Nd:YAG laser irradiation was found to be safe, and normal brain tissues had a tolerance for this laser.[12] Besides, in the microvasculature experiment, CO_2 laser irradiation caused vascular dilation and hemorrhage peripheral to coagulation or the edema zone, while the Nd:YAG laser irradiation caused avascularity or oligovascularity at the irradiated part and constricted the blood vessels with little hemorrhages.[13]

Safety in direct irradiation by the quartz fiber has been confirmed as mentioned above; however, there have been no reports on the effect of the laser rod yet. The laser rod has no sideward irradiation from the surface of the tapered conical portion, and all of the irradiation is from the distal end.[2] As the laser rod has little backscattering, as opposed to 30 to 40% of backscattering by the noncontact type, the output can be reduced about 20–30% as compared to the noncontact type.[2] Moreover, the angle of divergency is more than 100° at the distal end of the rod in contrast to 10° or less by the noncontact laser, which reduced remarkably the power density at the distance in a straight line. These facts have been shown experimentally by our results in vitro and in vivo.[3] A shorter extinction length, both in the vaporized and the edema zones, than that with the noncontact laser, enables the contact laser rod to be utilized the same as the conventional scalpel for surgery and the preservation of coagulative function, which is a primary characteristic of the Nd:YAG laser, makes it possible to control hemorrhage at the same time as cutting—an advantage the conventional scalpel did not possess.

Clinical Application

Procedures

Fifty-four operations using the laser rod have been performed at our hospital. Though it may be difficult to absolutely compare the conventional operation and this procedure, the time of operation and the amount of hemorrhage during the operation were generally evaluated by the same surgeon as "very helpful" (helpful both in time and hemorrhage), "not helpful" and "questionable benefits" (result shown in Table 22.1). It was very helpful for the solid extramedullary tumor, especially for the case that required coring in order to reduce the volume of tumor, because of an inclination to hemorrhage, firm accretion, and possible adhesion to the surrounding tissue in depth.

The case of meningioma which was most effectively operated on is described below. In cases of convex meningioma, it is not necessary to use the laser because the tumor can be removed by conventional microneurosurgical techniques without damaging the cortex. How-

TABLE 22.1. Experience with the contact Nd:YAG laser in 54 neurosurgical procedures

Result	Lesion	No. of cases
Very helpful	Meningioma	13
	Neurinoma	7
	Lymphoma	1
	Metastasis	1
	Chordoma	1
Helpful	Glioma	10
	Glioblastoma	6
	Pituitary adenoma	2
	Metastasis	2
	Lymphoma	1
	Epidermoid	1
	Craniopharyngioma	1
Not helpful	Glioma	2
	Lymphoma	1
Questionable benefits	Arteriovenous malformation	5

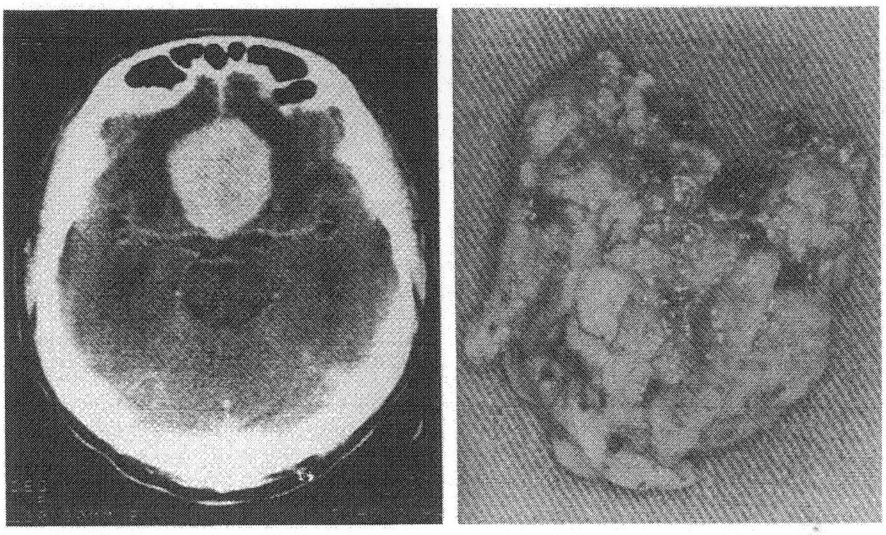

FIGURE 22.3. (*Left*) Preoperative CT scan with contrast enhancement showing olfactory groove meningioma. At the beginning, the attachment of tumor was resected in a wedge-like shape by the laser rod. Total removal of the tumor was then done without transfusion. (*Right*) Macrograph showing the tumor.

ever, in basal meningioma, especially in olfactory meningioma expanded bifrontally (Figure 22.3), or when hemorrhage is anticipated by firm attachment, for example, to the planum sphenoidale. For this operation the low power rod, 25 W, is used for slow excision of the lesion, either directly or wedge-shaped. If the rod is operated quickly, incomplete hemostasis may possibly cause excessive hemorrhage. After the initial treatment of the attachment, coring or enucleation is recommended for huge menigioma, and then detachment may be performed by conventional techniques.

In case the tumor is located at depth and a

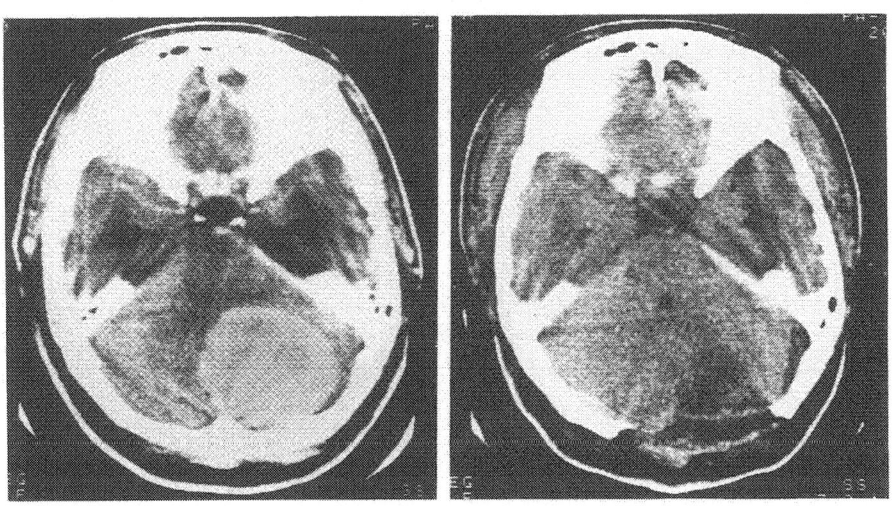

FIGURE 22.4. (*Left*) Preoperative CT scan with contrast enhancement showing tentorial meningioma. The huge tumor sat in the right cerebellar hemisphere and adhered to the transverse sinus and tentorium. The feeding artery was a tentorial artery. Total removal of the tumor was done by the coring method. Hemorrhage was easily controllable. (*Right*) Postoperative CT scan after 6 days.

feeder cannot be treated at the beginning, the capsule should be incised by the laser at 25 to 40 W, then coring should be done in advance of the detachment in order to reduce the volume of the tumor (Figure 22.4). In that case, detachment should not be done before the tumor volume is reduced sufficiently. This may spare unnecessary cortex damage by retraction. If the attachment is burned off after sufficient coring, the tumor may be resected easily. This method is also applied for detachment from the sinus or important vasculature.

When the tumor cannot be completely extirpated but is left partially, due to infiltration into the bony matrix or dura where the tumor cannot be reached, the remains are preventatively irradiated by the laser beam. However, further long-range follow-up and cumulative practices are required for satisfactory judgment as to whether this method inhibits the tumor from growing again.

Although the laser rod is also effective for the enucleation of a large acoustic tumor, an operation should be carefully done at the part where the facial nerve traverses. In soft and easily aspirated tumors, such as glioma, hemostasis possibly occurs by a low power output, but there is absolutely no better method than the conventional one.

Though the effectiveness of arteriovenous malformation has been reported,[16] it was evaluated as of "questionable benefit" from our experience: the detachment from normal tissue was easy but the tissue change was unknown.

Discussion

It was Rosomoff and Carroll[1] who reported the use of the laser in neurosurgical practice in 1966. But the safety and effectiveness of the laser beam was first confirmed in 1978 by Heppner,[14] Ascher,[15] and Takizawa.[7] The CO_2 laser was used mainly at that time. Clinical application of the Nd:YAG laser was first reported by Beck[5] in 1980, which showed superior effectiveness to the CO_2 laser for richly vascular meningioma in resection with a distinct decrease of transfusion. Takeuchi and co-workers[6] reported that it was efficacious for hard and hemorrhagic tumors with a shorter time of operation, easy manipulation of the flexible quartz fiber and safety to the operating team staff. Perceiving the coagulativeness which is a distinguishing characteristic of the Nd:YAG laser's wavelength, it is also applied for the extirpation of arteriovenous malformations.[16]

As the Nd:YAG laser does not damage tissue and has strong coagulative ability, hemorrahgic degeneration in deeper parts other than the vaporized zone found when the CO_2 laser was used, does not occur.[13] Clinical application has increased by these safety confirmations.

It has been said that the laser should have been operated a certain distance from the lesion for beneficial usage, but as the laser is used routinely, invasion of the tissue and dangers beyond the operation field are well-known problems. Some investigators require further development of the contact instrument, which is even more easily operable than the flexible quartz fiber.[5,9,16]

For the surgeon, especially the neurosurgeon who performs microsurgery, it may be essential that delicate operations be possible and instruments be controlled by himself touching the tissue directly for a safe operation. In this regard, the laser rod whose safety has been confirmed enables an incision of the tissue by the distal end of the rod at the same time as vaporization, and coagulativeness, a distinguishing characteristic of the Nd:YAG. Moreover, the thin distal end of the rod with 0.5 to 2.0 mm diameter and a Burnett type of handpiece are expedient for microsurgery.[2,3]

Detaching a deep tumor and controlling hemorrhage through a small space is a definite advantage compared to the conventional bipolar electric forceps or CO_2 laser. However, if the high power output is applied from the beginning, smoke may disturb visibility and the distal end of the rod may possibly melt.[2] The ultrasonic scalpel (CUSA) is useful for coring to reduce the content of the tumor, but its thick handpiece is unsuitable for microsurgery.

When operation on Sympson's types II and III meningioma is required, or in case of glioma, the effect of photoradiation therapy can be expected by radiating the remains.[5,6,9] However, the effect of the laser beam on inhibition of the growth of tumor cells has not been explained yet, and we expect further developments in this field in the future.

Conclusions

The Nd:YAG laser that was delivered by the artificial sapphire laser rod was used as a contact laser instrument.

1. The laser beam radiating from the distal end of the rod acts to histologically coagulate maintaining its characteristics as Nd:YAG laser. The depth of the effect in the tissue was shallower than that directly by the Nd:YAG laser delivery fiber and its safety was confirmed.
2. In clinical applications, it showed an effectiveness for the resection of solid and hemorrhagic tumors, especially useful in microsurgery.

The use of the contact laser in microsurgical procedures should increase, especially for the surgical resection and treatment of tumors.

Acknowledgment. We are grateful to Dr. Shiro Naoe M.D. Department of Pathology, Toho University Ohashi Hospital for his advice in pathological examination.

References

1. Rosomoff HL, Carroll F: Reaction of neoplasm and brain to laser. Arch Neurol 14:143–148, 1966.
2. Daikuzono N, Joffe SN: Artificial sapphire probe for contact photocongulation and tissue vaporization with the Nd:YAG laser. J Med Instrum 19:151–192, 1985.
3. Samejima H, Mizokami T, Ushikubo Y, et al: Clinical use of contact type Nd-YAG laser (laser rod). Nippon Laser Igaku Kaishi 4:117–118, 1984.
4. Beck OJ, Wilske J, Schonberger JL, et al: Tissue changes following application of lasers to the rabbit brain. Neurosurg Rev 1:31–36, 1979.
5. Beck OJ: The use of the Nd-YAG and the CO_2 laser in neurosurgery. Neurosurg Rev 3:261–266, 1980.
6. Takeuchi J, Handa H, Taki W, et al: The Nd:YAG laser in neurological surgery. Surg Neurol 18:140–142, 1982.
7. Takizawa T, Yamazaki T, Miura N, et al: Laser surgery of basal, orbital, and ventricular meningiomas which are difficult to extirpate by conventional methods. Neurol Med Chir 20:729–737, 1980.
8. Wharen RE, Anderson RE, Scheithauer B, et al: The Nd:YAG laser in neurosurgery. Part 1. Laboratory investigations: Dose-related biological response of neural tissue. J Neurosurg 60:531–539, 1984.
9. Edwards MSB, Boggan JE, Fuller TA: The laser in neurological surgery. J Neurosurg 59:555–566, 1983.
10. Saunders ML, Young HG, Becker DP, et al: The use of the laser in neurological surgery. Surg Neurol 14:1–10, 1980.
11. Halldorsson T, Rother W, Langeholc J, et al: Theoretical and experimental investigations prove Nd:YAG laser treatment to be safe. Laser Surg Med 1:253–262, 1981.
12. Yamagami T, Handa H, Takeuchi J, et al: Histologic study of normal rat brain tissue after neodymium-yttrium aluminum garnet laser irradiation. Surg Neurol 23:475–482, 1985.
13. Kuroiwa T, Matsutaira T, Takei H, Inaba Y: Effects of Nd:YAG and CO_2 laser on cerebral microvasculature. Study in normal rabbit brain. J Neurosurg 64:128–133, 1986.
14. Heppner F: The laser scalpel on the nervous system. In Kaplan I (ed): Laser Surgery II. Academic Press, Jerusalem, 1978, pp. 79–80.
15. Ascher PW: The use of CO_2 in neurosurgery. In Kaplan I (ed): Laser Surgery II. Academic Press, Jerusalem, 1978, pp. 28–30.
16. Wharen RE, Anderson RE, Sundt TM: The Nd:YAG laser in neurosurgery. Part 2. Clinical studies: An adjunctive measure for hemostasis in resection of arteriovenous malformations. J Neurosurg 60:540–547, 1984.

23
Nd:YAG Laser Surgery: Overview of Applications

Stanley M. Shapshay

Since its introduction into clinical medicine the neodymium:yttrium aluminum garnet (Nd:YAG) laser has found definite multispecialty use. The carbon dioxide (CO_2) laser is clearly established as the premier precision cutting device but is seriously lacking in endoscopic applications because of its inability to be transmitted through available fibers. Certain specialties, such as otolaryngology, gynecology, and neurosurgery, still use the CO_2 laser in preference to other laser wavelengths, since accessibility to the larynx, cervix, and brain is adequate without fiber technology. Good hemostasis with the CO_2 laser, primarily for capillary-size blood vessels (microvasculature), and the ability to predict its precise soft tissue interaction have made it ideal for such applications as excisional biopsy of early carcinoma of the vocal cord and control of carcinoma in situ of the cervix. However, treatment of malignancy originating in such vascular areas as the trachea or bronchus requires more reliable hemostasis. For control of blood vessels larger than capillary size the Nd:YAG laser is the ideal wavelength.

The first successful application of the Nd:YAG laser was in gastroenterology and bronchology through standard endoscopes available in these specialities.[1] The availability of flexible quartz fibers facilitated this application. Recently, the Nd:YAG laser has been applied as a macroscopic tool with unfocused quartz fibers in holders, with focused handpieces, or in a contact mode.

High- and Low-Power Applications

High-power applications of the Nd:YAG laser, namely, at 40 W or greater, usually with intermittent exposure settings, are most often used for volumetric heating of tissue to achieve coagulation, ablation, and control of hemorrhage. The 1060-nm wavelength of the Nd:YAG laser makes it ideal for heating a large volume of tissue below 100°C. This effect results from scattering of the Nd:YAG laser wavelength in tissue rather than absorption on the tissue surface as is characteristic of the CO_2 laser. In fact, in heavily pigmented soft tissue, such as that of the skin, liver, and spleen, scattering is about twice as great as absorption. This "cooking" effect with the Nd:YAG laser is ideal for ablation of malignant tissue with increased hemorrhagic potential. However, a problem associated with the scattering effect is the clinician's difficulty in judging the depth of penetration, particularly in pale-colored tissue. The surface appearance of the laser irradiated area is not necessarily indicative of the degree of underlying laser penetration. Under these conditions the less experienced clinician may cause serious tissue damage by continuing to irradiate the tissue without pausing intermittently to evaluate the effects and, more important, to allow cooling of the tissue. High-power Nd:YAG laser applications can be used for the following: thermal coagulation of neoplastic tissue, usually for palliation of tumor obstruction, such as in the tracheobronchial tree; ablation of neoplastic tissue, such as removal of superficial bladder tumors; and control of hemorrhage, in particular, gastrointestinal bleeding. In general, if a large amount of Nd:YAG laser energy is absorbed as heat, the result is immediate vaporization. Slightly lower energy levels may cause necrosis with subsequent sloughing of tissue. A still lower amount of laser energy may cause necrosis with some stimulation of an inflammatory response with subsequent healing with fibrosis. The primary hemostatic mechanism with laser application is thermal contraction of the blood vessel wall. Usually, the laser power is reduced if longer exposure is used to accomplish hemostasis.[2]

At low power the Nd:YAG laser has recently been used for photocoagulation of vascular lesions, such as angiodysplasia, telangiectasia (associated with Osler–Weber–Rendu disease), and cavernous hemangiomas.[3,4] In this application a power setting of 30 W or less is employed at short-interval exposures of less than 1 second to photocoagulate vascular lesions without disrupting overlying epithelium, either skin or mucous membranes. The success of treatment depends on the color selectivity or pigment concentration as well as the hemoglobin content of tissue. The purple color of a cavernous hemangioma is particularly good for selective absorption of the Nd:YAG laser wavelength.

A new and promising application of the Nd:YAG laser is in its contact mode utilizing artificial sapphire tips. The treatment relies on high-power density at the tissue contact site achieved by high-power output. This Nd:YAG laser technique developed by Joffe[5] has both endoscopic and macroscopic uses.

Applications by Specialties

Pulmonary Medicine, Otolaryngology, and Thoracic Surgery

Application of the Nd:YAG laser through rigid and flexible endoscopes has helped to create the exciting new area known as therapeutic endoscopy. Thanks to the pioneering efforts in France by Dumon et al.[6] and Toty and co-workers[7] and by others in the United States,[8] the Nd:YAG laser has been extremely successful for palliation of obstructing malignancy poorly treated by other therapeutic modalities. For the most part, such symptoms as dyspnea, hemoptysis, and obstructive pneumonitis have been palliated with minimal morbidity in this high-risk group of patients. Although lacking the precision of the CO_2 laser, the Nd:YAG laser with its superior hemostatic abilities and ease of application through flexible quartz fibers has proved indispensable to the bronchologist. Other uses for the Nd:YAG laser in bronchology appear to be palliation of benign tracheal stenosis limited to weblike scar formation and some miscellaneous applications, such as removal of granulation tissue and selected benign neoplasms, that is, hamartomas, chondromas, and papillomas.

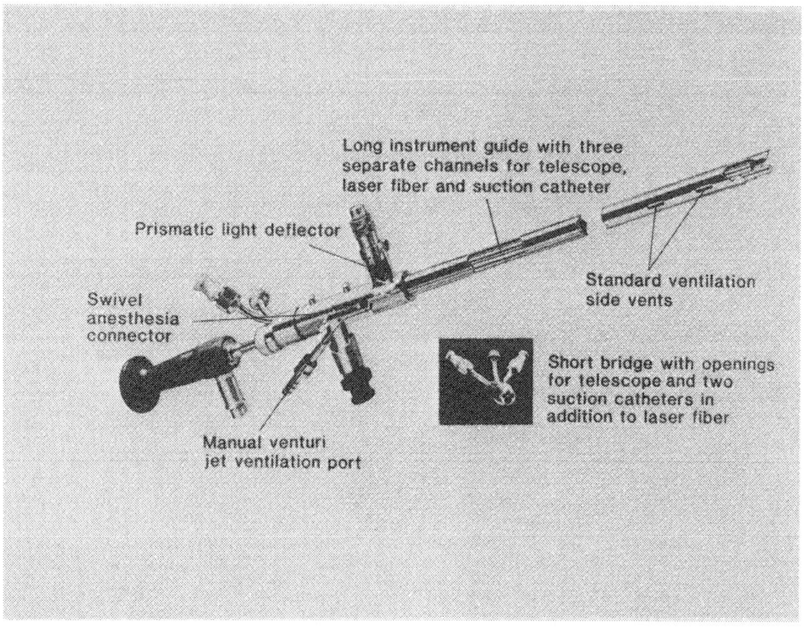

FIGURE 23.1. Shapshay laser bronchoscope. Illustration shows component parts of the rigid ventilating laser fiber bronchoscope. Inset shows proximal part allowing passage of a telescope (0°), suction catheter, and laser fiber. (Courtesy of Karl Storz Endoscopy, 10111 West Jefferson Boulevard, Culver City, CA.)

The new contact probes seem promising for precise removal of tracheal webs and scarring because less charring of surrounding tissue occurs than with the free, noncontact fiber mode. With the integration of newer endoscopic systems and primarily rigid bronchoscopes with special features for laser fiber application, Nd:YAG laser bronchoscopy has reached a stage of greater precision and safety (Figure 23.1).

Laryngeal applications of the Nd:YAG laser have thus far been limited to the treatment of vascular lesions, such as laryngeal cavernous hemangiomas. Isolated rare occurrences of these vascular malformations have been treated successfully with the Nd:YAG laser through a laryngoscope[4] (Figure 23.2). A low-power setting of 20 to 30 W at an exposure setting of 0.5 second permits photocoagulation of the hemangiomas without disruption of the overlying epithelium. Minimal bleeding and negligible morbidity have been associated with this type of application. Because of its lack of precision, however, the Nd:YAG laser has not challenged the secure role of the CO_2 laser in microlaryngoscopy.

In the field of thoracic surgery the Nd:YAG laser as well as the CO_2 laser has been used mostly experimentally for pulmonary resections and thoracoscopy. The latter application shows promise for sealing of lung defects in spontaneous pneumothorax or emphysematous blebs and for thoracoscopic lung biopsy. The Nd:YAG laser wavelength either delivered through a bare quartz fiber or by contact probe makes thoracoscopic lung biopsy possible, with sealing of the lung and adequate hemostasis.[9]

Gastroenterology

Upper Gastrointestinal Tract

The two major applications of endoscopic Nd:YAG laser therapy in the upper gastrointestinal tract are for control of hemorrhage and neoplastic disease. Treatment for the latter is

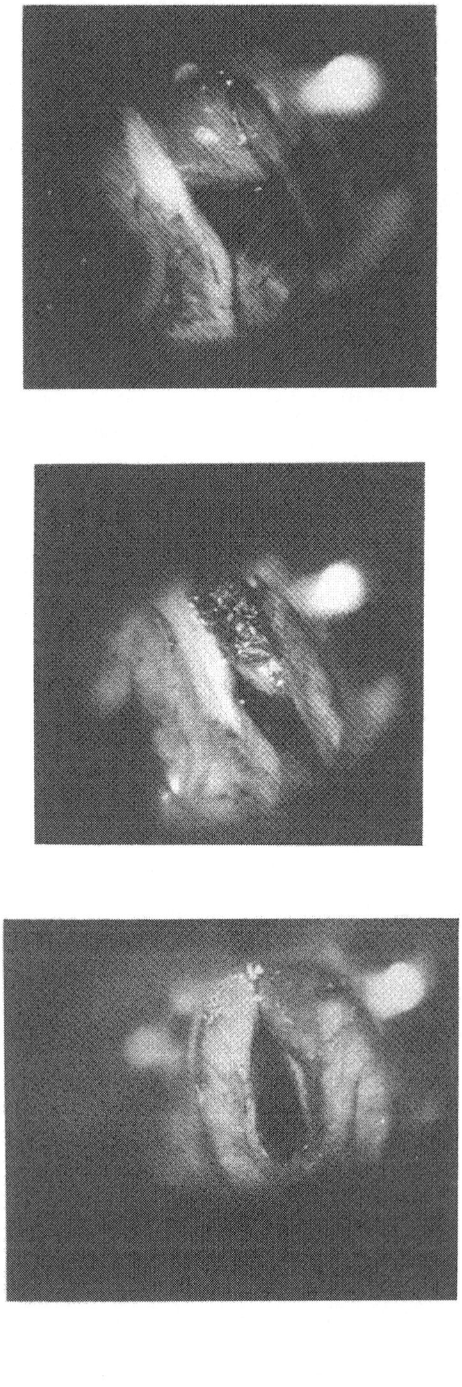

FIGURE 23.2. Treatment of hemangioma with the Nd:YAG laser. *(Top)* Endoscopic view shows cavernous hemangioma involving the superior surface of the right true vocal cord. The patient also had cavernous hemangiomas involving the oral cavity and oropharynx. *(Middle)* Result immediately after Nd:YAG laser photocoagulation at a power setting of 30 W and exposure setting of 0.5 second. Marked shrinkage of the hemangioma is seen with some crusting on the surface. *(Bottom)* Result two months after photocoagulation with the Nd:YAG laser. Fibrous tissue has replaced the hemangioma. The superior surface of the right true vocal cord can now be seen. (Courtesy of Marvin Fried, M.D., 398 Brookline Avenue, Boston, MA. Reprinted with permission of *Laryngoscope.)*

generally palliative to reduce symptoms of obstruction and to improve the quality of life. A departure from this approach has occurred in Japan where diagnosis of early gastric cancer is more commonly made and experience with application of the Nd:YAG laser for curative treatment is growing.[10]

Most endoscopists at present tend to agree that hemorrhage associated with nonvariceal lesions—particularly those that are discrete, such as ulcers and erosions—should be treated by Nd:YAG laser photocoagulation. Although the Nd:YAG laser has been used to stop variceal bleeding, endoscopic injection sclerotherapy seems to be utilized more commonly. The first reports of endoscopic laser therapy appeared in the middle 1970s with data from Nath et al.[1] Dwyer et al.[11] and Frühmorgen et al.[12] Nath et al.[1] reported the largest experience—994 acute bleeding incidents in 625 patients—and their overall success rate for achieving initial hemostasis was 94%. Considerable experience from several investigators both in Europe and the United States now suggests that endoscopic laser therapy effectively produces initial hemostasis for acutely bleeding lesions. However, few data are available from controlled studies. Therefore, controversy exists among gastroenterologists whether Nd:YAG laser therapy for hemorrhage is more effective than electrocautery or other methods for controlling gastrointestinal hemorrhage. Encouraging reports utilizing the Nd:YAG laser for angiodysplasia have appeared in the literature documenting good control of bleeding with decrease in transfusion requirements and hospitalizations. Both the argon and Nd:YAG lasers have been used for this purpose.

The Nd:YAG laser appears to have made a definite contribution for therapy of obstructing neoplasms in the difficult-to-treat upper gastrointestinal area. This endoscopic approach for the palliation of obstructing carcinoma obviates the need for surgery and general anesthesia with their attendant morbidity, diminishes the likelihood of systemic side effects, and may be performed under direct vision and applied repeatedly, since laser energy is nonionizing.[13] Both prograde and retrograde approaches for treating esophageal carcinoma have been utilized on an outpatient basis. Appreciable palliation with acceptable morbidity has been reported by several investigators. Standard flexible gastrointestinal endoscopes have been used making this technique available to well-trained endoscopists.

Lower Gastrointestinal Tract

The Nd:YAG appears to be the laser of choice for palliation of obstructing carcinomas of the colorectal area. Kiefhaber et al.[14] reported a series of 13 patients in whom unmodified colonoscopes were used for laser treatment of obstructing colorectal tumors. Lumen recanalization may be achieved obviating the need for a colostomy. Successful palliation is often obtained with one or more Nd:YAG laser phototherapy sessions. Again, acceptable morbidity is associated with this type of application. Recently, the contact laser endoprobes have been used effectively at low-power settings (10 to 15 W) to palliate obstructing colorectal neoplasms. Investigations are under way concerning applications of the Nd:YAG laser for benign mucosal lesions, such as familial polyposis syndrome, villous adenomas, adenomatous polyps, hemorrhoids, and condyloma acuminata. In treating condyloma acuminata, in the colorectal specialty and gynecology, both the CO_2 laser and the Nd:YAG laser have been found useful.

General Surgery

In general surgery, great interest has been stimulated by the development of the contact "laser scalpel." This device, developed for use with the Nd:YAG laser by Joffe,[5] promises to provide a hemostatic effect with partial resection of vascular organs, such as the liver, spleen, and pancreas. In addition, its endoscopic application in the hepatobiliary tract may prove helpful in the treatment of obstructing carcinomas of the bile ducts. Another possible application in an endoscopic mode might be destruction of bile duct stones utilizing continuous-wave or pulsed laser technology. The studies in this area are still experimental but appear promising.

Urology

The Nd:YAG is the most versatile and preferred laser for use in urology because it is easily adapted to standard cystoscopes, ureteroscopes, and nephroscopes and because the equipment can be used in a medium of water or urine. The

Nd:YAG laser provides the highest degree of tissue penetration and therefore permits transmural laser irradiation and destruction of lesions by thermal coagulation necrosis rather than excision, making it a superior hemostatic device for endoscopic application. The most successful uses of the Nd:YAG laser have been in patients with bladder cancer and, to a lesser extent, in patients with transitional tumors of the ureter and renal pelvis, urethral strictures, bladder neck contractures, and carcinomas of the penis.[15]

Bladder tumors up to to 3 cm have been treated effectively with the Nd:YAG laser. Typical dosimetry seems to be 40 W of power at 4- to 5-second pulses applied broadly so that one area is not overly treated. A conical area of necrosis 3 to 5 mm in depth is created with this technique. The largest series is from Hofstetter and Frank,[15] who reported 302 bladder tumors treated between 1976 and 1979. Local recurrence rate in a short-term follow-up period was 9% with standard electroresection techniques and 1% with the laser technique. Although results with early bladder carcinoma are encouraging, the initial reports from several investigators regarding urethral strictures are less optimistic. Restenosis after irradiation with the Nd:YAG laser appears to be common, and many groups of investigators have abandoned use of this laser for urethral strictures. External applications of the Nd:YAG laser in urology utilizing handheld devices were considered effective in a small series of patients with carcinoma of the penis in stages T1 and T2.[15] Equally encouraging results have been reported for condyloma acuminatum on the urethral caruncle and for condyloma of the vulva.

Gynecology

The Nd:YAG laser has been used more extensively than the CO_2 laser for lesions of the intrauterine area. In particular, the ablation of endometrium in women who wish to avoid hysterectomy for refractory menometrorrhagia appears promising.[16] Since the Nd:YAG laser can be used with a fiberoptic bundle in a fluid-filled medium, its particular wavelength appears well suited for this application. Otherwise, the CO_2 laser has certainly found more usefulness in gynecology because of its precise soft tissue interaction on the uterine cervix and vagina. Likewise, laparoscopic laser applications have been primarily with the CO_2 laser because of its precision in establishing tubal patency and in removing pelvic adhesions.

Dermatology and Plastic Surgery

The control of vascular lesions utilizing photoablation techniques with the Nd:YAG laser is a new development in dermatology and plastic surgery.[17] In particular, treatment of cavernous hemangiomas of the skin and mucosal surfaces of the head and neck, as reported by Shapshay and David,[4] is extremely promising. Extensive cavernous hamangiomas, bulky port-wine stains, and lesions associated with Osler–Weber–Rendu disease (intranasal and gastric telangiectasia) have been treated with success in a small number of patients with limited follow-up study. The laser is used with low-power settings of 20 to 30 W at intermittent 0.5- to 1.0-second exposures to photoablate these lesions without disrupting the overlying epithelial or skin cover. Since the depth of penetration of the Nd:YAG laser is limited to approximately 5 mm, glass slide compression and laser coagulation are used to permit deeper full-thickness coagulation of larger hemangiomas. Good healing with minimal bleeding has been observed in patients treated thus far. High-flow lesions, such as arteriovenous malformations, are not well treated with the Nd:YAG laser because of the excessive heat sink effect. Although most port-wine stains may be treated effectively with the argon laser, thicker raised port-wine stain lesions respond well with the Nd:YAG laser used in a photocoagulative mode.

Summary

The Nd:YAG laser has found multispecialty application because of its suitability for endoscopic transmission through currently available quartz fibers. When used appropriately as a photocoagulative instrument, this laser is effective on neoplastic tissue with a high hemorrhagic potential and can achieve excellent palliation in such areas as the gastrointestinal tract and tracheobronchial tree. In addition, its affinity for pigmented tissues rich in hemoglobin or melanin makes it an extremely attractive tool for selective ablation of vascular neoplasms, such as telangiectasia and cavernous hemangiomas. With the advent of effective contact probes for the Nd:YAG laser an entirely new area of application has emerged. High-power density laser scalpel effects on tissue have made possible the removal of vascular lesions and partial resection of vascular organs, such as liver, kidney, and spleen. In addition, precise endoscopic removal or coagulation of tissue may be achieved with contact probes.

The importance of the Nd:YAG laser in various medical specialties has been established but still needs to be defined with the help of carefully controlled studies. The burden of proof rests with the laser operator when the Nd:YAG laser is judged against more "conventional" modalities, such as electrocautery and the scalpel blade. Will this expensive new technology become the treatment of choice in many of the areas reviewed in this chapter? Will other laser wavelengths replace the Nd:YAG laser in some of these applications? Certainly, this new technology promises eventual cost-effectiveness in that it often obviates the need for external surgical approaches when used endoscopically. It is hoped that controlled studies and the test of time will provide the answers to these important questions.

References

1. Nath G, Gorisch W, Kiefhaber P: First laser endoscopy via fiberoptic transmission system. Endoscopy 5:208–213, 1973.
2. Bown SG: Tumour therapy with the Nd:YAG laser. In Joffe SN, Muckerheide MC, Goldman L (eds): Neodymium-YAG Laser in Medicine and Surgery. Elsevier, New York, 1983, pp 51–58.
3. Shapshay SM, Oliver P: Treatment of hereditary hemorrhagic telangiectasia by Nd-YAG laser photocoagulation. Laryngoscope 94:1554–1556, 1984.
4. Shapshay SM, David LM, Zeitels S: Neodymium-YAG laser photocoagulation of hemangiomas of the head and neck. Laryngoscope 97:323–329, 1986.
5. Joffe SN: Contact neodymium:YAG laser surgery in gastroenterology: A preliminary report. Lasers Surg Med 6:155–157, 1986.
6. Dumon J-F, Reboud E, Garbe L, et al: Treatment of tracheobronchial lesions by laser photoresection. Chest 81:278–284, 1982.
7. Toty L, Personne C, Colchen A, Vourc'h G: Bronchoscopic management of tracheal lesions using the neodymium yttrium aluminum garnet laser. Thorax 36:175–178, 1981.
8. Shapshay SM, Dumon J-F, Beamis JF Jr: Endoscopic treatment of tracheobronchial malignancy: Experience with Nd-YAG and CO_2 lasers in 506 operations. Otolaryngol Head Neck Surg 93:205–210, 1985.
9. Shapshay SM, Beamis JR Jr, Shahian DM: The use of lasers in thoracic surgery (editorial). Chest 87:706–707, 1985.
10. Mizushima K, Marada R, Namik M, et al: Endoscopic therapy of the YAG laser in early gastric cancer and gastric polyp. In Atsumi K, Nimsakul N (eds): Laser Tokyo 81. Inter Group Corp, Tokyo, 1981.
11. Dwyer RM, Yellin AE, Craig J, et al: Gastric hemostasis by laser phototherapy in man: A preliminary report. JAMA 236:1883–1884, 1976.
12. Frühmorgen P, Reidenbach H-D, Bodem F, et al: Experimental examinations on laser endoscopy. Endoscopy 6:116–122, 1974.
13. Fleischer D: Laser therapy of the upper GI tract. In Shapshay SM (ed): Endoscopic Laser Surgery Handbook. Marcel Dekker, New York, 1987.
14. Kiefhaber P, Kiefhaber K, Huber F, Nalb G: Endoscopic applications of Nd:YAG laser radiation in the gastrointestinal tract. In Joffe SN, Muckerheide MC, Goldman L (eds): Neodymium-YAG Laser in Medicine and Surgery. Elsevier, New York, 1983, pp 5–14.
15. Hofstetter A, Frank F: Laser use in urology. In Dixon JA (ed): Surgical Application of Lasers. Year Book Medical Publishers, Chicago, 1983, pp 146–162.
16. Goldrath MH, Fuller TA, Segal S: Laser photovaporization of endometrium for the treatment of menorrhagia. Am J Obstet Gynecol 140:14–19, 1981.
17. Landthaler M, Brunner R, Haina D, et al: First experiences with the Nd:YAG laser in dermatology. In Joffe SN, Muckerheide MC, Goldman L (eds): Neodymium-YAG Laser in Medicine and Surgery. Elsevier, New York, 1983, pp 175–183.

24
Applications of the Nd:YAG Laser in Otorhinolaryngology

Masaru Ohyama, Kouichi Yamashita, Shigeru Furuta, Takuo Nobori and Norio Daikuzono

Treatment of Head and Neck Tumors by Contact Nd:YAG Laser Technique

Masuru Ohyama

Recently, the clinical application of the Nd:YAG laser has begun to assume an increasingly important role, with a multidisciplinary approach to its uses. However, the conventional noncontact Nd:YAG laser system delivers irradiation at some distance, from the target tissue, and this beam spread at the quartz fiber tip causes backscatter and damage to adjacent tissue and vaporization and coagulation of soft tissue is limited.

The convergent Nd:YAG laser system has been made possible by using lenses like the carbon dioxide laser technique, but the target spot of the tissue irradiated by this high power laser beam, 40 to 60 W, becomes carbonized and generates smoke, which often disturbs the surgery. Additionally, the surgeon has to wear special eye glasses to avoid injury by the laser beam as it is reflected by the tissue or instruments.

In order to resolve these problems, we have attempted to devise a laser probe, constructed of a new ceramic, to be attached to the tip of the laser optical quartz fiber. This contact Nd:YAG laser technique would be capable of focusing the laser beam on a target spot, or otherwise diffusing it. Its low power requirement of 6 to 8 W allows a more precise excision of soft tissue, with less bleeding and minimal injury to uninvolved tissue (Figure 24.1). Also, the contact Nd:YAG laser scalpel requires no protection of the eyes from injury by the laser beam.

This chapter is concerned with clinical studies on the effectiveness of this laser treatment in head and neck tumors.[1–4]

Clinical Studies

In our department during the past three years, contact Nd:YAG laser surgery was carried out on 80 patients with head and neck tumors—23 benign and 57 malignant. Of the 23 benign tumors, 9 were in the larynx and oral cavity, 2 were in the nasal cavity, and 3 were in other sites. The histopathologic classification of these tumors showed 7 hemangiomas, 6 granulomas, 6 papillomas, and 4 others. Of the 57 malignant tumors, 23 originated in the oral cavity, 8 in the larynx, 7 in the maxillary sinus, 6 in the nasal cavity, 6 in the hypopharynx, 6 in the tonsils, and 2 in other sites. Histopathologic findings showed 52 specimens of squamous cell carcinoma and 5 specimens of malignant lymphoma and other neoplasms.

Figure 24.2A shows the views during contact Nd:YAG laser excision of tongue cancer (T2, N1, M0) and the resected tissue in a female patient, aged 52. Figure 24.2B indicates the macroscopic findings of a large papilloma in the tongue, the wound sutured with several stitches after removal of the tumor by contact Nd:YAG laser excision, and the extirpated tumor in a male patient, aged 72. Figure 24.3 shows microlaryngoscopic views of a laryngeal granuloma before and after contact Nd:YAG laser microsurgery. There was less bleeding during contact Nd:YAG laser surgery, and the surgical wound healed rapidly in most of the patients with head and neck tumors, especially tumors in the oral cavity, tongue, and larynx (Figure 24.4).

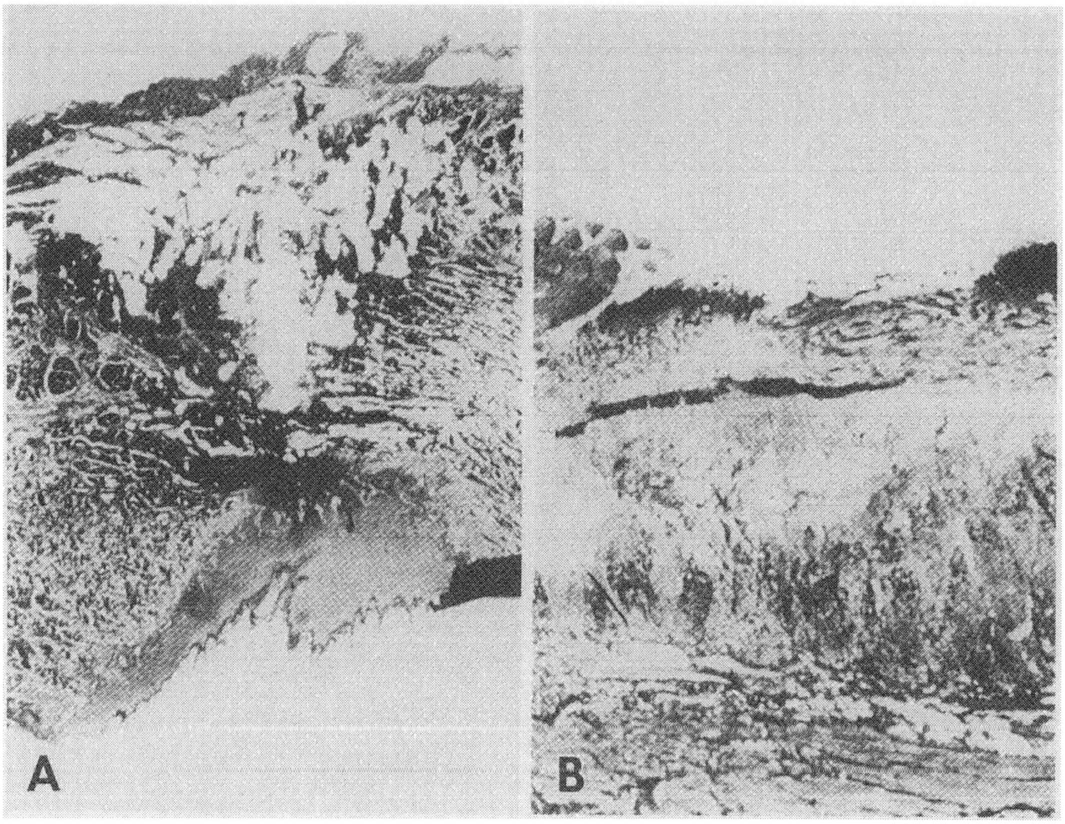

FIGURE 24.1. The histologic appearances of mice buccal mucosa after contact Nd:YAG laser surgery. (*A*) Azan staining immediately after. (*B*) The 3rd day after.

Discussion

The role of laser surgery in the management of head and neck cancer can be divided into the following three categories: (1) removal of the tumor by laser surgery alone, (2) the use of laser surgery as part of a multidisciplinary treatment, and (3) the use of laser irradiation as a palliative treatment.

In general, T1 cancers originating in the mucous membrane of the head and neck region are most suitable for contact Nd:YAG laser excision and may be curable only by this procedure. For T1 malignancies such as oropharyngeal or vocal cord cancer, radiotherapy has been used as the treatment of choice with successful results at many medical facilities. Nevertheless, radiotherapy requires treatment as long as six weeks or more, and furthermore, the possibility of radiation-induced cancer may become a grave problem. Laser surgery, on the other hand, requires only a limited number of operations and there is no risk of radiation-induced cancer.

We have also used the contact Nd:YAG laser technique as part of a multidisciplinary treatment of T2 cancer of the tongue and oral cavity. In hemiglossectomy, the tip of the tongue is threaded and pulled in the opposite direction to give tension. Contact Nd:YAG laser surgery should be performed by maintaining a sufficient safety margin from the cancer tissue. As the contact Nd:YAG laser scalpel touches the target tissue, we can incise, relying on the tactile sense, with a conventional surgical knife. Also, the contact Nd:YAG laser consumes one fifth the light required by the conventional system. At the same time it eliminates the danger of beam reflection for the surgeon because the laser beam is concentrated on the object, and thereby disperses the energy efficiently.

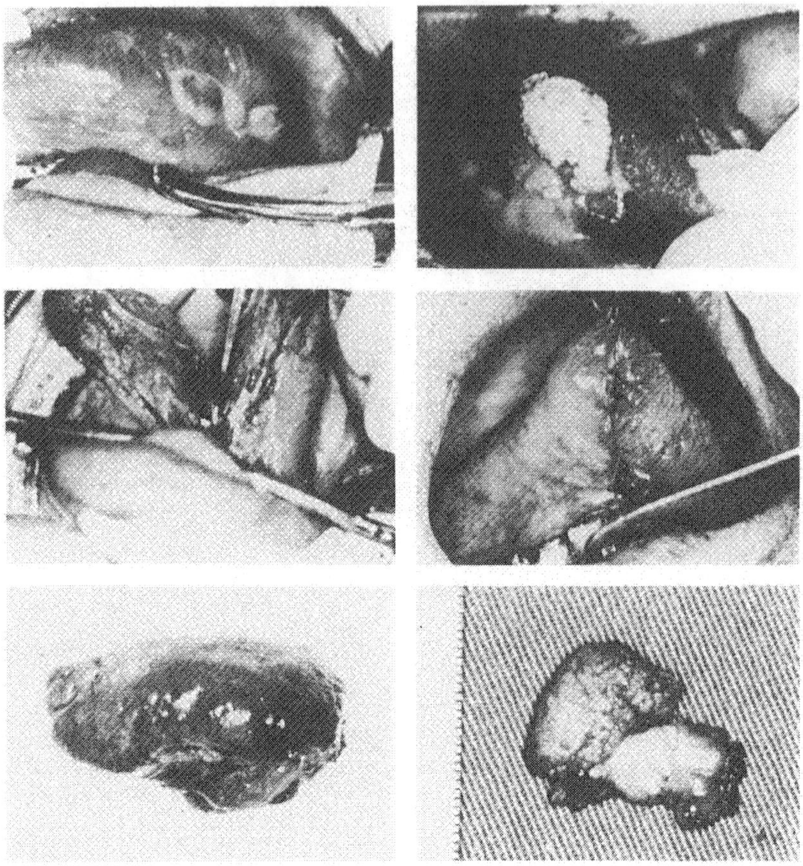

FIGURE 24.2. The photographs were taken during contact Nd:YAG laser surgery of tongue tumors. *(Left)* The upper view shows the preoperative state of tongue cancer (T2, N2, M0). The middle view indicates a shene of hemiglossectomy. The bottom view is the resected tongue tissue with cancer. *(Right)* The upper view shows the preoperative state of tongue papilloma. The middle view shows the sutured wound of tongue after the removal of tumor. The bottom view is the extirpated tumor specimen.

The contact Nd:YAG laser can be applied for skin and mucosal incisions in maxillary cancer. As the operating field in the nasal cavity is very narrow, there is a fear that the excessive bleeding accompanying a mucosal incision may disturb the process of operation visually. But the contact Nd:YAG laser can perform incision and hemostasis simultaneously without such adversity, which makes this technique unparalleled for this type of operation.

The blood vessels with a diameter of 1.5 cm are cut off after coagulation by pulse emission of the laser beam. Moreover, in cases where plastic surgery is necessary, this laser technique is very useful for incision of the skin or muscle. In conclusion, the contact Nd:YAG laser technique will probably be very beneficial in head and neck surgery, and its indications should be expanded through further study.

Summary

The advantages in clinical practice of the contact Nd:YAG laser system are summarized as follows:

1. This system can be performed at a low power of 6 to 8 W in contact laser incision of soft tissue.

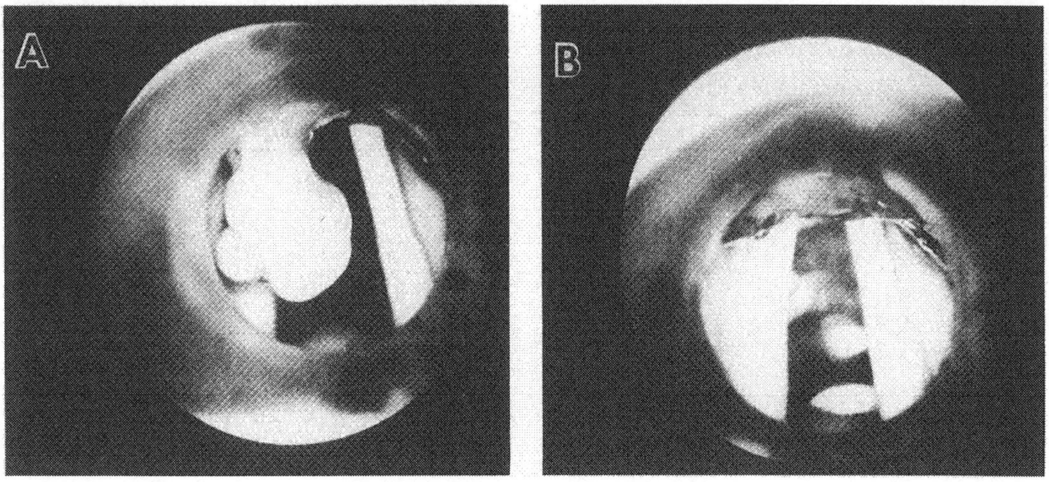

FIGURE 24.3. Laryngoscopic views of glottic granuloma. (*A*) Before contact Nd:YAG laser laryngomicrosurgery. (*B*) After contact Nd:YAG laser laryngomicrosurgery.

2. It permits accurate and precise incision because misshots of laser irradiation can be eliminated in the target tissue.
3. It causes less bleeding with minimal damage to adjacent tissue.
4. It has remarkably high controllability.
5. It causes only slight pain and edema and avoids the proliferation of granulation tissue or scar formation.
6. It may prevent metastasis of cancer cells by sealing up the lymphatic vessels.

On the basis of the results obtained, the contact Nd:YAG laser technique is very useful as one of the treatment modalities in head and neck surgery.

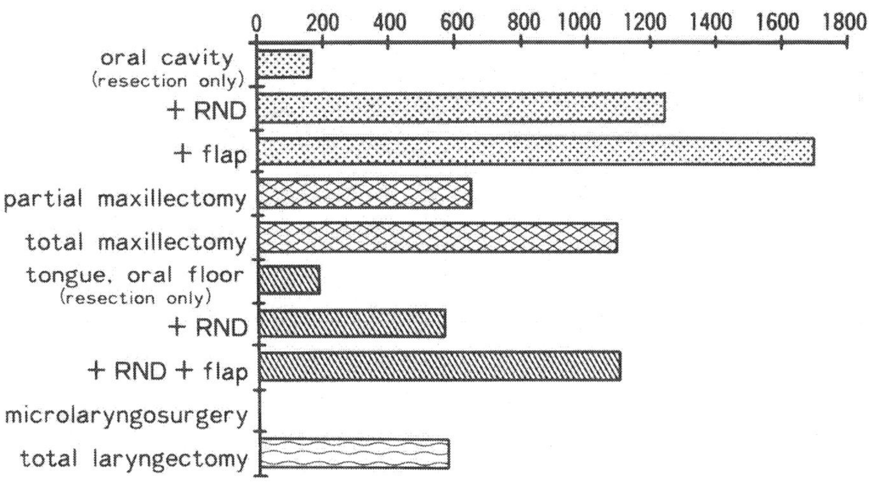

FIGURE 24.4. A comparison of the volume of bleeding in the different kinds of operation during contact Nd:YAG laser surgery.

References

1. Joffe A: Neodymium-YAG Laser in Medicine and Surgery. Elsevier, New York, 1983, pp. 216–239.
2. Ohyama M, Katsuda K, Nobori T, et al: Treatment of head and neck tumors by contact Nd-YAG laser surgery. Auris Nasus Larynx (Tokyo) 12 (Suppl II):S138–S142, 1985.
3. Ohyama M: Near future of laser medicine in otolaryngology and, head and neck surgery. J Jpn Soc Laser Med 6:21–25, 1985.
4. Ohyama M, Nobori T, Ueno K, et al: Contact Nd-YAG laser surgery for head and neck tumor. Pract Otol (Kyoto) 79 (suppl 3):1–9, 1986.

Tonsillectomy and Other Same-Day Laser Applications

Shigeru Furuta and Takuo Nobori

Tonsillectomy and conchotomy are common operative procedures in the practice of otorhinolaryngology. Sudden bleeding and other complications often compromise these operations. It was thought that cryotonsillectomy would resolve these problems, but this procedure has not been taken up enthusiastically throughout the world because it is extremely difficult to control the freezing range in cryosurgery. Another clinical modality, the argon-ion laser, has been reported by Lenz as very promising for tonsillectomy, but its reception has also been lukewarm.

The use of the conventional laser to coagulate, vaporize, or resect soft tissue requires the beam to travel a certain distance to reach the target. Although the Co_2 laser is useful for the vaporization or excision of tissues, it often produces a carbonized layer on the tissue surface. Furthermore, it cannot be used for fine dissection such as tonsillectomy and conchotomy.

On the other hand, the Nd:YAG laser beam may be scattered in the tissue even if the focus is concentrated on the target spot, thereby creating a dispersion of energy. The rise in temperature induced by Nd:YAG laser irradiation is slow and gradual, but the resultant coagulation is significantly more efficient than that produced by the CO_2 laser, with an equal volume of energy.

We have improved the Nd:YAG laser system with our innovation of a microtip or probe constructed from the new ceramic and attached to the tip of the quartz fiber. The probe is used to focus the beam on a target spot or to perform contact laser tonsillectomy and conchotomy. Recently, we have also developed a chisel probe for tonsillectomy.

The present study concerns the new modalities of contact Nd:YAG laser surgery and clinical applications in both tonsillectomy and conchotomy.[1–7]

Development of the Contact Nd:YAG Laser Probe

Figure 24.5 is a schematic representation of the beam pattern of the surgical rod used for general surgery or for conchotomy, and Figure 24-II.1B,C shows the chisel probe used for tonsillectomy. This procedure can be performed with no or minimal bleeding in tonsillectomy and conchotomy. Figure 24.6 shows histologic findings of the tonsil tissue excised with the contact Nd:YAG laser. These is no marked beam damage in the adjacent tissue after dissection by contact Nd:YAG laser irradiation.

Contact Nd:YAG Laser Tonsillectomy

Anesthesia

General anesthesia is usually administered in this operation. After local sterilization, the patient is placed in the supine position on the operating table. The surgeon stands at the cranial side of the patient's head, directly confronting him. Using a Davis mouth retractor, the surgeon opens the mouth wide, and depresses the base

FIGURE 24.5. Schematic drawing of *A*, a surgical rod, *B* and *C*, chisel probes, and their beam patterns.

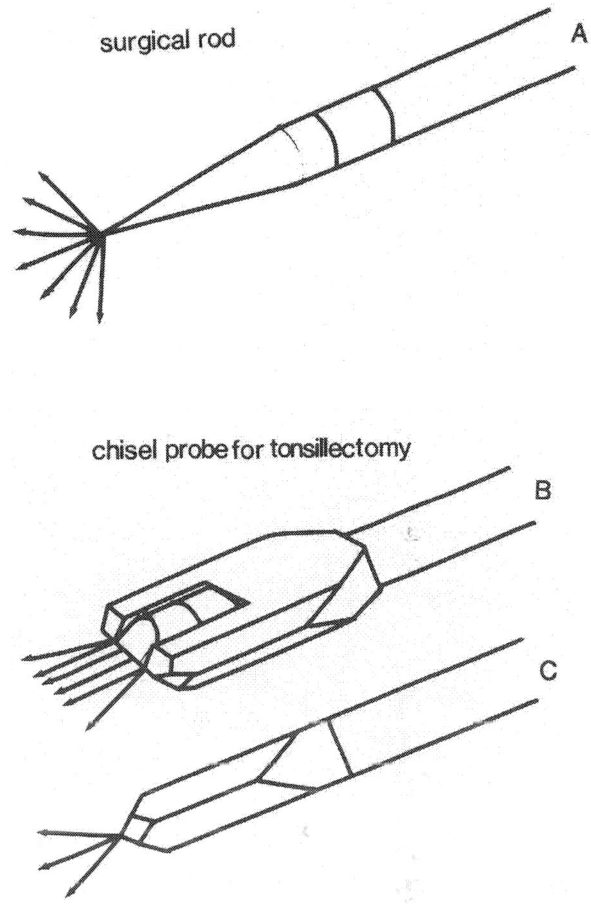

of the tongue and the endotracheal tube so that he has direct visualization of the fossa. Physiologic saline, in a volume of 4–6 ml, is injected into several peritonsillar submucosal layers, in order to prevent excessive parenchymal bleeding during the operation.

Surgical Technique

The surface tissue of the tonsil is grasped with a vulsellum or tonsil clamp and is retracted medially so as to place the posterior tonsillar pillar on a stretch. The saline is injected again into the submucosal layer at the posterior region of the tonsil. With the application of contact Nd:YAG laser irradiation, the pillar mucosa is superficially incised along its attachment to the tonsil.

The laser incision begins at the plica triangularis and then continues superiorly to the supratonsillar fossa. After confirming the tonsillar capsule the tonsillar tissue is prepared away from the surrounding soft tissues by medical retraction. The upper tonsillar pole then is exposed by blunt dissection, using the new chisel probe of the contact Nd:YAG laser. The tonsillar capsule is usually in loose contact with the constrictor muscle posteriorly. Consequently, an initial dissection may be started from this region; the tonsil can be easily enucleated from the fossa by low-power laser irradiation, 10 to 15 W, even if the connective tissue is compact as a result of a previous peritonsillar abscess. Care is taken in the dissection to preserve both tonsillar pillars and constrictor muscles, as well as to avoid penetration through the tonsillar capsule. The lingual tonsil near the base of the palatine tonsil can easily be removed by using a laser beam without scissors or raspatory. These steps are then repeated for removal of the other tonsil.

The fossa is then carefully inspected, and any bleeding is usually controlled by hemostasis

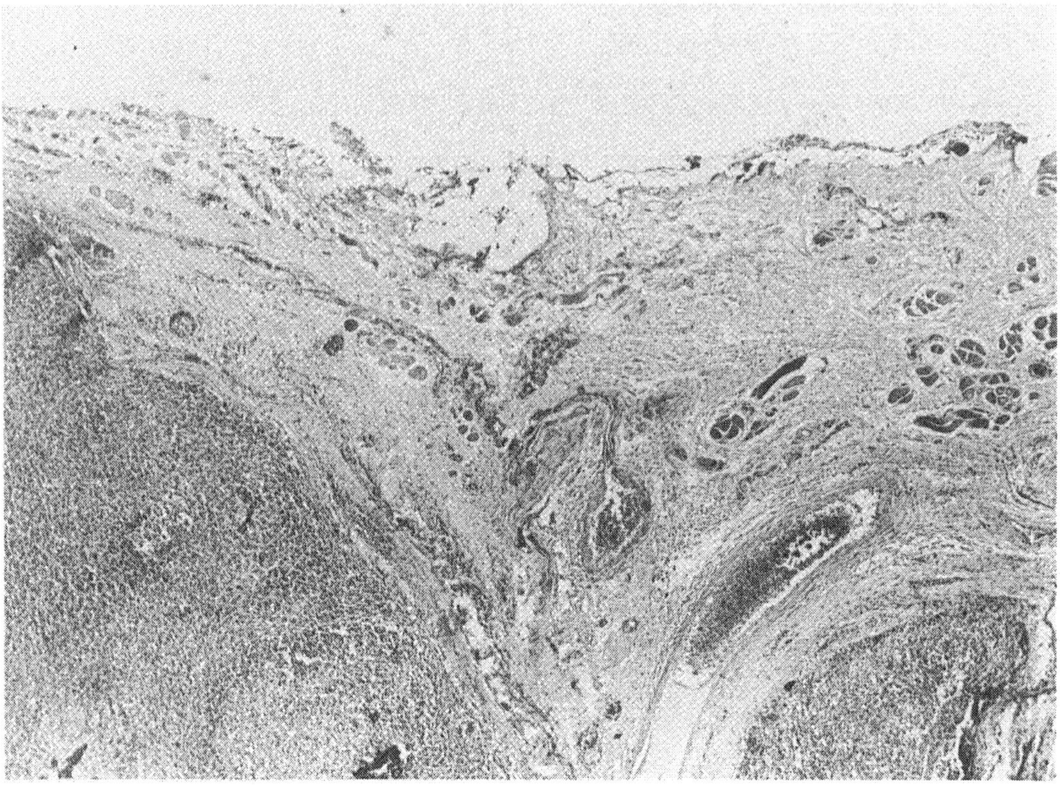

FIGURE 24.6. Histologic findings of a removed tonsil using the contact Nd:YAG laser technique. There is no marked evidence of a coagulated or carbonized tissue layer.

achieved by localized laser vaporization. However, excessive sponging or suction may disrupt retracted vessels or remove vital factors necessary for normal coagulation. Profuse bleeding from the vessel should be avoided because the internal carotid artery could be injured. After the bleeding is under control, topical thrombin should be applied; this powder expands within the tonsillar fossae and controls hemorrhage. In most instances, adequate hemostasis is the result of careful surgical dissection and direct control of bleeding vessels.

Postoperative Care

In the period immediately following a tonsillectomy under general anesthesia, the patient is taken to a recovery room and placed on his side. This allows easy removal of secretions from the mouth or pharynx, although care is taken not to injure the tonsillar fossae with a suction apparatus.

Diet and activity are gradually advanced as tolerated. Normal activities can be resumed with in two weeks. Generally speaking, local treatment of the oral region is necessary at one week, and medical follow-up is commonly one month after surgery. Various foods may be prohibited during the immediate postoperative period, primarily those foods with significant roughage that might injure the pharynx or induce bleeding. Periods of food prohibition vary from one to three days postoperatively, after which normal diets are resumed.

Clinical Results

Contact Nd:YAG laser tonsillectomy was performed in 10 patients—5 males, 5 females, aged 6 to 51 years—with chronic tonsillitis during the past 7 months. One patient had had a previous episode of peritonsillar abscess. For this application, the Nd:YAG laser was set at a low power of 10 to 15 W, in the continuous wave mode,

TABLE 24.1. Clinical evaluation of tonsillectomy using contact Nd:YAG laser with a new dissector

Case no.	Age (years)	Sex	Dissector	Ligation	Pain*	Diet**	Complications
1	14	M	Rod	—	1	1	—
2	33	M	Rod	—	2	5	—
3	23	F	Rod	—	7	8	—
4	29	F	Chisel	+	3	4	—
5	24	M	Rod	—	3	3	—
6	17	M	Rod and chisel	—	0	1	Infection
7	49	M	Rod	—	1	3	—
8	51	F	Chisel	—	1	2	—
9	6	F	Chisel	—	1	2	—
10	11	F	Chisel	—	2	3	—

*Duration of pain after the operation (days).
**Beginning of normal diet (days).

with a total delivered energy of 3000 to 6000 J. Table 24.1 indicates the clinical evaluation of tonsillectomy wtih the contact Nd:YAG laser and accessories. In 5 of our cases a surgical rod was attached to the laser, in 5 cases a chisel probe was affixed, and in 1 case we used both the rod and the chisel probe (Figure 24.7).

After this laser tonsillectomy the patients were relieved of chronic tonsillitis. They had sore throat for one to three days postoperatively. However, the laser wound did not heal as quickly as the wound produced by classical tonsillectomy procedures, and complete epithelization took about 14 days. A normal diet was resumed three days after surgery. One patient had a mild localized infection, which responded to oral antibiotics.

Contact Nd:YAG Laser Conchotomy

Anesthesia

Local anesthesia is administered for contact Nd:YAG laser conchotomy. After general sterilization, the patient is placed in a supine position on the operation table. The surgeon stands at the lateral side of the patient's shoulder. After stabilizing the nasal speculum, with the aid of a head mirror the surgeon inspects the nasal chambers. An anesthetic solution of 4% lidocaine with epinephrine (1:1000) is applied to the mucous membrane of the nasal cavity. Then, 4 ml of 0.5% lidocaine is injected into the submucosal layer of the inferior turbinate.

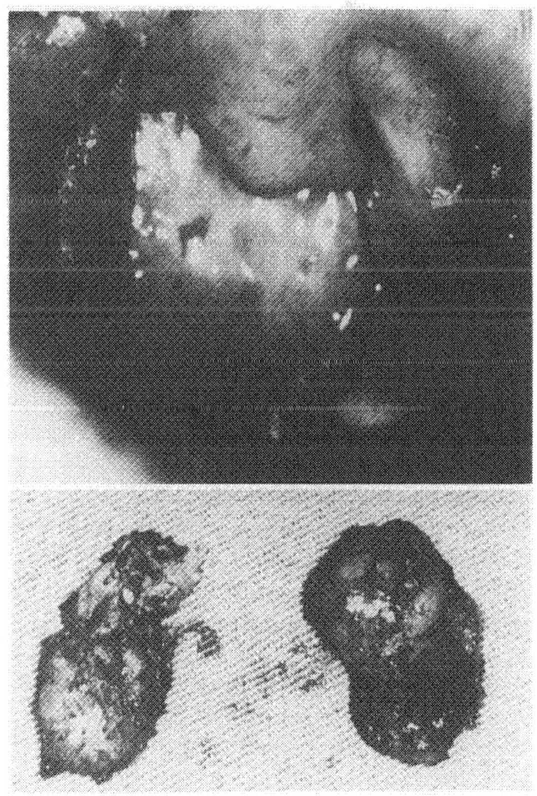

FIGURE 24.7. *(Top)* Postoperative tonsillar fossae. *(Bottom)* The removed tonsils in case 6 (see text and Table 24-II.1).

Surgical Technique

The surgeon stabilizes the nasal speculum with his left index finger. The surgical rod (Figure 24-II.1A) attached to the Nd:YAG laser is used

TABLE 24.2. Clinical evaluation of conchotomy using the contact Nd:YAG laser technique

Diagnosis	No. of Patients	Age (mean)	No packing	Complications
Allergic rhinitis	8	26.1	2	0
Hypertrophic rhinitis	7	31.8	0	0

to make an incision on the anterior point of the inferior turbinate. The turbinate mucosa is dissected through the turbinate periosteum by the irradiation of the contact Nd:YAG laser beam. Before surgery, it is necessary to prepare for postoperative blockage by using gauze with antibiotic ointment to suppress bleeding from the resection wound. After surgery, however, nasal packing is not required because there is no bleeding from the incision wound.

Clinical Results

During a period of two years, we performed contact Nd:YAG laser conchotomy on 15 patients, aged 12 to 58 years with allergic (8 patients) or hypertrophic (7 patients) rhinitis. Table 24.2 indicates the clinical evaluation of conchotomy with the contact Nd:YAG laser technique. Satisfactory results were obtained in all the patients with nasal obstruction. Postoperatively, two patients were free from the blockage of the gauze-applied ointment in the nasal cavity. Figure 24.8 shows pre- and postoperative views of the nasal cavity in a patient with allergic rhinitis. Seven days after the operation a fibrin mass and crust had formed on the surface of the inferior turbinate but in one month regeneration of the epithelium was good in the surgical fields.

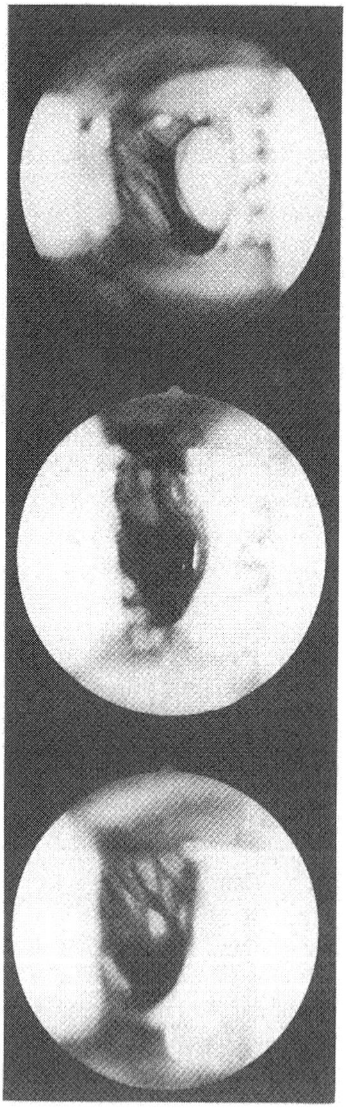

FIGURE 24.8. Postoperative findings in a conchotomy of the inferior turbinate, using the contact Nd:YAG laser technique on a patient with allergic rhinitis. (*Top*) Before the operation. (*Middle*) One week after the operation. (*Bottom*) Two months after the operation.

Discussion

A total removal of the tonsillar tissue with minimum bleeding and minimum trauma to adjacent tissues is the primary goal in tonsillectomy. A guillotine-type tonsillectomy as well as tonsillectomy are useful in children with extremely swollen tonsils, although dissection techniques using tonsil snares may be more common at the present time. On occasion, cryosurgical tonsillectomy has been performed successfully in selected patients. In other patients, electrocoagulation of the tonsils has been advocated. However, regardless of the method used in tonsillectomy, the skill and experience of the surgeon predict the technical success of the procedure. As previously noted, selected procedures are usually carried out in very young patients in whom even minimal blood loss results in significant whole-body fluid volume depletion. Selective procedures are also performed if excessive bleeding is encountered or if unexpected problems arise during surgery that necessitate rapid termination of the procedure. On the other hand, the carbonization caused by the CO_2 laser and the electrocoagulator hinder the surgeon from certifying the capsule of the tonsil. For this reason the tonsillar wound grows larger and larger, and there is a possibility that the surgeon will leave part of the tonsillar tissue at the site.

Nd:YAG surgery has been performed in otorhinolaryngology since 1981. The vaporization approach of noncontact laser surgery has been successfully carried out on lesions in this category. However, recently we developed a ceramic rod, which, attached to the contact Nd:YAG laser we have used in the surgery of head and neck tumors.

Our distress at the excessive bleeding concomitant with conventional tonsillectomy and conchotomy led us to new procedures. We developed two new dissectors, a ceramic rod and chisel probe, and attached them to the contact Nd:YAG laser. We have used these new accessories, both separately and in combination, very effectively in our recent tonsillectomies and conchotomies.

Summary

The advantages of the contact Nd:YAG laser technique for tonsillectomy and conchotomy are as follows:

1. It can be used at a low power of 10 to 15 W in the incision of mucous membrane or the dissection of soft tissue.
2. It has a remarkably high controllability.
3. It causes less bleeding, with minimal damage to adjacent tissue.
4. A normal diet can be resumed relatively soon after surgery because postoperative edema and pain are negligible.

On the basis of the results obtained, the contact Nd:YAG laser technique is clinically beneficial as one of the operative modalities for both tonsillitis and hyperthrophic or allergic rhinitis.

References

1. Joffe A. Neodymium-YAG Laser in Medicine and Surgery. Elsevier, New York, 1983, pp 216–239.
2. Ohyama M, Nobori T, Ueno K: Contact YAG laser surgery for the treatments of head and neck tumors. Pract Otol (Kyoto) 79(S3):1–9, 1986.
3. Ohyama M, Nobori T, Yamamoto M: Clinical evaluation of the contact YAG laser irradiation applied to the nasal and paranasal lesion. Pract Otol (Kyoto) 79: , 1986.
4. Ohyama M, Nobori T, Miyazaki Y, et al: Contact Nd-YAG laser surgery in the treatment of the head and neck tumors. In Laser / Optoelectronics in Medicine. Springer-Verlag, Berlin, 1986, pp 432–437.
5. Lenz H: Tonsillectomie mit einem Laserraspatorium. Laryngol Rhinol Otol 63:582–584, 1984.
6. Ohyama M, Katsuda K, Nobori T, et al: Treatment of head and neck tumors by contact Nd-YAG laser surgery. Auris Nasus Larynx (Tokyo) 12:s138–s142, 1985.
7. Almqvist U: Cryosurgical treatment of tonsillar hypertrophy in children. J Laryngol Otol (London) 100:311–314, 1986.

Flexible Fiberoptic Endoscopic Applications of the Nd:YAG Laser
A. Application in Chronic Sinusitis

Masaru Ohyama

Chronic sinusitis is a common rhinologic disorder. Severe cases of chronic sinusitis have gradually decreased during the past 20 years, but there are still a large number that require surgery. Many attempts have been made to assure satisfactory surgical treatment, but with limited success until now. The Denker-Watsuji and Caldwell-Luc radical sinuectomies are generally used for treatment of chronic sinusitis. With these techniques it is necessary to remove all of the pathologic sinus mucosa. At the end of the operation, a drainage hole is made in the inferior meatus, where the medial wall of the antrum has thick bone. Later, this drainage route often becomes blocked. In addition, the larger fenestration made in the canine fossa may be responsible for neuralgic pains and hypesthesia of the teeth and around the upper lip. Finally, the sinus mucosa is often removed unnecessarily.

To overcome this unsatisfactory procedure, we have designed a new surgical technique that produces minimal trauma and takes into consideration the physiologic anatomy of the nose and paranasal sinuses. Since 1983 we have performed Nd:YAG laser antrostomy, using a flexible fiberscope for chronic sinusitis.[1–3]

Pathophysiology of Chronic Sinusitis

The causes of mucosal pathology in chronic sinusitis are numerous. Great importance is attributed to the ostium, mucociliary function, and characteristics of sinus secretion.

Owing to such inflammatory factors as shown in Figure 24.9, there is often a blocked ostium due to local infection, trauma, or swelling of the nasal mucosa.

In the closed sinus, oxygen is absorbed and the pressure may fall. A blocked ostium facilitates transudation and mucous secretion, and consequently, provides a salutary environment for bacterial invasion or growth. In such cases, mucociliary function is disturbed by an engorged and suppurative mucous layer. A vicious circle thus commences, as illustrated in Figure 24.9.

Surgical Procedure

Local anesthesia is usually used for most of this operation. With the contact Nd:YAG laser technique a mucosal incision with a diameter of about 1.5 cm along the labiogingival line is made laterally from the root of the canine tooth. The incision is carried down to the bone and the soft tissue of the cheek and the periosteum are elevated.

A fenestration in the canine fossa is made just large enough to permit the access of instruments and general inspection of the antrum. This fenestration, with a diameter of 8 mm, is made with a bone drill using a perforating burr on the appropriate level of the sinus wall, as determined by x-ray examination. Through the hole, the sinus can be observed with the flexible fiberscope, and the Nd:YAG laser beam is used to vaporize the pathologic mucosa. The nonpathologic sinus mucosa is untouched and promotes reepithelization of the vaporized focus.

Figure 24.10 shows a flexible fiberscope with the Nd:YAG laser quartz fiber placed into a fenestration in the canine fossa. The Nd:YAG laser beam vaporizes the transmaxillary closed

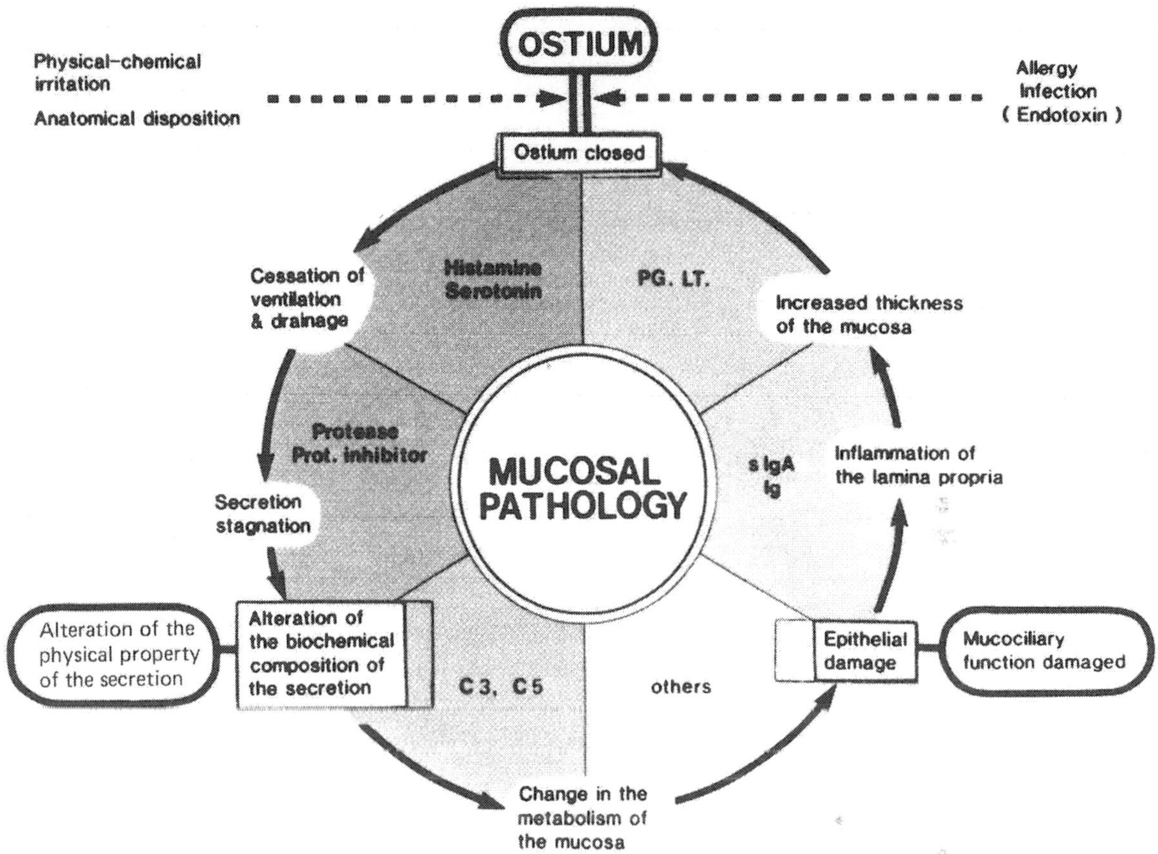

FIGURE 24.9. The relationship between the pathobiochemistry of the sinus mucosa and the vicious circle of sinus inflammation.

natural ostium so that a middle meatus can be widened and antrostomy can be carried out. Mucociliary transport inside the antrum is directed toward the natural ostium, and secretions are expelled out of the new large opening. Two silk sutures are used to close the mucosal incision.

Ethmoidal cells adjacent to the natural ostium are often diseased, and the removal of pathologic mucosal or nasal polyps is obligatory for the success of this operation, as infection in these cells may be responsible for creating edema and stenosis of the ostium.

Indications for the Operation

The indications for Nd:YAG laser antrostomy with a flexible fiberscope are as follows:

1. Chronic maxillary sinusitis
2. Antral polyps and cysts
3. Sinus bleeding
4. Localized tumor in the sinus

Clinical Results

Table 24.3 shows the efficacy of antrostomy with Nd:YAG laser irradiation using the fiberscopic technique. This operation was carried out in 98 patients with chronic sinusitis during the years 1983 to 1985. Based on the results of both subjective and objective findings, followed up over six months after the operation, 73 patients (74.5%) were markedly improved, 23 (23.5%) showed moderate improvement, while only 2 (2.0%) showed no improvement.

Figure 24.11 shows the comparative x-ray findings of healing conditions in the sinus for the Nd:YAG laser antrostomy on the right side and the Caldwell-Luc operation on the left side, at one week to six months after the operation. It can be seen that there is more remarkable

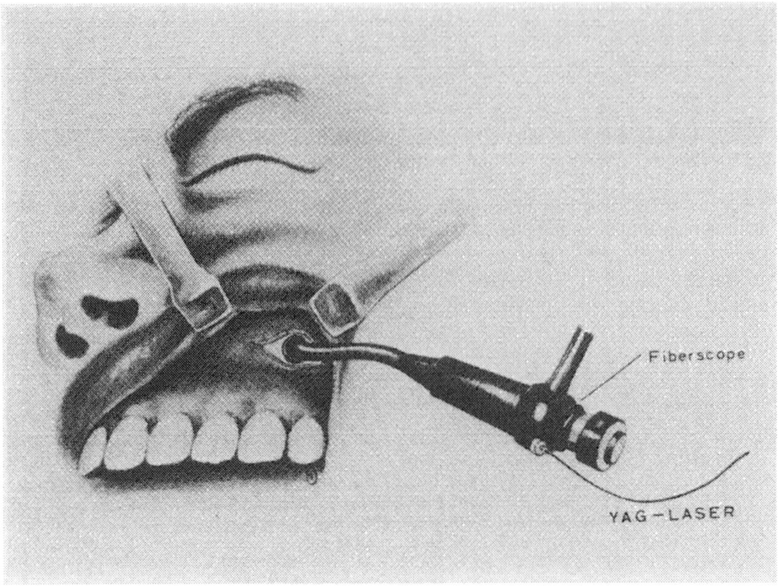

FIGURE 24.10. Schematic representation of the status of the flexible fiberscope with Nd:YAG laser optic quartz fiber introduced into the sinus bony hole.

evidence of aeration in the right antrum, showing the original sinus configuration.

TABLE 24.3. Clinical results based on both subjective and objective findings over 6 months after Nd:YAG laser antrostomy

Evaluation	Male	Female	Total	Rate (%)
Good	53	20	73	74.5
Fair	12	11	23	23.5
Poor	2	0	2	2.0
Total	67	31	98	100

Discussion

There have been various surgical treatments of paranasal sinusitis. The most popular operations for chronic maxillary sinusitis were developed by Caldwell and Luc and Watsuji and Denker. These operations resulted sometimes in unexpected trouble for patients owing to hyperplasia of granulation and inflamed remnants of the sinus mucosa.

To overcome these unsatisfactory procedures we have developed a new technique of Nd:YAG laser antrostomy using a flexible fiberscope for chronic maxillary sinusitis. This new approach to the surgical treatment of chronic sinusitis is based on anatomic, physiologic, and pathobiochemical considerations.

The advantages of this technique for maxillary sinusitis are summarized as follows:

1. The normal anatomic and physiologic relationships are restored.
2. Any pathologic changes involving the maxillary sinus can be observed by direct visualization.
3. Less bleeding and minimum mucosal damage during the operation are seen.
4. The severe sequelae of the conventional technique of sinus operation can be reduced or eliminated.
5. Postoperative care can be simple.

Nd:YAG laser antrostomy using a flexible fiberscope is therefore a promising new treatment for chronic maxillary sinusitis.

Summary

In 1983 we developed a new operation technique for chronic sinusitis: Nd:YAG laser antrostomy using a flexible fiberscope. This procedure was performed in 98 patients with chronic sinusitis during the years 1983 to 1985.

Better results and fewer complications were obtained by this new operation than with the conventional techniques such as the Caldwell-Luc or Watsuji-Denker operations.

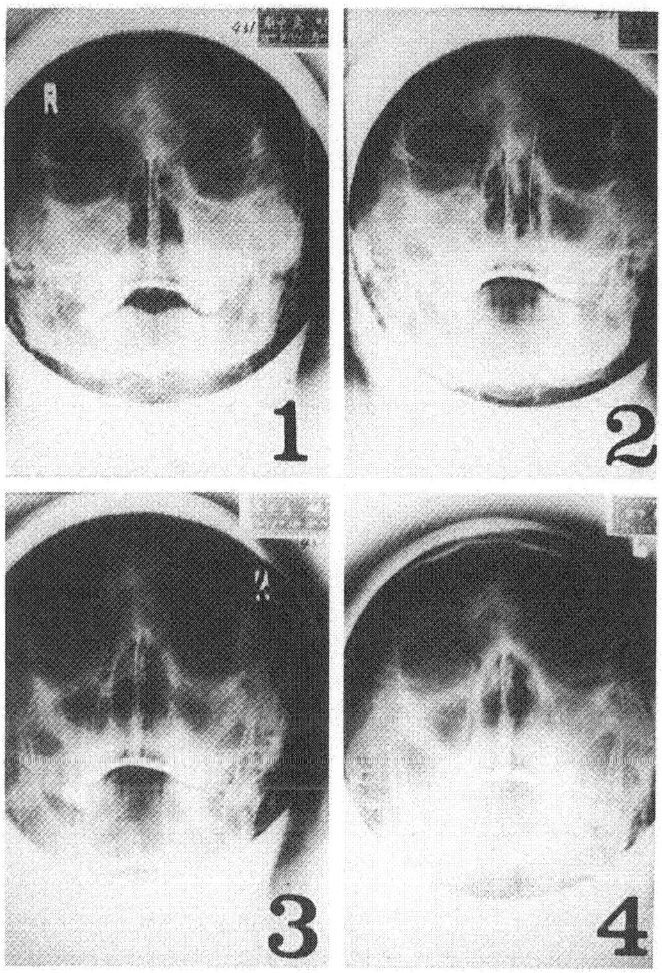

FIGURE 24.11. A comparison of x-ray findings of the postoperative sinus state by the Caldwell-Luc operation and by Nd:YAG laser antrostomy. (*1*) Preoperative x-ray findings of sinusitis. (*2*) X-ray findings of sinus one week after the Caldwell-Luc operation of the left maxillary sinusitis. (*3*) X-ray findings of sinus one week after Nd:YAG laser antrostomy of the right sinus, at an interval of one week following the left sinus operation. (*4*) X-ray findings of the sinus 6 months after the last operation.

References

1. Ohyama, M: Pathobiochemistry of Chronic Sinusitis. Shibundo, Kagoshima, 1984.
2. Ohyama, M: Laser treatment for sinus diseases. Pract Otol. (Kyoto) 79:694–697, 1986.
3. Matsune S, Miyazaki Y, Ueno K, et al: Histopathological study of nasal ostium in experimental sinusitis in rabbits. Oto Rhino Laryngol (Tokyo) 255–262, 1986.

B. Applications in Nasopharyngeal Diseases

Kouichi Yamashita

In otorhinolaryngology the CO_2 laser has been effectively applied for laryngeal diseases by use of the operating microscope and other accessible means from outside the body. However, application of the Nd:YAG laser through the flexible fiberscope is expected to lead to further efficiency of laser surgery in difficult-to-reach sites.

In the nasopharynx, the Nd:YAG laser through the flexible fiberscope inserted perinasally has no dead angles and all sites of the nasopharyngeal structure are accessible. Thus, Nd:YAG laser surgery is indicated as an efficient method to manage nasopharyngeal pathology.

Dissimilar Characteristics of Laser Beams

The CO_2 and Nd:YAG lasers are distinctly different. The CO_2 laser beam is totally absorbed on the tissue surface, therefore its effects are superficial and well-defined, resulting in direct evaporation of the tissue. The Nd:YAG laser beam can penetrate the tissue and coagulate it. The absorption of the Nd:YAG laser beam and the capacity to backscatter are contingent on the color of the tissue to which the beam is applied. The different characteristics of these beams must be taken into consideration when therapy is administered.

Method of Treatment

To introduce the Nd:YAG laser beam into the nasopharynx, a thin Teflon-coated quartz guide, 1.1 mm diameter, is used. The fiber guide is introduced through the instrumentation channel of the Olympus ENF-LB fiberscope, and irradiation is performed under visual control. The tip of the laser guide is usually protruded approximately 5 mm in length on irradiation. Since the diameter of the channel of the ENF-LB scope is 2 mm, the thicker laser guide with its air insufflation lumen cannot be applied. Therefore, air insufflation is made through the scope channel itself to remove smoke during coagulation. The 1.1-mm laser guide can also be used as a contact laser coagulator by itself.

To generate the Nd:YAG laser beam, the Nd:YAG laser coagulators of Molectron Model 8000, Olympus MYL-1, and Pentax SLY-1 have been used. The procedure is performed using a television monitor under general anesthesia. This way, the safety of the surgeon's eye and of the patient himself may be ensured (Figure 24.12).[1–3]

Indications and Cases

Indications for this procedure were selected as follows.

(1) Hypertrophied tubal tonsil on and around the tubal torus of the eustachian tube at the nasopharynx, which is considered to be the cause of tubal dysfunction in cases of persistent secretory otitis media or middle ear cholesteatoma.

Eighteen patients, ranging from 4 to 38 years of age, were treated for this disorder with the Nd:YAG laser and flexible fiberscope.

(2) Benign and malignant neoplasms of the nasopharynx. Nasopharyngeal angiofibroma, nasopharyngeal carcinoma, and malignant lymphoma are relatively common neoplasms in the nasopharynx, and lymphangioma, hemangioma, neurilemoma, paraganglioma, and papilloma are found less frequently. Because of the anatomic situation, nasopharyngeal neoplasms tend to be found at a rather advanced stage and larger size.

One patient with nasopharyngeal extension of glomus jugulare tumor and one patient with Stage III nasopharyngeal carcinoma were treated with the Nd:YAG laser and flexible fiberscope.

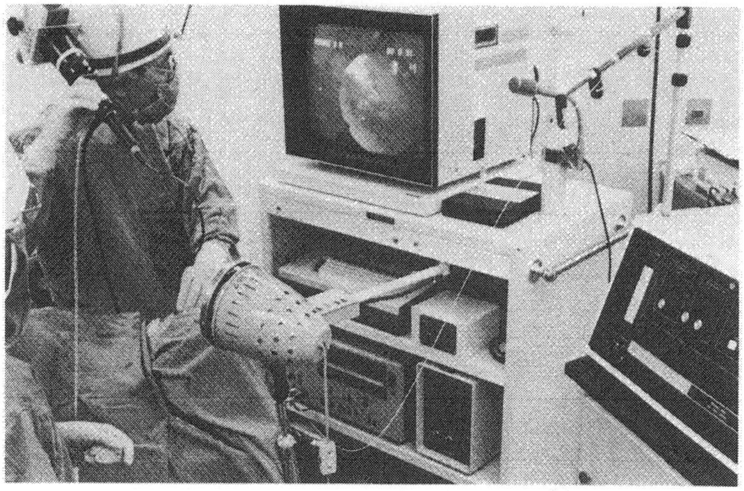

FIGURE 24.12. Nd:YAG laser surgery procedure with use of closed-circuit television.

Results and Discussion

Hypertrophied Tubal Tonsil Causing Tubal Dysfunction

The tubal tonsil is found on the tubal torus at its postrior half side and continues to the Rosenmüller fossa. In cases of markedly hypertropied tubal tonsil, it is also observed at the Rosenmüller fossa, filling the fossa and the anterior surface of the torus facing the tubal orifice. Since adenoid enlargement is also complicated in such cases, laser application follows adenoidectomy by the usual methods. Coagulation is not performed around the orifice to avoid a scarred stricture of the orifice after irradiation. The energy level of the Nd:YAG laser beam is limited to below 30 W to prevent too much penetration, which will result in destruction of the tubal cartilage underneath the torus. In this procedure, 15 to 25 W has proved to be sufficient.

It is characteristic that granulation formation after laser coagulation is minimal. The superposition of necrotic debris is observed for 1 week after irradiation. However, the wound heals completely after 3 weeks (Figure 24.13).

The results of 18 cases treated are shown in Table 24.4, classified by age. The best results were obtained in the group from 13 to 23 years old; yet 100% of the cases showed good results. In the age group below 10 years, 90% of the cases showed an improvement of tubal dysfunction. Less improvement in this age group may result

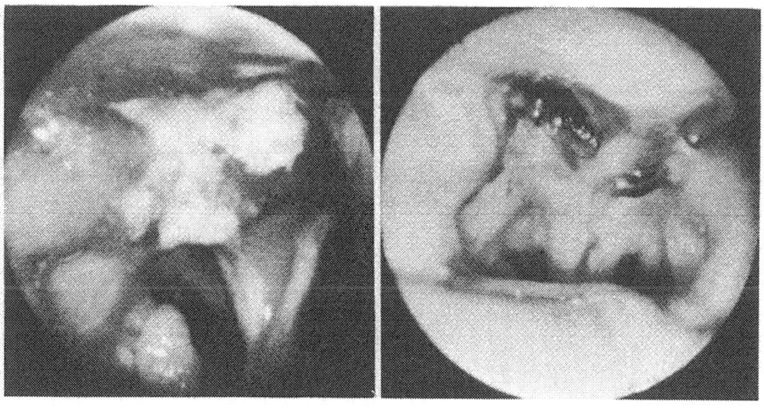

FIGURE 24.13. Pre- and postoperative (10 months) conditions of hypertrophied tubal tonsil, showing marked improvement around the tubal orifice after surgery.

TABLE 24.4. Patients receiving Nd:YAG laser treatment for tubal dysfunction due to tubal tonsil hypertrophy*

Case	Age (years)	Ear diseases	Duration of ear diseases (years)	Additional surgery	Imporovement of tubal function	Tympanogram Preop	Tympanogram Postop
1 KY	4	r. SOM	2		+	B	C
		l. SOM			+	B	B
2* MN	4	r. ate	3		+	B	B
		l. ate			+ +	B	C
3 YY	5	r. SOM	10 mos		+ +	B	C
		l. SOM			+ +	B	C
4 FH	5	r. cho	3		+ + +	B	A
		l. cho			+ + +	B	A
5 OT	6	r. cho	3		+ + +	B	A
		l. normal			Good condition	A	A
6 KT	6	r. COM	4	Myringoplasty	+ +	—	B
		l. normal			Good condition	A	A
7* OY	6	r. SOM	3	Tubing	+ + +	B	A
		l. SOM		Tubing	+ +	B	C
8 DS	6	r. COM	5		+	—	—
		l. SOM		Myringotomy	+	B	Cs
9 KA	6	r. SOM	2	Tubing	−	B	—
		l. SOM		Tubing	−	B	—
10 MK	8	r. SOM	4	Myringotomy	+ +	B	C
		l. SOM			+ +	B	A
11 TK	13	r. cho	6		+ + +	—	B
		l. cho		Tympanoplasty	+ + +	As	A
12 SA	14	r. ret	(1)	Tympanoplasty	+ + +	C	A
		l. SOM			+ + +	B	As
13 AH	14	r. SOM	10		+ +	B	C
		l. SOM			+ +	B	C
14 SK	16	r. ret	(1)		+ + +	A	A
		l. cho		Tympanoplasty	+ + +	B	Cs
15 SS	23	r. pos	7	Tympanoplasty	+ + +	—	Cs
		l. SOM			+ + +	C	A
16 NJ	31	r. ate	20	Typanoplasty	−	—	—
		l. pos		Tympanoplasty	−	—	—
17 IM	36	r. sca	20		−	A	—
		l. ate			−	B	—
18 MS	38	r. COM	10	Tympanoplasty	−	—	C
		l. COM		Tympanoplasty	−	—	C

*All the patients are male-except Case 2 and Case 7.
SOM: secretory otitis media, COM: chronic otitis media, cho: cholesteatoma, ret: retracted ear drum, pos: postoperative, sca: scarred ear drum, ate: atelectatic ear

from immaturation of the tubal function, which is not controlled by this procedure. Three patients over 30 years old showed no improvement of tubal function. In these cases, the tubal dysfunctions were considered to be of tubotympanal origin secondary to a long-standing pathologic condition of the tubal orifice area.

It can be concluded that the Nd:YAG laser surgery is one of the most effective and appropriate treatments against hypertrophied lymphoid tissue causing tubal dysfunction.

Benign and Malignant Neoplasms of the Nasopharynx

Since the Nd:YAG laser is regarded as a coagulator, when it is applied to neoplasms, the treatment is mainly palliative (Figures 24.14 and 24.15). Certain limited and circumscribed lesions of benign and also malignant neoplasms can be treated curatively. In a proliferative lesion, effective destruction is attained by an application of high-energy laser of 50 to 100 W.

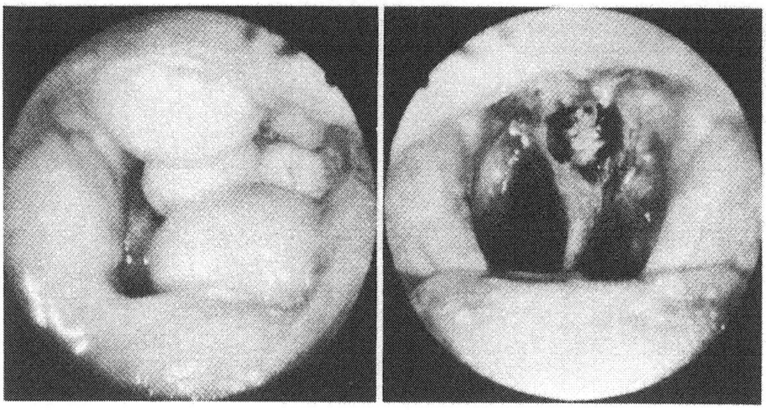

FIGURE 24.14. Nasopharyngeal extension of glomus jugulare tumor, pre- and postoperative. Surgery was performed palliatively for airway obstruction.

Bony tissue is relatively to the Nd:YAG laser beam and it plays a protective role in extending its effect to the posterior direction. However, the surgeon should take special care of the anatomy of the internal carotid artery, the internal jugular vein, and caudal cranial nerves that are just lateral to the nasopharynx in the parapharyngeal space. Therefore, in cases with nasopharyngeal malignant neoplasm, only limited lesions indicate sufficient need for Nd:YAG laser surgery. To investigate the indication in such cases, a high resolution CT of the nasopharynx and the parapharyngeal space provides indispensable assistance. When the Nd:YAG laser beam is applied to the nasopharyngeal cavity, the surgeon should also take care of the effect of the penetrated laser beam to the musculature underneath the mucous membrane at the soft palate, which may cause postoperative immobility due to cicatricial contracture of the tissue.

Conclusion

Nd:YAG laser surgery, with the flexible fiberscope attached, is appropriately applicable to nasopharyngeal pathology. It has been found that this is one of the most effective procedures against hypertrophied tubal tonsil causing longstanding tubal dysfunction, to which no appropriate and effective therapeutic procedure has been established.

Certain limited and circumscribed lesions of

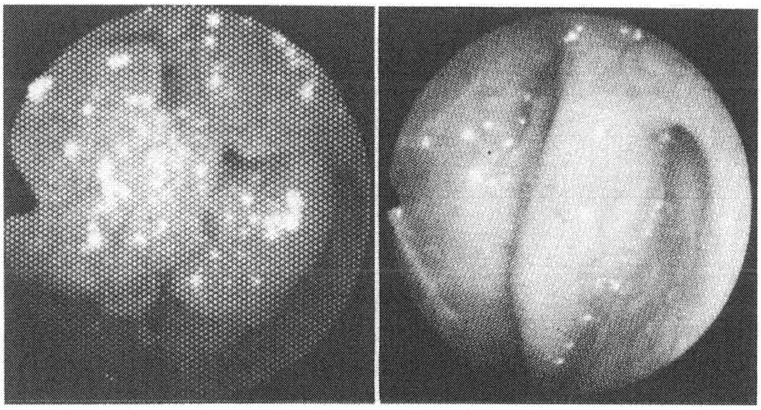

FIGURE 24.15. Nasopharyngeal cancer, pre- and postoperative. The extension of the tumor to the parapharyngeal space was not controlled by this procedure.

benign and malignant neoplasms in the nasopharynx are also good indications for Nd:YAG laser surgery.

References

1. Yamashita K, Ogawa A: The use of Nd:YAG laser in the management of nasopharyngeal pathology. J Jpn Laser Med 4:229–230, 1984.
2. Buiter CT: Endoscopic Nd:YAG laser therapy in the upper airways. In Clement PAR (ed): Recent Advances in E.N.T. endoscopy. Scientific Society for Medical Information Gent, Belgium, 1985, pp 197–205.
3. Yamashita K, Sakamoto M, Ogawa A, et al: Management of tubal tonsil hypertrophy by means of Nd:YAG laser. Jpn J Tonsil 24:70–76, 1985.

Clinical Trials of Interstitial Localized Nd:YAG Laser Hyperthermia on Head and Neck Malignancies

Masaru Ohyama and Norio Daikuzono

In recent years, remarkable progress has been made in thermotherapy. This technique has proven to be one of the most promising methods available for treatment of cancer. However, treatment using microwave or radiofrequencies has been limited to thoracoabdominal malignancies. There is little information on localized laser hyperthermia or on the conventional hyperthermia technique applied to head and neck tumors.

We have developed a ceramic probe to insert into tumor tissue and irradiate the laser omnidirectionally. This probe can heat a spherical range of 1.5 cm to 43°C. This is applicable as interstitial localized laser hyperthermia (laser hyperthermia).

This chapter concerns experimental and clinical studies on the effectiveness of laser hyperthermia using our technique in the head and neck regions.[1–4]

Experimental Studies

The Effects of Laser Hyperthermia on Normal Rabbit Mucosa

Morphologic and biochemical investigations were carried out on rabbit tongue and lip after laser hyperthermia. Figure 24-IV.1A shows the typical histopathology on the third day after treatment. There is no remarkable tissue damage in the heated area. Furthermore, immunohistochemical study by laminin staining (Figure 24.16) showed evidence of a steady regeneration of the basal membrane, and the blood vessels of the hyperthermic wounds were gradually healing and were completely healed one week later. Quantitative analysis performed immediately after laser hyperthermia, and again 3 days later, showed that lipoxygenase metabolites such as 5-HETE, 12-HETE, and 15-HETE and cyclooxygenase metabolites such as PGE_2, indicators of inflammation, had increased moderately; but after the seventh day these arachidonic acid metabolites had returned to normal levels (Figure 24.17).

These results and histologic findings revealed that the effect of laser hyperthermia on normal tissue is very slight, and, moreover, the concomitant inflammation is of relatively short duration.

Effects of the Combined Treatments of Laser Hyperthermia and Chemotherapy

It is known that cellular function is influenced by the environment, including, primarily, temperature, pH, osmotic pressure, and microcirculation.

All the reports regarding the effect of temperature on cellular metabolism agree that the

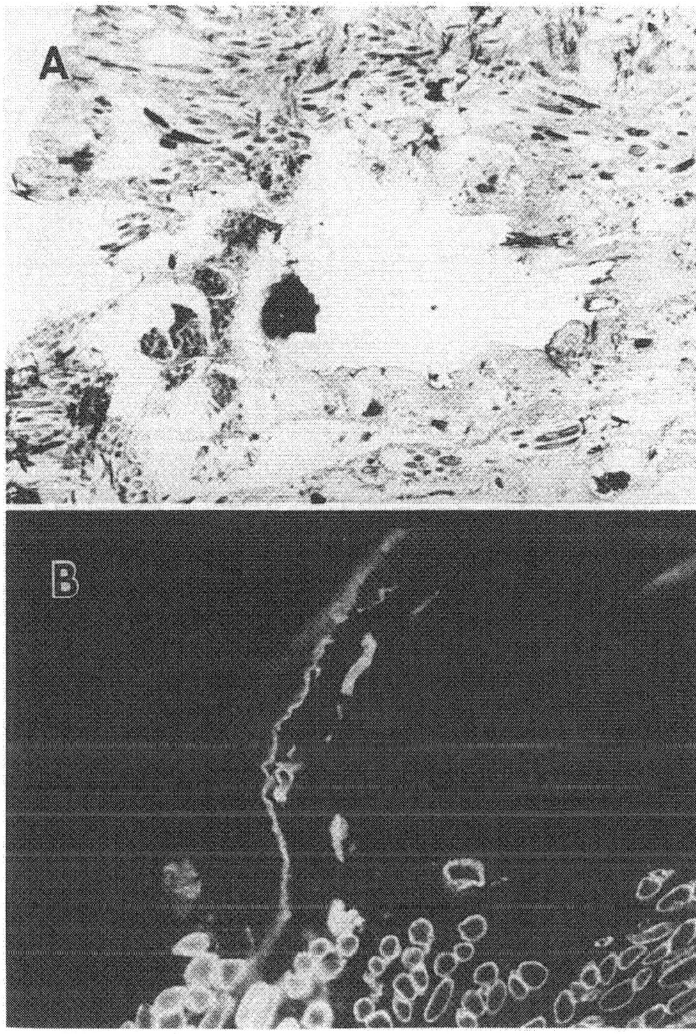

FIGURE 24.16. Morphologic findings of rabbit oral tissues after Nd:YAG laser irradiation. (A) The histologic appearance of rabbit tongue 3 days after laser hyperthermia. (B) Immunohistochemical findings in rabbit lip 7 days after laser incision. Evidence of basal membrane regeneration can be seen by laminin staining.

cellular function of malignant tumors is much more easily affected by high temperature. Above 43°C, the tumor cell would virtually fall into an irreversible failure. This is based on fundamental research concerning the cell-lethal effect. On the other hand, it was confirmed that, as a result of exposure to hyperthermia, an acceleration in the local microcirculation occurs through the ample blood vessels peculiar to the vicinity of tumor cells. On the basis of these works, the combined therapy with laser hyperthermia and cis-dichlorodiamine platinium (CDDP) injection was studied in nude mice implanted with human thyroid cancer cells.

The subjects were divided into four groups of five animals: the first group was treated with laser hyperthermia alone, the second received CDDP injection, the third received the combined therapy of laser hyperthermia and CDDP injection, and the last is the control group, receiving no therapy.

The results of this study indicated that the combination of laser hyperthermia and CDDP injection was the most effective treatment for these tumors (Figure 24.18). We believe that the combined modality of laser hyperthermia and antitumor chemotherapy may have some efficacy in the management of papillary adenocarcinoma of the human thyroid gland, even though this malignancy is known to be chemoradioresistant.

Clinical Study

On the basis of experimental studies, laser hyperthermia with chemoradiotherapy was applied to the advanced malignant neck mass in patients

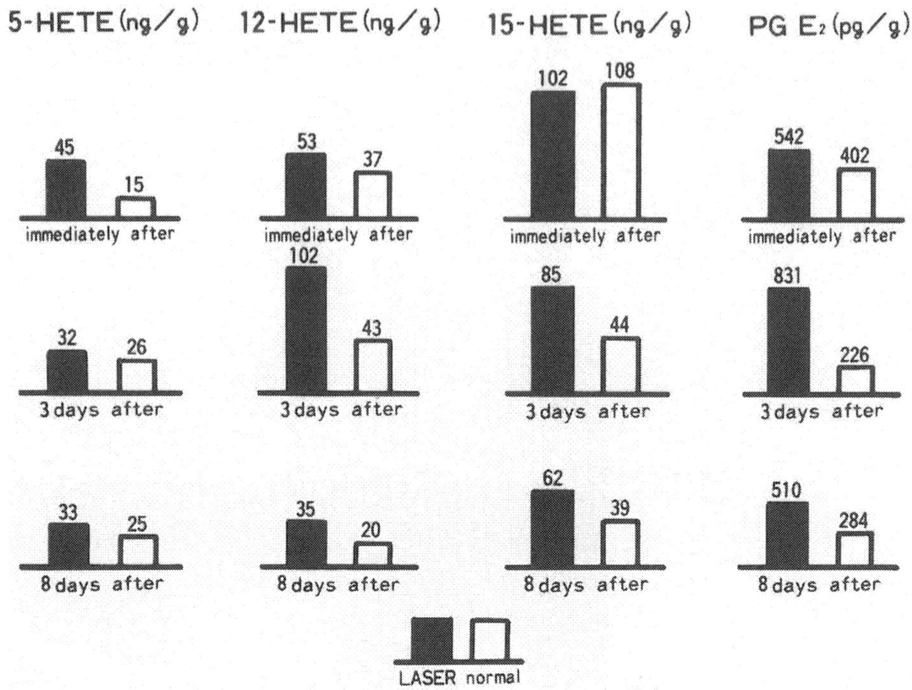

FIGURE 24.17. Changes of arachidonic acid metabolites in rabbit tongue after localized Nd:YAG laser hyperthermia.

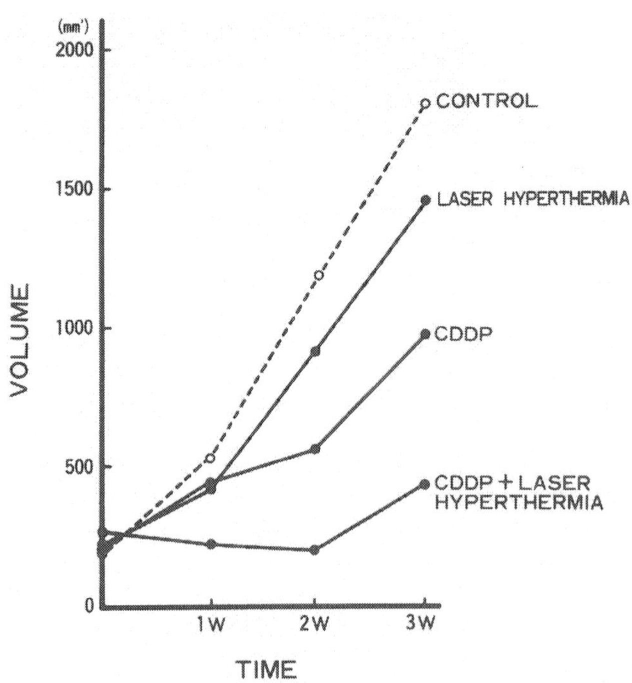

FIGURE 24.18. A comparison of the effects of the combined therapy of localized Nd:YAG laser hyperthermia and chemotherapy on human thyroid cancer transplanted in nude mice. (Subjects: 15 nude mice with tumors of 1.5 cm diameter.)

A laser beam of less than 3 W is sufficient for this laser hyperthermia. The center of the tumor is irradiated for 30 minutes at 43°C.

Temperature in the tumor and peripheral tissue is recorded by using a thermogram and is also monitored by a digital thermometer in order to maintain 42 to 43°C, the requisite temperature around the target tissue. The patient tolerated this therapy well and the neck tumor responded markedly after two treatments (laser hyperthermia once a week, combined with radiotherapy in a total dose of 40 Gy). After laser hyperthermia, radical neck dissection was usually performed in these cases.

Figure 24.19 shows a histologic specimen of a patient with tongue cancer who received laser hyperthermia two times combined with radiation therapy in a total dose of 40 Gy and Tegafur in a total dose of 20 g over 4 weeks.

Then a hemiglossectomy and radical neck dissection were performed, using the contact Nd:YAG laser technique. Although this tongue cancer had been classified as T2, N1, M0, a histologic examination of the excised specimen failed to find any evidence of cancer cells (Figure 24.19B). The combined therapy with laser hyperthermia and chemoradiotherapy was applied to 10 patients with advanced head and neck malignancies, and very good clinical results were obtained in 8 patients during the past two years.

Since hyperthermia modifies the response of tumors to ionizing radiation, it is lethal to radioresistant cells such as hypoxic cells or cells in the S-phase, it is synergistic with radiother-

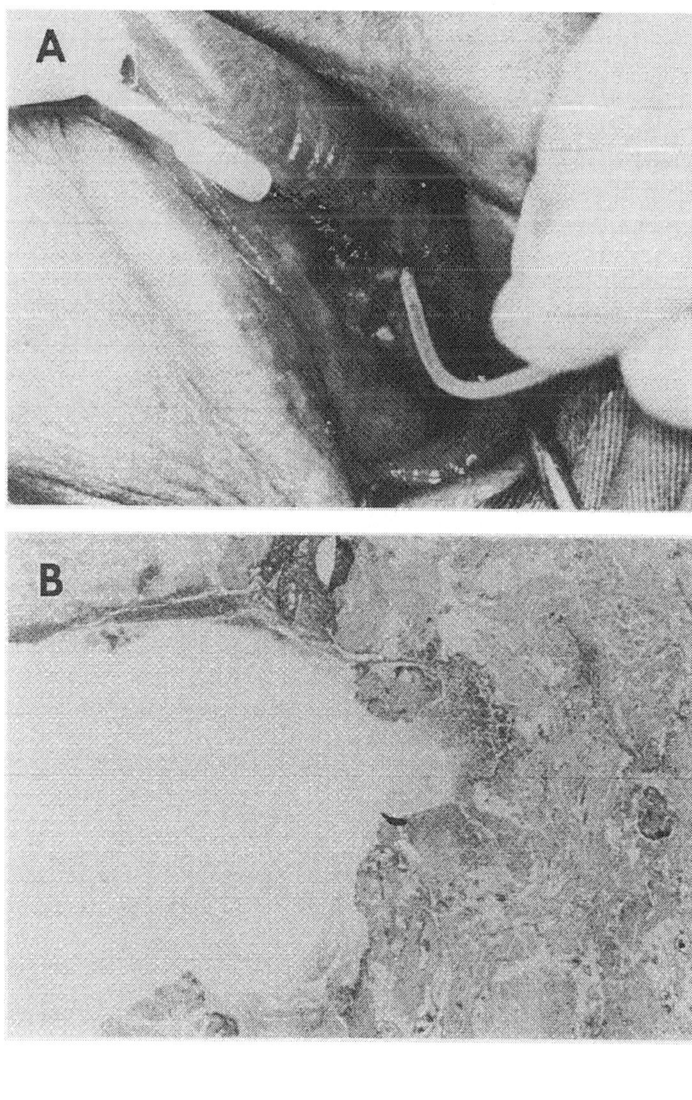

FIGURE 24.19. Localized laser hyperthermia in tongue cancer (T2, N2, M0). (*A*) Laser probe inserted in the left side and the tip of the thermocouple in the right side of cancer tissue. (*B*) Histologic findings of the resected cancer tissue. There is no evidence of vivid cancer cells.

apy, and it enhances the action of selected chemotherapeutic agents.

By continuing efforts to substantiate the application of laser hyperthermia to malignant tumors in the head and neck regions, this treatment may establish itself as one of the new multidisciplinary cancer therapies.

Further study on the relationship between laser hyperthermia and chemoradiotherapy will be necessary to confirm these interesting results, and a multichannel laser hyperthermia system should be developed.

Summary

Although most malignant tumors cannot be controlled by laser hyperthermia alone, the combined modalities of hyperthermia, chemotherapy, radiotherapy, and surgery could be highly useful for cancer treatment in the head and neck regions.

References

1. Brenne EJ, Yerushalmi A: Combined local hyperthermia and X irradiation in the treatment of metastatic tumors. Br J Cancer 33:91–96, 1975.
2. Hahn GM: Hyperthermia and Cancer. Plenum, New York and London, 1982.
3. Ohyama M, Nobori T, Ueno K, et al: Contact Nd-YAG laser surgery for head and neck tumor. Pract Otol (Kyoto) Suppl 3:1–9, 1986.
4. Ohyama M, Katsuda K, Nobori T, et al: Treatment of head and neck tumors by contact Nd-YAG laser surgery. Auris Nasus Larynx (Tokyo) 12(Suppl 2):S138–142, 1985.

25
Reconstructive Surgery for Head and Neck Tumors by Contact Nd:YAG Laser Technique

Goro Mogi, Yuichi Kurono, and Issei Ichimiya

Although the usefulness of laser power in surgery has been proven, its application using carbon dioxide (CO_2) or the Nd:YAG laser in the field of head and neck surgery has only recently begun. Usage of the Nd:YAG laser has a beneficial effect on hemostasis and coagulation. Its weakness, however, lies in the cutting and evaporation of tissue. The contact laser probe, made of ceramic, is a new form of the Nd:YAG laser delivery system that by means of contact irradiation, can be used in coagulation, vaporization, and cutting.

Reconstructive procedures using a pedicle flap have improved the cure rate of head and neck cancer because such procedures make it possible to resect a large part of the dissected lesion, including an adequate safety margin, and to provide acceptable, functional, and cosmetic rehabilitation. Particularly, it has been proven that the myocutaneous (MC) island flap is invaluable reconstructive material for head and neck cancer patients.[1–4] The one-stage operation, which consists of a composite resection of the primary tumor, radical neck dissection (RND), and subsequent reconstructive surgery, causes a large volume of blood loss due to the highly vascularized operation field, thus requiring a blood transfusion. Postoperative hematoma sometimes causes major flap necrosis.[4]

In order to compensate for the disadvantages of this procedure, contact Nd:YAG laser surgery, using a new SLT contact laser probe, was applied. It was chosen because the contact laser probes provide hemostatic abilities of the Nd:YAG laser and cutting proficiency of the CO_2 laser and because this surgery combines the precise control and tactile sensation of steel scalpel techniques.

Subjects and Methods

The contact Nd:YAG laser instrument employed was Model 130 YZ (Nippon Infrared Industries Co., Ltd, Tokyo). Two ceramic probes (Surgical Laser Technologies Japan Co., Tokyo), one with a 0.4-mm diameter tip (small), and the other with 0.6-mm diameter tip (large) were used. Both ceramic scalpels were 9 mm in length and attached to a holder (Model SRH 1, Surgical Laser Technologies Japan Co., Tokyo). The laser power output was 20 W for the large probe and 16 W for the small probe.

Seven patients were treated with contact Nd:YAG laser surgery. Four patients (3 male and 1 female) had a pharyngoesophageal cancer, and three had a cancer lesion in the oral cavity, tongue, or palatopharynx. All patients had unilateral or bilateral neck metastasis and were classified as stage 3 or 4. All patients underwent a composite resection of the primary tumor and RND after receiving Linac X-Ray radiation totaling 30 grays and 3000 mg of 5-Fu by intravenous or intraarterial infusion. Intraarterial infusion to the feeding artery was used for cancer of the tongue, oral cavity, and palatopharynx. Reconstructive surgery using the MC flap was performed immediately after the composite resection of the tumor lesion. A pectoralis major-MC flap was prepared as reported by Ariyan,[5] and the lattisimus dorsi-MC flap was made according to the method described by Morris et al.[6] The latter flap was used in the female patient with pharyngoesophageal cancer. Three of seven patients underwent bilateral RND, preserving the internal jugular vein on one side.

As shown in Figure 25.1a, a skin incision was made with the small contact probe, producing adequate tension on the skin. Dissection of the subcutaneous tissues and resection of the mucosal wall of the pharynx, esophagus, and tongue were carried out by use of the large contact-scalpel (Figures 25.1b and 25.2). All procedures of RND, except for the isolation, ligation, and cutting off of the internal jugular vein, were also performed using the large contact probe. The cut surface of the MC island flap was slightly resected by scissors to removed the burned skin layer.

Results

Skin Incision

Incisions of the skin could be made without bleeding. Figure 25.1d shows a skin incision made by the contact Nd:YAG laser (right half) and by a conventional surgical scalpel (left half). No blood is seen on the left half, whereas the right half is moistened with blood.

Dissection of Subcutaneous Tissue and RND

Dissection of the subcutaneous tissue and the procedure for RND were completed safely. This was because such tactile cues provided by steel scalpels can also be obtained by use of contact probes, and because the identification of blood vessels, nerve fibers, and other parts is easier with the contact Nd:YAG laser surgery than with conventional operating methods because of less bleeding (Figures 25.1b and 25.2b). Contact laser techniques can be used to detach the sternocleidomastoid muscle from its attached parts and to dissect it from scalenoùs muscles.

Cutting Off the Mucosal Wall and Tongue

During dissection of the skin and muscular layers, relatively large vessels in which bleeding does not stop when incised by the contact laser probe were easily identified and suture ligated (Figures 25.1b and 25.2b). Since the contact las-

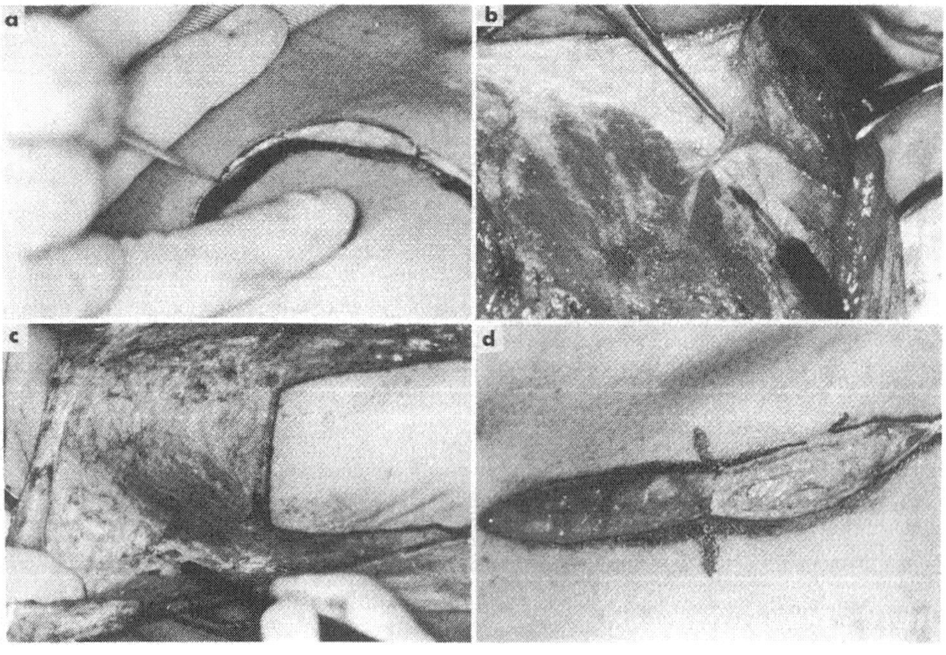

FIGURE 25.1. Skin incision and preparation of myocutaneous flap. (a) Skin incision using a ceramic probe with 0.4-mm diameter tip. (b) Dissection of the subcutaneous tissues during the preparation of the pectoralis major–MC flap. (c) Preparation of a lattissimus dorsi–MC flap. (d) Skin incision made by contact Nd:YAG laser (right half) and by a conventional surgical scalpel (left half).

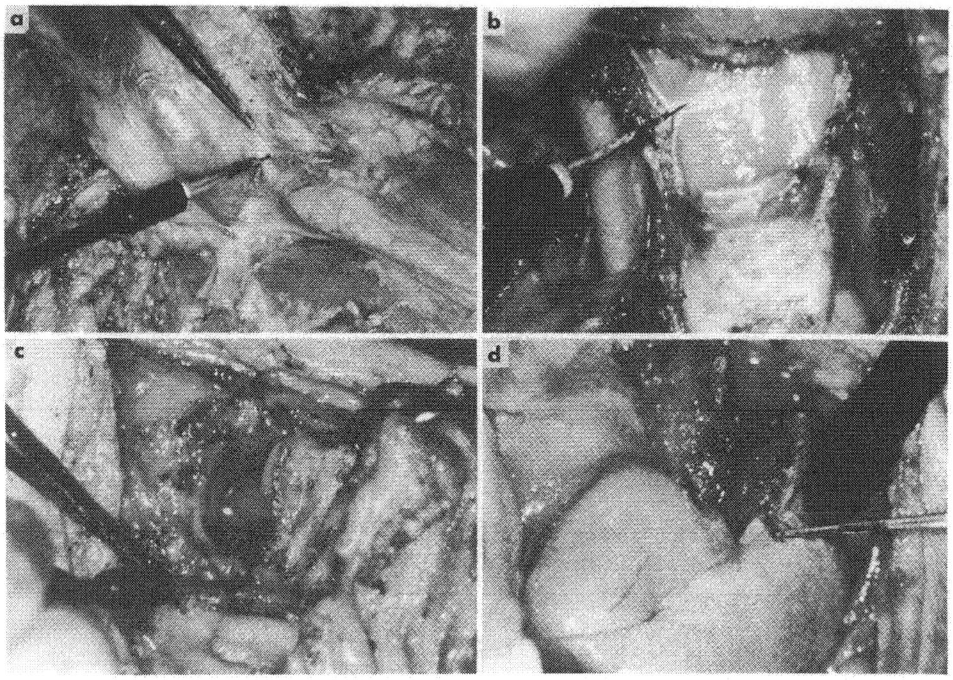

FIGURE 25.2. Dissection of the subcutaneous tissues and resection of the mucosal wall of the pharynx and tongue. (a) Separation of the radical neck dissected material from bifurcation of the common carotid artery. (b) Resection of the posterior wall of the pharynx. (c) Exposure of the hypopharynx by dissecting the suprahyoid space. (d) Resection of the tongue.

er scalpel differs from the electric knife, large muscular bundles were cut off without muscular spasm or contraction.

Blood Loss

The mean volume of blood loss during a composite operation with RND performed on 7 patients by use of the contact Nd:YAG laser was 98 ± 27 ml, whereas that of 110 patients operated on in our department by conventional procedures was 730 ± 351 ml. The making of the MC flap caused an average loss of 71 ± 46 ml of blood in 7 cases using contact laser surgery, whereas conventional procedures resulted in an average loss of 280 ± 134 ml in 28 operations. The mean volume of blood and exudate from negative pressure suction drains after contact laser surger was 92 ± 31 ml from the RND incision and 56 ± 51 ml from the donor's site of the MC flap. Using conventional surgery it was 206 ± 104 ml from the RND incision and 124 ± 39 ml from the donor's site of the MC flap. Only one patient received a blood transfusion due to preoperative anemia.

Results of Reconstructive Surgery

In one of the four patients who had pharyngoesophageal reconstruction, a fistula occurred at the lower attachment between the flap and recipient mucosa. All three patients who underwent reconstruction of the tongue and oral cavity had a dehiscience between the flap and donor's mucosa. However, this was probably due to an insufficient amount of remaining oral mucosa. The dehiscience closed spontaneously within 3 weeks in each case.

Conclusions

The results of the present study demonstrate that contact Nd:YAG laser surgery using SLT contact probes is extremely useful in head and neck tumor surgery and reconstruction. Moreover, this new method apparently surpasses conventional surgical procedures in many ways. Since contact laser surgery offers precise, controlled cutting and hemostasis, the surgeon is not troubled by bleeding from small vessels during the incision of the skin and mucosal wall and while dissecting subcutaneous tissue. It is easy to identify blood vessels, nerve fibers, and other anatomical parts which increase the operation's safety factor. If bleeding occurs, it can be stopped by use of the lateral surface of the probe. Contact ceramic probes are, of course, unable to control all bleeding. Experience indicates that vessels less than 0.5 mm in diameter are probably best controlled by contact laser scalpels. The cutting speed is slow with contact laser probes as compared to conventional surgery using steel scalpels. However, the operation is not prolonged in contact laser surgery because of the hemostatic capability.

The most notable merit of contact Nd:YAG laser surgery for one-stage operations of head and neck cancer is the remarkable reduction in blood loss, thus eliminating blood transfusions. Conventional one-stage operations cannot be carried out without blood transfusion, with all the inherent risks of hepatitis and AIDS.

Based on these results, we believe it is not an overstatement to say that contact Nd:YAG laser techniques are revolutionary in the field of head and neck surgery.

Acknowledgment. The authors greatly thank Professor Masaru Ohyama, Kagoshima University Medical School, for his kind invitation to publish in this book.

References

1. Biller MF, Baek S, Lawson W, et al: Pectoralis major myocutaneous island flap in head and neck surgery. Analysis of complications in 42 cases. Arch Otolaryngol 107:23–36, 1981.
2. Schuller, DE: Pectoralis myocutaneous flap in head and neck cancer reconstruction. Arch Otolaryngol 109:185–189, 1983.
3. Mogi G, Fujiyoshi T, Kurono Y, et al: Latissimus dorsi myocutaneous-iliac bone flap for massive defects of mandible and oral basis. Laryngoscope 96:171–177, 1986.
4. Mogi G, Fujiyoshi T, Kurono Y, et al: Reconstructive surgery of head and neck cancer using various pendicle flaps. Auris Nasus Larynx 12(Suppl 2):S24–S29, 1986.
5. Ariyan S: The pectoralis myocutaneous flap. Plast Reconstr Surg 63:73–81, 1979.
6. Morris RL, Given KS, McCabe JS: Repair of head and neck defects with the lattisimus dorsi myocutaneous flap. Am Surg 47:167–173, 1981.

26
Laser Conization of the Uterine Cervix

Ryozo Totani, Tesuro Karasawa, and Yozo Suzuoki

The optimum treatment for intraepitheial cervical cancer (carcinoma in situ, CIS) has been the subject of much controversy. For many years hysterectomy was the recommended therapy because a rather high incidence of recurrence of carcinoma was reported after conservative treatments such as conization or destruction of the uterine cervix.[1-3] Recently, focused CO_2 laser conization, which excises selected cervical tissue, enabled us to evaluate the histologic findings of the resected cone.[4,5] But we found that this method also has some serious deficiencies.

Today, we are more optimistic about the future of laser conization. A new ceramic scalpel has been designed for attachment to the Nd:YAG laser, which converts this laser into a surgical instrument that can cut as accurately and precisely as the CO_2 laser, without sacrificing any of the coagulative properties of the noncontact Nd:YAG laser.

In this report we present the details—subjects, methods, operational procedures, and results—of a conization study we implemented at our hospital, using the newest modality of Nd:YAG laser equipped with a synthetic sapphire laser scalpel. We also discuss the advantages of this technique for both the surgeon and the patient.

Subjects

Our study group consisted of 16 patients with abnormal cervical pap smears indicating CIN III (severe dysplasia and carcinoma in situ) or class IIIa (Table 26.3) who underwent laser conization between October 1984 and May 1985. Colposcopy was performed in all patients before the operation, and cases that did not reveal any suspicion of malignancy received laser conization for the purpose of treatment of the disease. Diagnostic laser conization was performed for the cases in which a deep cervical evaluation could not be obtained through preoperative colposcopical examinations. The mean age of the patients was 39.6 years, ranging from 22 to 54 years. The mean parity and gravity were 2.3 and 3.4, respectively. None of the women were pregnant at the time of conization. All patients who underwent conization were admitted to the hospital in expectation of likely complications, a precaution typically taken in Japan. The healing process of conization was checked daily, and cytologic examinations of the cervical area were performed every 2 weeks for a 6-month period, and then monthly. All cones were fixed in 10% formaldehyde and extensively sectioned for histopathologic analysis. The severity of the malignancy and the affected areas, as well as the distance from the edge of the cone to the affected area, were evaluated. When the edge of the cone was more than 5 mm from the affected area, the patient was considered cured. When the affected area was less than 5 mm from the edge of the cone, a hysterectomy was performed by either the vaginal or the abdominal route. Therapeutic conizations were performed on nine patients. From the colposcopic findings and the pathologic analysis of the punch biopsies, we were convinced that the malignancies had not advanced beyond carcinoma in situ. Of nine therapeutic conizations, additional hysterectomies were performed on two patients. One patient (Case 8) had an incomplete resection of the cone—its affected area was within 3 mm of the cone's edge. The second patient (Case 9) wanted to have a hysterectomy, although the cervical findings did not indicate it was necessary. Seven patients were followed-up for 10 to 20 months postoperatively.

Diagnostic conizations were performed on seven patients. Of these, four cases were diagnosed as carcinoma in situ by punch biopsy through colposcopy. But deep findings could not be obtained by this method. In order to procure a more precise diagnosis, laser conization was performed on these patients. This procedure enabled us to determine which surgical therapy was most appropriate: panhysterectomy, extended hysterectomy, or simple total hysterectomy with or without lymphadenectomy of the pelvic cavity.

The three remaining patients had diagnostic laser conization, although they were recommended to have hysterectomies because of larger than fist-sized myoma uteri. These patients were among many others having myoma uteri, and their screening pap smears and punch biopsies showed Class IIIa and mild dysplasia, which are inconclusive findings of further malignancy.

Methods

The Nd:YAG laser equipment we used was the Molectron Model 8000 (Molectron Industries, USA). The wavelength of the laser was 1.06 μm and the maximum power output was 110 W. The benefit of this equipment was that stable and accurate wattage was available from low power, 1 to 30 W. The ceramic laser scalpel was made of synthetic sapphire (aluminum oxide, $A1_2O_3$), which can center the laser beam at the tip of the scalpel.[6] (Figure 26.1).

This $A1_2O_3$ crystal scalpel (Surgical Laser Technologies, Malvern, PA and Japan, Tokyo), transmits a laser beam of more than 90% of the original power, and so greatly surpasses conventional artificial sapphire or quartz crystal scalpels. This SLT Laser Scalpel® is fixed at the tip of the holder and the Nd:YAG laser beam is delivered from the Molectron Model 8000 through several meters of optical quartz fiber.

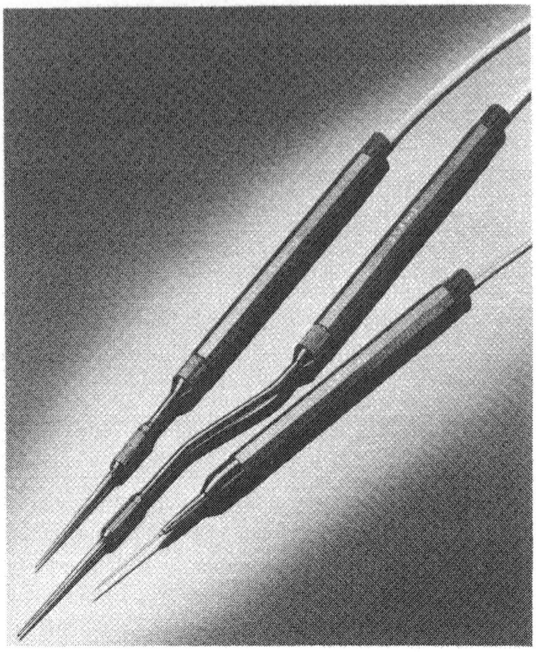

FIGURE 26.1. The synthetic sapphire-ceramic probes with laser handpieces—the SLT contact laser scalpels.

Preliminary examinations of clinical trials were done on the resected uterine cervix or just before the hysterectomy for myoma uteri or adenomyosis. Conization was attempted with several probe sizes with the laser scalpel and with varying laser wattage. The 0.6-mm scalpel probe with 30 W of power was found to be the most effective combination to conize the uterine cervix.[7] This SLT contact laser scalpel, used with the Nd:YAG laser, surpasses the noncontact focused CO_2 laser by allowing narrower and deeper incisions and by considerably reducing backscattering. It is also a distinctly safer procedure for the medical staff (Table 26.1).

Operational Procedures

Conization was performed under general anesthesia after colposcopy, which determined the size and shape of the cone. The operational procedures are as follows (Figure 26.2): (1) After the disinfection of the vaginal cavity and portio

TABLE 26.1. Comparison of Contact and Noncontact Procedures

Characteristics	Contact (Nd:YAG)	Noncontact (CO_2 focused)
Heat damage of marginal tissue	Minimal	Great
Incision width	Narrow	Wide
Laser power	Low	High
Backscattering of laser beam	Minimal	Great
Surgical procedure	Simple	Complex
Danger from laser exposure	Minimal	Caution required

vaginalis, four sutures are placed at 3, 6, 9, and 12 o'clock on the portio just outside the affected area, for the purpose of controlling the uterine cervix. The use of cervical forceps is not recommended because they frequently cause damage that later hinders the pathologic evaluation of the resected cone. (2) The rami descendens of the uterine artery on both sides of the cervix are sutured with 2-0 chromic catgut close to the lateral vaginal fornix. (3) The cervix is pulled out with the implanted sutures 2 or 3 cm, so that the tip of the laser scalpel can easily maneuver around the portio (Figure 26.3). The laser scalpel is carefully aimed to cut approximately 5 mm around the affected area before it is actually switched on for use with a foot pedal. The scalpel is hand-operated clockwise around the portio repeatedly with 5 mm incisions until the cone is finally resected (Figure 26.4). (4) Although this method of laser conization usually results in minimal bleeding of the incision site, additional laser therapy can be used to coagulate blood vessels not sealed off by the earlier incisions. (5) The weight and length of the resected cone are determined after removal of the cone from the cervix (Figure 26.5). The cone is vertically incised at 12 o'clock (Figure 26.6). (6) The opened cone is pinned to a small board and the affected area is again examined by the colposcope. More exact measurements of the cone are taken, and the specimen is then delivered to the pathologist for evaluation. Figure 26.7 shows the pathologic findings of one case (Case 6). Note that the malignant area is at a reasonably safe distance from the cone's edge, which is located both on the top of and on the right side of the photographed specimen. The black marks identify the boundaries of the affected area. A schematic representation of the stages of the operation are shown in Figure 26.8

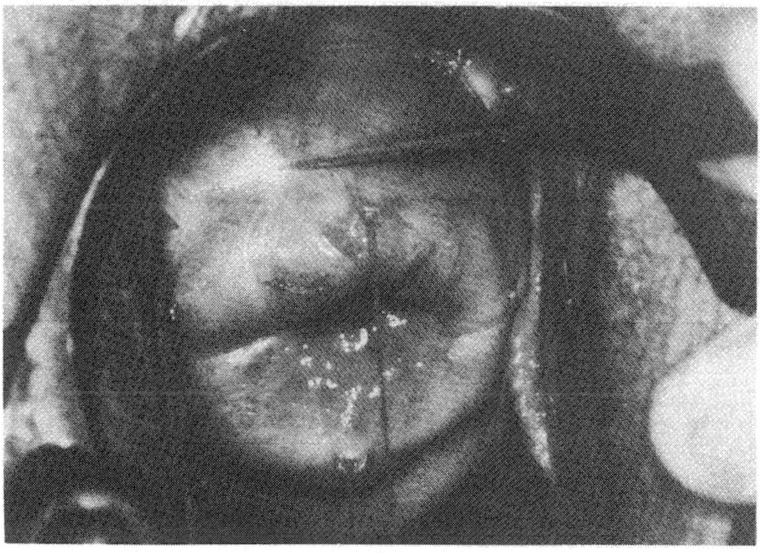

FIGURE 26.2. The tip of the laser scalpel is placed directly on the sutured portio at the beginning of the procedure.

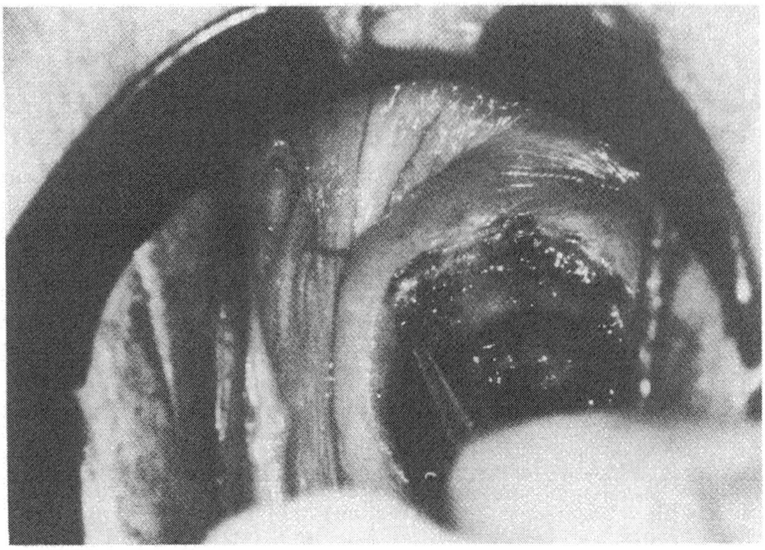

FIGURE 26.3. Repeated circular incisions are made at depths of 5 mm.

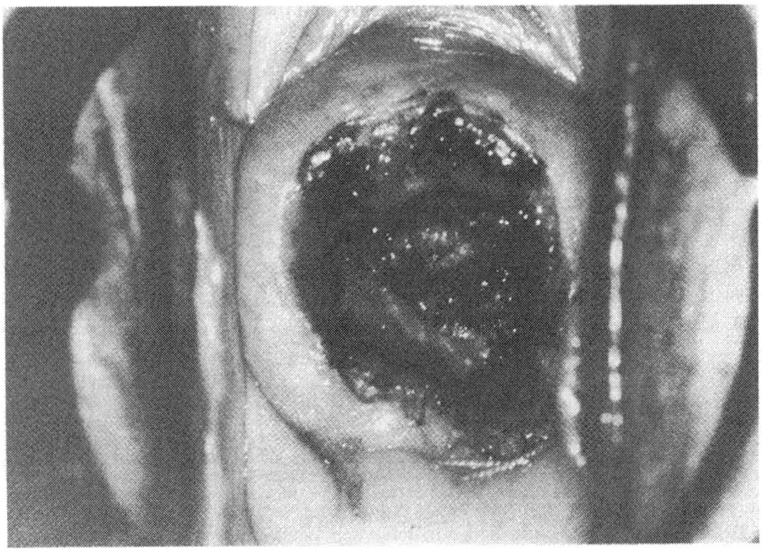

FIGURE 26.4. Hemorrhage is almost nonexistent after resectioning of the cone.

Results

Table 26.2 shows the surgical data of Nd:YAG laser conization of 16 cases. The mean operating time for each case was about 22 minutes, but the actual laser operational time was only about 8 minutes; disinfection, suturing of the portio to stretch the cervix, and observation time for postoperative hemorrhage took 14 minutes on the average. Of nine cases treated by conization, two cases were hysterectomized. Seven patients were followed-up for 10 to 20 months postoperatively. No abnormal findings on periodical pap smears were obtained. All seven patients who received diagnostic conizations were hysterectomized after full analysis of the pathologic data was obtained. Among the group treated by conization, only one postoperative diagnosis (Case 8) was more severe than its preoperative diagnosis, with a finding of severe dysplasia extending to carcinoma in situ (Table 26.3).

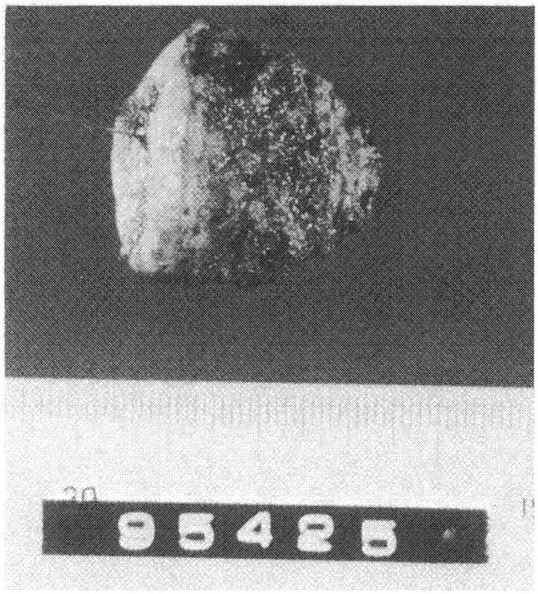

FIGURE 26.5. Cone resected by Nd:YAG laser conization.

Discussion

For all 16 cases, the affected areas were resected by laser conization, but hysterectomies were performed on 9 patients: 3 because of myoma uteri, 4 to determine the thermal effect of the laser on tissue of the remaining uterus, and 2 (Cases 4 and 8) because the edge of the affected area extended within 5 mm of the apex of the resected cone. Of the nine hysterectomies performed, however, postoperative examinations indicated that only two cases actually required the operation to forestall uterine malignancy.

According to Grundsell,[5] malignancy on the surface of the resected cone is not a reliable indicator of malignancy on the unoperated facing portion of the uterus. In fact, he reports that recurrence of cancer in such cases is limited.

Concerning the partial resection of the uterus as a treatment of early cervical cancer, the accuracy of the treatment is the most important factor because the uterus is not an indispensable organ for life. If some women have a recurrence of cancer after the conization of the uterine cervix, the responsibility of the medical staff is exceedingly serious. This explains why hysterectomy or extended hysterectomy is frequently performed in Japan. But owing to progress in the accuracy of preoperative diagnosis of this condition, the number of patients who have conization increases slightly every year[8] (Figure 26.9). The conization of the uterine cervix becomes a truly valuable operation when its postoperative recurrence ratio closely approaches that of the hysterectomy. Thus, the crucial criterion used in deciding whether to perform the hysterectomy is the extent of the malignancy it-

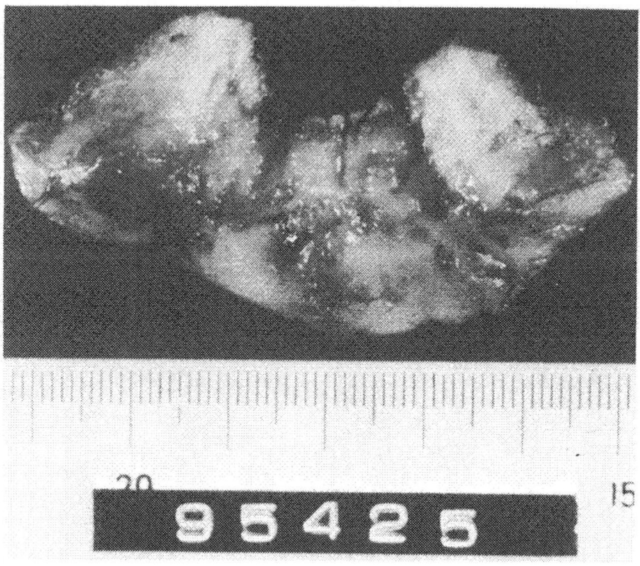

FIGURE 26.6. Cone resected at 12 o'clock and opened.

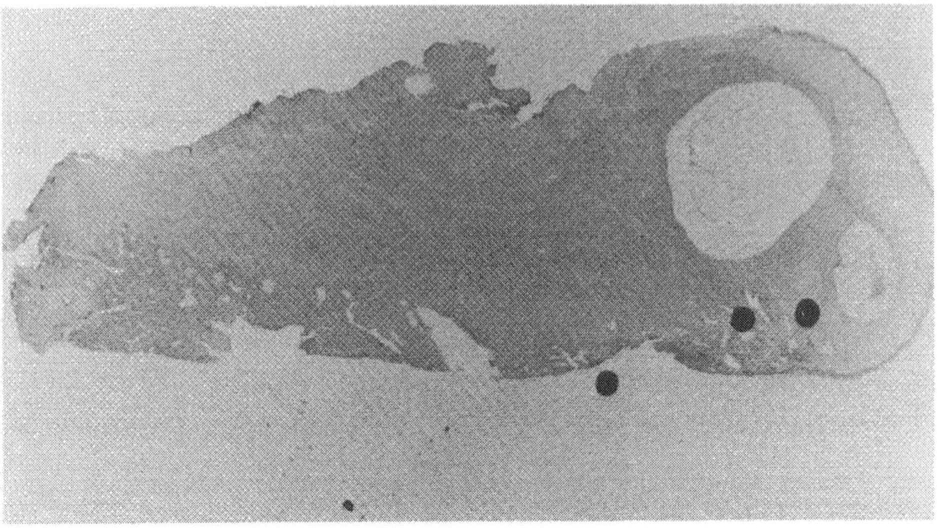

FIGURE 26.7. Pathologic specimen with edges of malignant areas marked by black dots.

self, that is, whether or not it extends to within 5 mm of the edge of the resected cone. Figure 26.10 shows the management scheme adopted for patients suffering form early-stage cervical cancer.

Besides the problem of tumor recurrence, insignificant bleeding from the operational site has been a reason for the popularity of conization. The uterine cervix is one of the hardest of the soft tissues in the human body, capable of dilating more than ten times its circumference at the time of delivery of the fetus. Although

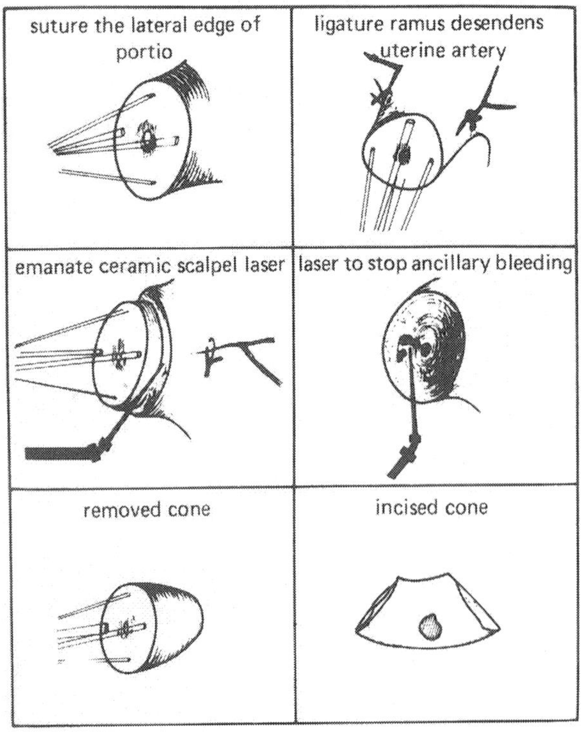

FIGURE 26.8. Schematic representation of the operative procedure of Nd:YAG laser conization using the synthetic sapphire scalpel.

TABLE 26.2. Surgical data of SLT contact Nd:YAG laser conization

Cases treated with Nd:YAG laser	16
Total operation time (min)	22.4 ± 4.0
Total laser joule (J)	11033.7 ± 4856.6
Total blood loss (g)	54.4 ± 47.9
Weight of removed cone (g)	9.3 ± 4.9
Length of removed cone (mm)	22.7 ± 7.6

bleeding from the conized cervix is negligible during or soon after the traditional operation, a few weeks later, when patients have already returned to their ordinary lives, they can suddenly, and unexpectedly, have a severe hemorrhage.

The third problem of traditional conization is the difficulty in detecting tumor recurrence at the operational site. The cervical tissue of the resected surface is usually scarred after the traditional conization, such as destructive procedures, Scott's open-cut edge operation, or Sturmdorff's well-known operation. When affected tissue remains under the scar of cervical tissue, or sometimes under the vaginal wall tissue, detection of the recurrence of the tumor is very difficult, and frequently it is discovered only after it has already developed to some extent.[3]

To resolve these difficulties of traditional conization, Nd:YAG laser conization applied with an synthetic contact sapphire scalpel was clinically evaluated. As for confirmation of the removal of the affected area, conization surpasses the destructive procedures such as cryosurgery, cauterization, or vaporization with CO_2 or Nd:YAG laser. It is also superior when compared to conization procedures with the cold-knife or CO_2 focused conization. The Nd:YAG contact procedure surpasses the others in its ease of use in cutting the hard tissue of the cervix more precisely; it allows a more accurate cutting of tissue at the top of the cone, in contrast to the CO_2 laser procedure.

There is much discussion as to the completeness of resection and how many millimeters of tissue from the affected area need be removed.[5, 10–12] Our experience with these cases is too limited to make any definite claims, but 5 mm of tissue beyond the affected area seems to be adequate. Some reports have indicated that even when isolated cancer cells remain after resection, these remaining cells rarely result in a recurrence of the tumor.[5]

Concerning the second problem of conization, bleeding, the focused CO_2 laser or Nd:YAG laser, used with adequate wattage, can coagu-

TABLE 26.3. List of the cases treated with SLT contact Nd:YAG laser conization

Case	Age	Pregnancy history	Purpose of conization	Pap smear	Colposcopic findings	Affected area at the portio (%)	Histologic diagnosis punch biopsy → cone specimen	Follow-up (months)
1	45	P(2) G(3)	D	Class IIIa	W	50 ↓	Mil.dys. → N.M.	STH[a]
2	43	P(2) G(2)	D	Class IIIa	W + AGO	50 ↓	Mil.dys. → N.M.	STH[a]
3	48	P(2) G(4)	D	Class IIIa	W	50 ↓	Mil.dys. → N.M.	STH[a]
4	42	P(2) G(5)	D	Class IV	W + AGO + P	50 ↑	CIS → Ia	EH
5	42	P(3) G(3)	D	Class IV	W	50 ↓	CIS → CIS	STH
6	48	P(2) G(3)	D	Class IV	W + M + aV	50 ↑	CIS → Ia	STH
7	43	P(2) G(2)	D	Class IV	W + M + P	50 ↑	CIS → CIS	STH
8	40	P(2) G(2)	T	Class IIIb	W + AGO	50 ↑	Sev.dys. → CIS	STH[b]
9	39	P(4) G(5)	T	Class IIIb	W + P	50 ↑	Sev.dys. → N.M.	STH[c]
10	22	P(1) G(2)	T	Class IV	W	50 ↓	CIS → CIS	17
11	54	P(2) G(3)	T	Class V	W + P + M	50 ↑	CIS → CIS	16
12	34	P(3) G(5)	T	Class IIIa	W	50 ↓	CIS → CIS	17
13	34	P(3) G(5)	T	Class IIIb	W	50 ↓	CIS → N.M.	10
14	31	P(2) G(2)	T	Class IIIb	W	50 ↓	Sev.dys. → N.M.	14
15	33	P(2) G(3)	T	Class IIIb	W	50 ↓	Sev.dys. → Mil.dys.	18
16	35	P(3) G(5)	T	Class IIIa	W + AGO	50 ↑	Sev.dys. → Mil.dys.	20

P, parity; G, gravity; D, diagnosis; T, treatment; Mil.dys., mild dysplasia; N.M., no malignancy; CIS, carcinoma in situ; Sev.dys., severe dysplasia; STH, simple total hysterectomy; EH, extended hysterectomy.

[a]Incomplete resection.

[b]Patient hope for operation.

[c]Hysterectomy for myoma uteri.

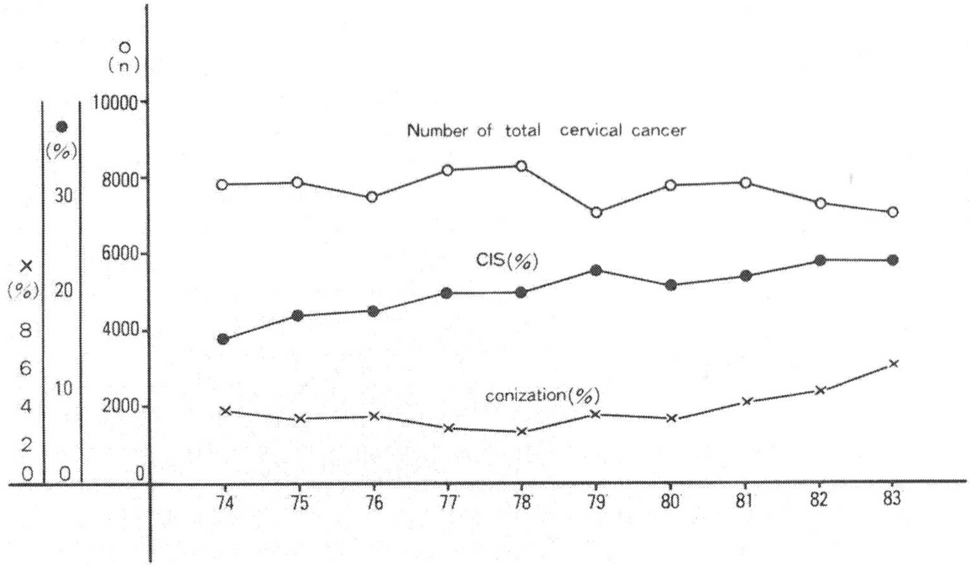

FIGURE 26.9. Increasing incidence of CIS (carcinoma in situ) and conization in Japan.

late the bleeding from arteries less than 0.5 mm in diameter. When the Nd:YAG lasers is used with the SLT contact scalpel attached, this technique for conization surpasses all other procedures.[4,6,13,14]

In our operative procedures we recommend suturing the ramis descendens of the uterine artery before laser conization. This step can probably be omitted, but as this procedure is simple and easy, it seems wise to simply reduce any risk of bleeding. However, there are very few reports of postoperative bleeding in laser procedures when compared to other operational procedures.[4]

Concerning the third point, the difficulty in detecting recurrence of cancer seems to remain even in Nd:YAG laser conization, although we have had not experienced any such recurrence. In most cases, we observed that the edges of the remaining cervical tissue turn inside gradually and fold upon themselves thus the neighboring vaginal tissue gathers at the cervical canal

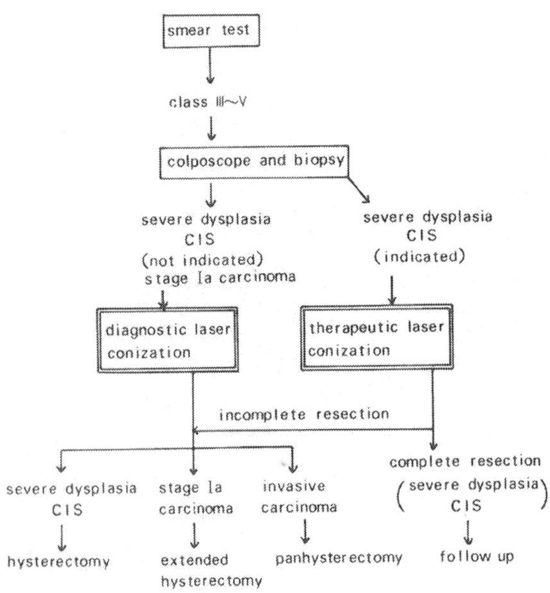

FIGURE 26.10. Management of early-stage cervical cancer.

TABLE 26.4. Indications for laser conization

1. Severe dysplasia or carcinoma in situ, which has been diagnosed by means of punch biopsy during colposcopy
2. The entire infected area is visable through colposcopic examination and the area of infection falls clearly within the bounds of cone removal
3. Patients whose postoperative follow-up can be reliably assured
4. Patients who are hoping for future pregnancies, or for other reasons desiring preservation of the uterine function

as is observed whenever a surgical procedure is used to remove the large cone.

We do not recommend conization for peri- or postmenopausal patients (Case 11) because follow-up reevaluation is extremely difficult owing to the wrinkling and shortening of the cervix that takes place at this time.

Conization of the cervix should be limited to patients who are still hopeful of a pregnancy or who have reasons for wanting to preserve the uterus. Although we had no pregnancies among our contact Nd:YAG laser conization cases, Shirodkar's operation of the cervical mucosa is strongly recommended to prevent premature delivery at 12 to 16 weeks of gestation (Table 26.4). Two pregnancies occurred in the noncontact vaporization of Nd:YAG laser conization that are not included in this report. Both resulted in full-term deliveries after Shirodkar's operation.

Clinically, there are many cases in which the severity of the affected areas of the cervical canal are not confirmed by colposcopy and also in which findings of the colposcope and the pap smears are at variance. In such cases, Nd:YAG contact conization is recommended to make a definite diagnosis.

Although conization has a long history, it is not commonly used in the management of early-stage cervical cancer because of the many difficulties with the operation itself, such as hemorrhage, and toughness of the tissue. We achieved some progress with our combination of the Nd:YAG laser and the synthetic SLT sapphire scalpel in cervical conization by simplifying the procedure and resolving some of the previous difficulties, especially hemorrhage, and by making reevaluation of the resected cone a possibility. The laser also allows cones of various sizes and shapes to be resected, in contrast to the earlier CO_2 and electrocautery conization procedures. It is hoped that this procedure will be widely used as both a diagnostic tool and as therapy in the near future.

References

1. Kirwan H, Smith IR, Naftalin NJ: A study of cryosurgery and the CO_2 laser in treatment of carcinoma in situ (CIN III) of the uterine cervix. Gynecol Oncol 22:195–220, 1985.
2. Nagell JR: Diagnostic and therapeutic efficacy of cervical conization. Am J Obstet Gynecol 124:134–139, 1976.
3. Ahlgrem M: Conization and treatment of carcinoma in situ of the uterine cervix. Obstet Gynecol 46:135–140, 1975.
4. Meandzija MP, Locher G, Jackson JD: CO_2 laser conization versus conventional conization: A clinico-pathological appraisal. Lasers Surg Med 4:139–144, 1984.
5. Grundsell H., Alm P, Larsson G: Cure rates after laser conization for early cervical neoplasia. Ann Chir Gynecol 72:218–222, 1983.
6. Dakiuzono N, Joffe, SN: Artificial sapphire for contact photocoagulation and tissue vaporization with the Nd:YAG laser. Med Instrum 19:173–178, 1985.
7. Totani R, Korasawa T, Suzuoki, Y: Application of newly-developed contact type surgical rod for Nd:YAG laser conization of uterine cervix. Laser Optoelectonics in Medicine Springer-Verlag, Tokyo, 1986, pp 495–501.
8. Japan Obstetrics and Gynecology Society. Annual Reports: Statistical Data of Cervical Cancer, 1974–1983.
9. Scott JW, Welch WB, Blake TF: Bloodless technique of cold knife conization Am J Obstet Gynecol 79:62 1960.
10. Baggish MS, Dersey JH: Carbon dioxide laser for combination excisional vaporization conization. Am J Obstet Cynecol 131:23–27 (1985).
11. Wright VC, Davies E, Riopella MA: Laser cylindrical excision to replace conization. Am J Obstet Gynecol 150:704–709 1984.
12. Lobraico RV: Lasers in gynecology. Med Instrum 17:411, 1983.
13. Schellhans HF, Weppelmann B: The neodymium:YAG laser in the treatment of gynecologic malignancies. Lasers Surg Med 3:225–229, 1983.
14. Larsson G: Conization for preinvasive and early invasive carcinoma of the uterine cervix. Acta obstet Gynecol Scand Suppl 114, 1983.

27
Endometrial Ablation

Theresa Zumwalt

History

The use of the high-energy Nd:YAG laser for endometrial ablation was recently approved by the Food and Drug Administration for endometrial destruction by vaporization and coagulation. Some years ago this technique was designed by Milton Goldrath[1,2] as a low-risk alternative to hysterectomy for the treatment of menorrhagia. To date he has completed 350 procedures, mainly in patients who are high risk for surgical hysterectomy.[3] The results are impressive: 50% of his patients now have hypomenorrhea, consisting of mild spotting, and the rest are amenorrheic.[2] Endometrial ablation has proven to be a safe, outpatient surgical procedure to correct menometrorrhagia, with an indirect result of amenorrhea and sterility.

Controversial Factors

Significant factors involved with this clinical application of the Nd:YAG laser are cost containment, painless convalesence, procedure success rates, patient selection and preparation, physician and surgical staff training, laser safety supervision, and future applications.

Today, the delivery of quality care appropriate to the presenting symptoms, with attention to the economic use of time, materials, and hospital beds, is influencing health care significantly. From an economic aspect, same day surgery is less expensive than a 4-day hospitalization. From the patient's point of view, she will lose only 3 days of work and will not undergo the standard 4- to 6-week physically uncomfortable and financially nonproductive convalesence. In fact, most patients experience only mild cramps and resume normal activities in 1 or 2 days.

The success rate of ablation is dependent on the technical expertise of the physician and proper patient selection. In the past, patient selection was based on medical contraindications for surgical hysterectomy; that is, cystic fibrosis, multiple lower abdominal surgeries, heart valve replacement, or coagulopathies. When evaluating a patient for endometrial ablation, the uterus should be examined, its depth determined, a Pap smear obtained, and a hysteroscopy with endometrial biopsy performed. Any malignancies should be triaged into a standard treatment protocol. Benign endometrial curettings should be obtained within 6 months of the ablation. The patient should have failed standard treatment for menometrorrhagia (dilatation and curettage, followed by cyclic progesterone therapy). Existing endometrial polyps should also be removed at the time of the initial office hysteroscopy. The use of a six-injection-point paracervical block will improve patient comfort during these procedures. Initially, the surgeon should select only a normal-sized uterus to ablate. The patient should be placed preoperatively on 4 to 8 weeks of Danazol 800 mg daily to achieve endometrial atrophy.[2,4] Patients on coumadin will need their dose adjusted. Depo-Provera should not be administered preoperatively.[4] Routinely, hysterograms are not needed. Laboratory screening should include a serum pregnancy test, blood count, type and screen, electrolytes, BUN and creatinine, and a coagulation screen. An investigational consent is no longer required by law but may be helpful for patient education. Patients have to be told that retreatment may be needed (6%).[2] The anesthesia used can be epidural, spinal, or general. Overnight cervical dilation with laminaria is currently done to avoid traumatic manual dilation.

Procedure for Endometrial Ablation

1. The patient is prepped and draped with a water salvage system taped under the buttocks on a table with leg rest (knee crutch) stirrups. The cystoscopy table is ideal.
2. A bimanual examination is done to remove the laminaria, lamicel, or dilapan artificial dilator. Straight mechanical dilation causes bleeding, which obscures the view. The cervix should be loose around the operating hysteroscope (20 French) to allow easy egress of the irrigant.[1] Either normal saline or Ringer's lactate is an excellent irrigation fluid.
3. A single-tooth tenaculum is placed vertically at 12 o'clock on the cervix. It is most comfortable to fix the tenaculum to the drape sheet, freeing the surgeon's hands to operate the hysteroscope. *Check to make sure that a Nd:YAG eye safety filter is firmly attached to the hysterscope.* Flush all air from the scope.
4. A red tape should be placed on the hysteroscope 4 cm from the end as a warning to the laser staff to turn the power off when the tape comes into view. Goldrath does not coagulate the lower 4 cm of the lower uterine segment and cervical canal because of the proximity of the uterine vessels (Figure 27.1).
5. The nursing responsibility is to manually irrigate the uterus under pressure to maintain a clear operative field. A continuous strict intake and output sheet must be maintained to monitor the intravenous fluid and the hysteroscope irrigant balanced against the urine, and vaginal irrigant output. Small, 5-mg doses of furosemide are given to avoid fluid overload.

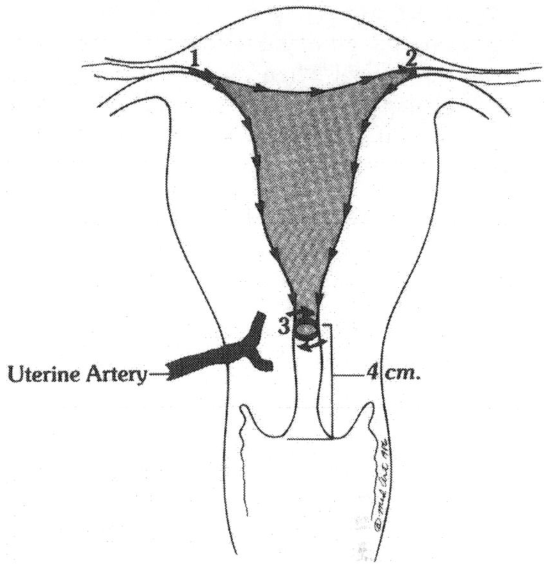

FIGURE 27.1. Uterine template. Initial marking lines to be traced on the endometrial surface outlining the limits of ablation.

6. A urologic quartz (0.6 mm) fiber is used at 50 to 55 W through an operating hysterscope with direct surface contact of the fiber on the endometrium. The Nd:YAG laser is set on continuous wave mode with foot control.
7. Goldrath ablates each tubal ostia initially. He then uses the laser to mark the lower limit of ablation and divides the surface of the uterus into anterior and posterior halves (Figure 27.1). He begins on the anterior or posterior work surface, completes it, and then does the remaining half.
8. Under direct visual control the quartz tip is passed over the endometrial surface at a rate of 0.25 cm/second. The operator can see the tip "mowing" off the endometrium by direct contact coagulation. A uniform field of tan vaporized myometrium should remain. The procedure is as tedious as "mowing the White House lawn with a hand mower." It is, therefore, important for the surgeon to position his/her back for maximum comfort. Also, the surgeon must be certain that he has the patience for this meticulous type of surgical discipline.
9. Start in the anterior or posterior superior fundus and gradually work down to the

cervical marked ring. During the procedure, occasional point coagulation of specific bleeders, seen when the water pressure is reduced, is helpful for maintaining a clear visual field and reducing postablation bleeding.

10. After completing the ablation, a reinspection for any pink viable areas of endometrium is needed. These pink areas are re-treated.
11. Finally, a strong sharp curettage to remove the burnt tissue and to assure scarificaton is performed.
12. At the close of the case fluid balance is noted and further adjustments in diuretic therapy are made if necessary. The patient is observed in the recovery room and may be sent home in a few hours.
13. Discharge medications can include Tylenol, Anaprox, Danazol, Depro-Provera, or antibiotics. Narcotics will only rarely be needed for the immediate postoperative cramping. The patient needs to be seen if she reports severe pain after discharge. Monthly, and then trimonthly, follow-up as previously requested by the FDA protocol[5] is indicated. Uterine sounding, endometrial biopsy, and office hysteroscopy are all useful in following the patient. Early in the surgeon's experience, hysteroscopy would be beneficial mainly in improving his own technical skills and completing his educational process.

Short-Term Complications

Air Embolization

Air embolization has occurred twice, once with a fatal outcome.[5] Both cases occurred when a sapphire tip had been attached to the gastrointestinal fiber, with gas probably being used as the distending medium. The gas was probably pushed directly into the venous system through the dilated uterine venous sinuses (Figure 27.2). The uterine venous sinuses function similarly to the prostatic venous plexus. These sinuses transfer whatever distending media is used, directly into the circulatory system.

The sapphire laser probe has been developed to decrease the power wattage required by focusing the laser energy. This probe increases the precision of the quartz fiber while attempting to decrease accidental perforation of thin-walled bronchi or esophageal tissue.[6] Designed for res-

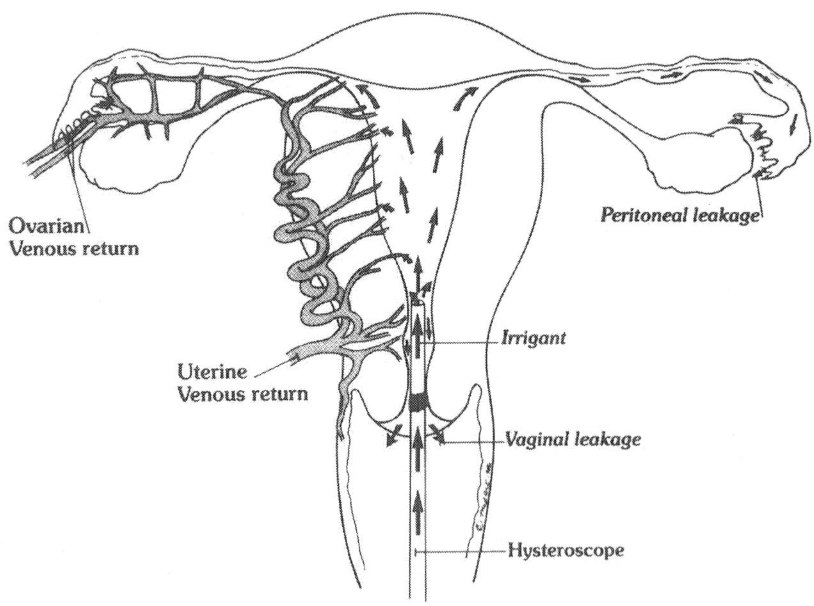

FIGURE 27.2. Irrigant absorption routes. **1,** Uterine venous sinuses transfer fluid to circulation; **2,** fallopian tubes to peritoneal cavity; **3,** cervix to vagina.

piratory and gastrointestinal work, it attaches to the end of the gastrointestinal laser fiber, which has an air or water purge channel alongside the quartz fiber. The air or water purging channel allows for tip cooling. Overheating the tip will render it nonfunctional especially at powers greater than 35 W. The sapphire probe as currently designed is not needed for endometrial ablation because it cannot deliver the 50–55 W of power necessary for adequate depth of myometrial coagulation.[7] The sapphire probe may prove helpful in intrauterine plastic surgery to remove polyps or small septae or to occlude tubes at its lower power settings.

Gynecologists and urologists should currently use the plain 0.6-mm quartz "urology fiber" through a hysteroscope or cystoscope—both instruments have their own fluid channels (Figure 27.1) without an air purge channel. Pulmonary and gastrointestinal surgeons use fibers with coaxial gas or fluid and a completely different technique. Saline or Ringer's lactate (*NOT AIR OR NITROUS OR CARBON DIOXIDE OR WATER*) is the safest irrigation medium. Gaseous insufflation should not be used for endometrial ablation in view of the risk of air embolization and death.

Fluid Overload

Patients will experience fluid overload (hypervolemia, pulmonary edema, and congestive heart failure) until you have developed and perfected your hydraulic system. This requires an ongoing, accurate, intraoperatively balanced charting of expended and recovered irrigating solution. Accurate fluid balancing is dependent on an informed, trained operating room staff. Currently, the ablation procedure is dependent on manual pumping of the irrigating solution. Several types of infusion pumps, ranging from cardiac bypass machines to Holters, have been tried without success. Goldrath[3] is currently testing a new hysteroscope which may eliminate this fluid overload problem.

1. Small incremental doses of furosemide 5 to 10 mg intravenously are frequently needed to maintain fluid balance during surgery.
2. An intraurethral Foley catheter to gravity drainage allows accurate recording of fluid balance and constant bladder decompression. Patients with aneuric renal failure may need to be dialyzed immediately after the procedure. The use of a limited volume of irrigant, a widely dilated cervix, an experienced laser surgeon, and an atrophic, well-prepared endometrium are crucial to proper care of these high-risk patients. Pre- and postoperative weighing, with the same bed scale for both weights, may be beneficial. Central venous pressure lines have been used for select patients.

Hemorrhage

Immediate Hemorrhage

During the procedure, bleeding occurs from venous sinuses unroofed by the laser's destruction of the endometrial gland layer. The positive intrauterine hydrostatic pressure that is necessary for adequate visualization (visual control) prevents intraoperative bleeding. Point coagulation of individual bleeding sinuses during laser vaporization is helpful to maintain clear fluid. Intractable uterine bleeding, which starts immediately after the ablation (after removing the hysteroscope) and is not changed by the curettage, may be awesome. Control of this is easily accomplished by Goldrath's intrauterine Foley technique.[8] Place a 28- to 32-gauge Foley catheter with a 30-cc balloon into the uterus and inflate the balloon with saline just until the bloody cascade stops flowing out of the uterus. The catheter can be left in place for 6 to 24 hours. Use of prophylactic antibiotics may be helpful if the catheter must stay in longer than a few hours. The catheter is ready to be removed when deflating the balloon does not restart the hemorrhage.

Delayed Hemorrhage Requiring Hysterectomy

In Goldrath's original series, he attributed delayed hemorrhage to delayed coagulation necrosis into the cervical artery. Goldrath's hysteroscope is marked with red tape at 4 cm, which correlates to this measured entry point of the cervical branch of the uterine artery into the myometrium. He avoids ablation of the last 4 cm of the endocervical canal to avoid this potential problem. No other cases have been reported to date (Figure 27.1).

Perforation

A good background experience in outpatient hysteroscopy will decrease the frequency of uterine perforation. An experienced hysteroscopist should be able to identify visually when perforation has occurred. He can then avoid further damage by stopping the procedure and completing it a week later. Continuing the ablation under laparoscopic guidance may rarely be indicated. The protective effect by the thickness of the myometrium against bowel burns has been tested experimentally and seen clinically.[1] Thus routine laparoscopic monitoring is not needed as it is when using a urologic resectoscope for endometrial ablation. Although the resectoscope may be faster, the control of resection depth is difficult, as well as the challenge to remove chips of resected endometrium, which orbit in the fluid-filled cavity. An attempted endometrial ablation with a resectoscope ended in total abdominal hysterectomy to control a broad ligament hematoma caused by multiple uterine perforations, which occurred when an experienced hysterocopist did not use laparoscopic guidance.

Long-Term Complications

Continued Menorrhagia

Patients must be informed by written consent, as well as verbally, of the 6% or greater need for repeat procedure. This is especially true when the uterus has a large cavity or fibroids. Strict attention must be paid to the cornual and superior fundal areas to avoid creating potential pockets of residual endometrium. The selection of small uteri (< 8 weeks) that do not contain fibroids or excessive adenomyosis, combined with practiced surgical skill, will greatly decrease the number of reoperations needed.

The surgeon should not attempt endometrial ablation on the large more symptomatic uterus (> 8 weeks) with its spacious cavity, until he is unconditionally accomplished in this procedure. He should be able to completely ablate a 4- to 6-week size uterine cavity in less than 1 hour. Larger cavities can take up to 4 hours to complete, especially at the early learning phases of his skill.

This procedure can be extremely backbreaking for the surgeon. His work can be greatly facilitated and enhanced if he administers Danazol preoperatively, to try to reduce the depth of the endometrial layer to less than 1 mm. This pretreatment course with Danazol takes 6 to 8 weeks or longer—to the endpoint of amenorrhea. On the other hand, to attempt to ablate a hypertrophic cavity stimulated by Depo-Provera is self-defeating.[2–4] The only failure in one of the investigator series was in a case pretreated with Depo-Provera for 2 to 3 months by a referring physician[4] (Figure 27.3). The hysterectomy specimen (removed for continual bleeding) showed persistent lush endometrium. Depo-Provera initially produces a pseudodecidual state with edema and engorgement of the endometrial stroma and glandular hypertrophy (Figure 27.4). Any chemical or mechanical manipulation that decreases endometrial depth preoperatively will enhance the ablation success

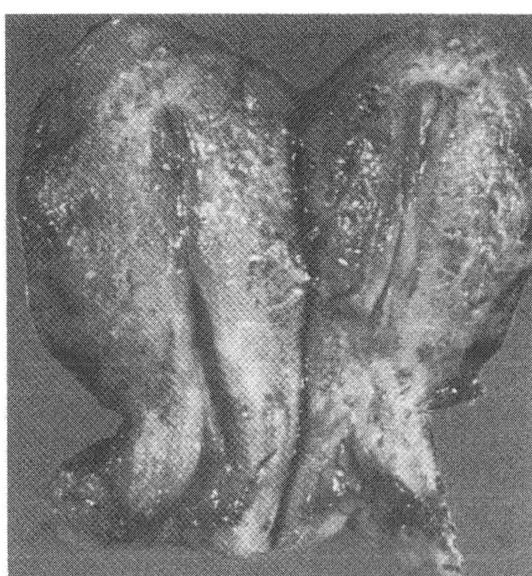

FIGURE 27.3. Hysterectomy specimen. After Nd:YAG laser ablation with Depo-Provera pretreatment. (Courtesy of G. Shirk, Cedar Rapids, IA.)

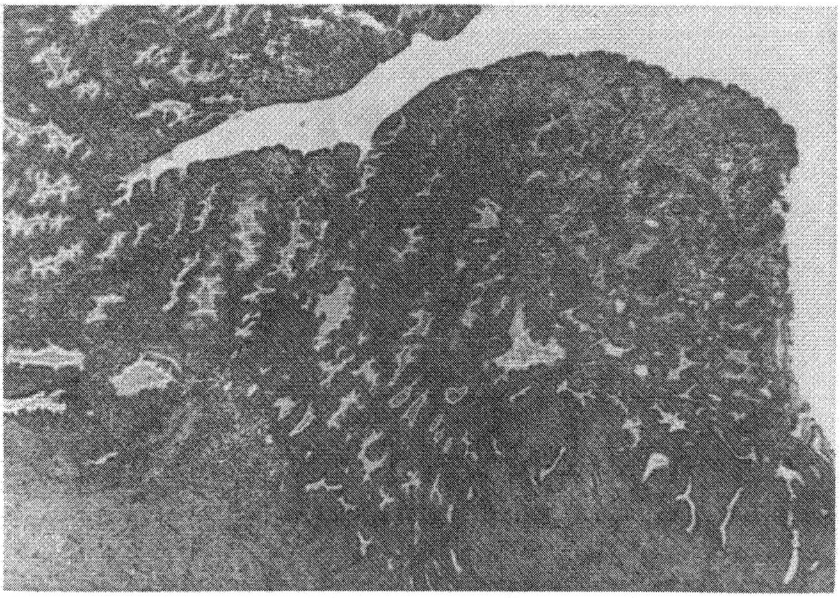

FIGURE 27.4. Microscopic specimen. Lush endometrium residual after Depo-Provera pretreatment. Nd:YAG laser ablation failure. (Courtesy of G. Shirk, Cedar Rapids, IA.)

rate by reducing the total volume of endometrium required to be removed. In the future, it may be possible to perform the procedure on patients whose endometrial mass has been diminished by the use of low-estrogen, combination birth control pills for a sufficient time. In these cases, the surgery could be timed for just after a withdrawal menses. At present, the procedure is only approved by the FDA for menometrorrhagia.

The preoperative evaluation, consisting of hysteroscopy and endometrial sampling, is done to diagnose possible malignancy and to learn the topography of the cavity. Knowing that fibroids, polyps, and septae are present is helpful in planning laser surgery after conservative medical therapy and polypectomy have failed. Thus prepared, the surgeon enters the operative cavity, knowing what he will find there. In larger referral services this initial preoperative workup may be done by the referring physician, who may not have performed a hysteroscopy. The surgeon's first examination of the cavity would be at the time of the surgery. The discovery of a large endometrial polyp, missed in the initial workup and the probable cause of the menorrhagia, allows the surgeon to choose one of several options: he can easily excise the polyp and stop the procedure, or he can perform both ablation and polypectomy. One wonders if the menometrorrhagia would have resolved initially, if a hysteroscopy had been performed to diagnose and properly remove the polyps at the time of the diagnostic dilatation and curettage. Was it really necessary to resort to more expensive laser surgery?

Hemorrhage

See "Delayed Hemorrhage" in the preceding section on Short-Term Complications.

Hysterectomy

In Goldrath's experience, hysterectomy after an ablation was required in 8 of 216 patients. Most of these hysterectomies occurred during his early experience and were indicated for continued bleeding associated with adenomyosis and submucous myoma, cervical bleeding, and an ovarian cyst.[2] To date, none of his patients, all screened preoperatively with biopsy and, when possible, hysteroscopy, has shown any evidence of malignancy. Goldrath has abandoned the routine laparoscopic tubal yoon ring occlusions and postoperative hysterograms that he did early in his study. He found that he was able to routinely obliterate the endometrial cavity and occlude the tubal ostia. The postoperative endometrial biopsy specimens contained only a minute amount of endometrial fragments. At one year he has shown bilateral tubal occulsion and endometrial cavity obliteration. This reflects Goldrath's compulsive attention to detail in ablating the endometrium.

Hematometria

Retention of blood in the ablated cavity can easily be diagnosed and treated by a routine 4-week postoperative Karman canula aspiration. At the same time, the depth of the cavity can be recorded. The frequency of hematometria in Goldrath's series was 7/216.

Urinary Tract Infections

During surgery an indwelling catheter is necessary to monitor fluid balance. It is also important to decompress the bladder to allow for adequate uterine mobilization needed to manipulate the hysteroscope for viewing the anterior uterine surface. Prophylactic oral antibiotics used for the laminaria insertion should be sufficient coverage for the short—4- to 6-hour—duration of Foley catheter use. The appropriate antibiotic is prescribed at the discretion of the surgeon.

Laser Training and Safety

Training

The 1060-nm Nd:YAG laser is one of the strongest lasers used in clinical medicine. It has the following characteristics: (1) backscatter, (2) absorption by the retinal maculae, and (3) deep (5–10 mm) transmission through fluids as well as solid tissue. These characteristics are completely different from those of the CO_2 laser well known to the gynecologist. The gynecologic CO_2 laser surgeon must have additional, specialized training in the use of the Nd:YAG laser and its physics, he must attend a gynecologic YAG laser course composed of didactic and laboratory experience, and, finally, he must acquire a preceptorship from a senior Nd:YAG laser gynecologic surgeon. A working expertise in outpatient hysteroscopy is needed. In vitro practice in the laboratory on excised specimens is necessary before attempting the procedure in vivo. Most important is hands-on experience—operating with a senior gynecologist to learn the visual changes that occur in the endometrium, practicing the manual dexterity required, and understanding the fluid insufflation system. The procedure is highly technical for both the surgeon and the operating crew, who must be completely familiar with both the Nd:YAG laser and the fluid insufflation-reclamation system. Training the operating room crew with a mock case, making sure the fluid system works and that the nurses have practiced the pump system, will reward with fewer complications the morning of your first endometrial ablation. Macular blindness will result if the eyes are not protected by 1060-nm filters. Goggles should be worn by the patient and the room crew. A hysteroscope lens filter is commercially available to protect the surgeon's eyes. Prescription glasses made from the 1060-nm filter glass can also be ordered.

Laser Safety

As laser surgery equipment is rapidly evolving with improved units and new devices are appearing daily, laser safety must be our first priority.[9] The Food and Drug Administration, Office of Device Evaluation, requires manufacturers to provide instructions that outline the operational mechanics of the device as well as the indications and contraindications for its use.[10] The Nd:YAG laser companies share the FDA's concern regarding informed, competent, compliant use of their equipment. The laser companies are prepared to provide extensive educational support for clinical and research purposes.[5] It is your responsibility to read the instructions carefully and to consult with surgeons who are more familiar with this technology before you use the new devices. Each hospital and surgicenter should employ a laser safety officer who is responsible for knowing everything about the devices, for teaching laser safety, for keeping the equipment running, and for monitoring its safe use in the operating theater. This person must assure safety to the patients as well as the staff.

Conclusion

Nd:YAG laser endometrial ablation may become the uterine surgery of the future. At this time the technique requires a surgeon attentive to fine details, precise and pedantic in his surgical training and technique, and compulsive in his preoperative workup and postoperative follow-through in this evolving procedure.

References

1. Goldrath MH, Fuller TA, Segal S: Laser photovaporization of endometrium for the treatment of menorrhagia. Am J Obstet Gynecol 104:14, 1981.
2. Goldrath MH: Hysteroscopic laser surgery. In Baggish M (ed): Basic and Advanced Laser Surgery in Gynecology. Appleton-Century-Croft, Norwalk, CT, 1985, pp 357–372.
3. Goldrath M: Personal communication. Chairman, Department OB/GYN Sinai Hospital, Detroit, MI, 1986.
4. Shirk G: Unpublished data. Licensed Nd:YAG laser clinical investigator, Cedar Rapids, IA, 1986.
5. Rose C: Personal communication. Director, Regulatory Affairs, Cooper LaserSonics, Santa Clara, CA, 1986.
6. Daikuzono N, Joffe S: An artificial sapphire probe for contact photocoagulation and tissue vaporization. Med Instrum 19:173–178, 1985.
7. Zumwalt T, Wesseler T, Joffe S: A comparison of artificial sapphire tip with the quartz tip in "in vitro" endometrial ablation. Colposc Gynecol Laser Surg 2:47, 1986.
8. Goldrath MH: Uterine tamponade for the control of acute uterine bleeding. Am J Obstet Gynecol 147:869–872, 1983.
9. Fisher J: Principles of safety in laser surgery and therapy. In Baggish M (ed): Basic and Advanced Laser Surgery in Gynecology. Appleton-Century-Croft, Norwalk, CT, 1985, pp 85–129.
10. Yin L: Personal communication. Director, Division of OB/GYN, ENT, and Dental Devices, Office of Device Evaluation, Food and Drug Administration, Silver Spring, MD, 1986.

28
Nd:YAG Laser Applications in Gynecology

Jack M. Lomano

Improved endoscopic techniques, coupled with advances in laser technology, have spurred an interest in using laser energy to treat gynecologic pathology. Laser therapy offers several advantages over other modalities, including the ability to produce precise tissue destruction, better hemostasis, and more rapid tissue healing. In addition, when combined with endoscopy, the laser increases accessibility to pelvic anatomy. Moreover, it achieves all of this at less expense and discomfort to the patient.

At the present time, the carbon dioxide, argon, potassium titanyl phosphate (KTP) twin crystal, and Nd:YAG lasers all have application to gynecology to treat intraabdominal, lower genital tract, and intrauterine disease. Specifically, these lasers have been used to treat pelvic endometriosis, cervical dysplasia, condyloma acuminata, pelvic adhesive disease, and premalignant diseases of the vulva and vagina.

The Nd:YAG laser can be used through the hysteroscope to treat chronic menorrhagia. Intraabdominally, it can be used through the laparoscope to perform ablation of pelvic endometriosis. Lesions of the lower genital tract are amenable to treatment with the Nd:YAG laser, either with direct application of the laser energy using a fiberoptic handpiece or with a focusing sapphire tip to perform excisional procedures. When passed through the hysteroscope, this same fiber can be used to excise intrauterine lesions.

Photocoagulation of the Endometrium to Treat Chronic Menorrhagia

Background and Rationale

Approximately 570,000 to 735,000 hysterectomies are performed in the United States each year, making it the most common major operation in this country and costing an estimated 1.7 billion dollars annually. Thirty to forty percent of these procedures are performed for chronic recurrent menorrhagia that is refractory to medical and surgical therapy. Although generally responsive to antibiotic therapy, morbidity occurs in 25 to 30% of hysterectomy procedures. Indeed, 600 deaths occur each year as a result of complications from the surgery. For all of these reasons, a more conservative procedure for the treatment of chronic menorrhagia has been sought.

Asherman's syndrome,[1] the development of uterine synechia secondary to uterine trauma, was first described in 1948. Although a significant problem for those women desiring pregnancy, it would be desirable for those seeking relief from heavy and prolonged menstrual flow. Accordingly, several investigators have applied various physical and chemical agents to the endometrium to intentionally create an Asherman's syndrome.[2,3] Most of these methods failed because of (1) inadequate destruction of the endometrial lining, allowing subsequent regeneration of the endometrium, or (2) complications resulting from the physical or chemical substance introduced into the uterine cavity.

In 1981, Goldrath and his colleagues[4] described the first cases of successful ablation of the endometrium with the Nd:YAG laser to create an Asherman's syndrome. Lomano[5] corroborated these findings in 1986 when he reported on 10 patients who had been treated with the Nd:YAG laser after being given the alternative of hysterectomy for the treatment of chronic menorrhagia. These patients had already undergone unsuccessful treatment, both with hormonal agents and diagnostic curettage. A multicenter study involving four centers was then carried out and 61 patients[6] were treated (including my first 10 patients). To date, over 200 patients have undergone the procedure, although not under this same protocol.

Patient Selection

Patients eligible for this treatment have a history of heavy menstrual flow, which has been refractory to surgical and medical management. All have had one or more dilatation and curettage and have been treated with hormones, including estrogen, progesterone, androgens, antiprostaglandins, or ergotrate derivatives. All patients are sterilized or willing to be sterilized, since the outcome of a pregnancy following this procedure has not been established.

Procedure

The goal of ablation of the endometrium with the Nd:YAG laser for the treatment of chronic menorrhagia is to obviate the need for hysterectomy and/or to provide complete amenorrhea. The treatment was removed from FDA protocols in March 1986. Two to four weeks prior to the procedure, patients are given danazol (800 mg/day) to decrease the thickness of the endometrial lining and to create the hypoestrogen state characteristic of Asherman's syndrome.

The procedure can be performed on an outpatient basis and takes from 20 to 45 minutes. A general anesthetic is used on most patients, although regional and paracervical anesthesia can be used in those patients where general anesthesia is contraindicated.

The photocoagulation process begins at one of the tubal ostia and then extends across the fundus of the uterus and finally down the side walls of the uterus to the level of the internal os, generally 4 cm above the external os. Two techniques of delivery have been described. In Goldrath's "dragging technique," the fiber is placed in direct contact with the endometrium and then is slowly dragged over the surface of the endometrial cavity. Approximately 40 to 60 W are required to achieve ablation by this method. Although the "dragging technique" allows the physician to observe a dramatic visual effect as the endometrium is destroyed, the buildup of carbonized particles on the fiber tip results in extremely high temperatures that can cause the tip to fracture. Consequently, it is often necessary to remove the fiber and repolish it one to three times during the procedure.

The so-called "blanching technique" is accomplished by bringing the fiber tip close to the endometrial lining without actually touching it. This requires approximately 10 W of additional power to penetrate the endometrium sufficiently (50 to 70 W). The operator observes the color of the endometrial surface, looking for a gradual change from pink to white. The "blanching technique" requires a much slower movement of the laser fiber than that required by the "dragging technique" to achieve temperatures high enough to cause protein coagulation and subsequent tissue death 4 to 5 mm below the surface. The disadvantage of this technique is poor visualization in the lower uterine segment. Because of the funnel-shaped contour of the uterine cavity, it is very difficult to place direct right-angle applications of the laser without actually touching the endometrial surface. To date, no controlled studies have been conducted to compare the clinical effectiveness of these two techniques.

Patients are discharged on the day of surgery. They may resume normal activity 2 to 3 days following the procedure.

Results of Treatment

Sixty-one patients were treated for chronic menorrhagia with the Nd:YAG laser under the

TABLE 28.1. Results of Nd:YAG laser ablation for the treatment of chronic menorrhagia (61 patients)

Menstrual flow	Pretreatment	Posttreatment
Duration (days)		
> 7	38 (62%)	0
4–6	18 (30%)	21 (34%)
1–3	5 (8%)	26 (43%)
0	0	14 (23%)
Amount (pads/menstrual period)		
> 40	19 (31%)	0
20–40	35 (57%)	0
< 20	7 (12%)	61 (100%)

multicenter protocol. Their ages ranged from 27 to 55 years. Table 28.1 compares menstrual flow of these patients before and after treatment according to duration and amount of flow. Prior to treatment, 38 patients (62%) reported menstrual flow of greater than seven days, 18 patients (30%) reported flow of 4 to 6 days, and 5 patients (8%) reported flow of 1 to 3 days. After treatment, no patients had flow lasting longer than seven days, 21 patients (34%) had flow lasting 4 to 6 days, 26 patients (43%) reported flow lasting 1 to 3 days, and 14 (23%) were totally amenorrheic.

When amount of flow was evaluated before treatment, 19 patients (31%) reported using more than 40 pads per menstrual period; 35 patients (57%) reported using 20 to 40 pads, and 7 patients (12%) used fewer than 20 pads. Following the procedure, all 61 patients (100%) were using fewer than 20 pads per menstrual period.

Complications

One of the 61 patients developed pulmonary edema, and three patients experienced edema during or following the procedure. All four were treated successfully with intravenous diuretics and no permanent complications developed. I[5] reported an average fluid absorption of 1930 ml in patients who had previous tubal ligations and an average of 2160 ml in patients using other kinds of contraception. Since this difference is not significant, it is theorized that the source of this fluid excess is direct intravenous fluid absorption through the veins of the endometrium. Loeffer[7] reported that his patients experienced less fluid absorption with the "blanching technique" than with the "dragging technique."

Difficulty with visualization in the uterine cavity continues to be a problem, especially in those patients who have not been sufficiently pretreated with danazol. As the intense burst of laser energy impacts onto the endometrium, it

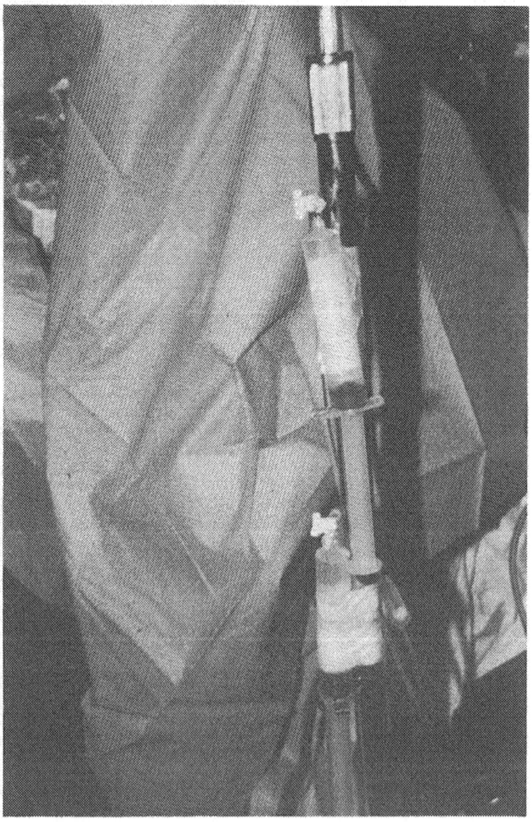

FIGURE 28.1. Nd:YAG laser ablation of the endometrium to treat chronic menorrhagia. To increase the pressure of irrigation during the procedure, 50-cc syringes are mounted in the main line from the irrigation solution to the hysteroscope to provide intermittent manual "flushing" of the endometrial cavity.

results in some clouding of the visual field. A rapid irrigation system, therefore, is essential to reduce these visualization problems. Several techniques have been described to increase the pressure of irrigation during the procedure. In the first technique, the urologic irrigation bag is raised on an intravenous infusion pole until the pressure of the irrigation approaches 100 mm Hg. A second technique is to mount 50-cc irrigating syringes in the main line from the irrigation solution to the hysteroscope to provide intermittent manual "flushing" of the endometrial cavity (Figure 28.1). A third option is to pressurize the urologic irrigation bag with either rapid blood infusion bags or gas cylinder pressure into the irrigation system. We are also evaluating a "balloon system," which would allow transmission of the Nd:YAG laser energy, but would seal off the endometrium to eliminate the possibility of clouding and intravenous absorption (Figure 28.2).

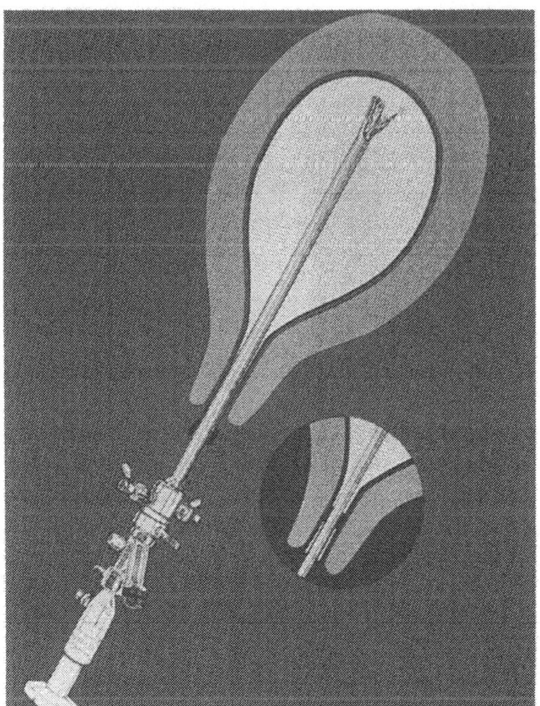

FIGURE 28.2. Experimental "balloon system" for use in ablation of endometrium to treat chronic menorrhagia. The system would allow transmission of the laser energy but seal off the endometrium to eliminate the possibility of clouding and intravenous absorption.

Ablation of Early Pelvic Endometriosis

Background and Rationale

Rokitansky described the first case of pelvic endometriosis in 1860.[8] In 1921, Cattell and Swinton[9] summarized the entire world's literature on the subject, consisting of 20 cases. Since then, the incidence of the disease has increased dramatically. This is particularly distressing, since it is occurring at a time when many women in the United States are choosing to postpone their age of childbirth.

The association between endometriosis and an inability to conceive has been recognized for years.[10] Premenstrual and menstrual pain caused by congestion of sclerosed ovaries and nodules in the uterosacral ligaments present a significant disability annually to thousands of women. Because of the increasingly young age at initial diagnosis, hysterectomy and bilateral salpingoopherectomy is an unacceptable treatment. Conservative treatment with oral contraceptive or danazol is expensive, and the side effects often prevent their long-term use.[11–14] Conservative surgery has been demonstrated to be effective in controlling the disease. However, sharp dissection of pelvic endometriosis is not only difficult but often results in bleeding, which can lead to adhesion formation, thus further compromising fertility. Another option, electrocautery, while providing excellent hemostasis, can produce thermal necrosis and perforation of underlying bowel, bladder, or ureter.

These problems led several investigators to treat endometriosis with laparoscopic laser surgery. Feste,[15] Martin,[16] Daniell and Pittaway,[17] and Kelly and Roberts[18] have reported on the use of the carbon dioxide laser. Keye and coworkers[19] has reported on treatment with the argon laser, and Daniell[20] has treated the disease with the KTP twin crystal laser.

I was first to report on photocoagulation of early pelvic endometriosis with the Nd:YAG laser.[21] It is an excellent treatment modality because of its inherent ability to penetrate tissue without vaporization of the serosa and its capability of being delivered through an optical fiber (easily manipulated through a laparoscope). Since the Nd:YAG laser is a coagulating rather than a vaporizing tool, a smoke evacuation system is not needed. The Nd:YAG laser also offers the advantage of color selectivity because its wavelength is selectively absorbed by the dark colors of pelvic endometriosis.

Patient Selection

Patients eligible for this treatment have shown signs and symptoms of early pelvic endometriosis, including pelvic pain, menstrual dysfunction, infertility, or suspicious pelvic examination. Since the procedure is still on FDA protocol, patients must sign an informed consent approved both by Grant Hospital's Human Experimentation Committee and the FDA. Patients who are discovered to have severe endometriosis, as defined by the American Fertility Society, are considered for open laparotomy, especially when the pelvic viscera are poorly visualized through the laparoscope.

Procedure

The Nd:YAG laser is placed in the operating room on a standby basis with the optical fiber sterilized. Patients undergo diagnostic laparoscopy under general anesthesia; if early pelvic endometriosis is found, the laser fiber is introduced through the operating channel of the laparoscope (Figure 28.3). A double-puncture technique is sometimes used so that additional instruments can be placed to facilitate the procedure. The fiber is placed approximately 1 cm from the observed lesion. A laparoscopic fiber deflector is used to direct the beam into difficult areas of the pelvis. Photocoagulation is performed at a 20-W setting until a blanching effect is achieved 1 to 2 mm beyond the border of the lesion. Intermittent 1- to 3-second exposures with a spot size of 2 mm are recommended to avoid the buildup of heat and subsequent vaporization of the serosa.[21] The procedure can be completed in approximately 10 to 40 minutes.

Patients are discharged on the day of surgery and resume normal activity within 1 to 2 days after surgery. They are followed postoperatively at 3-month intervals. Adjunctive therapy with oral contraception and/or danazol can be used following treatment.

Results of Treatment

Of 135 patients who underwent diagnostic laparoscopy at the Grant Laser Center during a three-year period, 61 were considered eligible for Nd:YAG laser photocoagulation of early pelvic endometriosis. Patients have been followed for an average of 22 months (range 1 to 34 months). There were no operative or postoperative complications. Symptoms improved following surgery in 45 patients (74%), worsened in 2 patients (3%), and did not change in 12 pa-

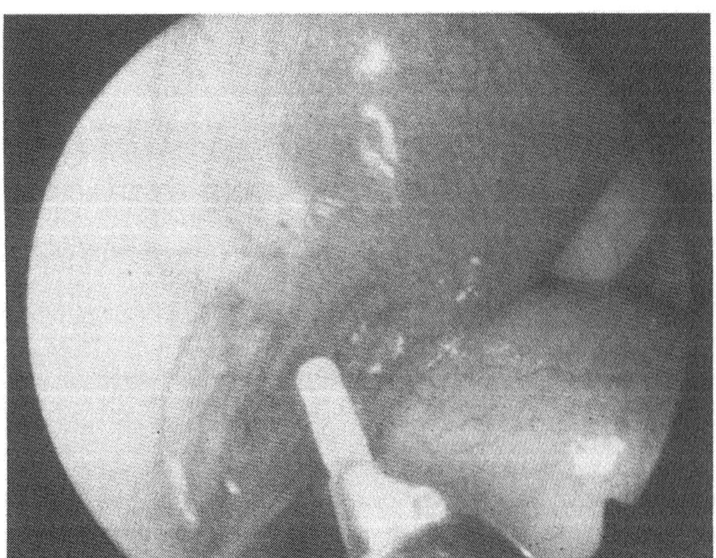

FIGURE 28.3. Nd:YAG laser ablation of early pelvic endometriosis. The sterilized optical fiber is introduced through the operating channel of the laparoscope.

TABLE 28.2. Results of Nd:YAG laser photocoagulation of early pelvic endometriosis (61 patients*; average follow-up 22 months)

Report of symptoms	No. of patients	%
Improved	45	74
Worsened	2	3
No change	12	20

*Two patients were lost to follow-up.

tients (20%). Two patients have been lost to follow-up (Table 28.2).

Currently, a multicenter study is underway to confirm the effectiveness of Nd:YAG laser photocoagulation in the treatment of early pelvic endometriosis.

Lesions of the Lower Genital Tract

Background and Rationale

Changing sexual attitudes have led to a younger age of first coital exposure and an increase in the number of sexual partners. This combination has resulted in a tremendous increase in sexually transmitted diseases. Papilloma virus types 16, 18, and 31 have been implicated in the etiology of malignant change in the lower genital tract, whereas types 6 and 11 have been associated with benign lesions. This virus has now been linked directly to cervical, vaginal, and vulvar intraepithelial neoplasia, as well as condyloma acuminata in the lower genital tract. If not eradicated prior to invasion of the basement membranes, these premalignant lesions have the potential of progressing to malignant disease. Thus, a conservative treatment modality is needed to eradicate these premalignant genital tract neoplasms.

Local excision, cryosurgery, cautery, and carbon dioxide laser vaporization have all been used successfully in treating cervical, vaginal, and vulvar intraepithelial neoplasia. The Nd:YAG laser has been used in the treatment of this disease process as well, but, as yet, results have not been as promising as those obtained with the carbon dioxide laser.

Colposcopic evaluation of the lower genital tract with selected biopsy of abnormal areas will provide a tissue diagnosis in 80% of suspected neoplastic lesions of the cervix, vulva, and vagina. In 20% of cases, however, diagnosis cannot be confirmed with colposcopic-selected biopsy. A need exists, therefore, for excisional biopsy in selected cases. The knife and carbon dioxide laser have been used for this purpose. Although both are effective, the knife can result in significant blood loss as well as potential scarring of the cervix, vagina, or vulva. The use of the colposcope with the carbon dioxide laser, on the other hand, allows procedures to be performed in a bloodless field. The recent development of sapphire tips for the Nd:YAG laser has allowed laser energy to be used as a cutting tool, making it a potentially effective excisional instrument.

Procedure

Direct Applications of Laser Energy

Nd:YAG laser destruction of lesions of the cervix, vagina, and vulva can be accomplished by placing the laser fiber over the lesion and then discharging the laser energy at a power setting of 20 to 30 W until a white blanching is visible 1 to 2 mm beyond the lesion. If intermittent 3-second exposures are applied, the depth of penetration will vary between 3 and 5 mm.

Excisional Procedures with the Sapphire Tip

Surgical Laser Technologies (SLT) (1 Great Valley Parkway, Malvern, PA 19355) has recently developed a sapphire tip for use with the Nd:YAG laser, which concentrates the laser energy into a small spot size and allows the laser to be used as a cutting modality rather than a coagulating one. Excisional procedures involving condyloma acuminata and vaginal, cervical, or vulvar neoplasia can be performed with the sapphire tip attached to the laser fiber in a manner similar to cold-knife excisions and excisions with the carbon dioxide laser. Since the sapphire-tipped Nd:YAG laser is more hemostatic than the carbon dioxide laser, it might have potential benefits in excisional procedures of the cervix (Figure 28.4). Comparison studies between the carbon dioxide and Nd:YAG lasers for this purpose are currently in progress.

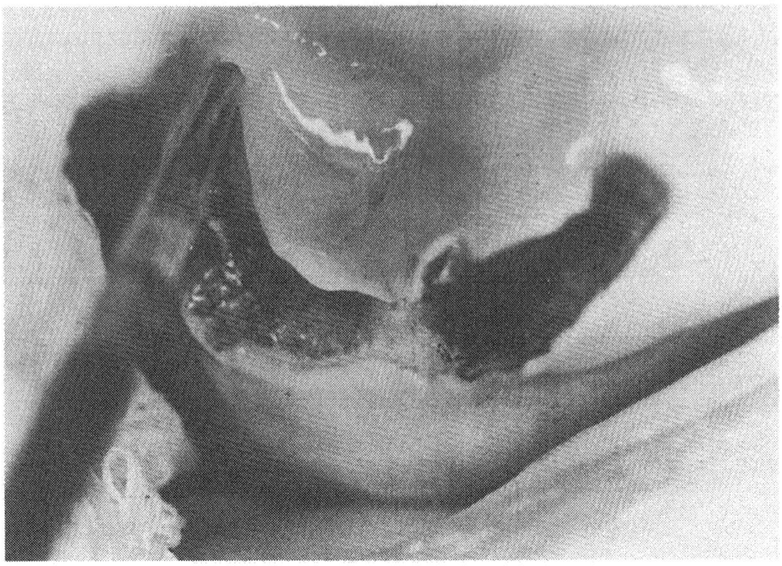

FIGURE 28.4. Nd:YAG laser cervical excision with sapphire tip.

Complications with Procedures Using Direct Application of Laser Energy

Because excisional procedures with the sapphire tip are just now under investigation, complications are as yet undetermined. Complications that have been reported involve procedures using direct application of laser energy. Specifically, as in cryosurgery, surgical excision, and cautery, the Nd:YAG laser does not allow for good control of the depth of penetration. In addition, the energy from the Nd:YAG often scatters well below the epidermis, causing damage that requires a longer period of tissue healing. The carbon dioxide laser, on the other hand, because of its vaporizing characteristic, allows precise removal of these lesions to a depth measurable with microsurgical calibers. Until newer techniques are developed, therefore, the carbon dioxide will likely remain the procedure of choice in these cases. Destruction of condyloma acuminata in the lower genital tract can be accomplished with the Nd:YAG laser, but once again, it is not possible to achieve a precise depth of destruction. Since the papilloma virus is located only in the epidermis, it is prudent for the operator to destroy only the epidermis and to leave the dermal layers of the skin undamaged. Thus, the carbon dioxide laser still remains the ideal laser for this procedure.

Intrauterine Excisional Procedures

Background and Rationale

Removal of uterine septa, submucous fibroids, and endometrial polyps and lysis of intrauterine adhesions can all be accomplished with laser hysteroscopy. The carbon dioxide laser must be used in a gas-distending media because it rapidly absorbs liquid materials. When used with incisional techniques, however, gas media has the potential to create a gas embolus. Fiberoptic lasers (Nd:YAG, argon, KTP twin crystals), on the other hand, are used in a fluid-distending media, thus eliminating the possibility of this risk.

Procedure

Excisional procedures with laser hysteroscopy offer very few advantages over those techniques that have been described using sharp dissection. The bare fiber or the sapphire tip of the Nd:YAG laser is placed directly against the lesion. If the bare fiber is used, very high temperatures can result in the destruction of the fiber tip. To prevent this, the fiber must be repolished several times during the procedure. When the sapphire tip is used, however, Nd:YAG laser excisional techniques offer the distinct advantage of precise tissue removal with a minimum of damage to surrounding normal uterine structures. In addition, these procedures can be accomplished with less bleeding and less risk of perforating the uterus than techniques using scissors or electrocautery. The fluid-distending media allows the laser tip to cool and permits irrigation of debris to facilitate visualization during the hysteroscopic excisional procedure.

Fiberoptic lasers used in combination with the focusing sapphire crystal must be limited to less than 20 W to avoid fracture of the crystalloid material. After the tissue is excised, the resultant debris is removed with a grasping forceps through the operating channel of the hysteroscope.

References

1. Asherman JG: Amenorrhoea traumatica (atretica). J Obstet Gynaecol Br Emp 55:23, 1948.
2. Droegemuller W, Greer B, David JR: Cryocoagulation of the endometrium at the uterine cornua. Am J Obstet Gynecol 131:1, 1978.
3. Droegemuller W, Greer B, Makowski E: Cryosurgery in patients with dysfunctional uterine bleeding. Obstet Gynecol 38:156, 1971.
4. Goldrath MH, Fuller TA, Segal S: Laser photovaporization of endometrium for the treatment of menorrhagia. Am J Obstet Gynecol 140:14, 1981.
5. Lomano JM: Photocoagulation of the endometrium with the Nd:YAG laser for the treatment of menorrhagia: A report of ten cases. J Reprod Med 31:148–150, 1986.
6. Lomano JM: Ablation of the endometrium with the Nd:YAG laser: A multicenter study. Colposc Gynecol Laser Surg Vol. 2, Number 4, 1986 pp. 203–207.
7. Loeffer F: Personal communication, May 30, 1986, Phoenix, AZ.
8. Kistner RW: Endometriosis. In Sciarra JJ, McElin TW (eds): Gynecology and Obstetrics, Vol. I. Harper & Row, Hagerstown, MD, 1977.
9. Cattell RB, Swinton NW: Endometriosis with reference to conservative treatment. N Engl J Med 214:341, 1936.
10. Naples JD, Batt RE, Sadigh H: Spontaneous abortion n rate in patients with endometriosis. Obstet Gynecol 57:409, 1981.
11. Seibel MM, Berger MJ, Weinstein F, et al: The effectiveness of danazol on subsequent fertility in minimal endometriosis. Fertil Steril (Suppl) 37:310, 1982.
12. Dmowski WP, Cohen MR: Treatment of endometriosis with an antigonadotropin, danazol: A laparoscopic and histologic evaluation. Obstet Gynecol 46:147, 1975.
13. Dmowski WP, Cohen MR: Antigonadotropin (danazol) in the treatment of endometriosis. Evaluation of post-treatment fertility and three-year follow-up data. Am J Obstet Gynecol 130:41, 1978.
14. Biberoglu KO, Behrman SJ: Dosage aspects of danazol therapy in endometriosis: Short-term and long-term effectiveness. Am J Obstet Gynecol 139:645, 1981.
15. Festy JR: CO_2 laser neurectomy for dysmenorrhea. Laser Surg Med 3:27, 1984.
16. Martin DC: CO_2 laser laparoscopy for the treatment of endometriosis associated with infertility. J Reprod Med 30:409–412, 1985.
17. Daniell JF, Pittaway DE: Use of the CO_2 laser in laparoscopic laser surgery: Initial experience with the second puncture technique. Infertility 5:15, 1982.
18. Kelly RW, Roberts DK: CO_2 laser laparoscopy: A potential alternative to danazol in the treatment of stage I and II endometriosis. J Reprod Med 28:638–640, 1983.
19. Keye WR, Matson GA, Dixon J: The use of the argon laser in the treatment of experimental endometriosis. Fertil Steril 39:26–29, 1983.
20. Daniell JF: Initial evaluation of the use of the KTP twin crystal laser in gynecologic laparoscopy. Fertil Steril Vol 46, Issue (3):373–7, September, 1986.
21. Lomano JM: Photocoagulation of early pelvic endometriosis with the Nd:YAG laser through the laparoscope. J Reprod Med 30:77–81, 1985.

29
Clinical Application of the Nd:YAG Laser in Dermatology and Plastic Surgery

K. Arai and T. Sato

Ever since Maiman developed the ruby laser in 1960, a series of newer laser devices have been developed and put to practical use, having shown great advances in a variety of fields.

At present, four lasers—ruby, argon, CO_2 and Nd:YAG—are used for therapeutic purposes in our field. As each of these lasers has distinctive features, frequently they are used for different and limited purposes. The Nd:YAG laser described in this chapter has more potential coagulability than the CO_2 laser and exerts a better hemostatic effect, while its ability for incision and vaporization is inferior to that of the CO_2 laser. Further, the Nd:YAG laser shows selectivity to some extent depending on the color of the object to which it is applied. Thus, the control of all functions by this device is somewhat difficult. Because of this setback, its usage had been greatly limited in the fields of plastic surgery and dermatology where precision and accuracy are important considerations.[1] However, during recent years a surgical probe made of a new ceramic has been developed for use with the Nd:YAG laser, which permits more accurate incisions and tissue vaporization, in addition to its hemostatic ability through coagulation.[2–4]

The principal surgical procedures required in the fields of plastic surgery and dermatology are incision, vaporization, hemostasis, and suture. With the exception of suture, favorable results can now be obtained with the Nd:YAG laser in all these procedures.

The following describes our clinical experience in the use of the Nd:YAG laser.

Instrument and Accessories

The Nd:YAG laser device we used was the Molectron Model 8000. For incision, vaporization, and coagulation, we used various SLT contact laser scalpels and SLT contact laser probes (Surgical Laser Technologies Co., Tokyo and Malvern PA). There are many different types of SLT contact laser probes, but we used mainly the SLT contact coagulation probe and SLT contact vaporization probe for dermatology and plastic surgery.

Functions of the Nd:YAG Laser Required in the Fields of Dermatology and Plastic Surgery

Noncontact Procedure

The coagulability properties of the Nd:YAG laser are used in noncontact procedures for the removal of pigmented nevus, verruca, neurofibroma, cavernous angioma, pachydermatocele in Recklinghausen's disease, and malignant skin tumors. For the spherical bulging pigmented nevus and verruca of 7 to 8 mm in diameter, the tip of the fiber is held 1 to 1.5 cm away from the lesion and irradiated for 1 second at 40 W. The carbonized coagulated layer induced on the skin surface is then removed with a sharp needle or a surgical scalpel. This process is repeated until the protrusion is removed. For neurofibromas, continuous irradiation at about 60 W is used to achieve coagulative necrosis without charring. The lesion is then removed with a scalpel and the site sutured. For cavernous angiomas, we use the Nd:YAG laser for protuberant lesions limited to the lip, tongue, fundus of oral cavity, buccal mucosa, and skin surface. For these lesions, we begin by first holding the tip of the fiber a distance away from the lesion and begin irradiation at about 60 W continuously and then bring the tip of the fiber closer to the surface of the lesion while carefully watching the surface condition. As soon as a slight change in the surface is observed, the tip is brought slightly closer to the lesion and held there for using continued irradiation to obtain a satisfactory coagulative necrosis. For cavernous angioma, charring or cracking of the lesion can frequently result in profuse bleeding. Therefore, caution is necessary in the use of the Nd:YAG laser for the removal of cavernous angioma and avoid charring. Following adequate coagulation a surgical scalpel or CO_2 laser is used to remove the coagulated tissue either entirely or as much as possible in those lesions on the skin surface or on the lip where the external appearance is important, and the site is then closed with sutures. Extensive lesions within the oral cavity are removed and sutured, but smaller lesions are left open. For the larger pachydermatocele of Recklinghausen's disease, a higher power output, around 70 to 80 W, is used. The same method as described above induces coagulative necrosis without charring, which is then vaporized entirely or the major portion removed with the CO_2 laser. However, if sinusoid large-diameter blood vessels are present in the pachydermatocele, it would be extremely difficult to control bleeding in this manner. For malignant skin tumors, if not too large, coagulative necrosis is induced at the site, including the peripheral area, by irradiation at about 60 W, followed by vaporization with the CO_2 laser. This step is repeated until the lesion is removed to the desired depth. In addition tissues around and beneath the tumor are also removed to ensure that no tumor cells remain.

Contact Procedure

Incision

SLT Contact laser scalpels of various diameters were tested in animal experiments. It was found that the scalpel with distal probe diameter of 0.2 mm operating at 7 to 8 W and moved at the same speed as the conventional scalpel, produced the best incision. Therefore, in the fields of dermatology and plastic surgery, where aesthetic features are important considerations, irradiation is conducted under the above conditions.

This procedure was used in clinical cases of pigmented nevus, atheroma, neurofibroma, and onychocryptosis (ingrown nail). Incisions must be made very carefully in order to terminate irradiation immediately on discontinuation of the incision. Otherwise, coagulative degeneration progresses, resulting in ugly scars.

As for bleeding during the incision, there is practically no bleeding in an incision of this depth. The small hemorrhage that may occasionally occur can be readily stopped by light touches with the laser scalpel.

In the case of removal of tissues such as tumors, an incision is made around the lesion. The tissue is lifted and the base is divided with the laser scalpel. If the removed tissue is of a relatively large size that does not allow suturing, the skin around the lesion is released to allow the skin to be brought together.

Vaporization

In the fields of dermatology and plastic surgery, small tumors are the major indication for treatment with contact vaporization. The most important point is to remove tumor tissue with a minimum damage to normal tissue. Based on the results obtained in animal experiments, the SLT Laser scalpel with a 0.2 mm tip diameter operating at about 5 W is best for vaporization.

It is important to maintain careful observation over the site of irradiation so that the laser beam does not extend outside the operating area. Furthermore, when the laser scalpel is held away from the target tissue, and not being used for surgery the laser should be turned off immediately. This is necessary to perform accurate vaporization and prevent damage to the scalpel. In experiments we found that a laser scalpel of 0.2 mm tip diameter can be damaged within 5 seconds if irradiated in the air at a power output of 8 W.

Hemostasis

The Nd:YAG laser provides excellent hemostasis by its powerful protein coagulation effect.

Because aesthetic considerations are important, the Nd:YAG laser has not been used frequently despite such excellent hemostatic effects, because of its widespread tissue damage when used in a noncontact manner. Furthermore it may be difficult to induce hemostasis once hemorrhage occurs. Considering these drawbacks, we prefer the SLT contact laser scalpel. With this scalpel, and a 0.2 to 0.4 mm tip diameter operating at about 5 W, a gentle touch with the probe can produce adequate hemostasis. However, when bleeding is serious, hemostasis with this procedure is impossible. Thus we investigated various hemostatic procedures for such bleeding. It seemed best to use quartz or sapphire to sandwich or compress the bleeding site (reported at the 123rd Tokyo Regional Assembly of the Japanese Academy of Plastic Surgery). We frequently use the coagulation probe (Surgical Laser Technologies) with favorable results. This probe is available on the market for endoscopic use.

To produce hemostasis, the oozing blood is cleared with a piece of gauze to determine the site of bleeding. The site is compressed with the coagulation probe and irradiated with the laser beam. There are currently two sizes of probes: 2.2 and 1.8 mm in diameter. Irradiation should be at 8 to 10 W for a duration of 0.3 to 0.5 seconds. For coagulation of exposed arteries or veins, the animal experiment showed that effective coagulation with the laser could be achieved in arteries of up to 1.5 mm in diameter and veins of up to 2 mm in diameter. The conditions for laser irradiation were the same as those used for the hemostasis of actively bleeding vessels. The important consideration here is to induce coagulatory degeneration of the target vessel with the probe operating at a suitable output and duration. If charring or cracking results from excessive output, hemorrhage may be aggravated.

Clinical Cases

The following clinical cases illustrate some of these points.

Case No. 1

Figure 29.1 shows an 18-year-old female with an extensive cavernous angioma on the tongue. Following the noncontact procedure previously described and using a power output of 60 W, coagulative necrosis was induced (arrow). The site was necrosed without charring. In cases such as this one, care must be taken to avoid

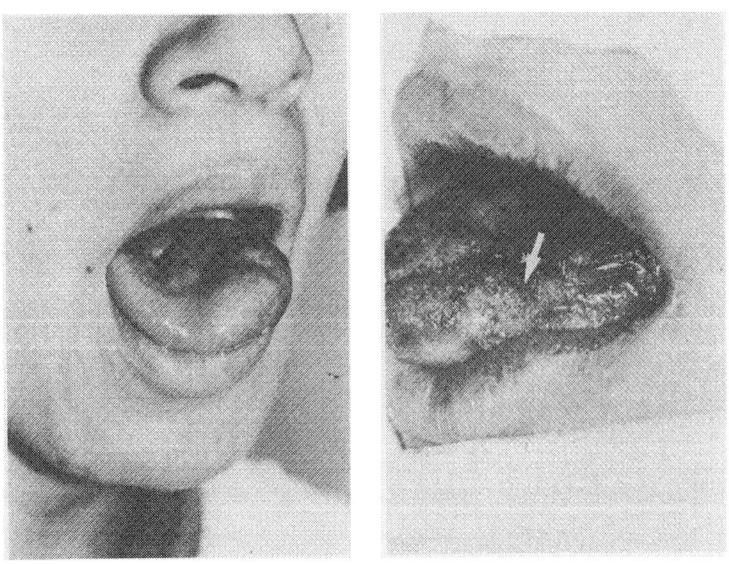

FIGURE 29.1. Case No. 1. *(Left)* Eighteen-year-old female with cavernous angioma on the tongue. *(Right)* Laser irradiation was performed at a power output of 60 W to induce coagulatory degeneration *(arrow)*.

charring, as it will result in cracking and can produce profuse bleeding.

Case No. 2

Figure 29.2 shows an 18-year-old female with cavernous angioma on the right side of the lower lip. By using noncontact continuous irradiation at 60 W, coagulative necrosis was induced, which was then removed with a conventional scalpel. Because of sufficient coagulation of the angioma, bleeding was minor, and the entire procedure took only about 30 minutes.

Case No. 3

Figure 29.3, top shows the ingrown nail of the right first digit of a 32-year-old male, with granulation tissue with infection. One fourth of the ingrown nail was removed first, followed by removal of the nail bed and root with the contact laser scalpel of 0.2 mm in tip diameter operating at 8 W. Particularly for the root of the nail, the laser scalpel with the power output reduced to 5 W was used for thorough vaporization to ensure complete removal of the root. If the conventional scalpel is used for this procedure, a considerable amount of bleeding would have occurred postoperatively and soaked the bandage; however, such is not be seen when the laser scalpel was used. The postoperative course was uneventful. Figure 29.3, bottom shows the operative site 1 month postoperatively.

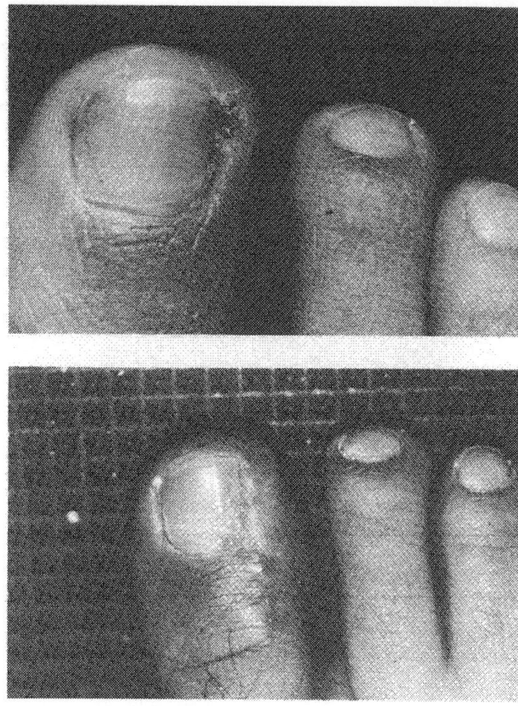

FIGURE 29.3. Case No. 3. *(Top)* Thirty-two-year-old male patient with ingrown nail on the right first digit. *(Bottom)* Condition 1 month postoperatively.

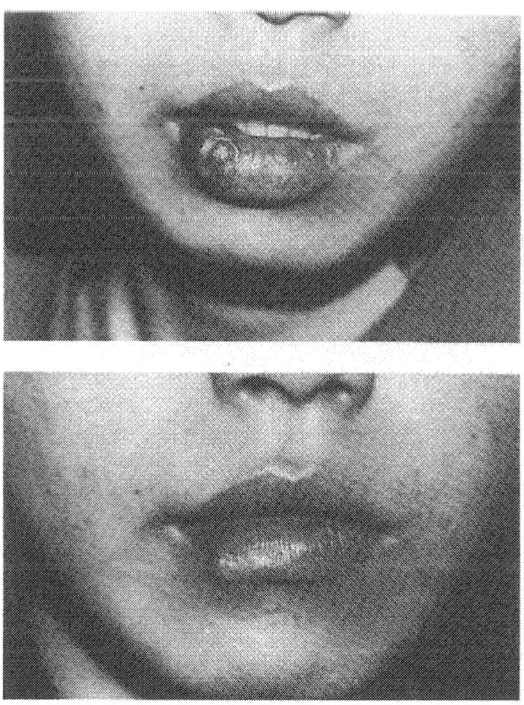

FIGURE 29.2. Case No. 2. *(Top)* Eighteen-year-old female patient with cavernous angioma on the lower lip. *(Bottom)* Coagulatory degeneration was induced with the laser operating at 60 W, followed by removal of the lesion with a conventional scalpel and closing with suture. This was taken 1 year postoperatively.

Case No. 4

Figure 29.4, top shows a 35-year-old male patient with two protruding pigmented naevi, which were vaporized with the contact laser scalpel and a probe 0.2 mm in diameter operating at 8 W; Figure 29.4, bottom was taken 4 months postoperatively.

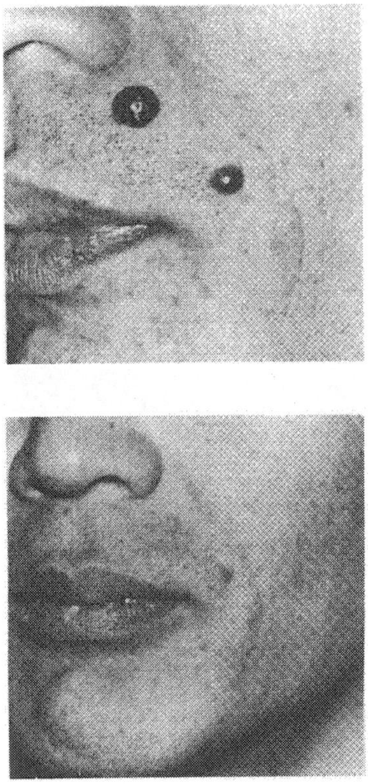

FIGURE 29.4. Case No. 4. *(Top)* Thirty-five-year-old male patient with 2 bulging pigmented nevi on the upper lip; 20 months before surgery. *(Bottom)* Vaporization was performed with a contact laser scalpel of 0.2 mm tip diameter; 5 months after surgery.

Past, Present, and Prospects of the Nd:YAG Laser in the Fields of Dermatology and Plastic Surgery

When the Nd:YAG laser characterized by excellent coagulating capability was first used clinically, its application in this field was extremely limited and it was utilized only for the removal of malignant skin tumors and cavernous angioma, or as a method to stop hemorrhage. The reason for such limited applications of the Nd:YAG laser was the lack of its ability to make incisions. With the recent development of a variety of SLT contact laser probes and SLT laser scalpels, the Nd:YAG laser now performs many functions necessary and important to the fields of dermatology and plastic surgery. These include ability to make incisions, vaporization, coagulation, and hemostasis, thus greatly widening the scope for application of the Nd:YAG laser. Unlike the supplementary role it played previously, it is now beginning to play a major role in surgery.

At present, only a single probe can be fitted to the Nd:YAG laser at one time. This may require frequent changing of the holder and probe according to the purpose for which it is used. This is cumbersome, involving a waste of time and effort. In view of the above, we are developing a Nd:YAG laser device that allows simultaneous use of multiple fibers that can meet different requirements during an operative procedure. With a multichannel fiber system, it is hoped that incision, vaporization, coagulation, and hemostasis can be performed quickly, as the need arises, permitting laser surgery with the Nd:YAG laser as a principal instrument.

References

1. Arai K, Waseda T, Ota H, et al: A preliminary study on clinical application of Nd:YAG laser to the face and head. Lasers Surg Med 3:231–239, 1983.
2. Washida H, Tsugaya M, Hirao N, Hachisuka Y: Experience using the laser rod in urological surgery. Acta Urol Jpn, 30(7):891–896, 1984.
3. Daikuzono N, Joffe SN: Artificial sapphire probe for contact photocoagulation and tissue vaporization with the Nd:YAG laser. Med Instrum 19(4):173–178, 1985.
4. Arai K, Sato T, Ito Y: On clinical application of surgical rod adapted YAG laser for benign tumor. J Jpn Soc Laser Med 6:505–508, 1986.

30 Study of the Benefits of the Nd:YAG Laser in Plastic Surgery

David B. Apfelberg and Teruko Smith

Lasers of various wavelengths have found increasing acceptance by plastic surgeons in the treatment of a wide variety of cutaneous and subcutaneous lesions. The CO_2 laser has been used the longest because of its versatility in providing hemostatic incision, photovaporization, photocoagulation, and photoablation.[1–4] This laser is widely accepted for excision of vascular tumors, vaporization of viral diseases such as warts, removal of tattoos, and the like. The argon laser provides photocoagulation of superficial vascular lesions due to the selective affinity of hemoglobin to the blue-green light. Multiple lesions such as port-wine hemangiomas, capillary/cavernous hemangiomas, telangiectasia, and the like are amenable to argon laser exposure.[5–9]

There exists the need to photoablate certain cutaneous lesions deeper than either the CO_2 or argon laser can achieve. In addition to photoablation, precise, hemostatic incision with sapphire focusing lens and scalpels has largely supplanted other lasers for surgical incision. Although scattered reports have appeared on the use of the Nd:YAG laser in plastic surgery, no detailed longitudinal report exists to describe the photocoagulation and photoablation capabilities of this laser. This chapter describes the results of the treatment of multiple categories of cutaneous lesions in 70 patients by the Molectron 8000 Nd:YAG laser.

Materials and Methods

Nd:YAG Laser Physiology

The Molectron 8000 Nd:YAG laser (Cooper LaserSonics) produces continuous wave power output of 1064 mm in the near-infrared light spectrum. This laser light is relatively unaffected by water, as is the CO_2 laser, or hemoglobin, as is the argon laser, and can produce tissue reactions to depths of 5–7 mm into the dermis. When Nd:YAG laser light encounters tissue, the result is a combination of backscatter (reflection), forward scatter, and absorption. The scattering effect around the incident laser beam within the tissue heats up a large volume and causes tissue coagulation and necrosis over a large volume of tissue without its removal. Tissue vaporization can be achieved by further heat generation of the coagulated and desiccated tissue with high-energy density over time. The Nd:YAG laser used in this study can produce outputs of 0.5–95 W, which may be transmitted through a fiberoptic handpiece to a specially designed dermal probe. The handpiece is held perpendicular to the treatment area with a focal length of 3–4 cm and a 1-mm spot size. Continuous or pulsed beams could be utilized.

Sapphire Contact Tips and Scalpels

Recently, the usefulness of the Nd:YAG laser has been dramatically extended by the use of ingenious peripheral devices based on synthetic sapphire technology. Due to the geometry and optic design of the synthetic sapphire probe, the laser scalpel combines excellent cutting properties with the coagulative ability of the Nd:YAG laser. Smaller diameter tips provide a sharp energy concentration for cutting and vaporization. Larger round or flat diameter tips give more diffuse energy distribution for greater hemostatic effect. These products are used with direct tissue contact as opposed to noncontact with other lasers. They greatly extend the hemostatic incision and vaporization capability of

TABLE 30.1. Summary of patients treated for lesions with Nd:YAG laser

Classification	No. of patients
Patients	64
Lesions	87
Categories	
Capillary/cavernous hemangiomas	13
Epistaxis (Osler–Weber–Rendu)	3
Port-wine hemangioma	8
Keloid/hypertrophic scar	12
Angiokeratoma	1
Granuloma faciale	2
Skin cancer/keratosis	2
Large cavernous hemangioma/lymphangioma	7
Superficial varicosity	16
Male/female	27/37
Average age	36.5 years (range 4 mo.–76 years)

the Nd:YAG laser very favorably in relation to standard argon and CO_2 laser usage. (Manufactured by Surgical Laser Technologies, Malvern, PA, USA).

Patient Data

Summary of Patient Group

The treatment group consisted of 64 patients with 87 different lesions (see Table 30.1). There were 27 males and 37 females with an average age of 36.5 years, ranging from 4 months to 76 years. Of the 37 female patients, 16 were treated by the Nd:YAG laser directly through a sapphire contact tip (Surgical Laser Technologies) for superficial varicose veins of the lower extremity. Of the remaining 48 patients, 12 were treated for keloid/hypertrophic scars, 13 for capillary/cavernous hemangiomas, 3 for epistaxis secondary to Osler–Weber–Rendu hereditary hemorrhagic telangiectasia, 2 for granuloma faciale, 2 for basal cell cancer/squamous cell cancer/keratosis, 1 for angiokeratoma, and 7 for port-wine hemangiomas. Of the 64 patients, 53 were treated as outpatients under local anesthesia in the office, while 11 patients required hospitalization and general anesthesia. Five hemangiomas and 2 lymphangiomas in 7 patients were excised utilizing contact sapphire laser tips/scalpels.

TABLE 30.2. Keloid/hypertrophic scars

Category	Quantity
Patients	12
Lesions	22
Male/female	4/8
Average age	37 years (range 16–76 years)
Location	
Chest/breast	3
Arm	5
Ear	2
Back/shoulder	2
Power density (irradiance)	6400 W/cm^2
Total average joules	2946 W · s
Energy fluence	6.8 J/cm^2
Immediate shrinkage	
Length	5–8%
Width	7%
Height	34%
Time to heal	43 days
Complications	0
Result	
Good flat	5/22 (steroid)
Recurrence	14/22 (nonsteroid)
Partial recurrence	3/22

Results

The results of various treatment groups are summarized in Tables 30.2–30.8.

Keloid/Hypertrophic Scars

Twelve patients with 22 keloid or hypertrophic scars were treated (Table 30.2). All patients served as their own controls in that they had long-standing keloids (over 2 years) that were resistant to other methods of treatment, such as surgery or steroid instillation. There were 4 males and 8 females with an average age of 37 years (range 16–76 years). The deltoid upper arm

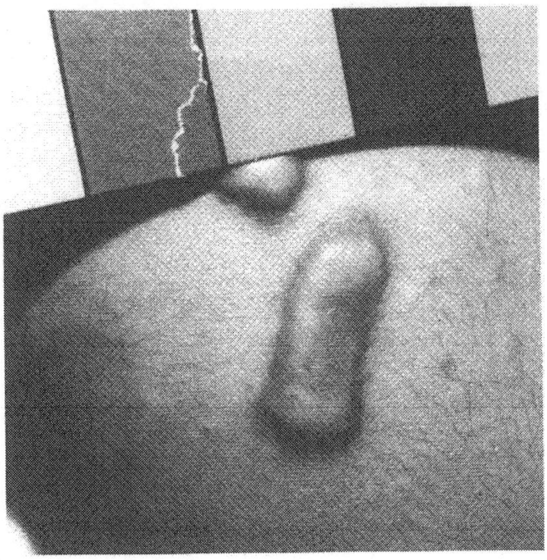

1A

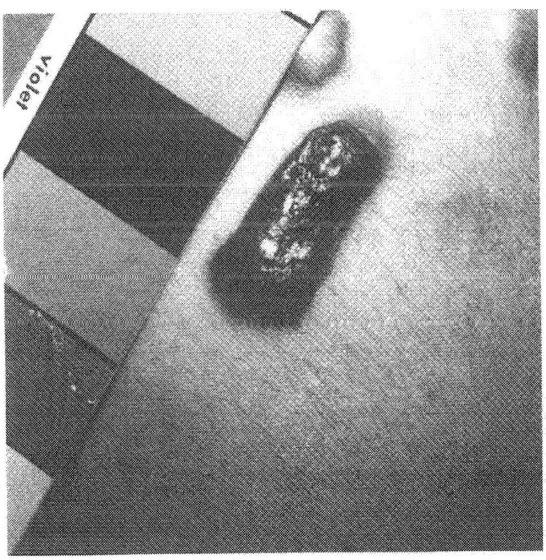

1B

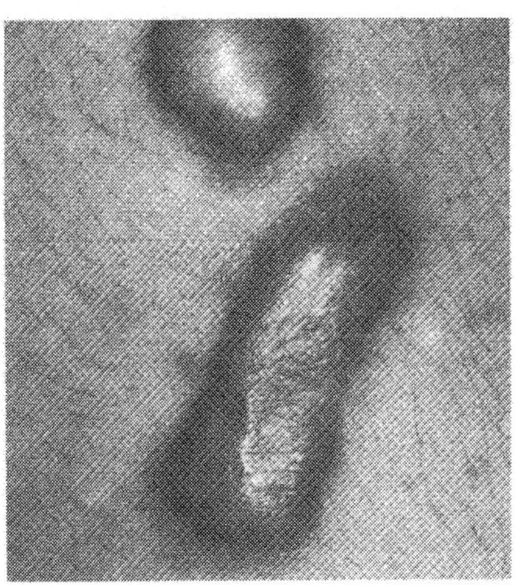

1C

FIGURE 30.1. (*A*) Keloid left deltoid pretreatment. (*B*) Escher and necrosis three weeks posttreatment. (*C*) Total recurrence after 4 months (no steroid adjunct). [From Apfelberg DB et al. Preliminary report on use of the neodymium:YAG laser in plastic surgery. Lasers Surg Med 7:189–198, 1987. Reprinted with permission of Alan R. Liss.]

was the most common area of treatment (5 patients), followed by the chest/breast in 3 patients and the back/shoulder or ear in 2 patients each. After treatment, immediate shrinkage was noted of 5–8% in length, 7% in width, and 34% in height, and the wounds averaged 43 days to healing. Early in the series, patients were treated with the Nd:YAG laser alone. Although the treatment resulted in marked shrinkage of the keloid, all keloids promptly recurred within the subsequent 3–4 months (Figure 30.1). Later in the series, the treatment areas were injected with intralesional steroid (Celestone Soluspan 1–3 cc) just before or immediately after epithelialization (average 4–6 weeks) and also treated with topical steroids (Diprolene 0.25%). This resulted in somewhat improved results (Figure 30.2). Of these 22 lesions, 5 showed good results with persistent flattening, 3 suffered minor recurrence, and 14 recurred to their original diameter or larger. There were no complications. Treatment of earlobe keloids in 2 black female patients was moderately successful at first but partial recurrence was seen with longer follow-up.

Capillary/Cavernous Hemangiomas

Thirteen patients with 15 capillary/cavernous hemangiomas were treated by photocoagulation (Table 30.3). There were 2 males and 11 females,

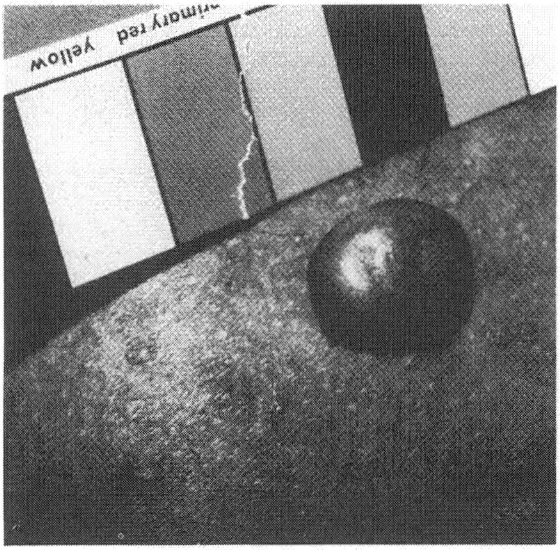

2A

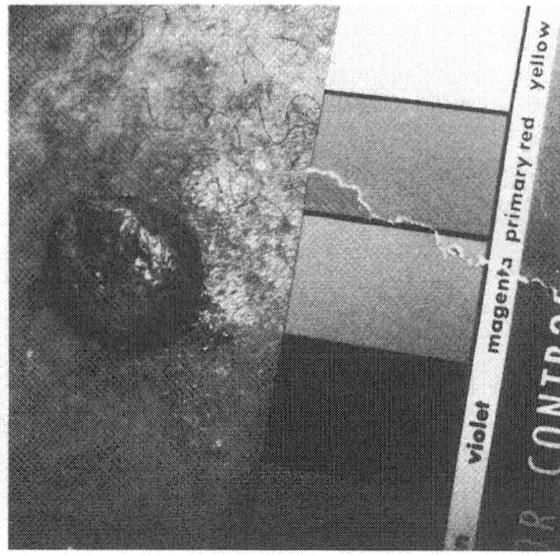

2B

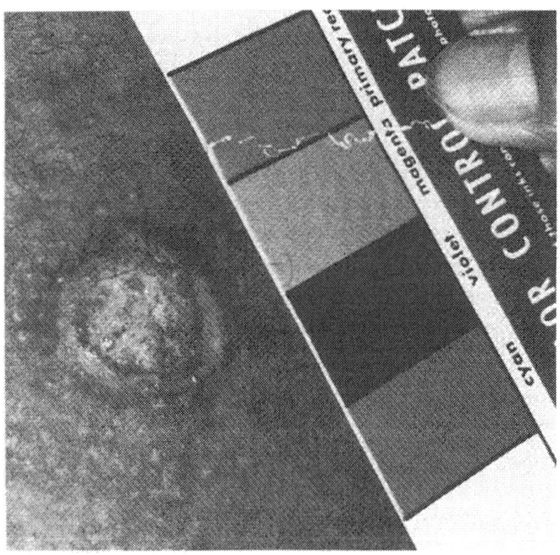

2C

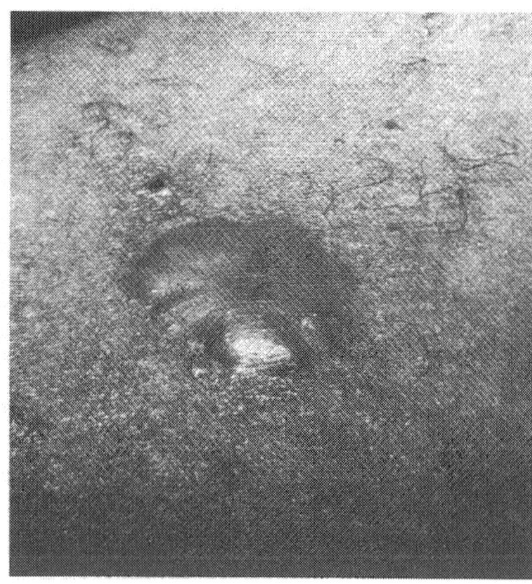

2D

FIGURE 30.2. (*A*) Keloid left scapula/shoulder measuring 3 cm wide, 4 cm long, and 2 cm high. (*B*) Immediately posttreatment and beginning eschar (50 W, 0.5-second pulse, 3394 W·s). (*C*) Intermediate stage at 5 weeks with flat granulating area (time of steroid injection). (*D*) Final result at 7 months—keloid is much flatter, 2½ cm wide, 3 cm long, only 5mm high, no recurrence. [From Apfelberg DB et al. Preliminary report on use of the neodymium:YAG laser in plastic surgery. Lasers Surg Med 7:189–198, 1987. Reprinted with permission of Alan R. Liss.]

average age of 16.6 years (range 2–45 years). Immediate shrinkage was noted to be 5–10% in length, 5% in width, and 32% in height, and healing averaged 19 days. Two patients' healing was complicated by minor wound infections rapidly responding to topical and systemic antibiotics. Treatment in 9 of 13 lesions resulted in complete disappearance and flattening, while 2 lesions (both capillary/cavernous hemangiomas of infancy) showed no significant response (Figures 30.3 and 30.4). Recently, the adjunct of intralesional steroid injection simultaneous with Nd:YAG laser photocoagulation has achieved a significant improvement in results (Figure 30.5). A further technical assistive maneuver is the compression of the hemangioma to a depth of 1 cm by pressure from a glass slide with application of the laser light through the glass. These adjuncts have markedly improved the results in capillary hemangiomas of infancy.

TABLE 30.3. Capillary/cavernous hemangioma

Category	Quantity
Patients	13
Lesions	15
Male/female	2/11
Average age	16.6 years (range 2–45 years)
Location	
Oral	8
Forehead	1
Chin	1
Scalp	2
Leg	1
Power density (irradiance)	3584 W/cm^2
Total average joules	2100 W · s
Energy fluence	3.9 J/cm^2
Immediate shrinkage	
Length	5–10%
Width	5%
Height	32%
Time to heal	19 days
Complications: Infection	2
Result	
Complete disappearance	9/13
No significant change	2/13
Progressive shrinkage	2/13

Sapphire Contact Scalpel Excision

Five hemangiomas and 2 lymphangiomas in 7 patients were excised under anesthesia as inpatients (Table 30.4). These hemangiomas were judged to be massive in size, frequently necessitating blood replacement. These vascular lesions required a hemostatic incision provided by the sapphire contact tips/scalpels and were either recurrent from traditional methods of surgery or had been rejected for surgery because of fear of exsanguinating hemorrhage. There were 3 males and 4 females with average age of 7 years (range 4 months to 24 years). Complete resection was achieved in all but 1 patient, with blood loss averaging 200 to 400 cc (Figure 30.6). One patient required transfusion. Resection of these lesions was significantly enhanced over traditional surgical modalities and in some cases made possible when traditional surgery had been either previously unsuccessful or judged to be incapable of resection without excess hemorrhage. One patient was unresectable by sapphire contact scalpel techniques due to a hemangioma that extended from the skin of the cheek all the way through into the oral mucosa. The resection of this lesion would have involved the removal of all structures in the entire right hemiface.

Epistaxis

Three patients (1 male, 2 females, average age 52 years) with severe recurrent epistaxis secondary to Osler–Weber–Rendu hereditary hemorrhagic telangiectasia were treated five times with the Nd:YAG laser (Table 30.5). Mucosa healed in 15 days, and all patients reported a marked diminution in nasal bleeding (infrequent bleeds lasting only a short time and easy to stop) for the first 4 to 5 months. At six months, the process returned to the original bleeding history, and repeat laser treatment became necessary. One patient who was treated with great difficulty because of intraoperative bleeding suffered the complication of septal perforation following her second treatment.

Miscellaneous Lesions

Granuloma Faciale

Two patients with granuloma faciale of the nose and cheeks (3 lesions, 1 male, 1 female, average age 64 years, healing time 44 days) were treated with good results in 2 lesions and hypertrophic scarring in 1 lesion (Table 30.6).

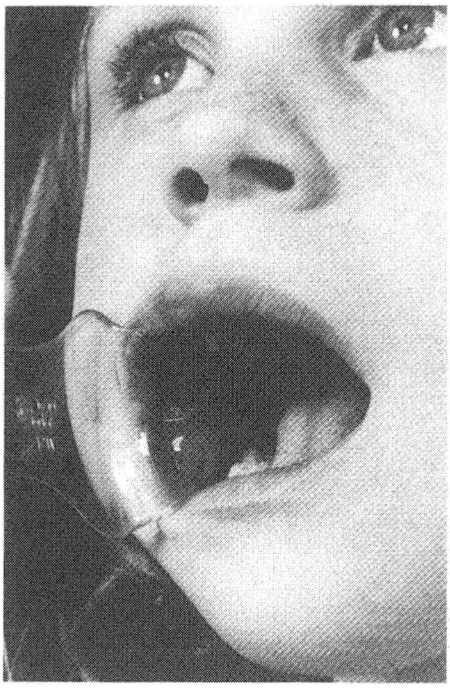

3A

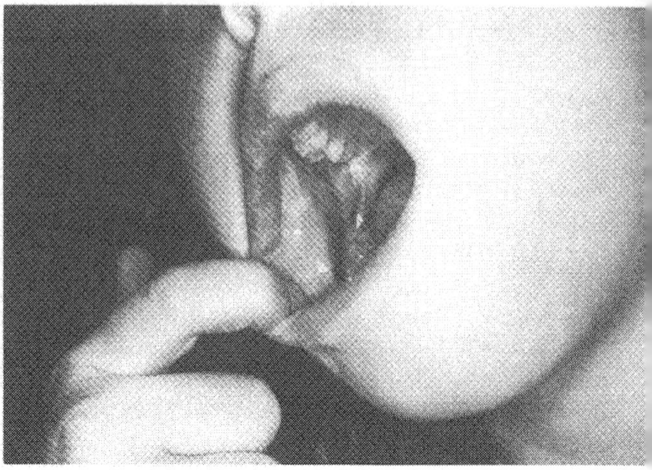

3B

FIGURE 30.3. (*A*) Pretreatment cavernous hemangioma right buccal mucosa. (*B*) Final healing with total disappearance of hemangioma and excellent healing of oral mucosa.

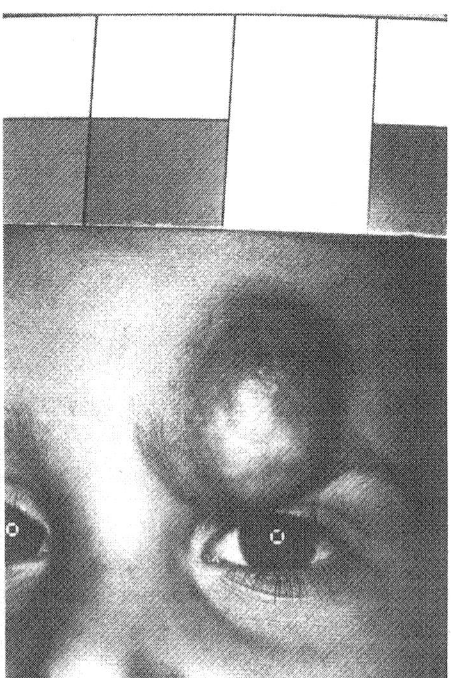

4A

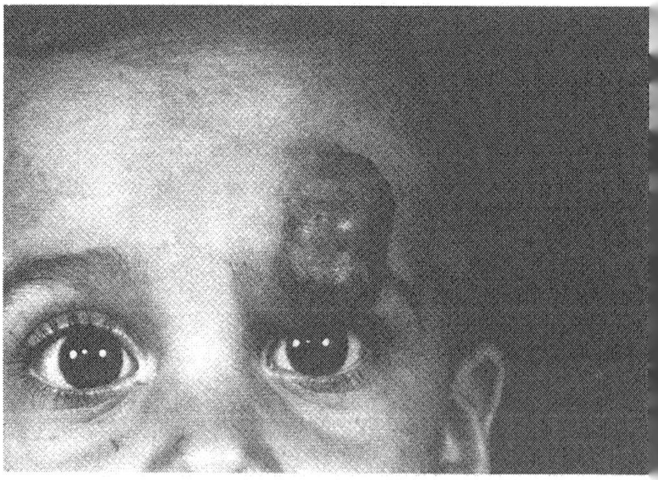

4B

FIGURE 30.4. (*A*) Capillary/cavernous hemangioma of forehead in 18-month-old infant. (*B*) Result 6 months after laser treatment, demonstrating minimal involultion and shrinkage (19–30 W, 0.5-second pulse, 3643 W·s). [From Apfelberg DB et al. Preliminary report on use of the neodymium:YAG laser in plastic surgery. Lasers Surg Med 7:189–198, 1987. Reprinted with permission of Alan R. Liss.]

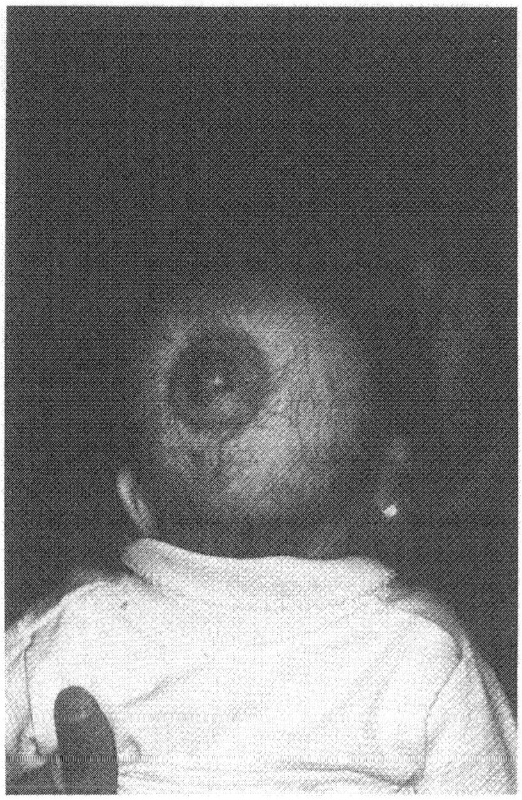
5A

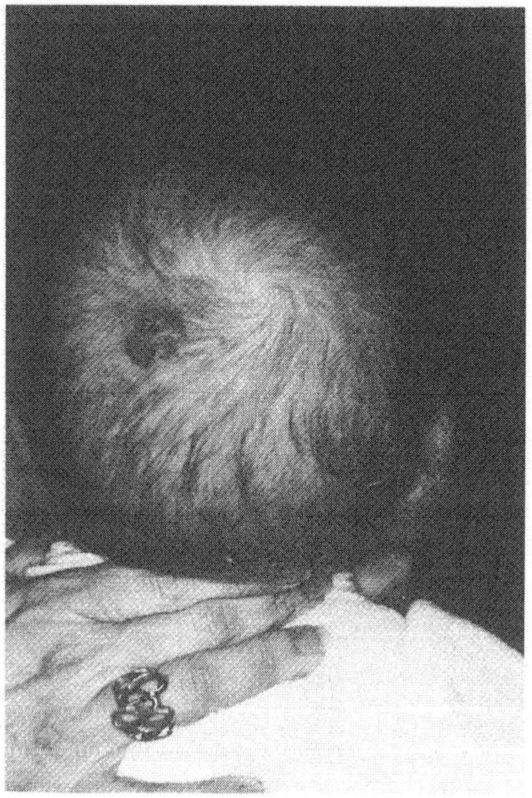
5B

FIGURE 30.5. (*A*) Large capillary/cavernous hemangioma of scalp prior to treatment. (*B*) Marked diminution in size of hemangioma following YAG laser photocoagulation plus steroid injection (Celestone Soluspan 3 cc).

TABLE 30.4. Sapphire scalpel excision

Category	Quantity
Patients	7
Lesions	
Large cavernous hemangioma	5
Lymphangioma	2
Male/female	3/4
Average age	7 years (range 7 months–24 years)
Location	
Face	5
Extremity	2
Time to heal	7–14 days
Complications: Dehiscence	1
Result	
Good	6
Unable to resect	1

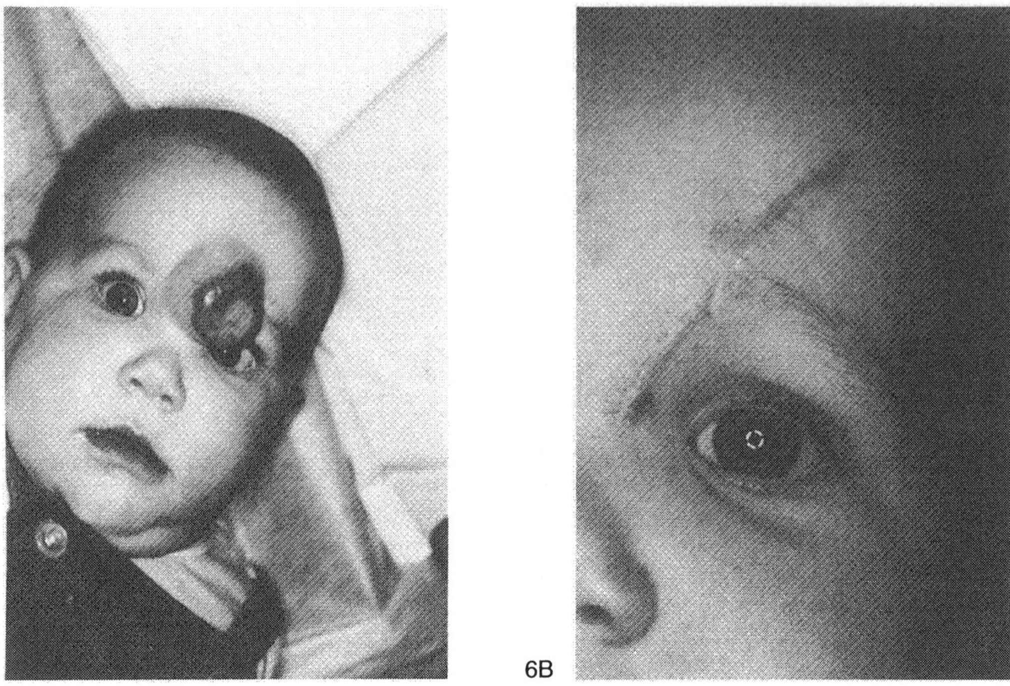

6A 6B

FIGURE 30.6. (*A*) Large capillary/cavernous hemangioma of eyelid and eyebrow obstructing vision. (*B*) Results after excision with Nd:YAG laser and sapphire scalpel accomplished with 50 cc blood loss.

Skin Cancer

Two male patients with 7 basal cell or squamous cell carcinomas or atypical keratosis (average age 62 years, healing time 41 days) were treated (Table 30.7). Six malignant lesions of the trunk, arms, or back completely disappeared without persistence or recurrence by clinical observation and random biopsy (Figure 30.7), and 1 scalp lesion resulted in a full-thickness skin loss exposing skull bone which necessitated flap closure (Figure 30.8).

TABLE 30.5. Epistaxis (Osler–Weber–Rendu)

Category	Quantity
Patients	3
Lesions	5
Male/female	1/2
Average age	52 years (range 43–66 years)
Location: bilateral septum	3
Power density (irradiance)	2688 W/cm^2
Total average joules	4320 W · s
Energy fluence	Unable to calculate
Immediate shrinkage	N.A.
Time to heal	15 days
Complications: Septal perforation	1
Result	
Minor bleeding	4–5 months
Recurrence at	6 months

TABLE 30.6. Granuloma faciale

Category	Quantity
Patients	2
Lesions	3
Male/female	1/1
Average age	64 years (range 62–67 years)
Location	
Nose	1
Cheek	2
Power density (irradiance)	2304 W/cm^2
Total average joules	1300 W · s
Energy fluence	6.1 J/cm^2
Immediate shrinkage	none
Time to heal	44 days
Complications: Hypertrophic scar	1
Result	
Good	2
Scar	1

Superficial Hemangiomas

One patient (female, age 14 years) with angiokeratoma of the ankle and 7 patients (3 male, 4 female, average age 50 years) with port-wine hemangiomas previously managed with the argon laser were treated (Table 30.8). The areas healed in an average of 27 days. The angiokeratoma involuted well. Port-wine hemangiomas undergo full-thickness injury and subsequent healing by secondary intention and scarring unless the treatment is broken up by "polka dot" or segmented treatment. In this method, 1- to 2-mm dots of laser photocoagulation are separated by 1 to 2 mm. Untreated interspaces are treated by similar dots when fading of the original set is obvious (usually averages 12 weeks). Although fading is slower and slightly variegated in appearance, scarring has been minimal (Figure 30.9).

Superficial Varicosities of the Lower Extremity

Sixteen patients with superficial telangiectasia of the lower extremity above the knee were treated as outpatients with only ice as anesthesia. Power of 0.5–0.8 W transmitted through

TABLE 30.7. Skin cancer keratosis

Category	Quantity
Patients	2
Lesions	7
Male	2
Average age	62 years (range 49–84 years)
Location	
Scalp	1
Trunk and arms	6
Power density (irradiance)	3712 W/cm^2
Total average joules	870 W · s
Energy fluence	9.87 J/cm^2
Immediate shrinkage	90%
Time to heal	41 days
Complications: Full-thickness loss	1
Result	
Complete disappearance	6
Full-thickness loss	1

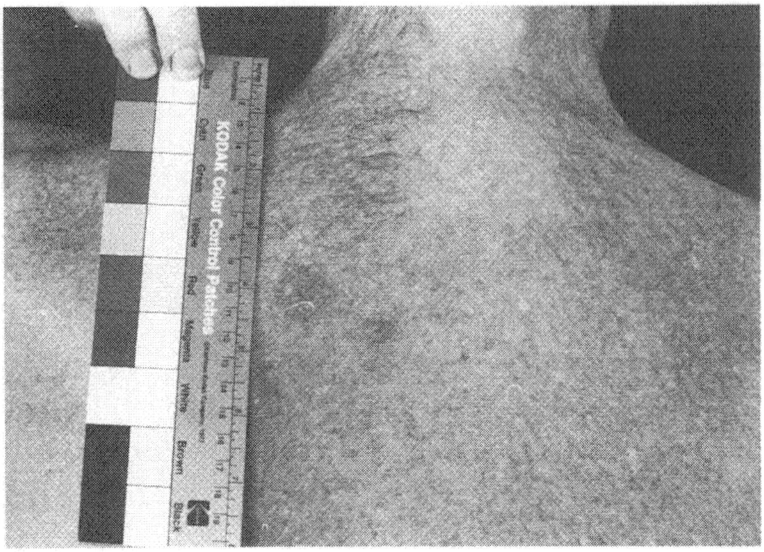

7A

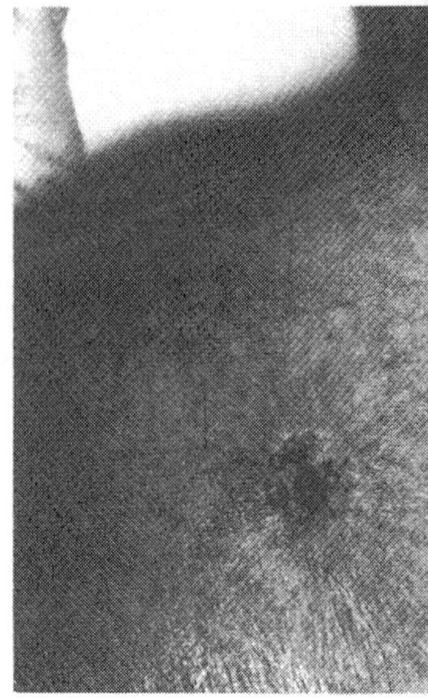

7B

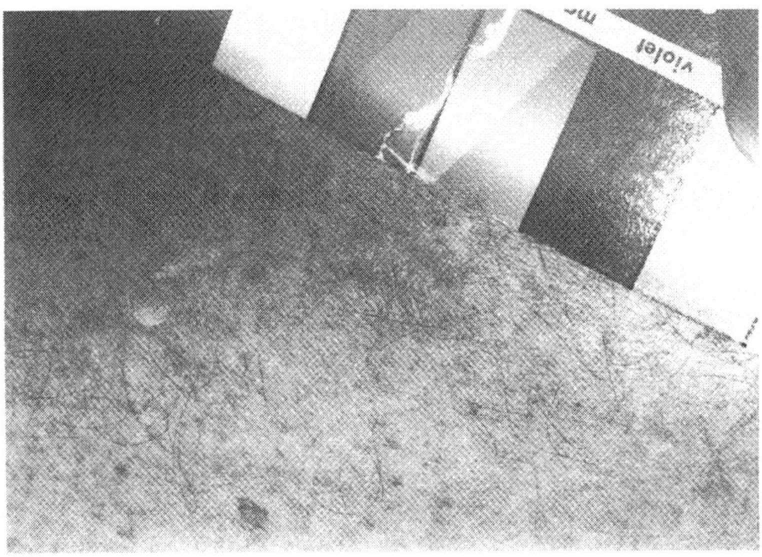

C

FIGURE 30.7. (*A*) Basal cell carcinoma of back/scapula. (*B*) Coagulation necrosis evident 2 weeks after treatment (30 W, 0.2-second pulse, 670 W·s). (*C*) Final healing at 6 months demonstrating satisfactory cosmetic result and no recurrence by biopsy. [From Apfelberg DB et al. Preliminary report on use of the neodymium:YAG laser in plastic surgery. Lasers Surg Med 7:189–198, 1987. Reprinted with permission of Alan R. Liss.]

a flat 15-mm vaporizing probe diffusing contact sapphire tip (Surgical Laser Technologies, Malvern, PA) was applied to produce blanching. All 16 patients were females between the ages of 27 and 58 (average age 43 years). Patients were evaluated every month until 12 months had elapsed. Only two patients demonstrated an excellent result (complete disappearance of vessels without scar or pigmentary changes). Eight patients achieved a good result (blanching of the majority of the vessels) and the remaining 6 patients achieved only fair or poor results. No complications were observed in this group of patients.

Discussion

Previous Reports

The Nd:YAG laser has been reported previously for treatment of cutaneous lesions. Landthaler et al.[10] reported its use in the treatment of skin tumors such as nodular basal cell carcinomas, superficial basal cell carcinomas, Bowen's disease, keratoses, and melanoma. Port wine hemangiomas were treated, but significant scarring was noted, and healing was prolonged to approximately 12 weeks. They concluded that only the most hypertrophic port wine hemangiomas

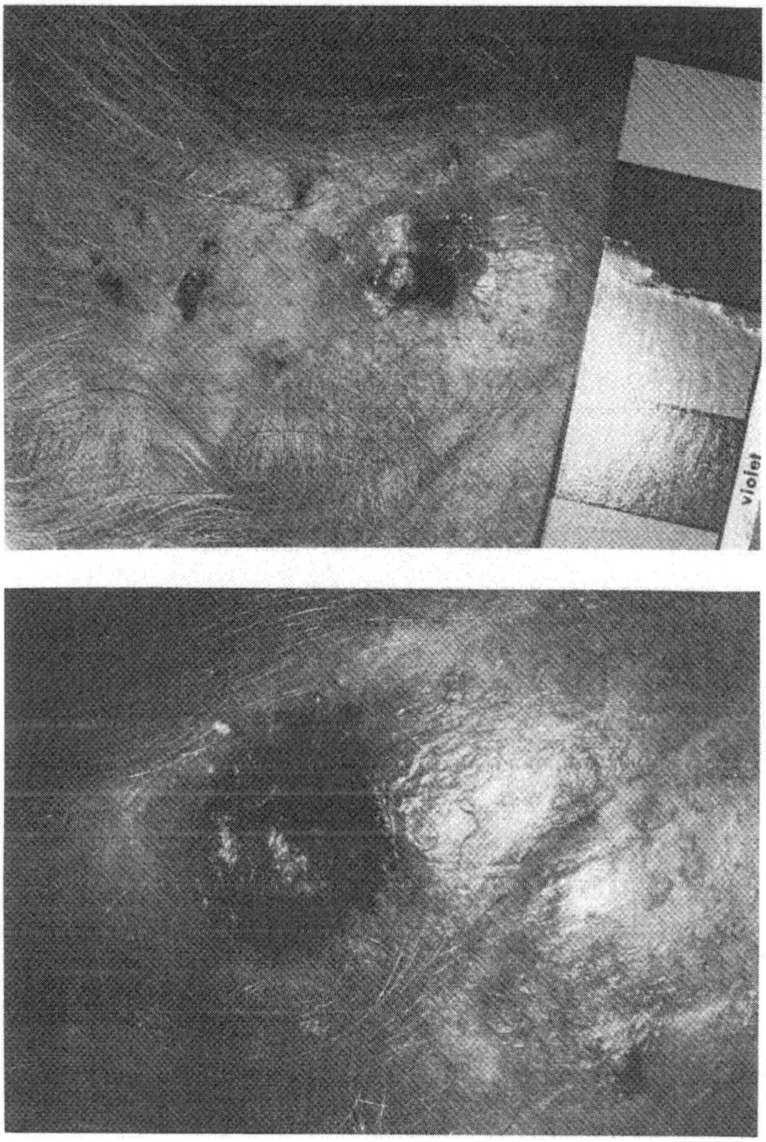

8A

8B

FIGURE 30.8. (*A*) Pretreatment dysplastic lesion of scalp. (*B*) Eschar produced 3 weeks after treatment (30 W, 0.5-second pulse, 2923 W·s). [From Apfelberg DB et al. Preliminary report on use of the neodymium: YAG laser in plastic surgery. Lasers Surg Med 7:189–198, 1987. Reprinted with permission of Alan R. Liss.]

were applicable for treatment. A later report by the same authors (Landthaler et al.[11]) has demonstrated the Nd:YAG laser's effectiveness only in the most thick nodular port-wine hemangiomas, deep capillary hemangiomas, and macrocheilia of the lip secondary to hemangioma. These authors also conducted in-vivo and in-vitro exposure experiments in human skin and concluded that coagulation necrosis in a hemispheric pattern can be produced as deep as 3.2 mm into the dermis. The same authors[12] demonstrated coagulation up to 5 mm in the dermis and that regions of the body with thin skin must be treated only with caution while safer application of the Nd:YAG laser occurs in thicker skin. This correlates with our study and the complications encountered. The keratosis of the scalp which was treated resulted in full thickness loss and exposure of the skull bone, and the port wine hemangioma previously treated by argon

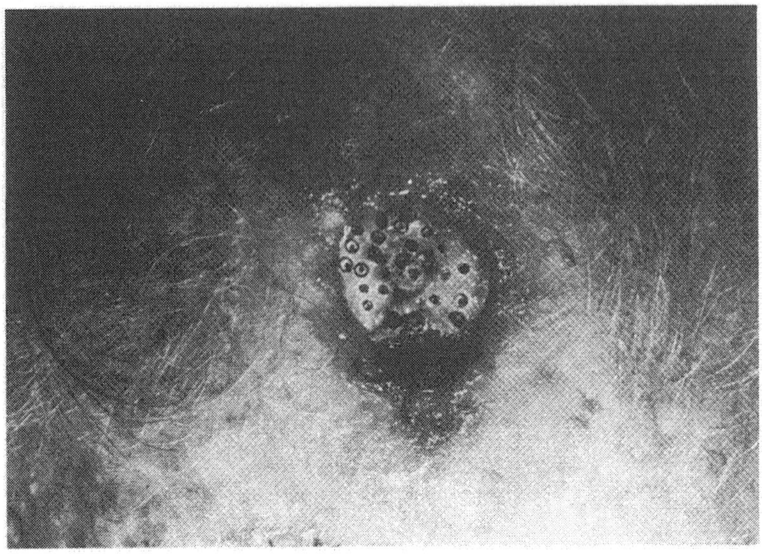

8C

FIGURE 30.8 (*C*) Full-thickness loss exposing skull bone which necessitated flap coverage (note CO_2 laser drill holes which failed to produce granulation).

laser which thinned the overlying epidermis also resulted in full thickness loss and scar. Nasal septal mucosa which is very thin may be perforated by prolonged bilateral exposure.

Nd:YAG Laser Physiology

Wound healing experiments in relation to the role of fibroblasts in hypertrophic and keloid scars have been conducted by Castro and coworkers[13] and Abergel and coworkers.[14] These authors have demonstrated beneficial effects of Nd:YAG laser exposure of keloids and hypertrophic scars in clinical patients and in fibroblasts in tissue culture. Rosenfeld[15] has reported treatment of a wide variety of vascular, keloid, and miscellaneous superficial lesions with the Nd:YAG laser. A recent study with wide clinical implications is the observation of Zimmerman et al.[16] on the ability of the Nd:YAG laser to interrupt lymphatic drainage in the urinary bladder, thus inhibiting the spread of tumor cells.

Conclusion

A wide spectrum of clinical lesions have treated under experimental protocol with the Nd:YAG laser. The following conclusions are offered.

1. The Nd:YAG laser is ideally suited for treatment of thick, deep capillary/cavernous hemangiomas, especially around the oral cavity of adults and produces excellent results without complications.
2. In infants with capillary/cavernous hemangiomas of infancy, no appreciable benefit could be obtained by laser alone, but significant shrinkage occurred with the simultaneous injection of steroids.
3. Nd:YAG laser exposure alone cannot control keloids or hypertrophic scars but may produce modest benefit when combined with posttreatment topical and intralesional steroid applications. Recurrence of keloid is seen frequently with longer follow-up.
4. Treatment of thin areas of skin such as scalp or skin previously treated by argon laser for port-wine hemangioma produces full thickness skin loss and deep necrosis resulting in scar. Port-wine hemangioma treatment may be safely accomplished by the "dot" method.
5. Treatment is effective for approximately 4 to 5 months for the nasal septal mucosa to control epistaxis in patients with Osler–Weber–Rendu hereditary hemorrhagic telangiectasia, but septal perforation may occur with overexposure.
6. Excisional surgery of major vascular or lymphangiomatous abnormalities has been greatly

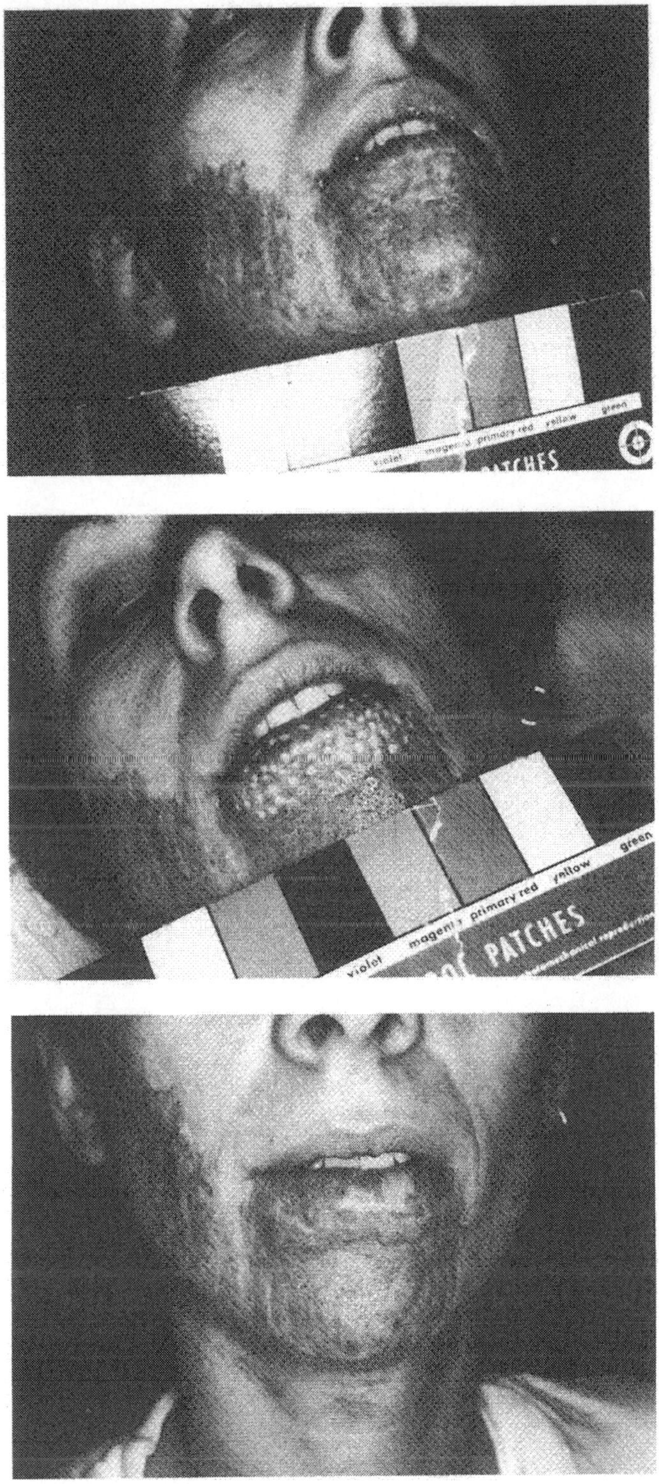

9A

9B

9C

FIGURE 30.9. (*A*) Port-wine hemangioma of face previously treated with argon laser demonstrating subtotal blanching. (*B*) Blanching of "polka dots" of segmental treatment. (*C*) Improvement of contour with blanching of port-wine hemangioma and no scarring.

TABLE 30.8. Angiokeratoma/port-wine hemangioma

Category	Quantity
Patients	8
Lesions	8
Male/female	3/5
Average age	32 years (range 14–50 years)
Location	
Face	7
Ankle	1
Power density (irradiance)	2304 W/cm^2
Total average joules	684 W · s
Energy fluence	5.17 J/cm^2
Immediate shrinkage	Minimal
Time to heal	27 days
Complications: scar	1
Result	
Scar	1
Involution and good fading	5
Fair fading	2

TABLE 30.9. Superficial varicosity lower extremity

Category	Quantity
Patients	16
Average age	43 years (range 27–58 years)
Location thigh	16
Time to heal	7–10 days
Complications	None
Result	
Excellent	2
Good	8
Fair/poor	6

enhanced and in some cases rendered possible by contact sapphire scalpel tips. The hemostatic incision and contact touch exceeds the CO_2 laser incision.

7. Treatment of superficial varicosities of the lower extremities with contact tips or diffusing lenses has been moderately successful.

The Nd:YAG laser definitely deserves a place in the clinical armamentarium of the laser surgeon treating cutaneous and subcutaneous lesions.

References

1. Apfelberg DB, Maser MR, Lash H: Review of usage of argon and carbon dioxide lasers for pediatric hemangiomas. Ann Plast Surg 12:353–361, 1984.
2. Apfelberg DB, Maser MR, Lash H, White DN: Efficacy of the carbon dioxide laser in hand surgery. Ann Plast Surg 13:320–327, 1984.
3. Apfelberg DB, Rothermel E, Widtfeldt A, et al: Preliminary report on the use of carbon dioxide laser in podiatry. J Am Podiat Assoc 74:509–513, 1984.
4. Apfelberg DB, Lash H, Maser MR, White DN: Benefits of the CO_2 laser for oral hemangioma excision. Plast Reconstr Surg 75:46–50, 1985.
5. Apfelberg DB, Maser MR, Lash H: Treatment of nevi aranei by means of an argon laser. J Dermatol Surg Oncol 4:172–174, 1978.
6. Apfelberg DB, et al: Pathophysiology and treatment of decorative tattoos with reference to argon laser treatment. Clin Plast Surg 7(3):Chap 9, 1980.
7. Apfelberg DB, Greene RA, Maser MR, et al: Results of argon laser exposure of capillary hemangiomas of infancy: Preliminary report. Plast Reconstr Surg 67:188–193, 1981.
8. Apfelberg DB, Maser MR, Lash H, Rivers J: The argon laser for cutaneous lesions. JAMA, 245:2073–2075, 1981.
9. Apfelberg DB, Maser MR, Lash H, Flores J: Expanded role of the argon laser in plastic surgery. J Dermatol Surg Oncol 9:145–151, 1983.
10. Landthaler M, Brunner R, Haina D, et al: First experiences with the Nd:YAG laser in dermatology. In Joffe SN (ed): Neodymium-YAG Lasers in Medicine and Surgery. Elsevier, New York, 1983, p 176–183.
11. Lanthaler M, Haina D, Brunner R, et al: Neodymium-YAG laser therapy for vascular lesions. J Am Acad Dermatol 14:107–117, 1986.
12. Brunner R, Landthaler M, Haina D, et al: Treatment of benign, semimalignant, and malignant skin tumors with the Nd:YAG laser. Lasers Surg Med 5:105–111, 1985.
13. Castro DJ, Abergel RP, Meeker CA, et al: Effects of the Nd:YAG laser on DNA synthesis and collagen production in human skin fibroblast cultures. Ann Plast Surg 11:214–222, 1983.
14. Abergel RP, Dwyer R, Meeker C, et al: Laser treatment of keloids: A clinical trial and an in vitro study with Nd:YAG laser. Lasers Surg Med 4(3):291–295, 1984.
15. Rosenfeld H, Sherman R: Treatment of cutaneous and deep vascular lesions with the Nd:YAG laser surgery. Lasers Surg Med 6:20–24, 1986.
16. Zimmerman I, Stern J, Frank F, et al: Interception of lymphatic drainage by Nd:YAG laser irradiation in rat urinary bladder. Lasers Surg Med 4(2):167–172, 1984.

31
Prevention of Dental Caries and Treatment of Early Caries Using the Nd:YAG Laser

Hajime Yamamoto and Teruo Kayano

It is well known that since the first laser made with a ruby crystal was built by Dr. Maiman in 1960,[1] the laser has been considered to be a potential tool in dentistry. The energy of high-power lasers can be concentrated in a short pulse. Many of the early studies on laser applications in dentistry first investigated the possibility of replacing conventional dental drills with lasers for restorative techniques in cavity preparation.[2, 3] However these attempts were unsuccessful because of too much damage to the tooth, especially to the dental pulp. Current investigations have turned to caries prevention and treatment by means of laser irradiation. The clinical application of lasers to the prevention and treatment of dental caries requires two important considerations[4]: First, minimum energy density is necessary to avoid damaging the oral soft tissue, especially the dental pulp, and, second, the laser beam must be easily guided with a flexible optical fiber to the restricted area of the tooth surface of the oral cavity. The ruby laser,[2, 3] the carbon dioxide laser,[6] and the Pockels cell Q-switched Nd:YAG laser,[7] all impart a degree of alteration that reduces subsurface demineralization to the enamel surface of the extracted human tooth. They cannot however be guided by a flexible optical fiber because of their wavelength in the infrared zone and their high peak power. But an acoustooptically Q-switched Nd:YAG laser beam can be easily guided by a single flexible optical fiber without transmission loss of laser energy.[4, 5] Remarkable acid resistance and reduced acid solubility are imparted not only to the enamel without caries but also to the enamel with incipient caries by irradiation of an acoustooptically Q-switched Nd:YAG laser with low energy.[4, 5, 8]

The studies considered in this chapter are related to the application of the Nd:YAG laser on the tooth not only for the prevention of primary dental caries and secondary caries associated with marginal closure of dental restorative materials, but also for the treatment of incipient enamel caries by means of Nd:YAG laser irradiation.

Prevention of Dental Caries by Nd:YAG Laser Irradiation

Dental caries is a disease of the enamel, dentin, and cementum of the tooth, producing progressive demineralization of the calcified component and eventual destruction of the organic component, with the formation of a cavity in the tooth.[9] The incipient phase of dental caries begins with subsurface demineralization of the enamel[10] by acids produced by oral microorganisms, especially some specific strains of streptococci.[9] A remarkable acid resistance is imparted to the enamel by some means, which seems to be effective in reducing its susceptibility to acids, and thereby preventing caries. It has already been pointed out that when the enamel surfaces of the extracted teeth were irradiated by laser beams, a degree of alteration was imparted to the enamel surface, resulting in reduced subsurface demineralization.[2, 6, 7] The Nd:YAG laser has been proved to be more effective for clinical application than other kinds of lasers[4] In this chapter, the different operational modes of Nd:YAG laser irradiation will be compared to determine their effectiveness in the prevention of dental caries.[4]

Dental caries will develop secondarily along the margin of the dental restorative materials where a narrow crevice is present.[9] The width of this crevice must be responsible for susceptibility to the secondary dental caries. One of the most important objectives is to close these crevices between the margin of the dental restorative materials and the enamel in order to prevent the secondary caries from developing. In this study, we also investigated the possibility of secondary caries prevention by means of Nd:YAG laser irradiation along the margin of the dental restorative materials.[11]

Prevention of Primary Enamel Caries

In Vitro Experiments

Different Modes of Nd:YAG Laser Irradiation[4]

POCKELS CELL Q-SWITCHED ND:YAG LASER IRRADIATION[7]: The enamel surface coated with a laser absorption black material (Chinese black ink) of the freshly extracted human permanent teeth without caries is irradiated by a Pockels cell Q-switched Nd:YAG laser. The irradiation conditions are as follows: peak power of 3 milliwatts, pulse width of 30 nanoseconds, repetition rate of 10 Hz, and total energy densities of 20 J/cm^2. In contrast to that of the control unlased enamel, the lased enamel shows no obvious structural change after being exposed for 7 days to a demineralizing culture system.[12] Because of its high peak power, this laser beam cannot be guided by a conventional optical fiber.

NORMAL-PULSED ND:YAG LASER IRRADIATION WITH OR WITHOUT AG(NH$_3$)$_2$F[13]: The enamel surface coated with Chinese black ink is exposed to a normal-pulsed Nd:YAG laser beam. The irradiation conditions are as follows: a repetition rate of 20 Hz, spot size of 2.5 mm, energy density of 3.4 J/cm^2 per pulse, and irradiation time of 3 minutes. The laser beam can be guided by a conventional optical fiber. The enamel reveals only a mild reduced subsurface demineralization and shows no obvious resistance to acid in a demineralizing solution of 6% hydroxyethyl cellulose and 0.1 *M* lactate buffered at pH 4.5[14] compared with the unlased enamel. But the enamel treated with the combination of the local application of Ag(NH$_3$)$_2$F on the enamel surface[15, 16] and this conditioned Nd:YAG laser irradiation showed a degree of acid resistance. But the lased enamel after treatment with Ag(NH$_3$)$_2$F is discolored in silver and brownish black, and a brown area remains even after cleaning the discolored enamel surface with pumice powder. Because of this cosmetic disadvantage and the complicated operational techniques, this method is inapplicable to clinical practice. However, some modifications have been proposed.[17, 18]

ACOUSTOOPTICALLY Q-SWITCHED ND:YAG LASER IRRADIATION[4, 5]: The enamel surfaces of the freshly extracted noncarious human permanent teeth are cleaned and dried in air, and the enamel surfaces are coated with Chinese black ink. Then the enamel surface is exposed to an acoutooptically Q-switched Nd:YAG laser. The irradiation conditions are as follows; a peak power of 100 KW with a pulse width of 100 nanoseconds, repetition rate of 1 KHz, average output of 10 W, spot size of 3.5 mm in diameter, and irradiation time of 0.4, 0.8, and 1.2 s, guided by a step index cylindrical quartz fiber of 300 μm in diameter. After irradiation, the laser absorption material coated on the enamel surfaces must be removed. The enamel surfaces exposed to this conditioned Nd:YAG laser show no gross changes after 4 days in the demineralizing solution.[14] but the boundary line between the lased and the unlased area becomes visible macroscopically on the dried enamel surfaces and the unlased enamel surfaces clearly appear white due to demineralization. Microradiograms demonstrate the difference in acid resistance of the enamel due to different laser irradiation times (Figure 31.1), and also reveal the best irradiation time for acid resistance of the enamel to be about 0.8 second.

CONTINUOUS WAVE BEAM OF ND:YAG LASER IRRADIATION[19]: Noncarious enamel surfaces of the freshly extracted teeth are exposed to a continuous wave beam of Nd:YAG laser at the same irradiation condition as the acoustooptically Q-switched Nd:YAG laser. A laser absorption black material must be coated on the enamel surface before irradiation. Acid resistance imparted by the continuous wave beam of Nd:YAG laser irradiation is less than that im-

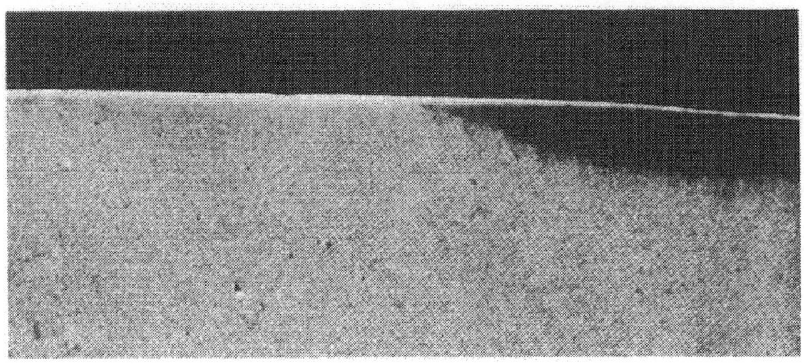

FIGURE 31.1. Microradiogram of the enamel exposed to an acoustooptically Q-switched Nd:YAG laser after 5 days of in vitro demineralization. No radiolucency at the left lased area and the clear subsurface radiolucency at the right unlased area.

parted by the acoustooptically Q-switched Nd:YAG laser irradiation.

Mechanisms of Caries Prevention by the Acoustooptically Q-switched Nd:YAG Laser Irradiation[4, 5, 7]

The incipient phase of enamel caries develops as subsurface demineralization.[9, 10] The acid solubility of the enamel is thought to be due to a degree of permeability of the enamel. Scanning electron microscopy reveals that the lased enamel shows a very smooth surface and the preexisting micropores disappear (Figure 31.2). These findings will be closely related to the reduced acid solubility of the lased enamel due to a decrease in permeability of acid into the enamel through the micropores and acid diffusion in the enamel. This is supported by the asymmetric electron spin resonance signal observed in the lased enamel.[4, 5, 20] According to the x-ray diffraction analysis, inorganic products other than hydroxyapatite are not formed in the lased enamel.[4, 5] Furthermore, the absence of significant changes in the lattice parameters of the lased enamel crystals suggests that the water may be loosely bound.[21] These findings suggest that the major contributing factors for acid resistance imparted to the lased enamel must be due to a physical alteration in acid permeability and acid diffusion in the enamel.[4, 5]

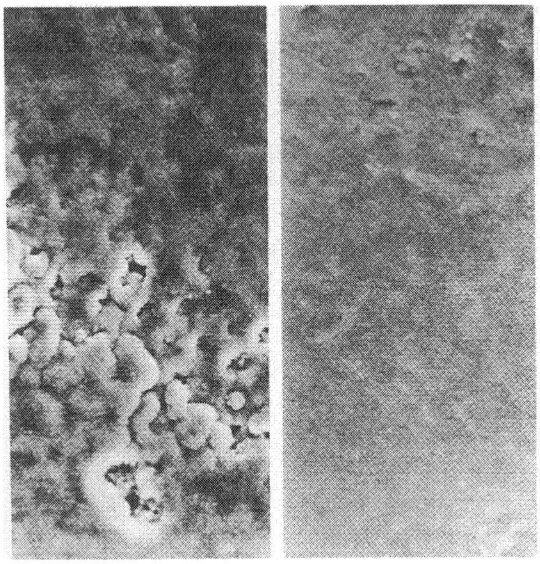

FIGURE 31.2. Scanning electron microscopy of the enamel surface before *(left)* and after *(right)* the acoustooptically Q-switched Nd:YAG laser irradiation. Micropores vanished and smooth surface was imparted by laser irradiation.

In Vivo Experiments

According to this series of in vitro experiments, an acoustooptically Q-switched Nd:YAG laser under the above-mentioned irradiation conditions is concluded to be the most effective in imparting the remarkable acid resistance to the enamel at a low-energy density without damaging the living dental pulp.[4, 5] Also, this operational mode of the Nd:YAG laser can be guided easily by a single flexible optical fiber without any transmission loss of laser energy. It is now necessary to clarify the effects of the acoustooptically Q-switched Nd:YAG laser irradiation on the tooth enamel in vivo.

Experiments in Rats[22]

Because rat teeth are smaller than human teeth, the irradiation time and spot size were calculated so that the energy density was approximately equal to that of the previous in vitro experiments using the extracted human teeth. Calculated irradiation time and spot size were 0.1 second and 2.0 mm, respectively. After coated with Chinese black ink, the first molars of the Wistar rats, weighing 140 to 160 g, were exposed to this conditioned acoustooptically Q-switched Nd:YAG laser guided by a flexible optical fiber. After irradiation, the rats were fed a cariogenic, low-casein diets.[23] Caries prevention of laser irradiation is clearly demonstrated after 70 days of experiment. At that time, no visible carious lesions were detected in the lased and the unlased teeth; however, the microradiogram of the unlased molar enamel revealed clear subsurface demineralization in the fissures. On the contrary, no demineralization was found in the enamel of the lased molars. After 200 days of experiment, severe carious decay developed macroscopically in the unlased molars, but no carious lesions were detected in the fissures of the lased molars. This operational conditioned acoustooptically Q-switched Nd:YAG laser showed only the slightest injury to the soft tissues such as the tongue and the skin of the rat where the Chinese black ink is coated. These injuries were healed within 2 weeks.

Experiments in Humans

TEST OF THE EXTRAORALLY IRRADIATED HUMAN ENAMEL PLACED IN THE HUMAN MOUTH[24]: In order to investigate the degree of acid resistance of the lased enamel in the human oral environmental influences, small pieces of the enamel of extracted sound deciduous human teeth irradiated by the acoustooptically Q-switched Nd:YAG laser for 0.8 second were embedded into several parts of human dentures or were set into fixed prostheses and were placed in the human oral environments for 3 and 6 months. Macroscopically, the unlased area of the enamel showed chalky white lesions by subsurface demineralization. On the contrary, no noticeable change was observed in the lased area and no subsurface demineralization was found on the microradiogram. No damage to the dental pulp occurred.

THE TEST OF LASER APPLICATION FOR CARIES PREVENTION OF HUMAN TEETH IN VIVO.[4,5] The occlusal surfaces of noncarious intact teeth of several volunteers were exposed to the acoustooptically Q-switched Nd:YAG laser after being coated with Chinese black ink. The irradiation time was 0.8 second for the permanent teeth and 0.4 second for the deciduous teeth, respectively. During the operation, some pain and discomfort was felt by the subjects. There developed no gross carious change in the lased area of the enamel even after a few years. Of course, this operational conditioned irradiation by the acoustooptically Q-switched Nd:YAG laser does not cause any injury to the human skin without the coating of Chinese black ink.

Clinical Application of Nd:YAG Laser for Caries Prevention

After numerous careful and prudent fundamental experiments, the first test of the laser application for caries prevention was performed successfully and safely.[4,5] These investigations have revealed some mechanisms of the acid resistance imparted by the acoustooptically Q-switched Nd:YAG laser irradiation. We have already de-

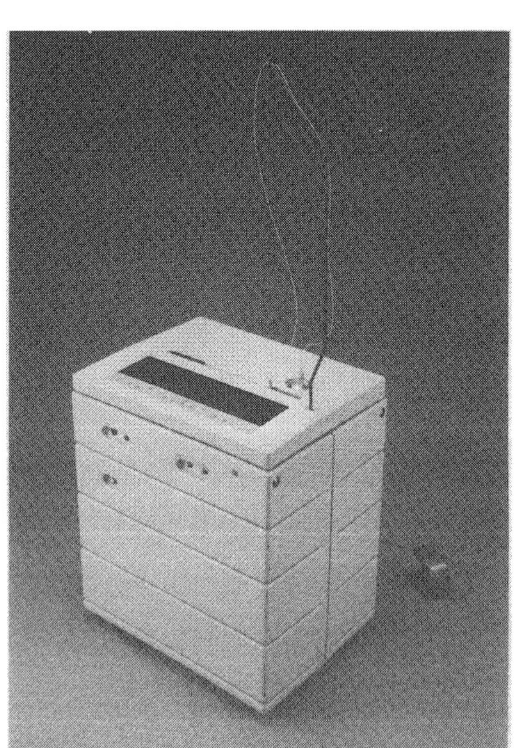

FIGURE 31.3. New model of Nd:YAG laser apparatus with newly developed laser manipulator for dentistry. Operational modes; continous wave beam of Nd:YAG laser/normal-pulsed Nd:YAG laser.

TABLE 31.1. Technical procedure for the prevention of dental caries using Nd:YAG laser irradiation

1. Clean the tooth surface.
2. Dry the tooth surface.
3. Coat black material (Chinese ink) on the tooth surface and dry it.
1′. Switch on the laser apparatus.
2′. Set the irradiation conditions and measure the average output.
3′. Select the irradiation time.
4. Irradiation.*
5. Remove the coated black material and clean the tooth surface.

The patient must be informed about this procedure before irradiation.
*Both the operator and the patient must wear protective eyeglasses during the irradiation process.

veloped the easily operable laser manipulator for the oral cavity, attached to the end of the flexible optical fiber, and also the clinical apparatus of the Nd:YAG laser for caries prevention (Figure 31.3). Persons who desire caries prevention by laser can have their teeth irradiated by the acoustooptically Q-switched Nd:YAG laser at the Pedodontics Clinic of Tohoku University Dental Hospital. The operational procedure is shown in Table 31.1.

Prevention of Secondary Enamel Caries and Marginal Closure of Dental Restorative Materials by Nd:YAG Laser Irradiation

Several in vitro experiments were carried out in order to examine the possibility of marginal closure and fusion between the dental restorative materials and the tooth enamel by means of Nd:YAG laser irradiation, to obtain resistance of teeth to acid and to prevent secondary caries.[11] Class V cavities were prepared on the buccal surface of the freshly extracted noncarious human teeth, and these teeth were restored by dental restorative materials, such as plastic filling materials and casted metallic inlays. Several kinds of resins and gold alloy inlays were investigated. The interface between the tooth enamel and the restorative materials was coated with laser absorption black material (Chinese black ink) and exposed to an acoustooptically Nd:YAG laser. The irradiation conditions were as follows; a peak power of 120 KW with a pulse width of 120 nanoseconds, repetition rate of 1 KHz, average output of 10 W, and spot size of 3.0 mm. The irradiation times were 0.1 to 0.3 second for resins and 0.8 to 1.5 seconds for inlays. The effects of a continuous wave beam of Nd:YAG laser were also examined. A scanning electron microscopy revealed that complete closure of the dental restorative materials and the tooth enamel was obtained by the acoustooptically Q-switched Nd:YAG laser irradiation at irradiation times of 0.2 second on margin of resin fillings (Clearfill®) (Figure 31.4) and 0.8 second on margin of gold alloy inlays. In the case of resin fillings, the same findings were obtained by the continuous wave beam of Nd:YAG laser irradiation. According to the microradiographic findings of the lased tooth samples after being placed in the demineralizing fluid[14] for 4 days, the sensitivity to acid in the irradiated areas decreased markedly. Although the effects of marginal closure by laser irradiation may depend on the irradiation conditions and physical characteristics of dental restorative materials, these preliminary results suggest a possibility of secondary caries prevention by laser irradiation.

Treatment of Incipient Enamel Caries by Nd:YAG Laser Irradiation: A Possible Clinical Application

In order to clarify the possibility of treatment of early enamel caries by Nd:YAG laser irradiation, we conducted in vitro experiments.[8] Artificial incipient enamel caries like lesions, that is subsurface demineralized lesions, were produced by exposure to the demineralizing fluid.[14] These lesions were exposed to an acoustooptically Q-switched Nd:YAG laser. The irradiation conditions were as follows; a peak power of 100 KW with a pulse width of 100 nsec, repetition rate of 1 KHz, average output of 10 W, spot size of 3.5 mm, and irradiation times of 0.4 to 1.2 second. A scanning electron microscopy of the acid-etched surfaces of the lased lesions showed reduced acid solubility of both the surface and subsurface enamel. After the lased lesions were exposed to the demineralizing fluid,[14] the acid resistance of the lased lesions was examined.

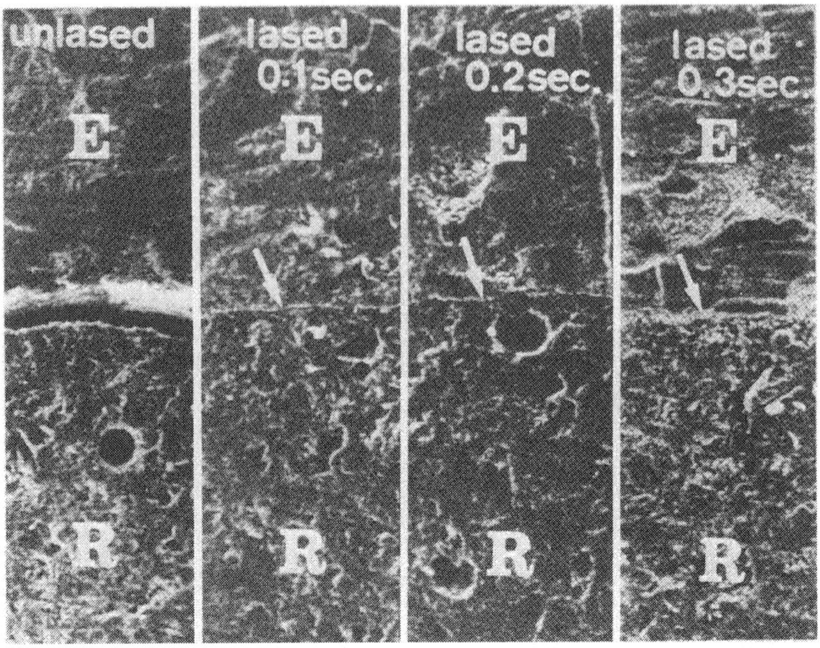

FIGURE 31.4. Scanning electron microscopy of the lased area at the margin of the dental restorative material (composite resin, Clearfill®). Complete closure *(arrow)* between the tooth enamel (E) and the resin (R) after the acoustooptically Q-switched Nd:YAG laser irradiation.

Fourteen days after demineralization, microradiographs of the lased lesions showed the appearance of radiodensity in the subsurface layer and a small amount of subsurface demineralization (Figure 31.5). Microradiographs of the lased lesions exposed to a remineralizing fluid[25] for 7 days revealed marked radiodensity in the subsurface layer where the subsurface demineralization was produced before the laser irradiation. These findings indicate that the acoustooptically Q-switched Nd:YAG laser irradiation to the artificial incipient enamel caries like lesions may not only prevent the demineralization from advancing but also accelerate remineralization. This mode of Nd:YAG laser may be effective for the prevention of the develop-

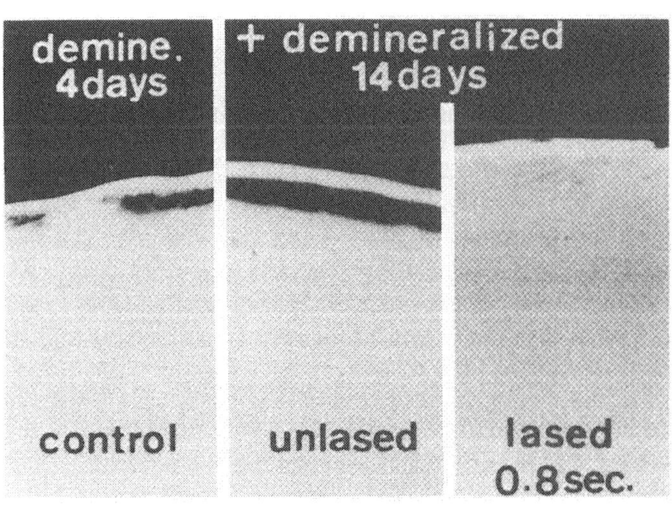

FIGURE 31.5. Microradiograms of 0.8 second irradiated incipient caries-like lesions (4 days demineralization) exposed to demineralizing fluid for 14 days. Subsurface demineralized lesion disappeared at the lased area.

ment of dental caries. The acoustooptically Q-switched Nd:YAG laser may have a advantage in treating small pit caries. When the focused laser beam is irradiated to these lesions, the pit lesions can be vaporized in a moment with the formation of a shallow crater. This crater can be easily restored by dental restorative materials such as an adhesive resin. These procedures may not need any more extensive cavity formation to prevent caries.[26]

Conclusion

It is clearly indicated that the acoustooptically Q-switched Nd:YAG laser might prove to be effective for clinical application for prevention of not only primary caries but also secondary caries. The latter is associated with marginal closure of the dental restorative materials. This laser may also be an effective tool for the treatment of incipient enamel caries. The irradiation conditions of these laser applications are a pulse width of 100 nanoseconds, repetition rate of 1 KHz, average output of 10 W, spot size of 3.5 mm, and irradiation time of about 0.8 second.

It is very important that these operational conditioned acoustooptically Q-switched Nd:YAG laser beams can be guided by a single flexible optical fiber. This property will make it possible for it to be developed into an effective tool easily operable in the small oral cavity for the prevention of dental caries and treatment of early caries.

Lasers may bring about a revolutionary strategy for the prevention and treatment of dental caries in the near future.

Acknowledgments. Collaborating with us in this series of studies were Prof. F. Inaba, Prof. K. Kamiyama, and Drs. K. Ooya, K. Sato, T. Ohkubo, Y. Tooya, S. Shoji, and K. Yamada.

These studies were supported in part by a Grant-in-Aid for Scientific Research from the Ministry of Education, Science and Culture.

References

1. Maiman TH: Stimulated optical radiation in ruby lasers. Nature 187:493, 1960.
2. Sognnaes RE, Stern RH: Laser effect on dental hard tissue. J South Calif State Dent Assoc 33:328–329, 1985.
3. Gordon JE: Single-surface cutting of normal tooth with ruby laser. J Am Dent Assoc 74:398–402, 1967.
4. Yamamoto S, Sato K: Prevention of dental caries by Nd:YAG laser irradiation. J Dent Res 59 (DII):2171–2177, 1980.
5. Yamamoto H, Sato K: Inhibition of dental caries by laser irradiation. In Atsumi K (ed): New Frontiers in Laser Medicine and Surgery. Excerpta Medica/Elsevier, Amsterdam, Oxford, and Princeton. pp 242–248, 1983.
6. Stern RH, Vahl, J, Sognnaes, RE: Ultrastructural observations of pulsed carbon dioxide laser effects. J Dent Res 51:455–460, 1972.
7. Yamamoto H, Ooya K: Potential of yttrium-aluminum-garnet laser in caries prevention. J Oral Pathol 3:7–15, 1974.
8. Sato H: Effect of acousto-optically Q-switched Nd:YAG laser irradiation on the artificial caries like lesion. Jpn J Oral Biol 24:913–925, 1982.
9. Shafer WG, Hine MK, Levy BM, Tomich CE: A Textbook of Oral Pathology. Saunders, Philadelphia, 1983.
10. Thewlis J: The calcification of enamel and dentin. Br Dent J 62:303, 1937.
11. Shoji S, Iiyama M, Ishikawa K, et al: Changes of boundary between dental enamel and restorative materials caused by Nd:YAG laser irradiation. J Jpn Soc Laser Med 4:265–266, 1984.
12. Gibbons RJ, Nygaard M: Syntheses of insoluble dextran and its significance in the formation of gelatinous deposits by plaque-forming streptococci. Arch Oral Biol 13:1249–1262, 1968.
13. Yamamoto H: The actual state and prospect of the laser application in the dental field. Dent J Iwate Med Univ 4:3–1, 1979.
14. Gray JA: Kinetics of enamel dissolution during formation of incipient caries-like lesions. Bri Dent J 120:461–471, 1966.
15. Yamaga R: Diamine fluoride and its clinical application. J Osaka Univ Dent Sch 12:1–20, 1972.
16. Suzuki T: Effects of diamine silver fluoride on tooth enamel. J Osaka Univ Dent Sch 14:61–72, 1974.
17. Sato H, Sato K, Toya Y, Yamamoto H: Effect of an acousto-optically Q-switched Nd:YAG laser irradiation on the fissure of the tooth in the presence of $Ag(NH_3)_2F$. Jpn J Oral Biol 23:401–406, 1981.
18. Tagomori S, Suzuki K, Morioka T: Combined effect of laser and fluoride on acid resistance. J Jpn Soc Laser Med 4(1):261–262, 1984.
19. Yamamoto H, Sato K, Ohkubo T, et al: Progress in caries prevention by laser irradiation. Dental Outlook 57:633–641, 1981.
20. Tochon-Danguy HJ, Very JM, Geofferoy M, Baud CA: Pramagnetic and crystallographic effects of

low temperature ashing on human bone and tooth enamel. Calcif Tiss Res 25:99–104, 1978.
21. Legeros RZ, Gilbert B, Legros R: Types of "H_2O" in human enamel and in precipitated apatites. Calcif Tiss Res 26:111–118, 1978.
22. Ohkubo T, Yamamoto H: Experimental study of laser inhibition of dental caries in rats. In Atsumi K, Nimsakul N (eds): Laser Tokyo '81. pp 12-5–12-8, 1981.
23. Onishi M, Ozaki F, Hamada M: Prevention of experimental rat caries III. Influences of casein contents in a cariogenic diet upon carious lesion of Pd-marked rats. J Dent Hlth 16:85–90, 1966.
24. Tooya Y: Acousto-optically Q-switched Nd:YAG laser resistence of human deciduous enamel to demineralization in vitro and in vivo. Jpn J Oral Biol 24:442–452, 1982.
25. Cate JM Ten, Arends J: Remineralization of artificial enamel lesions in vitro. Determination of activation energy and reaction order. Caries Res 12:213–222, 1978.
26. Yamamoto H, Kayano T: Laser and dentistry. Rev Laser Eng 13:549–558, 1985.

32
Nd:YAG Laser Therapy in Dental and Oral Surgery

Akinori Nagasawa

The laser has brought us numerous technical innovations in every scientific field since its invention in 1960.[1] Since then, lasers have elevated the level of traditional medicine and given us the benefit of modern advanced technology. The effect of light on tissues depends on the wavelength of the ray and since the coherent laser beam has a constant wavelength, an appropriate laser can be selected to achieve the best therapeutic result. The laser affords us the following therapeutic possibilities:

1. Selective treatment of the affected area is possible, based on the differences in optical characteristics.
2. Noncontact surgery is possible owing to the energy transference by laser radiation.
3. Noninvasive surgery is possible for deeply placed lesions by using optical fibers.
4. Various kinds of effects are possible to select.

Research on application of lasers to dentistry was started in 1964 by Goldman and coworkers[2] and other investigators, and numerous papers have been published with reports of these innovations that can change the method of traditional dentristy, still, various problems limit widespread applications of laser technology in dental practice, as previously reported. My coworkers and I have developed several therapeutic applications of lasers that are useful for medical treatment.[3–5] In particular, the Nd:YAG laser is clinically the most useful because of its high tissue penetration and high power output.

Fundamental Studies

Laser Effect on Tissue

Spectral Analysis of Tissues

The physical effect of light on tissue varies corresponding to the wavelength of the ray, and the effect of the coherent laser ray with a constant wavelength on tissue depends on the optical characteristics of the tissue at the wavelength of the laser. The analysis of the optical characteristics of tissues is most important to the development of laser technology. The effect of lasers on tissues can be estimated from the spectral analysis of the tissues.[6] Spectral analysis of dental tissues with the Nd:YAG laser shows the laser ray to be comparatively penetrable to the structures and, by scattering, it is minimally absorbed by them.[7] The reflectance on a tooth surface decreases with the wavelength, and therefore the surface of the tooth reflects the Nd:YAG laser much greater than CO_2 laser. Carious dentin has much greater absorptivity of Nd:YAG laser than intact dental structures and the difference in the optical characteristics can be applied to selective treatment of dental caries. Since these tissues generally consist of multistructures of different optical charecteristics, it is not easy to determine the laser effect on tissues exactly by spectrum analysis of a single structure.

Analysis of the Thermal Effect of Lasers

The accurate temperature measurement of lased tissues is very important in identifying the effects of the laser on these tissues. With such a tissue-penetrable ray as the Nd:YAG laser, however, there are some crucial problems in the temperature measurement of lased tissues. The direct effect of the laser on thermal sensors located in the tissue disturbs the accurate indication of the actual temperature of the lased tissue.

We devised an original system to measure the actual temperature of lased tissues.[8] The thermocouple probes for the temperature measurement of lased tissues have been coated on the surface with a very highly reflective material. An infrared thermometer provided the sensing wave band of 7 to 11 μm used for the measurement of the surface temperature of the lased tissues. Since the wavelength of the Nd:YAG laser is not detected by this thermometer, the actual temperature of the lased tissue can be measured accurately.

Observation of Laser Distribution in Tissues by Charge-Coupled Device Image Sensor

Nonvisible near-infrared laser distribution on and in tissues can easily be observed as visible images using a TV camera with a charge-coupled device (CCD) image sensor.[9] The CCD image sensor was developed in 1970 by W. S. Boyle.[10] The CCD has the following capabilities: (1) imaging, (2) signal transfer, (3) register, (4) reading out, and so is applicable an an excellent imaging sensor for TV cameras. Since the CCD image sensor is sensitive to the near-infrared ray of wavelength less than 1.2 μm, the laser distribution on and in tissues can easily be observed as a visible image using the TV camera provided with a CCD image sensor. Figure 32.1 shows the CCD TV image of the sectional plane of liver tissue exposed to a Nd:YAG laser on the surface of the liver. In these results, it is clearly observed that the Nd:YAG laser scatters spherically in the tissue. The exposure times of the laser are 1.0 0.2 second. Since the scattering areas are similar in these two cases, the CCD image sensor was proved to have high sensitivity to the Nd:YAG laser. The CCD TV image is too sensitive to the Nd:YAG laser of high power and can easily to go beyond the full range of detection. Therefore, some light reduction such as an iris or an optical filter proper to the laser intensity is required when measuring laser distribution of high resolution.

Measurement of Distribution of Laser Intensity in Tissue

It is also important to recognize the distribution of laser intensity in and on tissues for the study on therapeutic application of lasers. We have applied a pinhole scanning technique to this measurement[11] Figure 32.2a,b shows the vari-

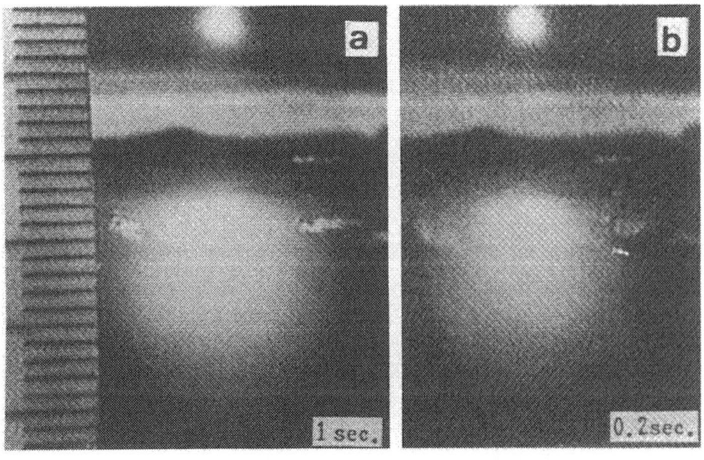

FIGURE 32.1. CCD TV image of the sectional view of liver being exposed to Nd:YAG laser (3 W) (a) 1.0 second, (b) 0.2 second (exposure time).

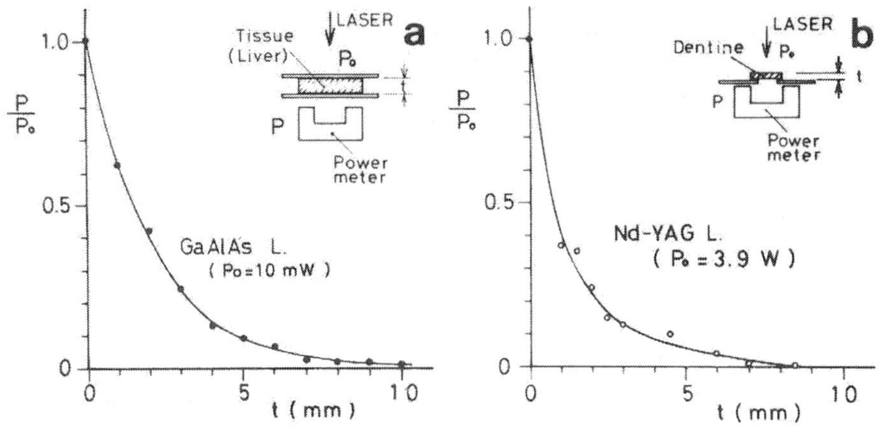

FIGURE 32.2. Power density rate of Nd:YAG laser in tissues. (a) Soft tissue (liver), (b) Dental tissue.

ation of the rate of a near-infrared laser intensity to the depth along the beam axis in a lased tissue in the case of liver tissue and in a dental structure.

Development of Clinically Available Laser Instruments

Laser Handpiece with Variable Beam Direction

A new laser handpiece provides a unique method of varying the exposing beam direction, as shown in Figure 32.3[12] This handpiece has a rotary reflective mirror at the top of the shaft. The reflector has a multicoating surface with extremely high reflectance to the Nd:YAG laser. Therefore this handpiece is practical and applicable to use with a 30-W Nd:YAG laser in the continuous wave mode for over 30 minutes without any problems. This handpiece is useful for laser surgery in a narrow field such as oral cavity.

Quartz Fiber Probe for Laser Endodontic Therapy

It is clinically impossible to apply sufficient laser energy to pulp tissue in treating a root canal by transmitting laser irradiation on the tooth surface because of decreased laser energy in the dental structure. In order to achieve a sufficient treatment effect on the root canal and a pulp tissue the laser beam must be guided only to the root canal for local treatment. Recently, ceramic surgical laser probes for contact laser therapy have been developed by Surgical Laser Technologics Inc (SLT) in the USA & Japan and are being used frequently. Fine needle-ceramic type probes have been used in laser root canal treat-

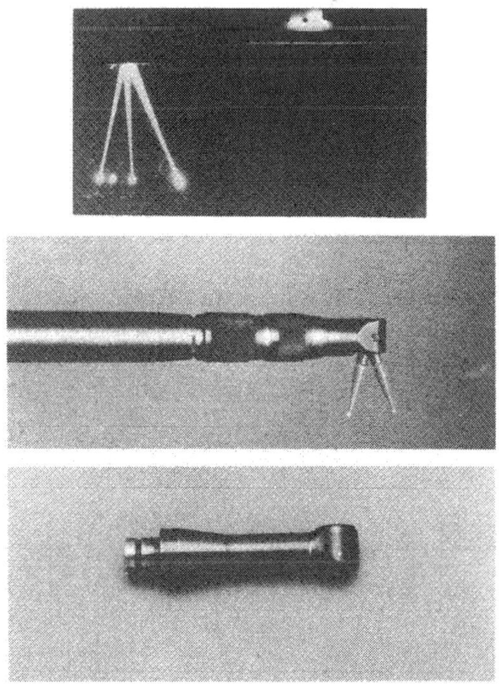

FIGURE 32.3. Laser handpiece of variable exposing beam direction. (Morita, Japan).

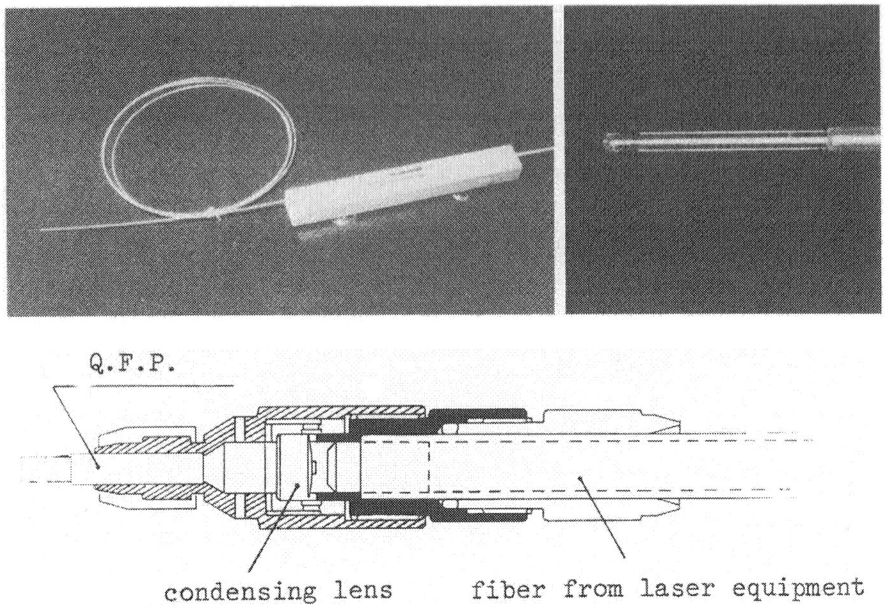

FIGURE 32.4. Quartz fiber probe system for endodontic therapy.

ment, but they can break particularly when they come into contact with the dental structures.

An endodontic quartz laser probe as developed, improving the commercially available quartz fiber, for laser waveguide with a core diameter of 0.6 mm.[13] This quartz fiber probe system is connected to the wave-guide fiber of the laser using a connecter (Figure 32.4). This probe is not easily broken. Even when the tip of the probe breaks off during use, it can be easily repaired. This probe is also easy to insert into the root canal previously enlarged with a root canal reamer, since it has a thin diameter of 0.6 mm and a slight flexibility.

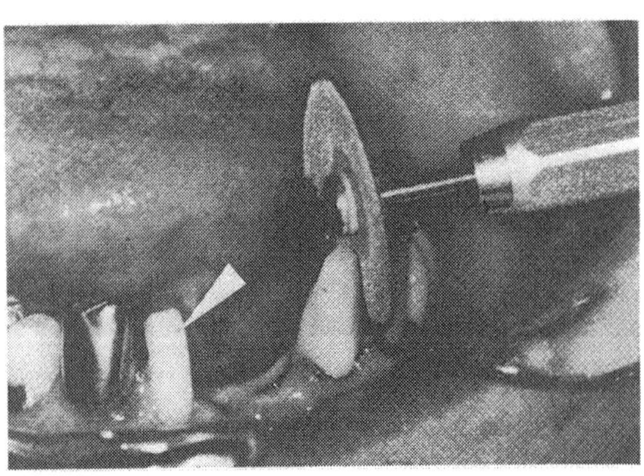

FIGURE 32.5. Clinical application of Nd:YAG laser analgesia on tooth (2|3).

Other Laser Instruments

In addition to the above, we have developed laser protectors[14] to safeguard the healthy parts of the body except for the treatment site; a laser irradiating system which can follow a moving target, and other equipments useful for dental laser surgery.

Therapeutic Effects of the Nd:YAG Laser in Dental and Oral Surgery

Analgesic Effect on Teeth in Dental Treatment

The Effect and the Technique

There is an analgesic effect produced on teeth exposed to the Nd:YAG laser.[15] The outline of this technique is as follows: A pain threshold can be elicited in a patient when a Nd:YAG laser is applied to the crown surface of a tooth. When a patient's tooth crown is exposed to pulsed. Nd:YAG laser under the pain threshold, for example, 10 to 20 W in fiber power output, 0.1-

second pulse width, 10 mm exposure distance (100 to 200 mW/cm^2), the patient has some tolerable sense. When the tooth is exposed repeatedly to the Nd:YAG laser under the pain threshold it becomes insensitive to the laser shot. At this stage the tooth is sufficiently anesthetized for cutting. It is now possible to increase the threshold dose of the laser beam on the tooth to induce pain in a staged technique and the analgesic effect on the tooth can be further increased. After such pretreatment the tooth can be cut without feeling pain.

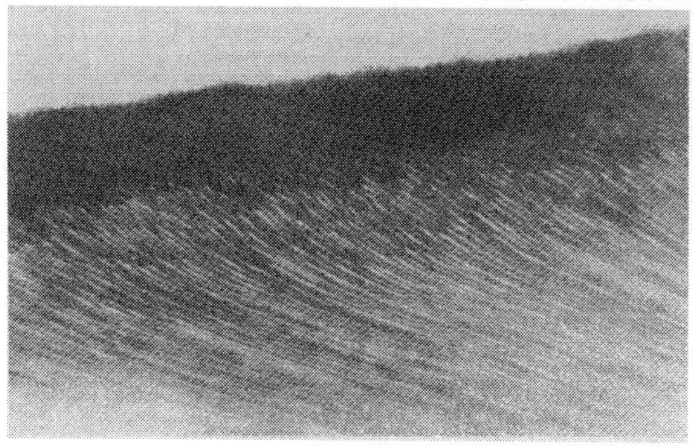

FIGURE 32.6. Microphotogram of a tooth exposed to the Nd:YAG laser.

Clinical Application

Figure 32.5 shows an example of a clinical application of laser dental analgesia. After the analgesic treatment of the Nd:YAG laser under the technique discussed earlier, the vital teeth 2|3 underwent the preparation for a jacket crown by cutting with a high-speed turbine instrument without any sense of pain, up to injuring just a corner of pulp of the tooth 2|(indicated with an arrow). As a result of the clinical application of this laser analgesia, more than 95% of cases were effective without any damage to the pulp and the surrounding tissue.

Discussion

Figure 32.6 shows a microphotogram of the dental structure of a tooth exposed the Nd:YAG laser. The dentin canal of the surface layer is observed to have disappeared. This layer is presumed to block the conduction of sensory stimulation to the pulp and provides the mechanism for laser dental analgesia. The argon laser has been found to have a greater analgesic effect on teeth than the Nd:YAG laser. The degenerative layer in the dentin canal of the tooth exposed to the argon laser is thicker than that exposed to the Nd:YAG laser.[16]

The roentgenographic survey and the long-term follow-up with electric pulp examination of the teeth exposed to laser analgesia have resulted in no problems. The safety of the pulp and the surrounding tissues in this technique has been confirmed by our thermal examinations.

Freedom from severe pain in dentistry has long been an earnest desire of patients. Therefore this laser analgesia that offers painless dental treatment with simple and safe technique is one of the most useful laser applications in dentistry.

Reactive Secondary Dentin Formation in Pulp

The Phenomenon

We observed, in the pulp tissue of lased rat teeth, the interesting phenomenon that the secondary dentin formation grows reactively toward filling the whole pulp cavity and the root canal of the tooth within a few months after exposure to the argon laser or the Nd:YAG laser, as shown in Figure 32.7.[16]

Results of Exposure of Human Teeth In the Nd:YAG Laser

Figure 32.8 shows a microphotogram of a milk tooth C| extracted 4 months after exposure to 400 J in total energy of Nd:YAG laser. In the case of human teeth exposed to the Nd:YAG laser, similar histologic changes to these experimental results in rat teeth have also been observed. The permanent adult teeth are weaker than the milk teeth in the secondary formation by exposure to the Nd:YAG laser.

Discussion

Thermal effect is well known as a stimulator to induce secondary dentin formation in dental pulp, and the thermal effect of the CO_2 laser is even greater on dental tissues, in that secondary dentin has been observed in the pulp of lased teeth. The secondary dentin formation in the

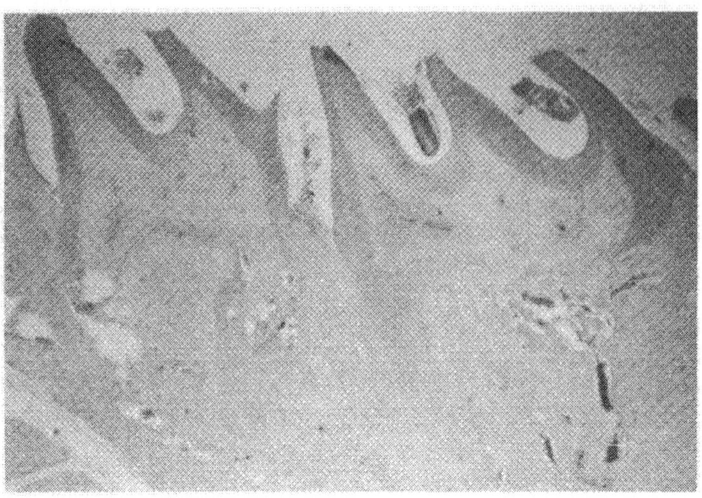

FIGURE 32.7. Microphotogram of a rat molar 3 months after exposed to 10 J of the argon laser.

pulp induced by the CO_2 laser, or mainly by thermal effect is, however, limited to the area that receives the thermal effect. This is different from the chainlike reaction of secondary dentin formation induced by the argon or the Nd:YAG laser. In addition to this, we have succeeded in producing similar reactive changes using the argon-dye laser in the pulp of the rat teeth exposed to such a low thermal effects as to be negligible after pretreating the rats with the photosensitizer hematoporphyrin derivative, as shown in Figure 32.9.[17] These results suggest that the laser-induced reactive secondary dentin formation is contingent not only on thermal effects but also on photodynamic effect of lasers. These result will hopefully suggest to lead to development of an epock-making laser dental application of biological endodontic therapy or biological root canal filling in the near future.

Bone Repair Activation Effect

The Effect

In the clinical application of the Nd:YAG laser to dental treatment we have identified interesting therapeutic effects on bone focuses as well as improving the mobility of loosened teeth and the inflammation of soft tissue. Roentgenographic survey for these cases proved that the laser activated the repairing process of the damaged bones.[18] The results of experimen-

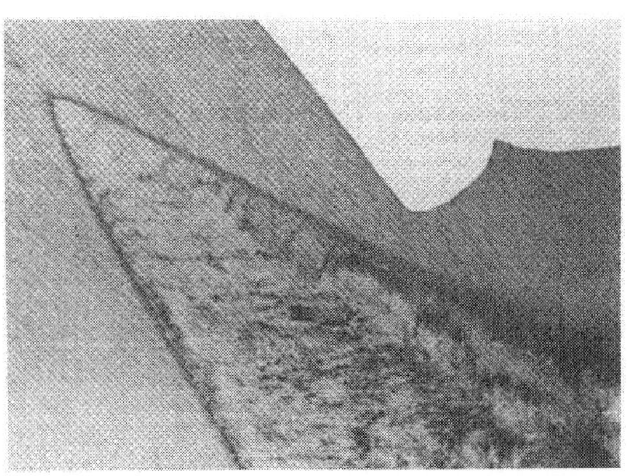

FIGURE 32.8. Microphotogram of extracted milk tooth C4 months after exposure to 400 J of Nd:YAG laser.

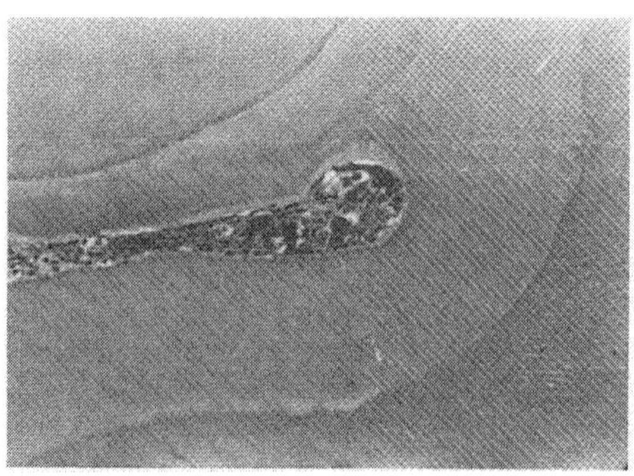

FIGURE 32.9. Microphotogram of a rat molar 3 months after exposure to 10 J of argon-dye laser after hematoporphyrin derivative premedication.

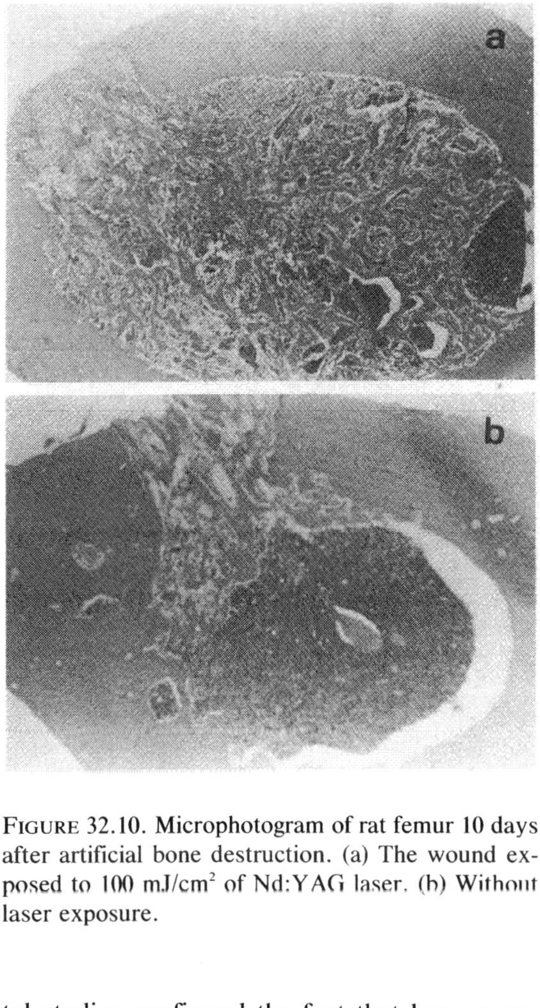

FIGURE 32.10. Microphotogram of rat femur 10 days after artificial bone destruction. (a) The wound exposed to 100 mJ/cm^2 of Nd:YAG laser. (b) Without laser exposure.

tal studies confirmed the fact that low-energy laser exposure was also effective in activating the repairing process of the artificial bone destructions. Figure 32.10 shows the microphotograms of rat femur 10 days after the bones were partially destroyed artificially by drilling. In Figure 32.10a, the artificial wound was exposed to a Nd:YAG laser of 100 J/cm^2 just after bone injury. Figure 32.10b shows the control femur, without any laser exposure. Comparative observation of the results shown in Figure 32.10a and b are summarized as follows: (1) New spongy bone formation with multiple bone trabecula in the bone marrow around the wound in case a is far superior to that of case b. (2) As for the adhesion of the newly produced bone tissue to cover the bone defect and the original bone wall in the wound, case A is much closer than case b. (3) Partial secondary calcification in the newly produced bone is observed in case A, but very little in case B. These results from this experiment prove that the laser activates the bone repair process for destroyed bone.

Clinical Application

Therapeutic Techniques

ENDODONTIC THERAPY. Root canals are firstly widened completely by the conventional technique. Then the quartz fiber probe used in root canal therapy, 0.6 mm diameter, is inserted as deep as possible. The Nd:YAG laser is irradiated from the tip of the quartz fiber probe in the root canal toward the root apex. Exposure conditions are 2 to 5 W power output at the tip of the probe in the tip the quartz fiber probe, 0.5 to 1 second in duration. Repeating the lasering, the quartz fiber probe is pulled up step by step toward the pulp chamber (Figure 32.11). Complete sterilization of the root canal after this laser treatment has been confirmed by bacterial culture, and more than 98% of the cases have been successfully cured.

PERIAPICAL OPERATION. The appropriate sizes the needle-shaped SLT ceramic surgical probe (CSR) is inserted on the gingiva to a periapical bone focus or a periodontal bone focus, and the Nd:YAG laser fired at 3 to 10 W in CSR tip, 0.5 to 1.0 second in duration, and is repeated to destroy the area. The destroyed structure flows out around the CSR, and the rest is cleaned up by curettage and washing. The periodontal bone focus is thus healed without cutting the gingiva or the alveolar bone.

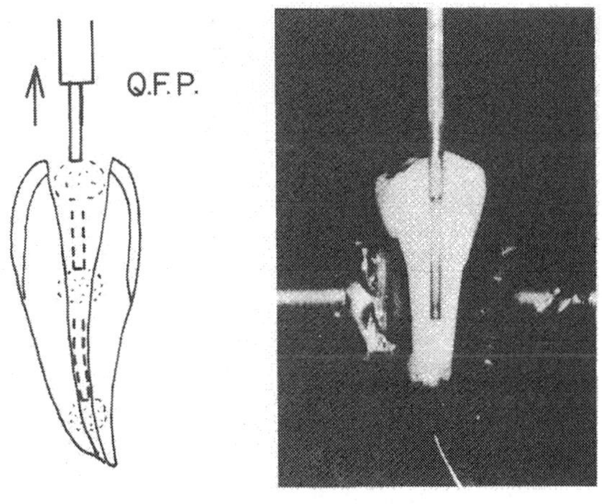

FIGURE 32.11. Nd:YAG laser endodontic therapy using quartz fiber probe.

PERIODONTAL OPERATION. First of all, a CSR of 0.4 mm apex diameter is inserted into the gingival pocket and Nd:YAG laser is irradiated in it. The gingival attachment is cut moving the SLT contact probe with irradiating a few watts of continuous wave Nd:YAG laser. Minimal bleeding occurs. After curettage on the inner surface of the gingival flap and the root surface of the teeth, the gingival flap is sutured to reattach to the root surface. Even severe cases of alveolar pyorrhea of hard gingivitis have been completely cured without recurrence for long periods.

Results of Clinical Application

CASE 1. CHRONIC ALVEOLAR OSTEITIS (6|), 22Y, F. As shown in the roentgenogram before treatment (Figure 32.12a), the remarkably progressed granulomatous bone destruction is observed widely spreaded over the two roots. This tooth suffered a serious gingivitis and percussive pain. It was remarkably loosened with high mobility and could not be used to chew any food.

In this endodontic therapy complete enlarging of the root canals was impossible because of their stricture with curved apex. Then Nd:YAG laser therapy was applied to this case by the technique discussed earlier. The laser exposure in this treatment was as follows: 10 W, 0.5 second 37 times, and 10 W, 1 second 23 times, total energy: 415 J. In spite of the incomplete result of this root canal filling, the severe gingivitis was improved soon after the laser treatment, and the tooth mobility was also improved gradually to recover normal mastication ability. No problems have occurred in this patient for 18 months after laser treatment. Figure 32.12b,c,d show roentgenograms after laser treatment (b: 2 months after, c: 5 months after, and d: 10 months after). These roentgenograms prove that bone repair in this large bone focus progresses to the stage of complete recovery.

CASE 2: ALVEOLAR PYORRHOA |4 59Y. F. This is a case of extremely severe alveolar pyorrhea of the upper teeth (3+4) with a hard inflammation in the palate, as shown in Figure 32.13a. In particular, the left upper first molar (|4) had a remarkable mobility and percussive pain and was difficult to use for chewing. The alveolar bone around the whole root was widely absorbed and destroyed as shown in the roentgenogram before treatment (Figure 32.14a). This

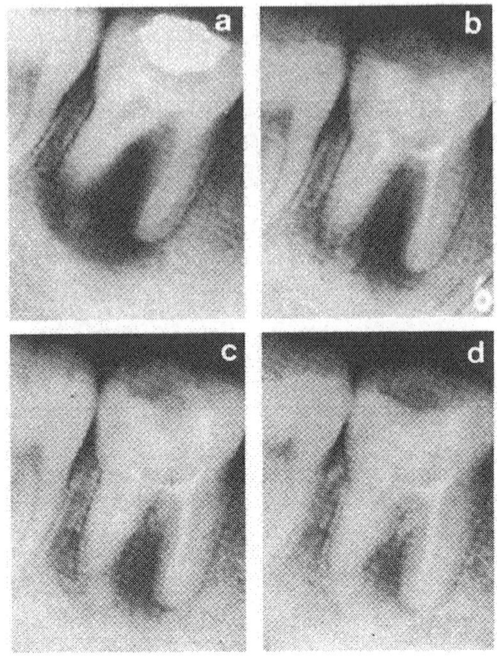

FIGURE 32.12. Roentgenograms in Nd:YAG laser endodontic therapy (chronic alveolar ostitis 6|). (a) Before treatment. (b) 2 months after laser root canal treatment. (c) 5 months after laser root canal treatment. (d) 10 months after laser root canal treatment.

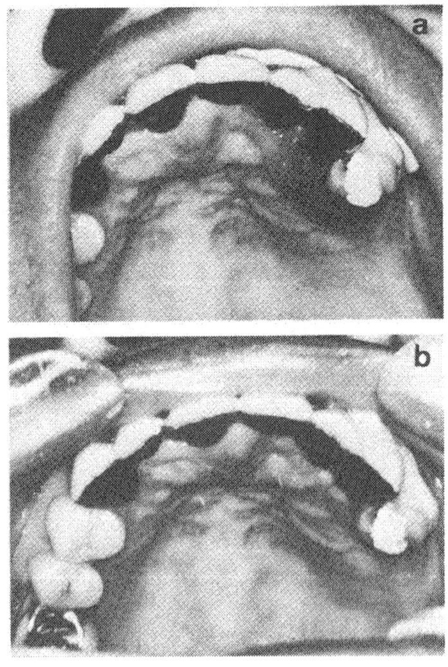

FIGURE 32.13. Alveolar pyorrhea of upper teeth (3+4). (a) Hard inflammation in the palate. (b) After laser operation.

case was difficult to cure by conventional treatments (Figure 32.14b). Thus the periodontal operation using the contact Nd:YAG laser was tried. As shown in Figure 32.13b the hard inflammation of the palate improved soon after laser operation. The remarkable tooth movement and other problems in this tooth have also improved gradually and the mastication has recovered normally. The roentgenograms 3 months after operation (Figure 32.14c) and 12 months after operation (Figure 32.14d) shows that the bone destruction has progressively being repaired. This case has been problems free 2 years after surgery.
The noteworthy findings in dental laser treatments are summarized as follows:

Roentogenographic Findings

1. The destroyed alveolar bone is activated to repair.
2. The affected bone tissue structurally improve.
3. The bone repairing effect occurs in the apical or periodontal bone damaged areas.

Clinical Findings

1. Mobility of loosened teeth improves.
2. Severe gingivitis and tooth pain, usually difficult to treat can be improved.
3. The mastication ability of the affected teeth recover.

The therapeutic effects in such laser dental surgery are summarized based on the above therapeutic findings.

1. Activation of bone repair
2. Antiinflammatory and sterilization effect.
3. Mastication recovery.

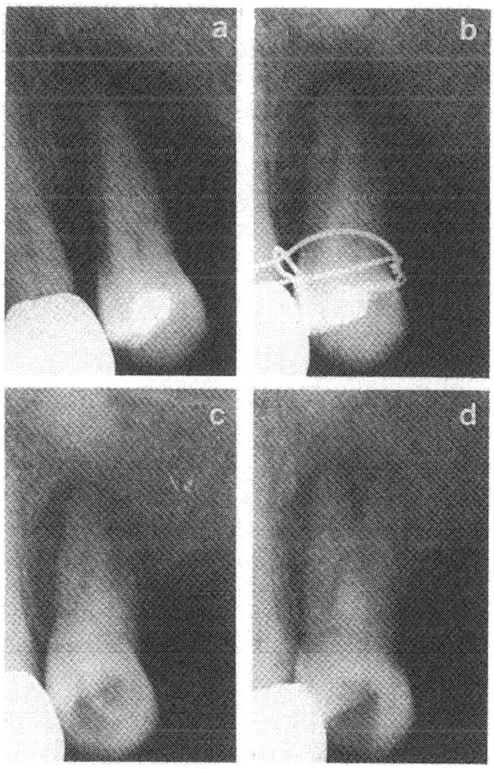

FIGURE 32.14. Roentgenograms in Nd:YAG laser operation (alveolar pyorrhea |4). (a) Before operation. (b) 3 months after conventional operation. (c) 9 months after laser operation. (d) 12 months after laser operation.

Discussion

The Physical Viewpoint

The Nd:YAG laser ray decreases its intensity at increased depth in the tissue, becoming quite weak or negligible in the deeper areas. Since the needle-shaped contact probe has a comparatively large exposure beam angle at the apex, the decrease in the laser intensity in deep tissues is much more remarkable than that of fiber exposing instruments. Therefore the bone repair is stimulated by low-energy lasers, which activate tissue metabolism. This theory has been confirmed by the results of the following experiment.

Figure 32.15 indicates the results of experiments on rat bone damages using the Ga-Al-As-diode laser or the He-Ne laser at milliwatt power output which are similar to experiments using the Nd:YAG laser, as shown in Figure 32.10. In each case the bone injury is exposed to the same laser energy density of 100 J/cm^2, but intensity of the lasers was different. In the experiment using the Nd:YAG laser, 4 W of exposure power was delivered, the Ga-Al-As laser delivered 40 mW, and the He-Ne laser delivered 6 mW. In the case of these low power lasers similar result of bone healing to Nd:YAG laser were obtained as shown in Figure 32.10. This bone repair appears also to be activated by using even extremely low power laser of milliwatt level as shown in these cases. These results confirm that the bone repair effect of lasers is contingent on photostimulation[19] for tissue activation.

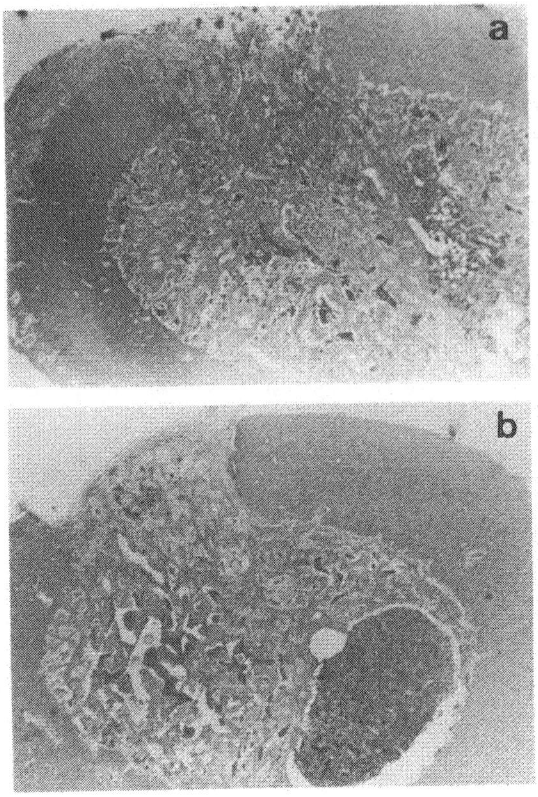

FIGURE 32.15. Microphotogram of rat femur 10 days after artificial bone destruction. (a) The wound exposed to 100 J/cm^2 of 40 mW Ga-Al-As laser. (b) The wound exposed to 100 J/cm^2 of 6 mW He-Ne laser.

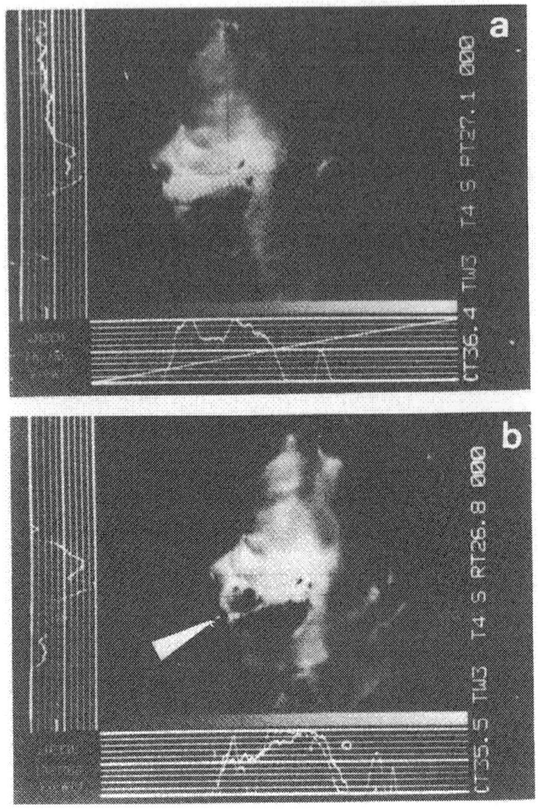

FIGURE 32.17. Thermographic survey for the therapeutic effect of the Nd:YAG laser on cancer of cheek. (a) Before treatment. (b) 1 day after exposure to Nd:YAG laser (indicated by arrow).

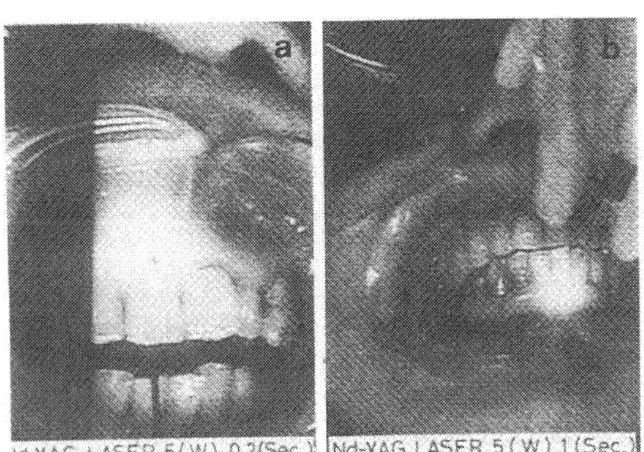

FIGURE 32.16. Charge-coupled device TV image of a mouth during irradiation of the Nd:YAG laser. (a) Root canal treatment, 5 W, 0.2 second. (b) Surgical operation for a case of alveolar pyorrhea, 5 W, 1 second.

Observation of the Light Scattering into a Tissue in the Laser Treatment

The area of light scattering into a tissue in these laser treatments can be easily observed as a visible image on TV by using a charge-coupled device (CCD) TV camera. Figure 32.16A is the CCD TV image of a mouth during irradiation of the Nd:YAG laser into the pulp of a tooth in the root canal treatment. The laser light can be observed widely spreading over the periodontal tissue and the effects can be seen. Figure 32.16B shows another case of the CCD image of a mouth during irradiation of the Nd:YAG laser into the periodontal pocket using a CSR of 0.4 mm apex diameter in the surgical operation for a case of alveolar pyorrhea. The laser light, in this case, scatters widely, spreading over the periodontal bone and, the gingiva also.

Other Therapeutic Effects

Therapeutic Effects of the Nd:YAG Laser on Malignant Tumor

We have developed a laser system for malignant tumors, combining the Nd:YAG and CO_2 lasers.[20] The destructive effect of the Nd:YAG laser on malignant tumors can be evaluated using thermography, as shown in Figure 32.17. Malignant tumors have a high temperature as shown in Figure 32.17A, but the cancerous area exposed to Nd:YAG laser changes to low temperature immediately after the laser therapy as shown in Figure 32.17B.

Laser Welding for Mucousa Flap

Vascular anastomosis[21] using weak lasers is now available for practical use.[22] The mechanism of this laser anastomosis is believed to be the entangling of the collagen fiber activated by laser stimulation. We attempted to weld the incised mucosa flap edges using Nd:YAG laser exposure. Figure 32.18A shows the histologic image of rat skin successfully applied with a Nd:YAG laser to weld the skin incision. Figure 32.18B shows a clinical example of successful welding of incised oral mucosa in oral surgery. This technique holds great promise for the future.

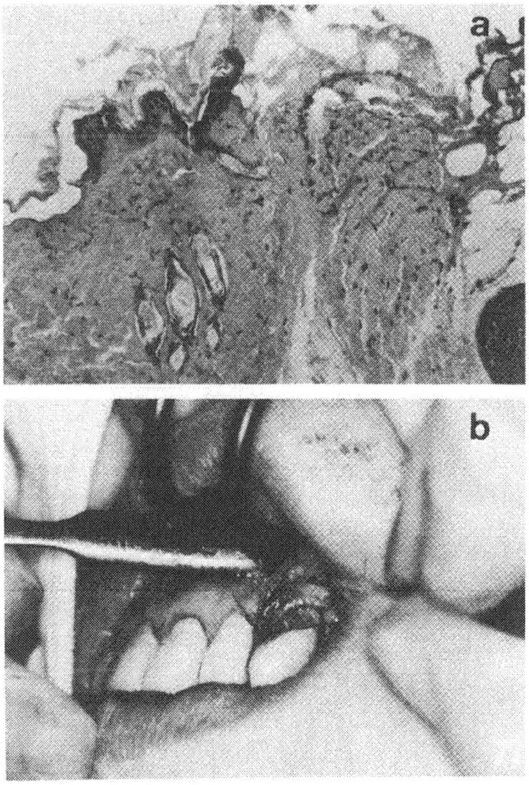

FIGURE 32.18. Nd:YAG laser welding on the incised flap. (a) Rat skin. (b) Human oral mucosa.

Others

The Nd:YAG laser is theoretically the most useful laser for tissue coagulation and it is very useful for controlling bleeding in oral surgery. Further application of the Nd:YAG laser to dental and oral surgery has been pursued.

Conclusion

Technical innovation is necessary in dentistry, particularly in the areas of intractable dental pain, endodontic therapy, avoidance of tooth extraction and in progressive alveolar diseases.

Several interesting therapeutic effects of the Nd:YAG laser have been presented. Almost all of them have been successfully used and the results indicate that these new therapeutic applications of the Nd:YAG laser could fulfil the desire of patients for improvement in traditional dentistry.

References

1. Maiman TH: Stimulated optical radiation in ruby. Nature 187:493, 1960.
2. Goldman L, et al: Impact of laser on dental caries. Nature 203:417, 1964.
3. Nagasawa A, et al: Survey of applicability of CO_2 laser to dental and oral surgery. Jpn J Med Biol Eng, 17(Suppl):672, 1979.
4. Nagasawa A: Laser in dental and oral surgery. In Atsumi K (ed): Clinical Laser. Medical Planning, Sappolo, 1981, pp. 233–273.
5. Nagasawa A: Nd:YAG laser therapies in dental and oral surgery. Proceedings of the 2nd International Nd:YAG Laser Conference 1985, pp 483–489.
6. Nagasawa A, et al: Optical characteristics of dental structures and the difference of the effect of lasers on them. Jpn J Med Biol Eng 18 (Suppl):178, 1980.
7. Spitzer S, et al: The absorption and scattering of light in bovine and human dental enamel. Calcif Tiss Res 17:129, 1975.
8. Nagasawa A, et al: Actual temperature measurement of tissues by using improved thermocouples J Jpn Soc Laser Med 3(1):195–200, 1982.

9. Nagasawa A, et al: Pilot study on application of CCD image sensor to survey near infrared laser distribution in tissues. BMTH (Jap), 6(1):12–15, 1986.
10. Boyle WS, et al: Charge coupled semiconductor devices Bell Syst Tech J 49:587, 1970.
11. Nagasawa A, et al: Optical characteristics and difference of effects on teeth in various kinds of lasers. Jpn J Med Biol Eng, 18(Suppl):178–179, 1980.
12. Nagasawa A, et al: Fundamental study on exposing beam direction variable laser handpiece and exposing beam angle variable laser handpiece, Med Instrum 53(Suppl):145–147, 1983.
13. Nagasawa A, et al: Effective Nd-YAG laser techniques for endodontic therapy. Jpn J Sci Laser Med 6(3):251–254, 1986.
14. Nishikawa K, et al: CO_2 laser protectors applied to laser surgery. The 4th Congress of the International Society for Laser Surgery (Tokyo), Feb. 21–24, 1981.
15. Nagasawa A, et al: The anesthetic effect of Nd-YAG laser in dental treatment. Jpn J Med Biol Eng 22(Suppl):830–831, 1984.
16. Nagasawa A: Histological changes in dental pulp exposed to argon laser. Jpn J Med Biol Eng 19(Suppl):319, 1981.
17. Nagasawa A, et al: (1985) Reactive changes in the pulp tissue of lased teeth. Proceedings of the 14th International Congress on Medical and Biological Engineering, 1985, pp. 1107–1108.
18. Nagasawa A, et al: Alveolar bone repair effect of Nd:YAG laser in dental surgery. Jpn J Med Biol Eng 24(Suppl):179, 1986.
19. Mester E, et al: (1981) The biostimulative effect of laser beam, Proceedings of the 4th Congress of the International Society for Laser Surgery (Tokyo), 1981, 22-4–22-7.
20. Nagasawa A, et al: Combined YAG laser and CO_2 laser therapy to malignant tumor. Proceedings of the 4th Congress of the International Society for Laser Surgery (Tokyo), 1981, 11-38–11-41.
21. Beck OJ: The use of Nd:YAG and CO_2 laser in neurosurgery. Neurosurg Rev 3:261, 1980.
22. Jain KK: Nd:YAG laser in Microneurosurgery: Chapter 15, Elsevier Science Publishing Co. Inc., 132–140, 1983.

33 Laser Hemorrhoidectomy

M.Y. Sankar

Hemorrhoids have afflicted mankind since ancient times: there is a record of the disease on Egyptian papyrus[1] and surgical treatment was reported in ancient Rome and Greece.[2] The disease may be asymptomatic at times, often detected on routine rectal and proctoscopic examinations. The incidence of hemorrhoids increases with age and affects at least 50% of people over 50 years old. Hemorrhoids occur in males and females of all ages, although men are more commonly affected.

The word hemorrhoid is derived from the Greek adjective *haimorrhoides*, meaning bleeding (*haima*–blood, *rhoos*–flowing), which places the emphasis on the prominent symptom of bleeding. The term "piles" is derived from the Latin word *pila*, meaning "a ball," which refers to a swelling around the anus during some stage of the disease. The terms hemorrhoids and piles are often used synonymously.

Classification of Hemorrhoids

Hemorrhoids are divided into *internal* and *external* types. The internal type arises in the upper two thirds of the anal canal, which is lined by columnar epithelium. External hemorrhoids arise in the lower third of the anal canal, which is covered by squamous epithelium of the skin. This type of classification may fit the description in the early stages, but later, when the hemorrhoids have enlarged sufficiently, the internal hemorrhoids may present externally at the anus.

According to Graham-Stewart,[3] internal hemorrhoids can be further divided into two categories:

1. Vascular hemorrhoids that consist mainly of distended vessels and are seen in the younger age group
2. Mucosal hemorrhoids that are composed of thickened mucosa and encountered in older patients

In the very early stages, the internal hemorrhoids protrude slightly into the anal canal as congested veins. These are called first-degree hemorrhoids. With the passage of time, they become larger and descend toward the anal orifice. The piles then may be found externally, especially on straining at defecation, and spontaneously regress into the anus at the end of the effort. These are second-degree hemorrhoids. Later, the internal hemorrhoids protrude not only during defecation but may stay prolapsed until they are digitally reduced and are called third-degree. Finally, long-standing piles, especially in the elderly, become very large, covered by skin and remain prolapsed permanently outside the anal canal. These irreducible masses are known as fourth-degree or complicated third-degree hemorrhoids and are seen as interoexternal hemorrhoids.

Shafik[4] suggests that there is no true anal canal but rather a continuity of the rectum to the perianal skin. The failure of remodeling and the persistence of an anorectal band results in a narrowing of the lower rectal neck, which initiates the hemorrhoid disease. An increase in rectal neck pressure and straining during defecation eventually lead to a prolapse of the rectal mucosa and venous congestion.

Clinical Features of Internal Hemorrhoids

The prominent symptoms of internal hemorrhoids are *bleeding* and *prolapse*. Apart from these two main symptoms, the patient may suffer from a discharge leading to soiling of underclothing, anal irritation, and symptoms of secondary anemia. Severe pain is present only in complicated cases of irreducible prolapse or with an associated perianal fissure. A history of slight pain was elicited by Bennett et al.[5] in 86% of 138 patients suffering from hemorrhoids and was the presenting complaint in 18% of these cases.

On clinical examination, proctoscopy is the essential step in confirming the presence of internal hemorrhoids. Barium enema followed by sigmoidoscopy and/or colonoscopy are mandatory in patients over 40 years of age with rectal bleeding.

Treatment of Internal Hemorrhoids

The treatment of internal hemorrhoids include the following major categories.

Conservative Treatment

A conservative treatment is useful for first-degree hemorrhoids, especially when discovered during a routine examination. The treatment consists of regulation of bowel habits, administration of mild laxatives, and advice regarding inclusion of a high-fiber diet. Suppositories and ointments used locally for symptomatic relief probably have negligible value.

Injection Treatment

In selected cases, injection therapy is of great value. The two important effects are as follows:

1. Fibrous tissue is formed, which surrounds, constricts, and obliterates blood vessels in the submucosa.
2. The fibrosis increases the fixation of the hemorrhoid and the mucosa to the underlying tissues, thus preventing prolapse.

Beneficial results are obtained with first- and second-degree bleeding hemorrhoids. Third- and fourth-degree hemorrhoids cannot be cured by injection treatment. The procedure is done in the office and can be repeated as necessary. The fibrous reaction that occurs after repeated injections makes further injections more difficult. During the injection therapy of scleroscent agents (e.g., phenol in almond oil, sodium tetradecyl), the patient may experience some discomfort. Late necrosis of the injection site may lead to ulcer formation and other rare complications, including submucous abscess formation, hematuria, prostatic abscess, and portal vein embolism.

Operative Treatment

The multiple operations available for the treatment of hemorrhoids include the following (see Table 33.1):

1. Ligation and excision[6–8]
2. Submucosal hemorrhoidectomy[9]
3. Excision of individual hemorrhoid with primary suture[10,11]
4. Excision of the entire pile-bearing area with suture[12]
5. Clamp and cautery technique[13]
6. Rubber-band ligation[14,15]
7. Maximum dilatation of the anus[16]
8. Cryosurgery[17,18]
9. Infrared coagulation[19]
10. Laser hemorrhoidectomy

The increasing number of techniques mentioned above for dealing with hemorrhoids attests to the lack of universal satisfaction with those currently available. Under these circumstances, the management is not only selected with a view to tailor the requirement to the individual patient's specific problem, but also with regard for other factors, such as associated morbidity (e.g., pain, bleeding), long-term complications (e.g., incontinence, recurrence, stricture), hospital stay, and cost-effectiveness.

Lasers in Surgery

The first reports on the use of lasers in medicine appeared in the early 1960s[20] at that time the

TABLE 33.1. Hemorrhoidectomy: Summary of review of various procedures, results, and postoperative complications

		Postoperative								
Mode of therapy	Anesthesia	Pain	Bleeding	Discharge	Urinary retention	Wound healing	Anal incontinence	Anal stricture	Recurrences	Return to work (average)
Injection therapy	—	+ (≃ 2 days)	+/++[a]	+	—	Good (7 days)	—	+[b]	*/**	Immediate. (repetition of procedure in most cases)
Rubber banding	—	+/++ (≃ 2 days)	++/+++[c]	+	—	Good	—	—	*/**	Immediate. (repetition of procedure in some cases)
Maximum dilation of the anus	General/local with IV sedation	++/+++[d]	±	±	—	Good	++/+++	—	**	7 days
Cryosurgery	Local with IV sedation	++/+++ (≃ 7 days)	+/++[c]	−+/+++	—	Good (14 days)	—	—	*/**	7–10 days
Infrared coagulation	—	+ (≃ 2 days)	+/++[c]	++	—	Good	—	—	*/**	3–7 days
Formal conventional hemorrhoidectomy	General/spinal/regional local with IV sedation	++/+++ (≃ 7 days)	++/+++[c]	+/++ (after 1st week)	+/++	Good (21–28 days)	±/++	+++	*/**	5 days as inpatient; 15–21 days home recuperation
Laser hemorrhoidectomy										
CO_2 laser	Local with sedation	+/++ (≃ 5–6 days)	±	±	—	Good (14–21 days)	—	—	*	Within 5 days
Nd:YAG laser										
Noncontact	General (short)/regional or local with IV sedation	+/++ (≃ 5–6 days)	±	±	±	Good (21 days)	—	±	*	Within 7 days
Contact	General (short)/regional or local with IV sedation	+ (≃ 2–3 days)	—	±	—	Good (7–14 days)	—	—	Being assessed	2–3 days

+ = mild/minimal; ++ = moderate; +++ = severe; — = nil or none.
* = occasional; ** = sometimes; *** = frequent.
[a] Injection ulcer.
[b] Temporary.
[c] Secondary/reactionary hemorrhage.
[d] With subsequent daily passage of large anal dilator.

CO_2 laser scalpel was used in general surgery. In 1973, the first flexible laser waveguide was developed, which made the use of lasers possible during fiberoptic endoscopy.[21] Lasers produce an intense beam of light of uniform wavelength and color that can be precisely focused to deliver high levels of energy to small areas. The most important interaction between laser radiation and tissue is the absorption of light and conversion of the light energy into heat. In performing a laser hemorrhoidectomy, both the CO_2 laser and the Nd:YAG laser have been tried with varying degrees of enthusiasm. The CO_2 laser, operating at a wavelength of 10,600 nm and with an energy output of 100 W, is effective in cutting, but not very adept in performing coagulation. On the other hand, the Nd:YAG laser, operating at a wavelength of 1064 nm and with energy output up to 150 W, can vaporize tissues at higher powers and coagulate bleeding points at relatively low powers, including blood vessels up to 2 to 3 mm in diameter. Current Nd:YAG laser light transmission systems use a flexible quartz fiber, which delivers laser energy at a distance of 0.5 to 1.5 cm from the tissue. This noncontact system has distinct disadvantages regarding beam irradiation, backscatter, and damage to the quartz tip should it come into contact with tissue or blood. Furthermore, the Nd:YAG laser, due to its depth of penetration into tissue in its noncontact mode, is used primarily for coagulation but has poor cutting capabilities and may cause excessive tissue damage resulting in perforation.

Recently, a synthetic sapphire crystal has been developed, which is easily attached to the end of the quartz fiber, with a universal metal connector allowing contact irradiation. The geometric shape of this contact synthetic sapphire provides the desired effect of coagulation of bleeding points and/or vaporization, as well as precise incision of tissues.[22] Furthermore, the contact probes prevent backscattering of Nd:YAG laser light, reduce the depth of tissue damage, and allow for much lower powers of laser energy to be used. A longer probe attached to a handpiece, the laser scalpel, allows for open surgery to be performed with ease. The power density at the tip of the contact probe is related to the distal probe diameter and the results obtained are comparable to the average power density values of different spot sizes and power levels found with CO_2 laser beam. The contact cutting probes thus combine the coagulating properties of Nd:YAG laser with incising capabilities previously only seen with CO_2 laser.

Laser Hemorrhoidectomy

In the United States, at present, over 150,000 conventional type of hemorrhoidectomies are performed each year, with an average inpatient hospitalization stay of 5.9 days. The laser offers an alternative method of treating hemorrhoids as an outpatient procedure under local, regional, or short general anesthesia.

CO_2 Laser

Eddy and colleagues[23] have performed 150 procedures using the CO_2 laser, and they claim that the incidence of postoperative pain was considerably reduced, and therefore narcotics were seldom needed. Complications such as urinary retention and constipation were not seen even in the elderly and poor-risk patients. Mokhniuk and colleagues,[24] in the Proctological Division of the Kiev Medical Institute in Russia, treated 352 patients suffering from hemorrhoids between 1976 and 1980. Of these, 281 were women. In 80%, a modified Milligan-Morgan procedure was performed. In the other 9% of patients, they vaporized the hemorrhoids with the CO_2 laser, employing a power of 60 W in a continuous wave mode with a focused beam diameter of 0.2 mm. Epidural anesthesia was administered and a clamp or hemostat was applied to the base of each hemorrhoid before removing it. After removal of the hemostat, no bleeding was observed. In the immediate postoperative period, edema was minimal and appeared much less than that observed following the conventional ligation and excision operation for hemorrhoids. Pain was almost absent, and no discharge was noted from the operated site. The laser may have sterilized the wound surface, preventing infection during the postoperative period. In cases of hemorrhoids with thrombosis, Mokhniuk and colleagues[24] recommend cryosurgery, but without supporting evidence. Rausis[25] has also used the CO_2 laser and found less pain in the postoperative period. Of their 21 proctologic procedures using the CO_2 laser, 12 were for third-degree hemorrhoids. The laser hemorrhoidectomy followed the same principles as the Milligan-Morgan procedure, and there was a decrease in postoperative complaints, normal bowel movements, and negligible postoperative bleeding. Healing was complete after 2 or 3 weeks. No incontinence of flatus or feces was observed nor anal stenosis. The follow-up of 1 to 5 months is too short for evaluating recurrences.

Denis and Lemarchand[26] have carried out 150 hemorrhoidectomies using the CO_2 laser, 150 cases by conventional operative methods, and 47 cases by electrocautery within a period of one year. Results showed very little difference at the statistical 5% level between the CO_2 laser and the conventional type of hemorrhoidectomy when factors like postoperative pain and wound healing are taken into consideration. On the other hand, electrocautery caused severe postoperative pain, requiring high analgesic consumption. Furthermore, with electrocautery, wound healing was delayed, and the consequent severe scarring inevitably led to anal stricture and stenosis. The initial postoperative bowel movements were similar in producing discomfort in all three groups. Denis and Lemarchand concluded that conventional surgery of hemorrhoids by high ligation and excision was just as effective as the laser.

In support of CO_2 laser hemorrhoidectomy, the advantages include faster healing, less scarring and fibrosis, decreased recurrence, fewer postoperative complications, and excellent patient acceptance.[27] Zadeh[28] performed CO_2 laser hemorrhoidectomy on 350 outpatients (70% male) in just over a year. In this group, 27% had second-degree hemorrhoids, 39% third-degree, and 34% fourth-degree. The majority received a local infiltration of anesthetic drug with intravenous sedation. The hemorrhoidectomy was performed in about 20 minutes at a power density between 38,200 and 47,000 W/cm^2 in the continuous wave mode. Pain was classified as none (6%), minimal (29.8%), moderate (41.3%), and severe (22.9%), and the average duration of postoperative pain was 5–6 days. Zadeh concludes that both routine and difficult cases can easily be treated on an outpatient basis, using the CO_2 laser, thereby enhancing the cost-effectiveness and convenience of patient care.

Nd:YAG Laser

The Nd:YAG laser has been used for hemorrhoidectomy with success though the techniques described are different.

Noncontact Nd:YAG Laser Technique

Eddy[29] applies the laser energy directly over the target tissue by the noncontact method. The patient is placed in the lithotomy position, as this seems to be better than the jackknife position. General anesthesia was administered in 95% of cases, in response to the particular request of these patients, although he feels the procedure can be done as effectively under local anesthetic infiltration with intravenous sedation. Eddy prefers a low power of 25 W for a short duration of 0.8 seconds, as opposed to a high power for longer duration. An important step is to leave a normal area of tissue between the lasered sites, as this seems to give better results. The total operation time may take about 1 hour. During the postoperative period, mild swelling, a little discharge and bleeding, and a feeling of slight pressure could be experienced by the patient. The complications that might occur are urinary retention, especially in the older age group, and bleeding, but not more than a cupful including clots. In Eddy's series of 350 cases, the healing of the wound has taken about three weeks. The other possible complications are fistula formation, excessive scarring, and sphincter damage. According to Eddy, the Nd:YAG nontouch laser technique is a "hot knife," which is similar to the "cold knife," but definitely more advantageous. Less pain is involved with this technique, and the patient returns to work sooner. Also, as is true of all laser hemorrhoidectomy, it can be performed as an outpatient procedure, which has two important benefits: Patients are not exposed to nosocomial infections, and the procedure is cost-effective.

Dwyer,[30] at the University Center of Los Angeles, uses the Nd:YAG laser noncontact technique through a flexible fiberoptic colonoscope, which is retroflexed in the rectum to visualize the internal hemorrhoids. The flexible laser guide is introduced through the operating channel, and the hemorrhoidal veins are lasered from the proximal to the distal areas.

Shude and Fengzao,[31] at the Laser Research Unit in Beijing, China, have treated 156 cases of hemorrhoids using the Nd:YAG laser noncontact technique under local anesthesia. In this group also the same advantages were apparent: It is a safe and simple procedure that can be used on an outpatient basis. The patients are able to return to work much earlier therefore it is cost-effective. Finally, there are fewer postoperative complications.

Contact Nd:YAG Laser

Since 1985, at the University of Cincinnati Medical Center, laser hemorrhoidectomy has been performed using Nd:YAG laser with the contact technique. To date, 23 cases have been treated (17 males), aged 31 to 76 years. A detailed study, including postoperative complications, cost-effectiveness, incidences of recurrence, and long-term results, is currently in preparation.

Technique of Contact Laser Hemorrhoidectomy

For two days before surgery the patients are on a low-residue diet, and take golytely preparation in adequate quantities on the previous afternoon before surgery. On the morning of the third day they report to the surgicenter on an empty stomach. One of the following anesthetics is used, as indicated: epidural, caudal, short general, or local with intravenous sedation. The patient is placed in the lithotomy position, and the anorectal region is examined. Flexible fiberoptic sigmoidoscopy/colonoscopy is performed to confirm or exclude associated chronic lesions. The nature and position of the internal hemorrhoids are noted on anoscopy.

First- and second-degree internal hemorrhoids are coapted by using the SLT *flat contact probe* or SLT *coagulation probe* (Surgical Laser Technologies, Inc., Malvern, PA), which is applied around the hemorrhoid to begin with and finally onto it directly (Figure 33.1). The power used is between 5 and 10 W for a duration of 2 to 3 seconds with coaxial water. Successful coapting is indicated by blanching the tissue, and the blood loss is nil. Care is taken not to use higher power levels, causing vaporization of the mucosa, which leads on to prolonged discharge per rectum. Local infiltration of a long-acting local anesthetic is carried out at the end of the procedure.

Third- and fourth-degree internal hemorrhoids are treated by submucosal hemorrhoidectomy using Nd:YAG laser contact technique (Figures 33.2–33.4). A Fansler proctoscope is inserted and the hemorrhoid to be operated on is brought under direct view. No dilatation of the anus or infiltration of norepinephrine is carried out. The hemorrhoid is grasped and pulled toward the operator with gentle traction. A linear incision, using the SLT Laser Scalpel (Surgical Laser Technologies, Inc., Malvern, PA) with a tip diameter of 0.2/0.4 mm, is made from the base of the pedicle outward. The power used is in the range of 10 to 15 W in the continuous wave mode

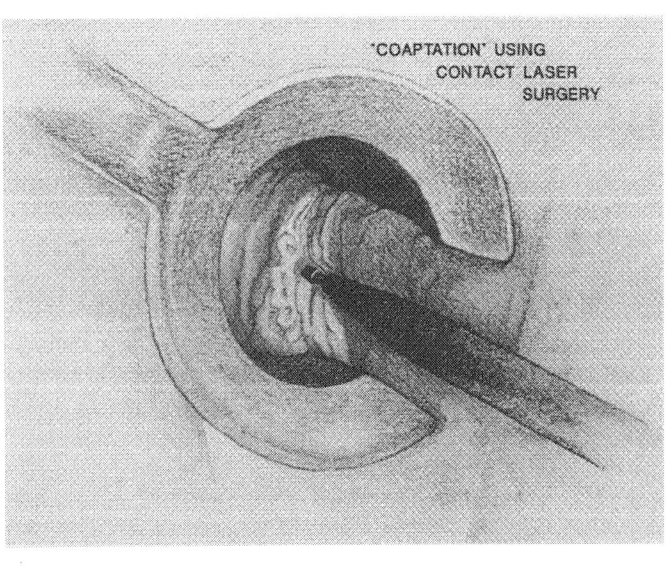

FIGURE 33.1. Internal hemorrhoids (second-degree): coaptation, using contact laser surgery technique.

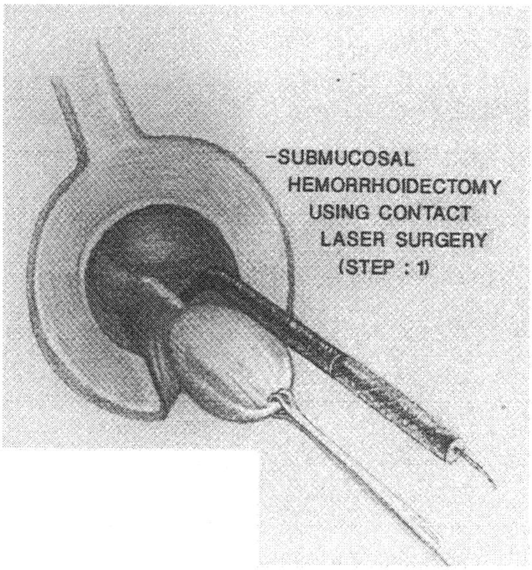

FIGURE 33.2. Internal hemorrhoids (left lateral, third-degree): submucosal hemorrhoidectomy, using contact laser surgery technique (step 1).

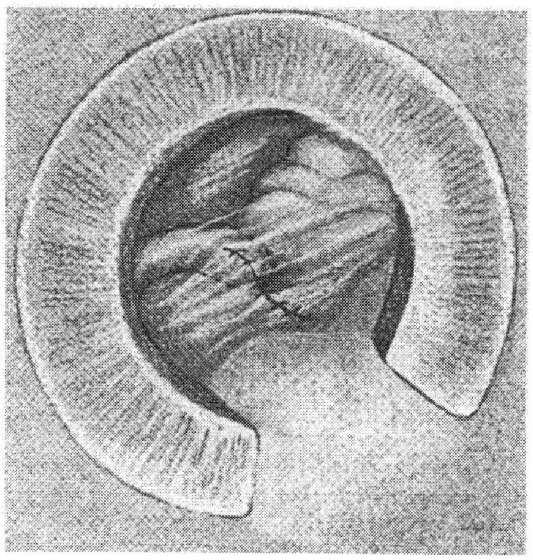

FIGURE 33.4. Internal hemorrhoids: submucosal hemorrhoidectomy, using contact laser surgery technique (step 3).

controlled by the foot pedal. The hemorrhoid is separated up to the pedicle and a high ligation is carried out using 0 chromic catgut/dexon suture. The pedicle is then "lased" distal to the ligature, leaving a comfortable sleeve, thus preventing any possible slipping of the ligature. Following this, any bleeding points are lased and a dry field almost invariably results. The mucosal incision is approximated together without tension using 2/0 chromic catgut. The procedure is repeated on the other hemorrhoids by laser excision of third- and fourth-degree hemorrhoids or coapted if they are first- or second-degree. At the end of the procedure, 0.5% Marcaine (bupivacaine) (10 ml) is injected around the sphincter region and the area is gently massaged, and an anal tampon is inserted. A dressing is applied and the patient is taken back to the day care center. The total blood loss during the submucosal hemorrhoidectomy by the YAG laser contact technique is less than 10 ml. The average duration of the procedure is less than 30 minutes. Patients are advised to take analgesics (acetaminophen) if and when they feel any discomfort. They are further advised to go on a high-fiber diet from postoperative day 1. Each patient is seen in 1 week as an outpatient.

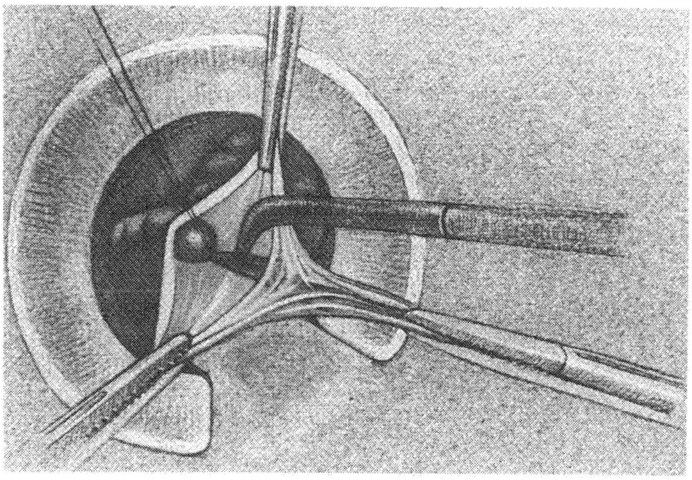

FIGURE 33.3. Internal hemorrhoids: submucosal hemorrhoidectomy, using contact laser surgery technique (step 2).

Evaluation of Contact Laser Hemorrhoidectomy

Pain

The surgical treatment of hemorrhoids carries with it a notorious reputation for severe postoperative pain. Following contact laser hemorrhoidectomy, in accordance with the scoring system of Watts,[32] all patients were in the B category—less than average pain. The first night after the operation, all were able to sleep upon taking 1 to 2 tablets of acetaminophen. All patients felt some discomfort during the first bowel movement, which ranged from a burning sensation to pain. This was of short duration and they were able to go about their daily chores without any further problem.

Retention of Urine

Urine retention, requiring catheterization, has not occurred in our small number of cases. This may be partially related to the avoidance of local infiltration of norepinephrine before the procedure.

Hemorrhage

Postoperative bleeding, either reactionary or secondary, has not occurred.

Wound Healing

The lesions produced in the anal canal cannot be visualized in the first week after surgery because of the pain, discomfort, and apprehension associated with the introduction of an anoscope. This method does not produce an actual wound over the skin area. Inspection at 15 days to 3 months will show a healed wound without fibrosis.

Anal Incontinence

No incontinence of flatus or feces with soiling of the underclothing has been observed. The risk of anal incontinence is decreased because maximal dilatation of the anus is avoided during contact laser surgery for hemorrhoids.

Formation of Skin and Mucosal Tags

Any skin tag that is found during the laser operative procedure is excised with the contact laser scalpel. No new skin or mucosal tags have been observed after the laser procedure.

Recurrence of Piles

The first contact laser hemorrhoidectomy was performed in our center in November 1985. To date, there have been no recurrences of internal hemorrhoids, but the follow-up period is too short. One patient returned with pain at 6 months due to the formation of a posterior fissure-in-ano associated with severe constipation and external hemorrhoids. Neither were present at the first visit.

Conclusion

The main advantage of the submucosal hemorrhoidectomy as outlined by Parks[9] and modified by Goligher[33] appears to be the decrease in postoperative pain. The reason for this is that the ligature does not include any anal mucosa, which is particularly sensitive. Furthermore, fibrosis or stricturing does not occur, as neither the mucosa nor the skin is excised. The disadvantage of this operation is that it is difficult to dissect the mucosa off the hemorrhoid because of bleeding, which may be troublesome and time-consuming. The use of the Nd:YAG laser contact technique in performing this operation eliminates this disadvantage. Thus, this method of contact laser hemorrhoidectomy may become the preferred treatment, replacing the other standard procedures. Further information and follow-up studies are required.

References

1. Banov L: The Chester Beatty medical papyrus: The earliest known treatise completely devoted to anorectal diseases. Surgery 58:1037–1043, 1965.
2. Parks AG: De Haemorrhoids. Guy's Hosp Rep 104:135, 1955.
3. Graham-Stewart CW: What causes hemorrhoids? A new theory of etiology. Dis Colon Rectum 6:333, 1963.
4. Shafik A: A new concept of the anatomy of the anal sphincter mechanism and the physiology of defecation, treatment of hemorrhoids: Report of a technique. Am J Surg 148:393–398, 1984.
5. Bennett RC, Friedman MHW, Goligher JC: The late results of hemorrhoidectomy by ligature and excision. Br Med J 2:216, 1963.

6. Lockhart-Mummery JP: Diseases of Rectum and Colon, 2nd ed. Bailliere, London, 1934.
7. Milligan ETC, Morgan C, Naunton Jones LE, Officer R: Surgical anatomy of anal canal and operative treatment of hemorrhoids. Lancet 2:1119, 1937.
8. Miles WE: Rectal Surgery. Cassell, London, 1939.
9. Parks AG: Surgical treatment of haemorrhoids. Br J Surg 43:337, 1956.
10. Mitchell AB: A simple method of operating on piles. Br Med J 1:482, 1903.
11. Ferguson JA, Heaton JR: Closed hemorrhoidectomy. Dis Colon Rectum 2:176, 1959.
12. Whitehead W: Surgical treatment of hemorrhoids. Br Med J 1:149, 1882.
13. Anderson HG: The after results of the operative treatment of hemorrhoids. Br J Med 2:1276, 1909.
14. Blaisdell PC: Prevention of massive hemorrhage secondary to hemorrhoidectomy. Surg Gynecol Obstet 106:485, 1958.
15. Barron J: Office ligation of internal hemorrhoids. Am J Surg 105:563, 1963.
16. Lord PH: A new regime for treatment of hemorrhoids. Proc R Soc Med 61:935, 1968.
17. Lewis MI: Diverse methods of managing hemorrhoids: Cryohemorrhoidectomy. Dis Colon Rectum 10:175, 1973.
18. Lloyd-Williams K, Haq IU, Glem B: Cryodestruction of hemorrhoids. Br Med J 1:666, 1973.
19. Leicester RJ, Nicholls RJ, Mann CV: Infrared coagulation in the treatment of hemorrhoids. Gut 22:436, 1981.
20. Goldman L, Hornby P, Long E: Effect of the laser beam on the skin. Transmission of laser beams through fiberoptics. J Invest Dermatol 42:231–234, 1964.
21. Nath G, Gorish W, Kiefhaber P: First laser endoscopy with a fiberoptic transmission system. Endoscopy 5:203–218, 1973.
22. Daikuzono N, Joffe SN: Artificial sapphire probe for contact photocoagulation and tissue vaporization with Nd:YAG laser. Med Instrum 19:173–178, 1985.
23. Eddy HJ, Yu JC, Eddy EC: Dual laser hemorrhoidectomy. (Abstract). Lasers Surg Med 6:201, 1986.
24. Mokhniuk YN, Baltaitis YV, Maltsev VN, et al: Comparative evaluation of methods of treatment of patients with hemorrhoids. Clin Surg 2(494):1–4, 1983.
25. Rausis C: Surgery of hemorrhoids by means of CO_2 laser (Chirurgie des hemorroides avec le laser CO_2). Schweiz Rundschauc Med (Praxis) 71:177–180, 1982.
26. Denis J, Lemarchand N: The present day treatment of hemorrhoids (Etat actuel due traitement des hemorrhoides). Rev Infirm 3:49–51, 1985.
27. Riedlinger J: The surgical treatment of hemorrhoids by means of CO_2 laser. Laser Tokyo '81 23:30–31, 1981.
28. Zadeh AT: Three hundred and fifty hemorrhoidectomies using the CO_2 laser. Lasers Surg Med 5:145, 1985.
29. Eddy HJ: Personal communication, 1986.
30. Dwyer R: The technique of gastrointestinal laser endoscopy. The Biomedical Laser. Springer-Verlag, New York, 1981, pp 255–269.
31. Shude Z, Fengzao MA: Hemorrhoidectomy and fistulectomy with neodymium:YAG laser. Personal communication, 1986.
32. Watts JM, Bennett RC, Duthie HL, Goligher JC: Healing and pain after different forms of hemorrhoidectomy. Br J Surg 51:88, 1966.
33. Goligher J: Haemorrhoids or piles. In Surgery of the Anus, Rectum and Colon, 5th ed. Bailliere Tindall, London, 1984, pp 123–125.

34
Splenic Resection with the SLT Contact Nd:YAG Laser System®: A Comparison of Contact Nd:YAG with the CO_2 Laser

John Foster, Tom Schroder, Kim A. Brackett, and Stephen N. Joffe

The spleen has important physiologic and immunologic functions and should be surgically conserved whenever possible. Morris and Bullock[1] in 1919 showed that splenectomized rats had an increased susceptibility to infection and in 1952, King and Shumacker[2] reported a significant increase in fatal aepsis in children following splenectomy. Subsequent studies have confirmed an increased morbidity and mortality of 50 to 200 times normal in patients of all ages, at various times following splenic removal, and have therefore advocated surgical alternatives to total splenectomy.[3–9] Splenic repair with adequate hemostasis is difficult due to the highly vascular and extremely fragile splenic tissue.

Lasers are ideally suited for use in surgery, especially in highly vascular organs such as the kidney, liver, and spleen, where cutting and simultaneous coagulation of small vessels are possible.[10–12] Both the CO_2 and Nd:YAG lasers have been used to undertake splenic resections using a noncontact method of directing the beam at the target tissue. However, the CO_2 laser achieved poor hemostasis while the noncontact Nd:YAG laser provided inadequate cutting.[13–17] Other disadvantages included the inability to coagulate larger vessels and the need for high-power levels leading to unnecessary tissue necrosis and excessive smoke production.[18–20]

The concept of laser contact probes has been previously proposed.[21] The idea is now practical, with the development of an effective and inexpensive synthetic sapphire probe, which allows the laser energy and simultaneous coaptive pressure to be applied to a desired point with little effect on adjacent tissue.[22] The conventional fiber optic delivery system of commercially available Nd:YAG laser systems lends itself to this application. Experiments comparing the noncontact with the contact Nd:YAG laser in liver and pancreas surgery have achieved superior results with the contact probes, with lower requirements of laser power, power density, reduced bleeding, less smoke production, and decreased tissue damage.[23,24] This study showed the advantages in splenic surgery of the new contact Nd:YAG laser over the noncontact CO_2 laser, the conventional laser modality.[13,15,16]

Instrumentation

For the noncontact method a directed energy 25-W CO_2 laser was used with 25-millisecond pulses and a spot size of 0.5 mm. For the contact method a Cooper Lasersonica 8000 Nd:YAG continuous wave laser (1.06 μm wavelength) was used, operated at 10 W. The beam was directed through a 600-μm quartz fiber to the hand-held contact saphire probe. A Surgical Laser Technologies (SLT) 1.2-mm Frosted Laser Scalpel probe was used for cutting the tissue and achieving hemostasis (Figure 34.1).

Surgical Procedure

Ten fasted dogs were divided into two groups. Under general anesthesia, the abdomen was opened with a midline incision and the would edges retracted. The spleen was identified and transected through its vascular bed into approximately two equal portions, each connected to its vascular pedicle, which was not clamped

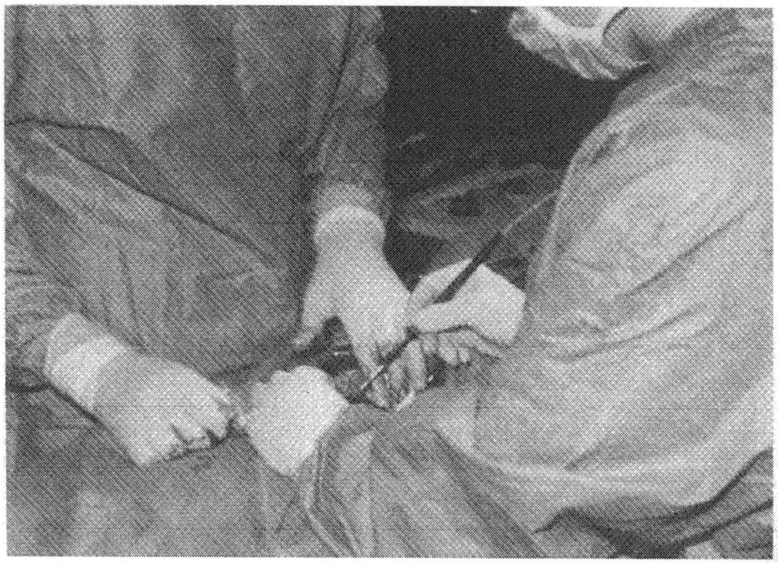

FIGURE 34.1. SLT Contact laser scalpel probe.® The hand-held scalpel assembly is seen here during splenic division. The SLT frosted scalpel contact probe ® is in use in the operative field. Note the fiberoptic delivery system entering the rear of the assembly.

during the procedure (Figure 34.2). One group of animals underwent splenic division with the noncontact CO_2 laser and the other with the contact Nd:YAG. Any residual bleeding was controlled with 3 0 chromic ties. The abdominal cavity was closed and the animals returned to their cages with free access to food and water.

Analysis of Results

Operative data included operating time (in minutes), blood loss (in milliliters), the number of ligatures used and amount of smoke production (graded semiquantitatively from 0 to 4+). Preoperative blood samples were taken on days 1,

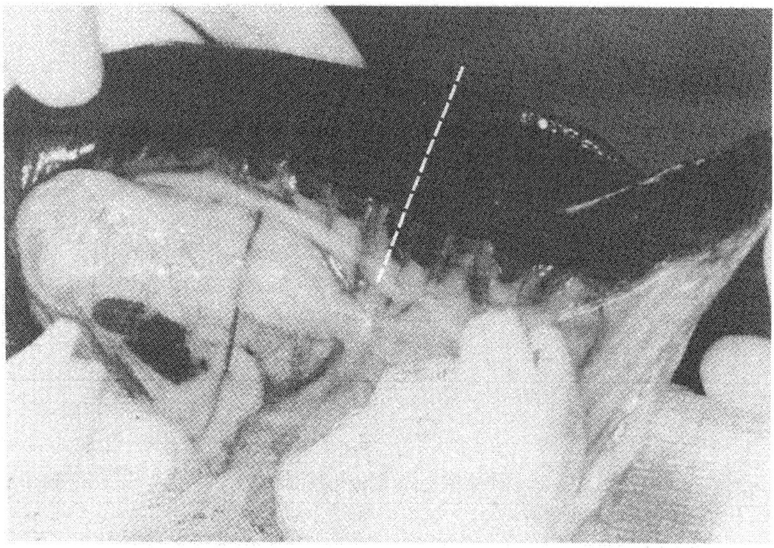

FIGURE 34.2. Isolated canine spleen and path of division. The spleen has been isolated and elevated from the abdominal cavity. The dashed line shows the approximate site of division, separating the spleen into two approximately equal sections and dividing the vascular bed between two adjacent vascular arcades.

4, and 14 and were analyzed for leukocyte count, hemoglobin, hematocrit, and platelet count. All animals were sacrificed on day 14. Histologic samples of the cut splenic edge were taken postoperatively and on day 14 and were used to measure the lateral penetration and depth of tissue necrosis from the laser energy. Values are given as means ± standard deviation. the statistical evaluation of the data used the analysis of variance method. A value of $p < 0.05$ was considered significant.

Experimental Results

There were no intraoperative deaths. Operative results are shown in Table 34.1. Operating time from the initial incision of the splenic capsule until hemostasis was achieved averaged only 13.2 ± 2.9 minutes with the SLT contact Nd:YAG laser scalpel, as compared to 23.6 ± 8.2 minutes with the noncontact CO_2 laser ($p < 0.05$).

The CO_2 laser energy was absorbed by any blood on the splenic surface, preventing penetration of the laser beam to the underlying tissue and necessitating constant suctioning and sponging with frequent operating delays. This prevented achieving hemostasis with even moderate-sized vessels as the issuing blood would prevent penetration of the laser energy to the vessel walls. Suture ties were needed frequently as a result.

The SLT Nd:YAG laser scalpel had none of these problems. Tissue cutting was easily achieved even in the presence of blood, and hemostasis was usually adequate, leaving a sealed splenic surface (Figure 34.3). Even the largest vessels were usually sealed with repeat application of energy from the froated sides of the laser scalpel. In three animals a chisel-shaped probe was also used to achieve adequate hemostasis, as it provided better coagulating properties than the scalpel probe alone.

TABLE 34.1. Operative data for splenic resection with the Nd:YAG laser.

Category	Noncontact CO_2	Contact Nd:YAG
Operating time	23.6 ± 8.2 min	13.2 ± 2.9 min
Blood loss	103.8 ± 30.2 ml	50.2 ± 31.9 ml
Suture ties	6.4 ± 2.3	0.2[a]
Smoke production	3+	1+

[a]Only one animal required one tie.

With the noncontact CO_2 laser, blood loss averaged 103.8 ± 30.2 cc and an average of 6.4 ± 2.3 ties were needed, with a minimum of four ties per animal (Table 34.1). Blood loss occurred throughout the operation from oozing at the cut parenchymal surface, requiring multiple treatment with the laser beam to achieve hemostasis. Larger vessel bleeding was frequent and was rapidly controlled with suture ligatures. With the contact Nd:YAG laser scalpel, blood loss averaged 50.2 ± 31.9 cc ($p < 0.05$), which was 52% less than the CO_2 group, with only one animal requiring one tie, giving a mean of 0.2 ties per animal ($p < 0.01$). Bleeding occurred as the tissue was divided but was rapidly controlled by the laser energy without residual bleeding. Larger vessel bleeding was rare (2 to 3 sites per operation) and hemostasis was usually achieved with repeat application of the frosted laser scalpel or use of the chisel-shaped probe.

Noncontact CO_2 laser resection at 25 W was associated with moderate to large amounts of malodorous smoke (3+ to 4+), requiring a large suction device for its removal. Contact Nd:Yag laser resection produced only minimal amounts of smoke (1+), and suctioning was not required.

All animals survived till 14 days and neither group showed any evidence of intraabdominal abscess or bleeding. Both groups showed minimal peritoneal adhesions that were easily separated from the cut splenic surface.

Hematologic studies showed no significant differences between the two laser modalities, and there were no major differences between preoperative and day 14 values. Several of the day 1 samples from the Nd:Yag animals were hemolyzed and the data were lost. With accurate values from only two animals, day 1 values are included for reference only but were excluded from any statistical analysis. In both groups there was a slight postoperative increase in the hemoglobin content (Figure 34.4A) and hematocrit (Figure 34.4B) that persisted for the full observation period. However, only in the hematocrit values from the Nd:YAG animals did this achieve statistical significance ($p < 0.05$). Both groups showed a similar increase in the postoperative white blood cell count that resolved by day 14 (Figure 34.4C).

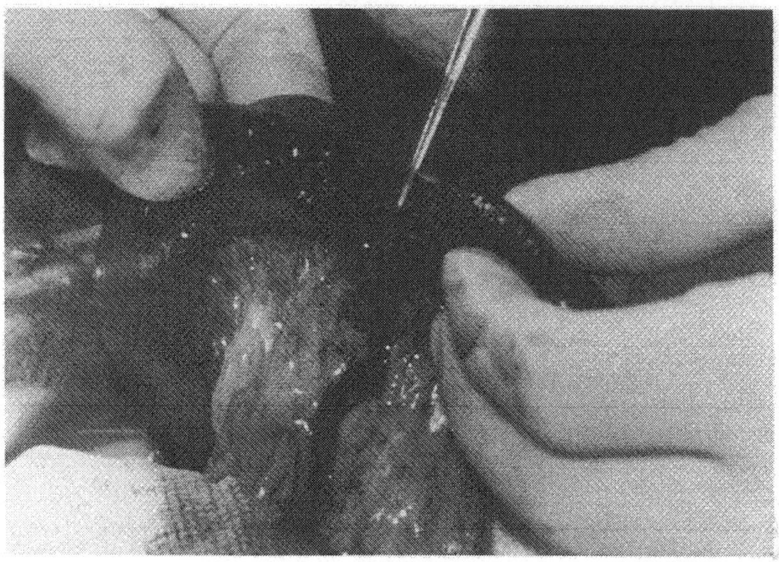

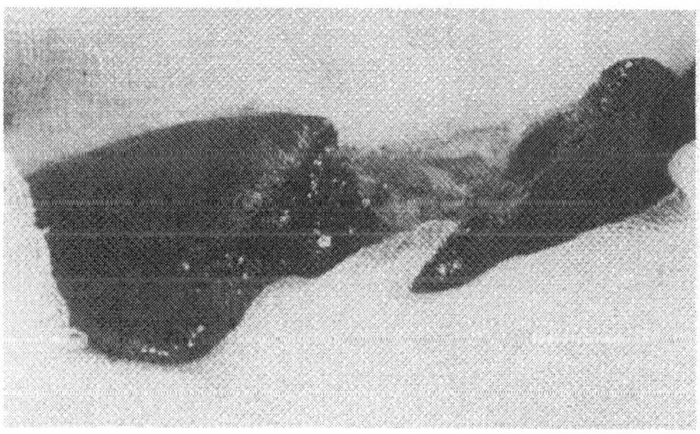

FIGURE 34.3. Division of the spleen with the SLT laser contact probe.® (*A*) The splenic parenchyma is being divided using laser energy focused through the sapphire contact probe. The frosted edges scatter some energy to the sides, aiding in achieving hemostasis. Note the minimal bleeding from the cut surfaces. No ties have been used in this division. (*B*) Appearance of cut splenic surfaces after division. Both sections are well supplied with their existing vascular pedicles but the division is complete. Note the absence of bleeding only moments after the division and the carbonized "sealed" cut surfaces. The actual tissue damage extends less than 0.8 mm into the splenic prenchyma.

In both groups the platelet count slowly increased postoperatively, but returned to baseline by day 14 (Figure 34.4D).

Histologic sections showed minimal necrosis and tissue damage that was equivalent between the two laser modalities by day 14 (Figure 34.5). Table 34.2 summarizes the histologic results. The Nd:YAG animals showed a larger initial tissue damage of 0.8 ± 0.3 mm compared to the CO_2 damage of 0.35 ± 0.05 mm. However, by day 14 the CO_2 damage had increased to 0.8 ± 0.4 mm and was equal to the Nd:YAG laser-induced damage, which remained at 0.8 ± 0.3 mm. In all cases the tissue damage was limited to 0.8 mm from the cut parenchymal edge.

Discussion

For over 20 years the importance of preserving splenic function has been recognized. In children especially, but in adults as well, the incidence

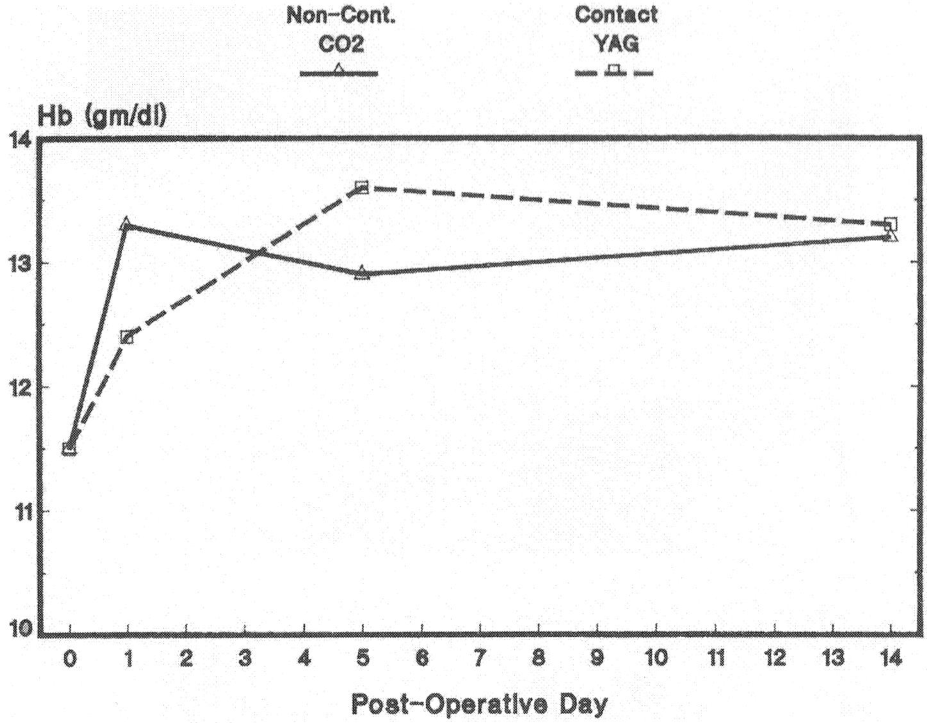

A

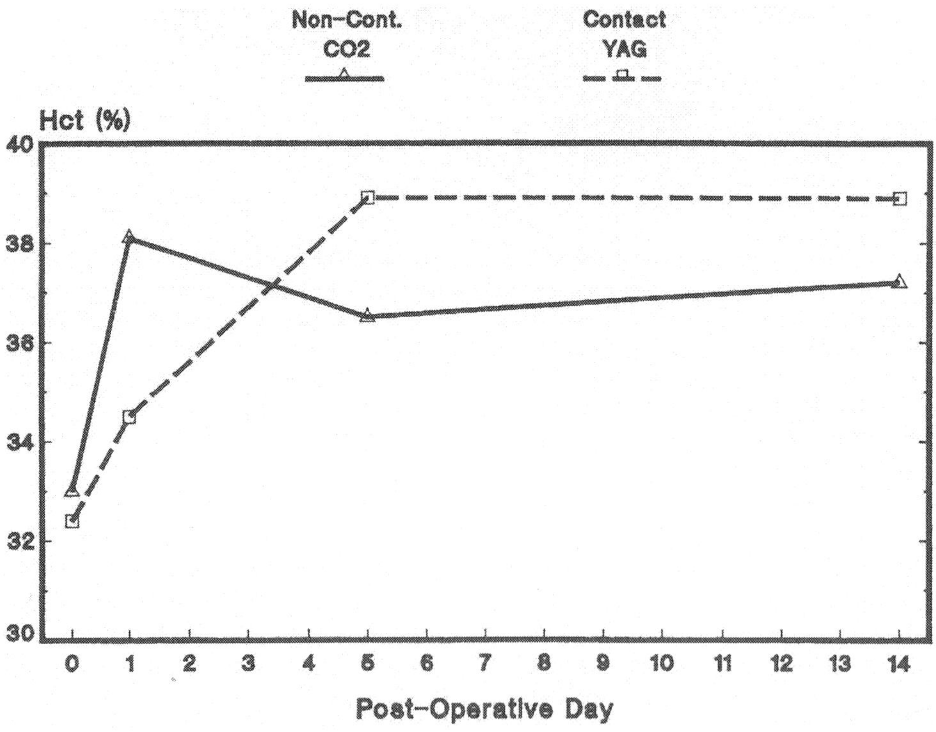

B

FIGURE 34.4. Comparison of hematologic parameters as measured preoperatively, and on days 1, 5, and 14. Day 1 values were not included in the statistical analysis and are included for reference only. Solid line = noncontact CO_2 laser; dashed line = contact Nd:YAG laser. (*A*) Hemoglobin levels. (*B*) Hematocrit levels.

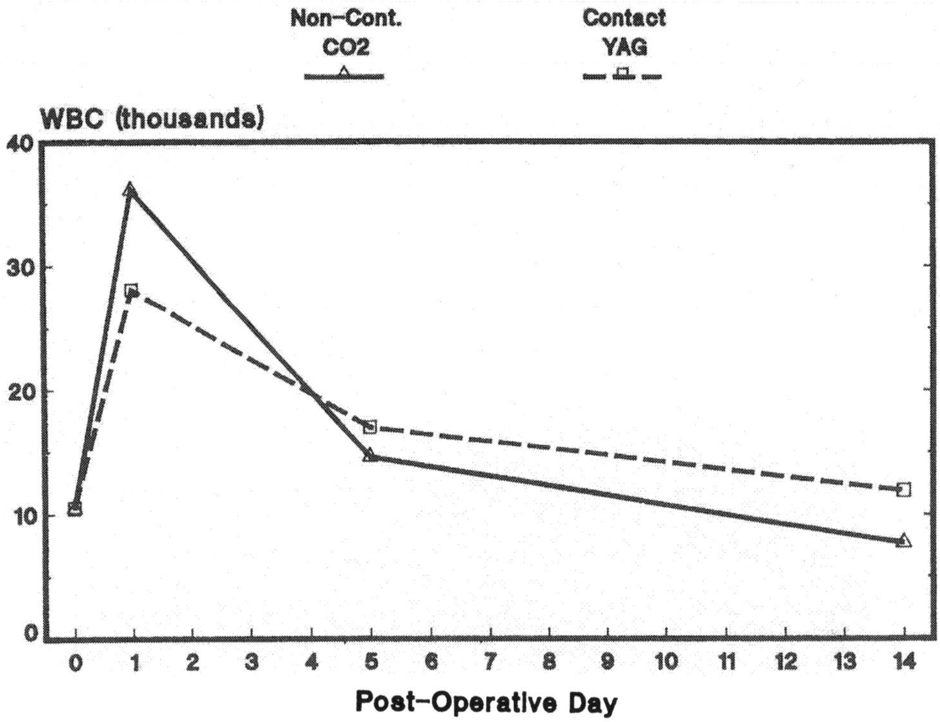

C

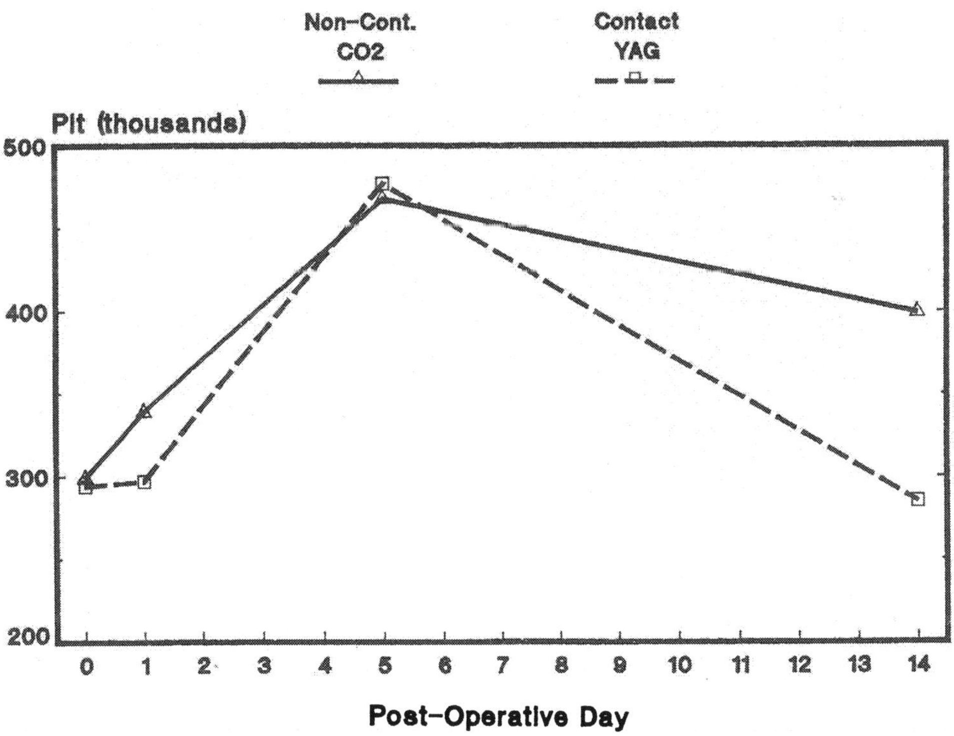

D

FIGURE 34.4 (*continued*). (*C*) White cell counts. (*D*) Platelet counts. With both laser modalities there were no statistically significant differences between the preoperative and day 14 values for any of the hematologic parameters studied.

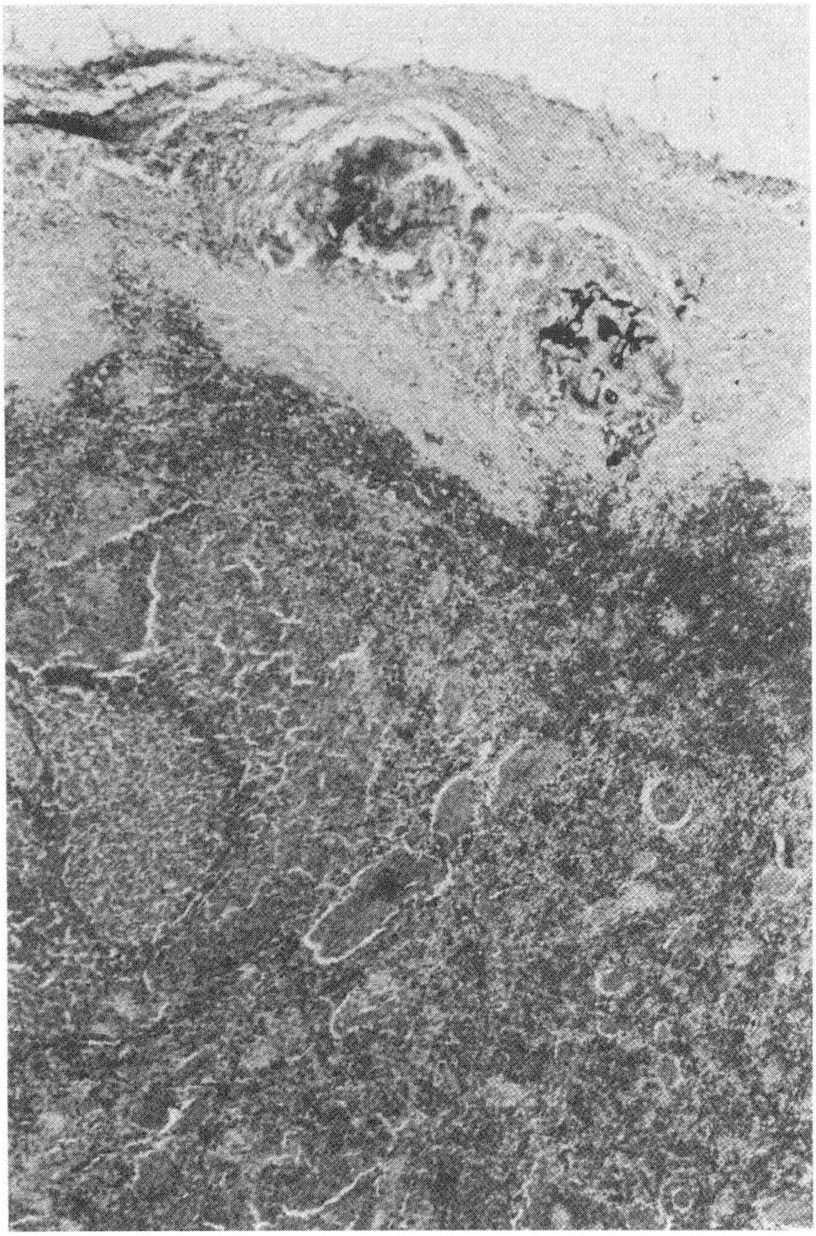

FIGURE 34.5. Resected spleen, 14 days postoperatively. The resected surface of the sample is covered by a layer of dense connective tissue, approximately 0.8 mm thick, containing small islands of carbonized debris. This appearance was the same for all samples regardless of whether resection was by CO_2 or contact Nd:YAG laser.

TABLE 34.2. Tissue damage (μm) in splenic resection.

Day	Noncontact CO_2	Contact Nd:YAG
0	350 ± 46	781 ± 326
14	756 ± 379	763 ± 253

of fatal sepsis and other fatal infections is markedly increased after splenectomy. Often splenectomy is performed when viable splenic tissue should have been preserved due to the difficulty in achieving hemostasis by conventional methods.

Noncontact lasers have been used in splenic surgery for some time with demonstrated improvement in achieving hemostasis, decreased intraoperative blood loss, and decreased operating time. The noncontact CO_2 laser has had the greatest application due to its excellent cutting properties. The CO_2 laser is limited by its inability to penetrate water or blood, making work in a bloody field quite difficult with significant blood loss. In the spleen this is often compensated for by cross-clamping the splenic artery while the parenchymal vessels are sealed in a bloodless field. However, this can allow ischemic or thrombotic events to occur and can damage the splenic artery.

The noncontact Nd:YAG laser is able to penetrate water and blood to reach the parenchyma, and can seal bleeding vessels with great efficiency, but is unable to match the cutting properties of the noncontact CO_2 laser. The 1.06-μm Nd:YAG wavelength is absorbed diffusely by tissue with a deeper penetration and wider distribution than the CO_2 wavelength, which is largely absorbed at the surface. This leads to a greater depth of tissue necrosis and decreased cutting ability.

The SLT contact Nd:YAG laser has the hemostatic characteristics of Nd:YAG energy with precise energy focusing and tissue penetration. This allows excellent hemostatic and cutting properties, even in a bloody field, with minimal tissue damage and necrosis. The synthetic sapphire scalpel probes sharply focus the energy directly in front of the crystal with a high angle of diffusion. This provides maximal energy density over a very limited area with rapid diffusion and minimal unwanted penetration. With the "frosted" tips a portion of the energy is scattered diffusely from the roughened lateral sides of the probe, allowing for better coagulating properties. Adequate coagulation is actually possible when only the energy from the frosted sides of the tip is used.

In our study, the SLT contact Nd:YAG laser showed a significant advantage over the noncontact CO_2 laser for splenic resection in the dog. We decided to compare the contact Nd:YAG with the noncontact CO_2, as the noncontact CO_2 laser is currently the most widely used laser modality for splenic resection.

The SLT contact Nd:YAG showed a significantly decreased blood loss (52%) and decreased operating time (44%) over the noncontact CO_2 laser as well as greater ease of handling and use. During the SLT contact Nd:YAG resection the field remained virtually dry, except when large vessels were encountered. These were almost always controlled with repeat application of the scalpel probe, first circumferentially, then with pressure on the vessel itself. No suture ties were needed in four of the five animals and the fifth required only one tie to achieve hemostasis.

With the noncontact CO_2 laser constant bleeding occurred, which required continuous suctioning, sponging, and repeat applications of the laser energy. Multiple ties were always needed due to the inability of the CO_2 laser to stop large-vessel bleeding. These factors led to twice the blood loss, almost twice the operating time, and the need for increased tissue manipulation when compared to the Nd:YAG group.

With both laser modalities tissue penetration and damage, as measured by depth of necrosis, was minimal. The contact Nd:YAG was not significantly different from the noncontact CO_2 with its surface-level absorption properties. Tissue necrosis was equivalent at day 14 and was <0.8 mm with both modalities.

Hematologic parameters varied equivalently with both laser modalities, and there were no significant differences between the preoperative baseline and day 14 values. None of the animals had postoperative complications, and in all animals adhesions were minimal and equivalent between the two groups.

One significant qualitative parameter was the ease of operation with the SLT contact Nd:YAG. In addition to the decreased blood loss, decreased number of ties, and decreased surgical manipulation, the entire operative procedure was subjectively much simpler and more effective. The hand-held laser scalpel was simple to use while providing tactile sensation and precise control to the user. The resection procedure involved simply cutting through the parenchymal tissue with the scalpel using variable direct pressure to assist in cutting and hemostasis. The CO_2 laser, however, was large and cumbersome and required balancing the laser unit manually while aiming the beam at the target tissue. There was only visual feedback from the aiming beam and tissue observation to assess beam penetration, depth of cut, and cutting characteristics of the tissue. No direct pressure could be applied to the tissue to aid in hemostasis. During the operation a great deal of effort was applied to suctioning and sponging the tissue surface to allow cutting to proceed. With the CO_2 laser, the entire operative field and all instrument surfaces had to be covered with wet gauze to prevent damage from stray beam penetration. This was not necessary with the SLT contact probe, as the energy is focused immediately in front of the scalpel tip.

Conclusion

Splenic resection in the dog proved to have decreased blood loss, decreased operating time, and decreased surgical manipulation when the SLT contact Nd:YAG laser with the SLT contact synthetic sapphire probe was used, in contrast to the noncontact CO_2 laser. Tissue damage and hematologic changes were minimal and equivalent between both laser sources. The overall ease of use and operating technique were subjectively better with the SLT contact Nd:YAG laser, and the danger of stray beam damage is eliminated. The SLT contact Nd:YAG laser with the synthetic sapphire probes offers a significant advantage over the noncontact CO_2 laser in the resection of splenic tissue.

References

1. Morris DH, Bullock FD: The importance of the spleen in resistance to infection. Ann Surg 70:513–521, 1919.
2. King H, Shumacker HB: Splenic studies. I. Susceptibility to infection after splenectomy performed in infancy. Ann Surg 136:239–242, 1952.
3. Dretzka L: Rupture of the spleen. A report of twenty-seven cases. Surg Gynecol Obstet 51:258–261, 1930.
4. Morgenstern L: Experimental partial splenectomy: Application of cyanoacrylate monomer tissue adhesive for hemostasis. Am Surg 31:709–712, 1965.
5. Bisno AL, Freeman JC: The syndrome of asplenia, pheumococcal sepsis, and disseminated intravascular coagulation. Ann Intern Med 72:389–393, 1970.
6. De Boer J, Sumner-Smith G, Downie HG: Partial splenectomy. Technique and some hematologic consequences in the dog. J Pediatr Surg 7:378–381, 1972.
7. Buntain WL, Lynn HB: Splenorrhaphy: Changing concepts for the traumatized spleen. Surgery 86:748–760, 1979.
8. Boerma EJ, Klopper PJ, Van Der Heyde MN: Save the spleen—An experimental study on the effects of three tissue adhesives on deep wounds of liver and spleen. Neth J Surg 33:10–13, 1981.
9. Barrett J, Sheaff C, Abuabara S, Jonasson O: Splenic preservation in adults after blunt and penetrating trauma. Am J Surg 145:313–317, 1983.
10. Meyer HJ, Haverkampf K: Experimental study of partial liver resection with a combined CO_2 and Nd:YAG laser. Lasers Surg Med 2:149–154, 1982.
11. Benderev TV, Schaeffer AJ: Efficacy and safety of the Nd:YAG laser in canine partial nephrectomy. J Urol 133:1108–1111, 1985.
12. Rosemberg SK: Clinical experience with carbon dioxide laser in renal surgery. Urology 25:115–118, 1985.
13. Giler S, Ben-Bassat M, Gassner S, Kaplan I: The CO_2 laser in surgery of the spleen—An experimental study. In Kaplan I (ed): Laser Surgery II, Vol 2. OT-PAZ POB 6048, Tel Aviv, 1979.
14. Dixon JA, Miller F, McCloskey D, Siddoway J: Anatomy and techniques in segmental splenectomy. Surg Gynecol Obstet 150:516–520, 1980.
15. Snider WR, Li S: Partial splenectomy with CO_2 laser: An experimental study. Lasers Surg Med 1:357–360, 1981.
16. Orda R, Wiznitzer T, Bubis JJ, Alon R: Hemisplenectomy using a hand-held CO_2 laser. An experimental study. J Pediatr Surg 17:163–165, 1982.
17. Van der Werken C, Goris RJA, Van der Sluis RF, et al: Comparison of sapphire infrared coagulation and YAG-laser in the surgery of parenchymatous organs: An experimental study. Neth J Surg 36:130–133, 1984.
18. Hall RR, Beach AD, Baker E, Morrison PCA: Incision of tissue by carbon dioxide laser. Nature 232:131–132, 1971.
19. Ben-Bassat M, Ben-Bassat M, Kaplan I: A study of the ultrastructural features of the cut margin of skin and mucous membrane specimens excised by carbon dioxide laser. J Surg Res 21:77–84, 1976.
20. Brackett KA, Sankar MY, Joffe SN: Effects of Nd:YAG laser photoradiation on intra-abdominal tissues: A histological study of tissue damage versus power density applied. 6:123, 1986.
21. Durtschi MB, Stothert JC, Ashleman B, et al: Laser scalpel for solid organ surgery. Am J Surg 139:665–668, 1980.

22. Daikuzono N, Joffe SN: Artificial sapphire probe for contact photocoagulation and tissue vaporization with the Nd:YAG laser. Med Instrum 19:173–178, 1985.
23. Joffe SN, Brackett KA, Sankar MY, Diakuzono N: Liver resection with the Nd:YAG laser: A comparison of a new contact probe, the laser scalpel, with the conventional non-contact method. Surg Gynecol Obstet , 1986.
24. Schroder T, Brackett K, Joffe SN: Proximal Pancreatectomy: A comparison of electrocutery with the contact and non-contact Nd:YAG laser techniques in the dog. Am J Surg In Press, 1987.

35
Liver And Pancreatic Laser Surgery

T. Schröder and Stephen N. Joffe

Pancreatic operations are often associated with technical difficulties due to the anatomy of the pancreas and its blood supply.[1] Clinical operations are time-consuming and blood loss can be considerable.[2] Blood vessels are commonly ligated and pancreatic tissue incised either with a scalpel or electrocautery.[3] There are only a few reports on the tissue effects of the various lasers on the pancreas.[2,3]

The trend in recent years for the treatment of pancreatic carcinoma, and occasionally for pancreatitis, has been toward total pancreatectomy. Furthermore, the pancreas is now being harvested for transplantation. Sutherland et al.[4] report recent clinical experience with living related pancreatic transplantation and Rossi et al.[5] call for refining the technique of total pancreatectomy with duodenal preservation and the use of total pancreatectomy in cases of chronic pancreatitis. Preservation of the duodenum during pancreatectomy is important in experiments designed to study the interaction of gut hormones in the apancreatic animal with intact biliary and gastrointestinal tract. Any operative technique that can reduce operating time, blood loss, and associated morbidity and mortality would be advantageous.[6]

In a recent study, pancreatic resections were done with the use of a noncontact Nd:YAG laser in dogs.[7] In that study the operative technique and the operative results were compared, using the noncontact Nd:YAG and a conventional multiple ligature technique. The study demonstrated that the laser and the conventional technique both caused minimal blood loss, but the operative time was significantly shorter in the laser group. All animals survived, and there were no differences in severe complications between the groups.

With the development of contact laser surgery and the contact probes (Surgical Laser Technologies, Malvern, PA) the Nd:YAG laser is now introduced into general surgery. The SLT contact probes provide a precise incision and dissection and the good coagulation properties of the Nd:YAG laser.[8] In a recent study the new SLT contact Nd:YAG laser technique was compared with the old noncontact method and with the conventional electrocautery technique.[9] In this study a proximal pancreatectomy was done in 15 mongrel dogs. The head of the pancreas was removed and only a small portion of the pancreatic tail was left in situ. The electrocautery ("bovie") technique was used, which is a modification of the conventional ligature technique. The small vessels were coagulated, and vessels too big to coagulate were ligated. Both the bovie and the contact Nd:YAG laser were technically superior to the noncontact Nd:YAG. The latter was slower and caused more bleeding and smoke than the other two methods.

The thermal injury to the pancreas by the contact Nd:YAG was less than in the noncontact group. When the pancreas was dissected with the contact laser, hemostasis was achieved immediately. After cutting with the two other devices, extensive coagulative energy had to be applied to the resected surface to stop bleeding. This resulted in a thick necrotic surface on the pancreatic stump, which was probably the reason for hemorrhagic pancreatitis resulting in death in two of the animals. Histologic samples were taken from the cut surface at the day of operation and three weeks later at sacrifice. From the acute samples the damage to the pancreas was determined by the depth of thermal injury seen at microscopy. The deepest damage was caused by the noncontact Nd:YAG and the most superficial by the bovie. The acute changes are shown in Figures 35.1 to 35.3. Two dogs died of acute necrotizing pancreatitis in the noncontact laser and bovie groups. All the other dogs showed degradation of acinar tissue and fibrosis of the pancreatic tail at autopsy as seen in Figure 35.4.

A recent report on performing a distal pancreatectomy in dogs using either the bovie, CO_2 laser, or steel scalpel showed that the laser caused much less damage to the pancreas than the bovie.[3] The authors found hemostasis to be difficult on the resected surface when using the bovie. However, the bovie was faster than the laser, which in turn was more rapid than the scalpel and suture method. There are no studies available to compare to the contact Nd:YAG laser to the CO_2 laser in surgery of the pancreas. However, the good cutting properties and the excellent coagulation properties of the contact Nd:YAG will probably make the Nd:YAG laser the superior laser in surgery of the pancreas.

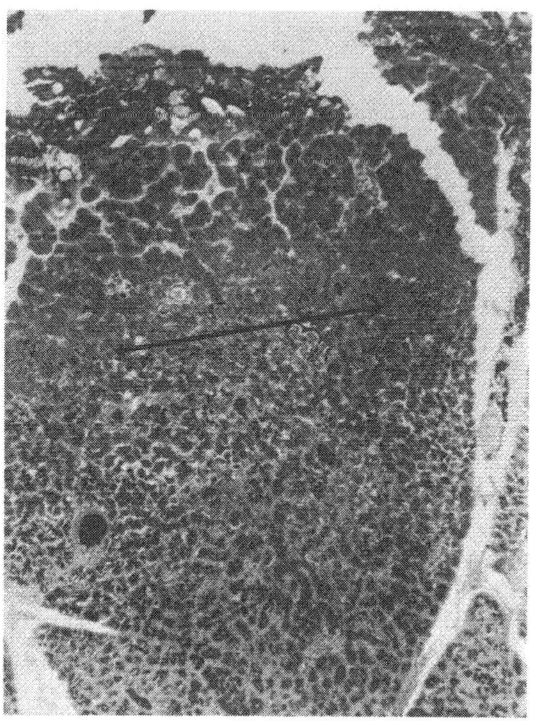

FIGURE 35.1. Acute effect on the pancreas following bovie resection. Surface is coated by a carbonized and coagulated layer of protein. Arrowed region represents plane of transition from acidophilic, necrotic cells to normal tissue. ×64, Masson's Trichrome.

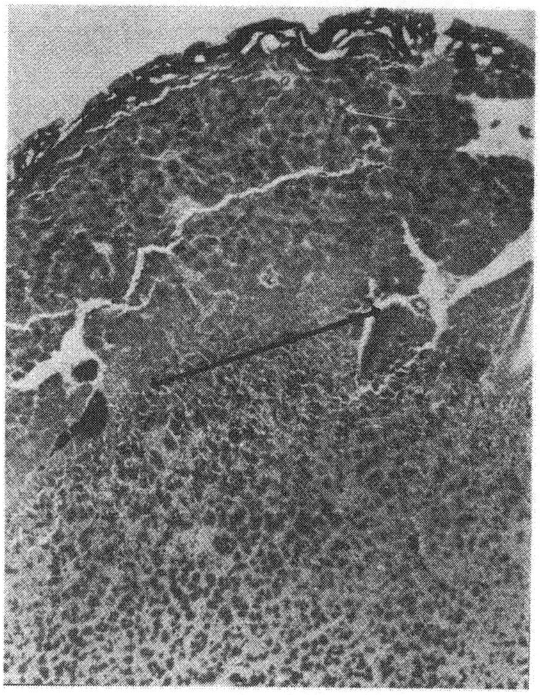

FIGURE 35.2. Acute effect on the pancreas following contact Nd:YAG laser resection. Coagulated surface followed by a more developed zone of cavitation of the tissue. Arrowed region represents transition from acidophilic zone to normal tissue. ×64, Masson's Trichrome.

Two patients with pancreatic disease treated with the Nd:YAG system have been reported.[10] One was a young male patient who was diagnosed as having insulinoma at the junction of the body and neck of the pancreas, and the other one was a young female having protracted pancreaticobiliary problems due to chronic pancreatitis. Both the patients underwent a pancreatic resection (50% and 80%, respectively) with preservation of the head of the pancreas and the duodenal loop. After lifting the pancreas from its inferior border, the dissection of the superior border was found to be relatively easy and safe using the Nd:YAG laser with the noncontact technique. The power density used was between 60 and 70 W for 1–2 seconds duration.

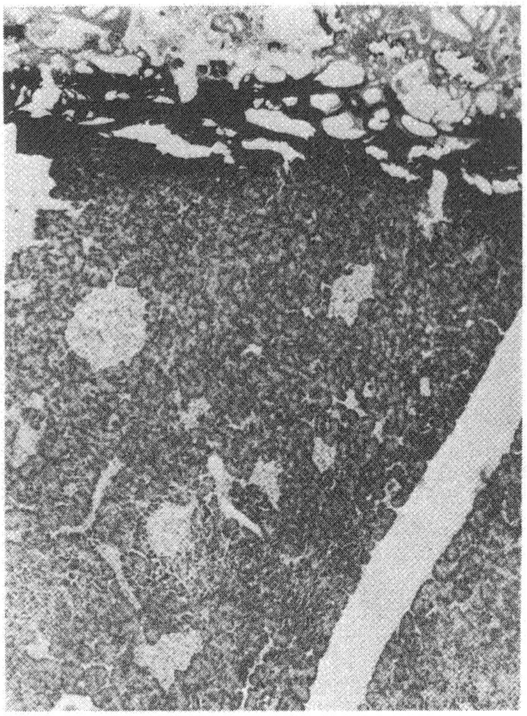

FIGURE 35.3. Acute effect on the pancreas following noncontact Nd:YAG laser resection. A comparatively broad area of coagulation and cavitation is seen on the surface of the specimen. Acidophilic zone of thermal damage extends below the bottom of this field. ×64, azure A-eosin B.

The postoperative period was uneventful in both patients. The acute histologic appearances of the resected human pancreas were similar in all respects to that of pancreas in experimental animals, with the exception of the depth of penetration of the acidophilic cells in zone 3, which reached a depth of 3.5 mm.

The Nd:YAG laser using the contact probe may relatively easy resect the head of the pancreas with preservation of the duodenum. No clinical data on this procedure have yet been reported.

Other innovative procedures include drainage of pancreatic pseudocyst by performing an endoscopic laser cystogastrostomy and endoscopic papillotomies, but more studies have to be done before the evaluation of these methods can be done.

The use of the contact Nd:YAG system in pancreatic surgery provides the surgeon with a new tool for precise dissection and coagulation with good preservation of normal surrounding tissue. This is especially important in the surgery of the pancreas since the procedure involves delicate dissection from the vitally important surrounding vessels.

Laser Surgery of the Liver

Despite well-standardized techniques for liver resection, operative mortality rates ranging from 4 to 20% have been reported in recent studies. Postoperative complications include liver failure, bleeding, infection, and sepsis. These complications are related to interoperative bleeding, amount of necrotic liver tissue, and bile leakage. The techniques used in liver resections are an important factor for preventing inter- and postoperative complications. The laser was first introduced for liver surgery by Dr. Fidler in 1975.[11] He used the CO_2 laser for exsanguinating liver injuries. In 1982 Meyer et al.[12] reported and experimental study of partial liver resection with a combined CO_2 and Nd:YAG laser system. They found this system effective in cutting as well as coagulating liver parenchyma. In 1985 another combination technique using the CO_2 and Nd:YAG laser simultaneously was reported by Sultan et al.[13] This report presents 15 patients who have undergone liver resection by laser, 10 by the use of a CO_2 laser alone, 1 with the Nd:YAG laser alone, and 4 with combined use. The CO_2 laser provided good cutting effects, but hemostasis was always difficult. This led the authors to using the Nd:YAG laser which provided better coagulation. With the Nd:YAG alone the necrotic zone of the liver surface was 5–6 mm, but when the Nd:YAG was combined with the CO_2 the damage was decreased to 1.6–1.8 mm. The authors used a prototype combined handpiece with the CO_2 and the Nd:YAG laser in the same instrument. The Nd:YAG was most effective when used at 100 W and the CO_2 at 80–90 W, which blended the hemostatic properties of the Nd:YAG laser with the cutting qualities of the CO_2 laser.

A recent study compared an ultrasonic dissector (CUSA) and a noncontact Nd:YAG laser with a conventional blunt dissection technique.[14] The CUSA was superior to the "finger fracture" technique by causing less postoperative tissue damage and reduced bleeding. The noncontact

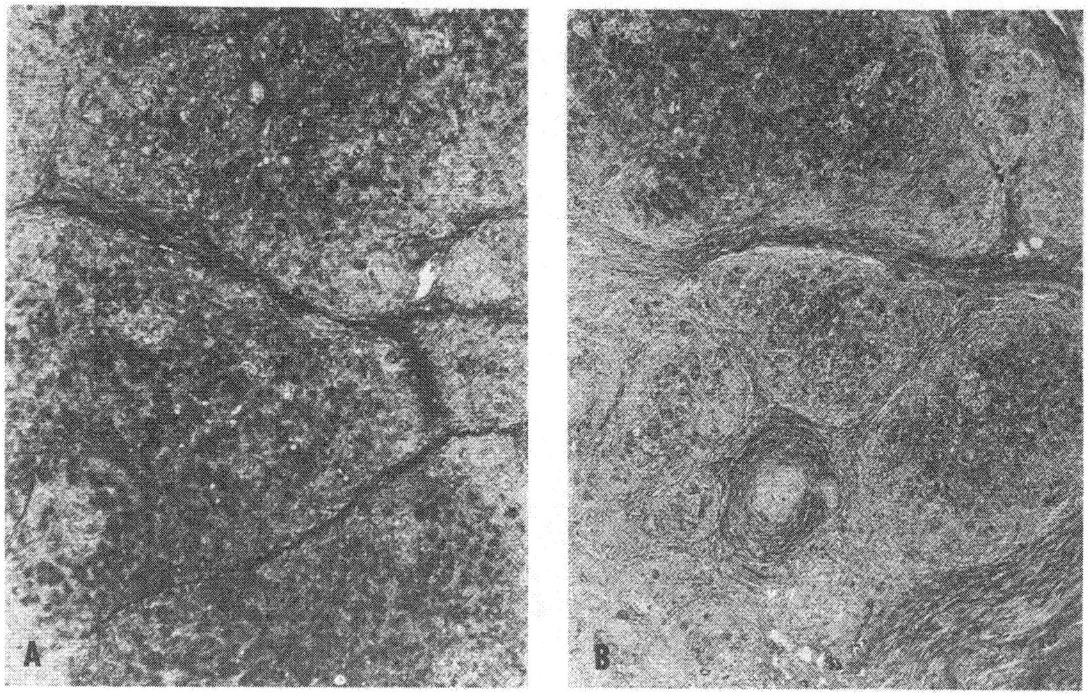

FIGURE 35.4. (A) Chronic bovie resected pancreas. (×62, Masson's Trichrome). (B) Chronic contract Nd:YAG laser resected pancreas. Extensive acinar necrosis and collagen infiltration of the parenchyma of the organ have occurred. ×64, Masson's Trichrome.

Nd:YAG laser had poor cutting properties, and, although it produced hemostasis the depth of tissue, damage was considerable.

Recently, the SLT contact Nd:YAG laser scalpel, with a synthetic sapphire, has been developed.[8] This device has proven to be effective and safe in general surgery. An experimental study comparing the contact Nd:YAG laser with the CUSA and a so-called "suction-knife" showed the inexpensive "suction knife" to be as effective as any of the new sophisticated methods. The problem with the contact Nd:YAG laser in major liver surgery was the difficulty in identifying the major central hepatic veins before a partial venotomy. The contact laser was able to coagulate 80–85% of the vessels. This finding was followed by the development of a totally new technique for laser liver resection.[15] In this technique a disposable plastic "strapper" was used to give control to the large hepatic vessels. The proximal resection surface was compressed by the "strapper," and then the liver parenchyma was resected with the SLT contact laser system. This gave complete control of blood loss and the resection could be completed in a few minutes. Thereafter all large vessels could be visualized and ligated during a gradual release of the "strapper." Histologic studies showed that this method did not cause more hepatic damage to the resected surface than the earlier reported contact laser method.

Liver resections are usually technically difficult and associated with problems in control of bleeding. The laser techniques are not yet optimal. All new techniques need to be critically evaluated and the use of a "strapper" looks promising. Clinical studies need to evaluate its application in liver surgery in a larger number of patients.

References

1. Traverso LW, Tomkins RK, Urrea PT, Longmire WP, Jr: Surgical treatment of chronic pancreatitis. Ann Surg 190:312–319, 1979.
2. White TT, Slavotinek AH: Results of surgical treatment of chronic pancreatitis. Ann Surg 189:217–224, 1979.

3. Orda R, Bara J, Orda S, Wiznitzer T: Partial distal pancreatectomy with a hand-held CO_2 laser. Arch Surg 115:869–873, 1980.
4. Sutherland DER, Goetz FC, Rynasiewicz JJ, et al: Segmental pancreas transplantation from living related and cadaver donors: A clinical experience. Surgery 90:159–168, 1981.
5. Rossi RL, Breasch JW, O'Bryan EM, Watkins E Jr: Segmental pancreatic autotransplantation for chronic pancreatitis. Gastroenterology 84:621–626, 1983.
6. Munda R, Berlatzky Y, Jonung M, et al: Studies on segmental pancreatic autotransplants in dogs. Arch Surg 118:1310–1315, 1983.
7. Berlatzky Y, Muggia-Sullam M, Munda R, Joffe SN: Use of Nd:YAG laser in pancreatic resections with duodenal preservation in the dog. Lasers in Surgery and Medicine 5:107–517, 1985.
8. Daikuzono N, Joffe SN: An artificial sapphire probe for contact photocoagulation and tissue vaporization. Med Instrum 19:173–178, 1985.
9. Schröder T, Brackett K, Joffe SN: Proximal pancreatectomy: A comparison of electrocautery with the contact and noncontact Nd:YAG laser techniques in the dog. Am J Surg, 1987.
10. Joffe SN, Sankar MY: Lasers in hepato-biliary and pancreatic surgery. In Shapsay SM (ed): Endoscopic Laser Surgery Handbook. Marcel Dekker, New York, 1986.
11. Fidler JP, Hoeter RW, Polyani TG, et al: Laser surgery in exsanguinating liver injury. Ann Surg 181:74–80, 1975.
12. Meyer H-J, Haverkampf K: Experimental study of partial liver resection with a combined CO_2 and Nd:YAG laser. Lasers Surg Med 2:149–154, 1982.
13. Sultan RA, Fallouh H, Lefebvre-Vilardebo M, Ladouch-Badre A: Separate and combined use of Nd-YAG and carbon dioxide lasers in liver resections: A preliminary report. Lasers Med Sci 1:101–105, 1986.
14. Tranberg K-G, Rigotti P, Brackett KA, et al: Liver resection. A comparison using the Nd:YAG laser, ultrasonic aspirator, or blunt dissection. Am J Surg 151:368–372, 1985.
15. Schröder T, Sankar MY, Bracket KM, et al: Major liver resection in the pig using contact Nd:YAG laser—A new technique. International Nd:YAG Laser Symposium, Tokyo, November 1–3, 1986.

36
Contact Laser Applications in Ophthalmology

Jay L. Federman and Fumitaka Ando

It is not by chance that light energy has been utilized therapeutically in ophthalmology for over four decades. The human eye has evolved into a complex sense organ that can convert minimal amounts of light into a chemical reaction to begin the visual process. Its anatomic structure is designed to focus light energy onto the photoreceptor cells of the retina and adjacent retinal pigment epithelium (RPE). The intensity of light reaching these structures is critically controlled by the lids and pupil. Too much light focused on the retina and the retinal pigment epithelium (RPE) can cause damage resulting in a chorioretinal scar. Clinically, light-induced chorioretinal lesions can be seen in patients after an eclipse of the sun,[1] arc welding,[2] and during exposure to microscope light source during cataract surgery.[3]

Light energy was harnessed early in ophthalmology to produce highly controlled chorioretinal burns in the treatment of various ocular disorders. In the mid-1940s, Dr. Gerd Meyer-Schwickerath[4] developed a device to focus sunlight into a fine beam, which he controlled and directed into the patient's eye for photocoagulation of the retina. Xenon arc photocoagulation was then developed as a more reliable light source.

Over the past two decades, as laser use in ophthalmology progressed, only a few wavelengths have survived. Argon and krypton are used for their coagulation effects on the retina and RPE, while the mechanical disruptive effects of Q-switched Nd:YAG are used on the posterior lens capsule.

All of our clinical experience with laser energy has been with noncontact slit lamp laser delivery systems; that is, the laser beam must pass through a medium, for example, air, aqueous, or vitreous, before reaching its target tissue. The development of contact laser probe made of sapphire ceramic crystal, first introduced by Joffe and Daikuzono,[5] offers new applications for lasers in the field of ophthalmology.

The use of contact laser delivery as a technique is in its infancy in ophthalmology. The laser energy is transmitted through a quartz fiber into the sapphire crystal probe. The laser probe is then applied either to the surface of the eye to affect inner adjacent tissue layers, or directly to target tissue during surgery. Experimental studies in pigmented rabbits show that the thermal effects of both Nd:YAG and argon wavelengths can be effectively delivered to target tissue sites with contact laser probes, and that the probes work well for both coagulation and cutting of ocular tissues.

With 2.2-mm flat or rounded probes applied to the surface of the conjunctiva, transcleral photocoagulation to both the retina and ciliary body has been accomplished experimentally.[6] Using argon laser energy, (1 W, 1 second duration) this technique caused photocoagulation burns at the level of the RPE and outer retinal layer in pigmented rabbits. The argon wavelength can penetrate the thin sclera of the rabbit eye with enough energy reaching the sensitive RPE to produce a chorioretinal lesion with minimal effect to the sclera. The clinical appearance of the lesion is identical to that seen with noncontact slit lamp delivery (Figure 36.1). Within one week this lesion begins to become pigmented, and there is a firm adhesion between the retina, RPE and choroid. Similar results have

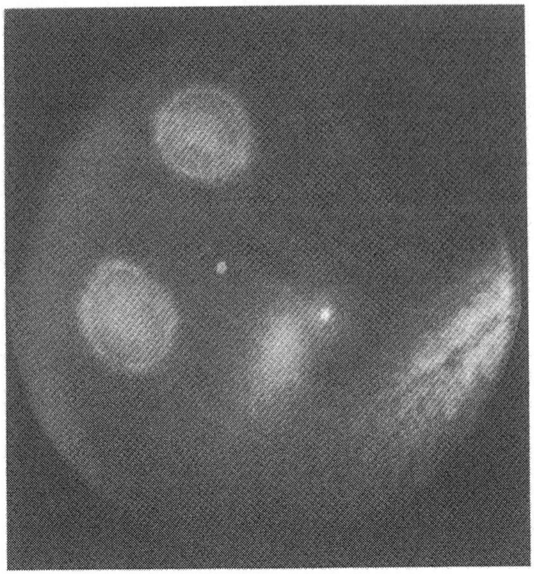

FIGURE 36.1. Fundus photograph of retinal burns immediately after transcleral laser coagulation in pigmented rabbit.

been attained using continuous wave Nd:YAG. However, since this wavelength is absorbed by all tissue layers, theoretically one would expect more scleral reaction. Although we have seen increased cellularity within the sclera (Figure 36.2), this does not appear to alter its integrity and strength. The contact laser could be employed for the peripheral retinal areas not easily reached with noncontact slit lamp laser delivery. We believe this technique can be used clinically for transcleral laser coagulation of the peripheral retina—for example, in coagulation of peripheral retinal tears; or for peripheral retinal ablation—instead of the traditional transcleral cryoretinopexy.

Using the same technique, experimental lesions produced in the ciliary body[6] result in increased pigmentation within the ciliary body and areas of destruction of the ciliary epithelium (Figure 36.3). The integrity of the sclera was maintained in pigmented rabbit studies, in spite of destructive lesions to the adjacent inner layers. Using this transcleral approach, contact laser probes may be important in glaucoma as a highly controlled method of causing focal destruction of the ciliary body epithelium. Theoretically, this technique should be more accurate, with less anterior segment reaction than is seen with cyclocryopexy or the currently used method of noncontact free-running Nd:YAG cyclodiathermy.[7]

Over the past few decades there has been a revolution in microsurgical techniques, providing direct access to all intraocular tissues. Ex-

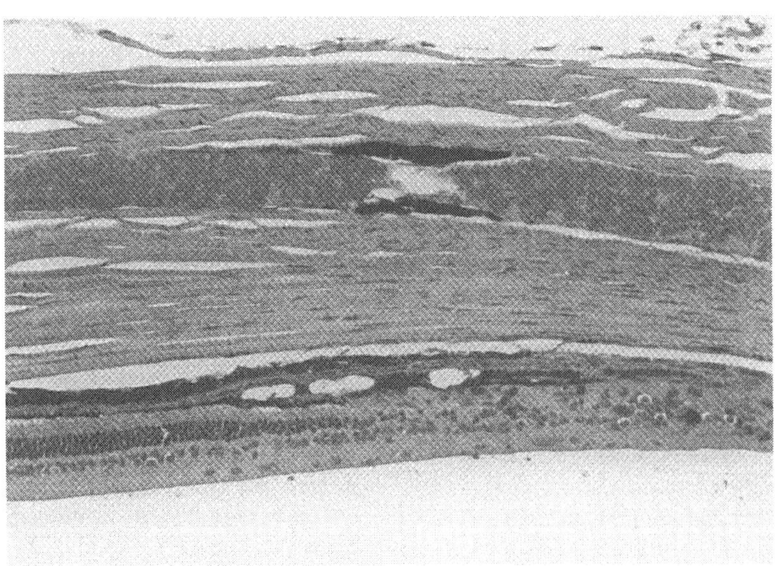

FIGURE 36.2. Histologic section through transcleral laser coagulation lesion showing firm adhesion of retina, RPE, and choroid with increased cellularity of sclera (3-month lesion). H&E.

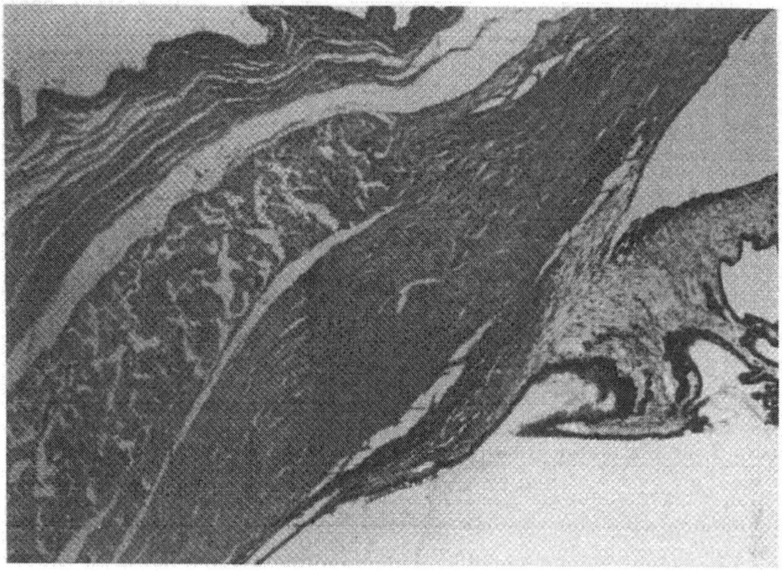

FIGURE 36.3. Histologic section through ciliary body showing increased cellularity, in a triangular shape, of sclera and increased pigmentation of ciliary body after transcleral laser coagulation (1 week lesion). H&E.

perimental work is ongoing with laser probes, 1 mm in outside diameter and 2.5 cm in length, developed for cutting and coagulation of target tissues by direct contact during various intraocular surgical procedures (Figure 36.4). The sapphire crystal probe is brought into the vitreous cavity through a sclerotomy, as in multiple incision vitrectomy procedures. Utilizing a 0.2-mm conical tip, retinotomies have been successfully performed with good hemostasis in incising the retina in the rabbit eye.[8] At low energy levels, using continuous wave Nd:YAG with the tip at the retinal surface, incisions have been made through all retinal layers. In the early experiments with attached retina, cuts in the inner scleral fibers were seen. At present, tip configurations are being designed to avoid this, but, since retinal cutting will be done predominantly on detached retina, this should not present a significant problem. With continuous wave Nd:YAG laser delivered through contact probes, retinal cutting can be performed without bleeding. With argon laser energy, using the same probes, initial studies do not show a cutting effect. However, when working with a 0.4-mm tip, focal, well-defined endophotocoagulation burns can be made to the attached retina and RPE with both continuous wave Nd:YAG and argon

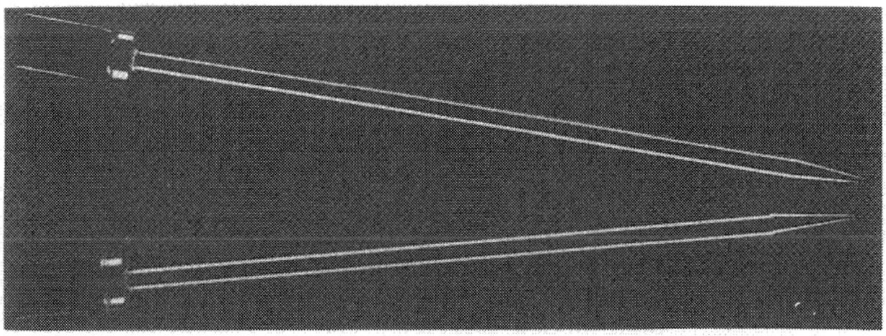

FIGURE 36.4. Sapphire ceramic cystals 2.5 cm in length and 2 mm in diameter for intraocular surgery. These tips have 0.1-mm and 0.2-mm points and have been used as laser scalpels for retinotomies in pigmented rabbit studies.

wavelengths. These burns appear to cause an immediate fusion of the retina with the RPE and choroid. This is important for detachment work as the laser coagulation may cause immediate fixation of the retina, RPE, and choroid.

A sapphire crystal has been used experimentally as a laser scalpel during ocular wall resections.[9] Full-thickness cuts can be made through sclera, choroid, and retina from an external approach. With appropriate technique, good hemostasis can be maintained during cutting. The laser scalpel should be helpful in preventing the complications of hemorrhage and retinal detachment seen with the present technique of ocular wall resection for choroidal tumors and biopsies.

Another area where contact laser probes may be beneficial involves anterior segment surgery for glaucoma. A tip can be passed across the anterior chamber to make a hole through the angle structures into the subconjunctival space for filtration of aqueous. This should be an improvement over present methods to produce an atraumatic permanent filtering fistula. Contact laser probes should also be most helpful for oculoplastic procedures.

We remain very enthusiastic about the many possible applications for contact laser probes, and feel this technology marks the beginning of a new era for lasers in ophthalmology. Continued experimental studies will supply the necessary data on the tissue effects of contact laser surgery as this technology makes its entrance into clinical ophthalmology.

References

1. Verhoff FH, Bell L, Walker CB: The pathological effects of radant energy on the eye. Proc Am Acad Arts Sci 51:630–818, 1916.
2. Naidoff MA, Sliney DH: Retinal injury from a welding arc. Am J Ophthalmol 77:663, 1974.
3. Boldrey EE, Ho BT, Griffith, RD: Retinal burns occurring at cataract extraction. Ophthalmology 91:1297–1302, 1984.
4. Meyer-Schwickerath G: Versl Dtsch Ophthal Ges Heidelberg Ber 55:256, 1949.
5. Daikuzono N, Joffe SN: Artificial sapphire tip for contact photocoagulation and tissue vaporization with the Nd:YAG laser. Med Instrum 19:173–178, 1985.
6. Federman JL, Ando F, Schubert HD, and Eagle, RC: Contact laser for transcleral photocoagulation. Ophthalmic Surgery 18:183–184, 1987.
7. Schwartz LW, Moster MX: Neodymium:YAG laser transcleral cyclodiathermy. Ophthal Laser Ther 1:135–141, 1986.
8. Ando F, Federman JL, Daikuzono N, Osborn J: Contact laser scalpel for intraocular surgery. Am J Ophthalmol 102:663–664, 1986.
9. Federman JL, Ando F, Peyman, GA, Schubert, HD: Contact laser scalpel for ocular wall resection. Ophthalmic Surgery 18:(4)305–306, 1987.

37

The Short-Pulsed Nd:YAG Laser in Ophthalmology: A Review of Current Clinical Techniques

Carmen A. Puliafito and Roger F. Steinert

The Q-switched and mode-locked Nd:YAG lasers rapidly entered the ophthalmic surgical armamentarium as the tool of choice for discission of the posterior capsule.[1–3] The large shift in the past decade from intracapsular to extracapsular surgery generated a widespread need for safe and effective techniques to manage both intact posterior capsules that opacify postoperatively and visually significant capsular fragments that remain after primary surgical capsular discission. The Nd:YAG laser also has proven to be a major tool in the management of postoperative complications, such as pupillary block and malignant glaucoma, vitreous incarceration in the wound, synechiae formation, and residual anterior capsular fragments.

Posterior Capsulotomy

Postoperative opacification of initially clear posterior capsules occurs frequently in patients after extracapsular extraction of senile cataracts. In adults, the time from surgery to visually significant opacification varies from months to years.[4] In younger age groups, almost 100% opacification occurs within 2 years after surgery; in adults, the rate declines with increasing age.[5]

Clinically, optical degradation of initially clear posterior capsules takes several forms. Fibrosis connotes a gray white band or plaquelike opacity that usually is recognized in the early postoperative period. *Fibrosis* present in the first days to weeks postoperatively probably most often represents cortical lamellae left at the time of surgery. Fibrosis that develops months to years postoperatively is caused by multiple layers of anterior lens epithelium that have migrated and undergone fibrous metaplasia.[6]

Migration of epithelial cells with formation of small *Elschnig's pearls* and *bladder cells*, the second major form of opacity, occurs months to years after surgery. Pathologic examination indicates that the proliferating anterior epithelial cells originate at the site of apposition of the anterior capsular flaps to the posterior capsule.[6] This finding explains the inability of polishing of the capsule at surgery to delay the onset or reduce the frequency of late capsular opacification[4,7] because polishing of the posterior capsule cannot remove the epithelial cells from the anterior capsular flaps.

Capsular wrinkling can have two manifestations. Broad undulations of clear capsule are particularly common in the early postoperative period before the capsule becomes tense. Posterior chamber lens haptics may induce these broad wrinkles along the axis of the haptic orientation. Conversely, a posterior chamber lens may tend to flatten broad wrinkles if the optic body or a YAG spacer bar or tab presses on the capsule. Broad undulating wrinkles of clear capsule rarely are visually disturbing to the patient; an unusual patient may perceive linear distortions or shadows that correspond to the wrinkles and are relieved by capsulotomy.

Fine wrinkles or folds in the capsule, in contrast, can result in marked optical disturbance.

All figures and portions of the text are reproduced with permission from Steinert, RF, and Puliafito, CA: The Nd:YAG Laser in Ophthalmology: Principles and Clinical Applications of Photodisruption. Saunders, Philadelphia, 1985.

These fine wrinkles are caused by myofibroblastic differentiation of the migrating lens epithelial cells, which acquire contractile properties, resulting in the wrinkles.[6]

Technique for Nd:YAG Laser Posterior Capsulotomy

Preoperative Assessment of Capsular Opacity

Judging the contribution of a capsular opacity to the patient's overall visual deficit may be difficult. Table 37.1 lists useful techniques. Some capsular opacities are impressive in oblique slit-lamp illumination but are insignificant when viewed against the red reflex. In general, these opacities cause little visual difficulty. The single most reliable technique for assessing capsular opacity is direct ophthalmoscopy. Retinoscopy and the red reflex seen at the slit lamp or with a direct or indirect ophthalmoscope also reveal significant optical disturbances.

The laser interferometer and the Potential Acuity Meter should penetrate mild to moderate capsular opacity and indicate macular function. Both instruments may give false-positive ("good") acuity prediction in the presence of cystoid macular edema,[8] which is the most likely cause of postcataract visual impairment besides capsular opacity itself, and may give false-negative predictions where the capsular opacity does not have clear "window" zones for penetration of the testing beam.

Unless the capsule is extremely dense, adequate visualization may be present for fluorescein angiography or angioscopy. For patients in whom the capsular opacity seems inadequate to explain the quality of vision, cystoid macular edema (CME) should be anticipated and documented, so that unnecessary and possibly deleterious capsulotomy can be avoided.

TABLE 37.1. Assessment of optical significance of capsular opacity

Direct ophthalmoscopic visualization of fundus structures
Retinoscopy
Red reflex evaluation by
Slit lamp examination
Direct ophthalmoscopic examination
Indirect ophthalmoscopic examination
Hruby lens view of fundus
Laser interferometer evaluation
Potential Acuity Meter evaluation
Fluorescein angiography or angioscopy

Preparation of the Patient for Laser Capsulotomy

Dilation of the pupil facilitates visualization of the capsule over a broad expanse. Except in the case of an iris-clip lens, dilation is very helpful for a surgeon inexperienced with laser capsulotomy. In the absence of a miotic pupil, however, dilation may be omitted. If the pupil is to be dilated, the landmarks of the pupillary zone of the capsule should be sketched beforehand. Inattention to the pupillary zone results in an eccentric capsulotomy and may necessitate a second session at the laser or induce the surgeon to perform an overly large capsulotomy to prevent this possibility. If the laser is available, the patient can be brought to the laser before dilation, and a single "marker" shot can be placed in the capsule near the middle of the pupillary axis. For routine dilation, weak agents are recommended to avoid inadvertent iris capture of a posterior capsule intraocular lens (PC IOL), which may be difficult to reposition properly.

Particularly after a surgeon becomes comfortable with the technique of laser capsulotomy, optimally sized capsulotomies can be achieved without dilation. As the patient looks up, down, left, and right, the laser can be applied to capsular edges behind the sphincter, so the capsulotomy can be both adequately sized and perfectly centered. The slit-lamp illumination should be with a narrow beam, angled obliquely, to minimize miosis and indicate average pupillary size with ambient lighting.

The surgeon should remind the patient that the procedure is painless. The patient may hear small clicks or pops, but he must simply maintain steady fixation.

No anesthesia is generally required for capsulotomy unless a contact lens is employed. In that case, a drop of topical anesthetic is applied to the cornea immediately before the beginning of the procedure. In rare circumstances, such as nystagmus, a retrobulbar injection for akinesia may be helpful. If topical anesthetic is applied in advance of the procedure for examination or instillation of painful mydriatics and

TABLE 37.2. Preparation of the patient

Before the treatment session
Complete ophthalmic history and examination.
Discussion of proposed procedure, including risks, benefits, and alternatives; signing of informed consent form
Pupillary dilation (optional)
Determination of visual axis and normal pupillary size: sketch and preliminary laser marker shot
Weak mydriatics and cycloplegics: 2.5% phenylephrine or 0.5% or 1% tropicamide
At the laser
Review of the procedure, the expected pop or click, and the importance of fixation
Application of topical anesthetic if contact lens is to be used
Adjustment of stool, table, chin rest, and foot rest for optimal patient comfort
Application of head strap to maintain forehead position
Darkening of the room (optional)
Provision of fixation target for fellow eye (illumination of target if room is darkened)

cycloplegics, the patient should be instructed to keep the eyes closed during the interval while waiting for the laser treatment, in order to maintain the surface integrity and optical quality of the corneal epithelium.

Table 37.2 summarizes the steps in patient preparation.

Contraindications for Laser Capsulotomy

Attempted Nd:YAG laser capsulotomy is contraindicated if corneal scars, irregularity, or edema preclude adequate visualization of the target or degrade the laser beam optics to prevent reliable and predictable optical breakdown. The procedure is also contraindicated if the patient proves unable or unwilling to fixate adequately, with the threat of inadvertent damage to adjacent intraocular structures.

The presence of a glass intraocular lens is a relative contraindication. The merits of surgical discission in this instance should be carefully weighed. Laser capsulotomy should be approached with extreme caution and only by an experienced Nd:YAG laser operator under ideal conditions, because of the possibility of causing a complete fracture in the glass optic.[9]

Known or suspected cystoid macular edema is a relative contraindication, given current evidence regarding a possible beneficial effect from an intact posterior capsule and in view of rare cases of clinical CME that apparently occur after Nd:YAG laser capsulotomy.[10]

Unlike the situation with surgical discission, the only data available to date do not show a difference in the rate of complications depending on the interval between cataract surgery and laser capsulotomy.[10] However, given the overall low incidence of long-term complications, recognition of such a trend may require an even larger study.

No data exist on laser capsulotomy in eyes at high risk for retinal detachment. As a minimal precaution, the least amount of energy and the lowest number of shots should be used that can accomplish the capsulotomy, and only a small opening should be made.

Capsulotomy Technique

The minimal amount of energy necessary to obtain breakdown and rupture the capsule is desired. With most lasers, a typical capsule can be opened by using 1 to 2 mJ per pulse.

The capsule is examined for wrinkles that indicate tension lines. Shots placed across tension lines result in the largest opening per pulse, since the tension causes the initial opening to widen. Figure 37.1 shows an actual capsulotomy photographed sequentially and drawn from the photographs, showing the opening as it develops and the location of the next laser shot. Table 37.3 outlines the basic technique. The usual strategy is to create a cruciate opening, beginning superiorly near the 12 o'clock position and progressing downward toward the 6 o'clock position. Unless a wide opening has already developed, shots are then placed at the edge of the capsule opening, progressing laterally toward the 3 and 9 o'clock positions. If any capsular flaps remain in the pupillary space, the laser is fired specifically at the flaps to cut them and cause them to retract and fall back to the periphery.

The goal is to achieve flaps based in the periphery and inferiorly. Free-floating fragments should be avoided because these may remain and cause interference. Cutting in a circle, "can-opener style," should be avoided because this tends to create large fragments that may not settle or that may settle against the endothelium or angle structures.

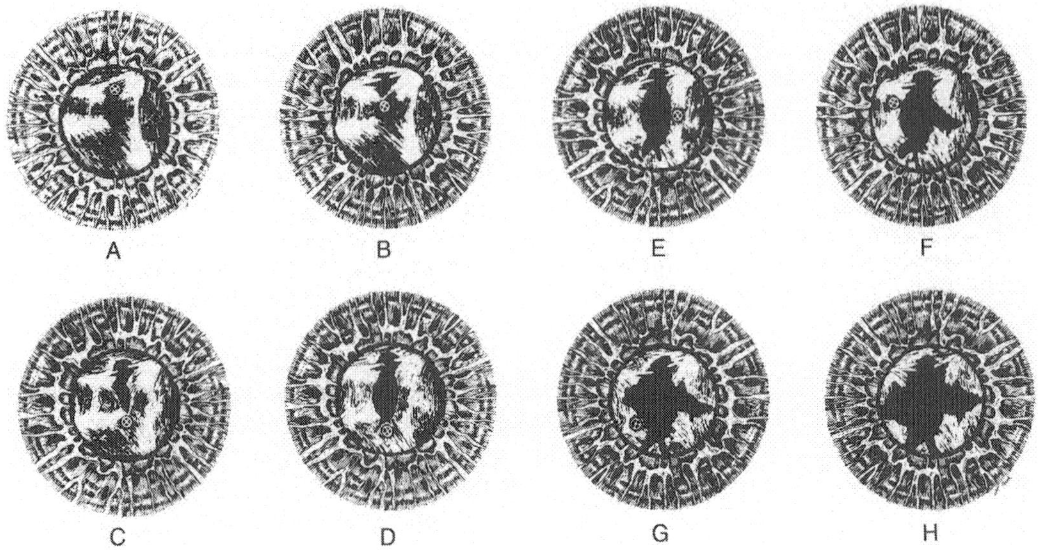

FIGURE 37.1 Artist's drawing based on sequential capsulotomy photographs. The capsulotomy is developed in a cruciate pattern. (*A*) The first shot is made superiorly in the location of some fine tension lines. (*B*) The second shot is aimed inside the inferior edge of the initial opening. (*C*) The next shot again is made at the 6 o'clock position of the capsulotomy border. (*D*) The fourth shot is made across inferior tension lines to allow the capsulotomy to widen. (*E*) The opening is nearly 3mm wide. It is widened by a shot at the 3 o'clock capsulotomy margin. (*F*) The opening now needs to be directed to the left, with a shot at the 9 o'clock position. (*G*) The cruciate opening has been accomplished, but a triangular flap extends into the pupillary space from the 7:30 o'clock region in the left inferior pupil. A shot is applied to the flap, to both cut it and push it toward the periphery. (*H*) The capsulotomy is complete, and the pupil will be clear of capsule when the dilation wears off.

An IOL may be marked in the course of the capsulotomy. This is particularly true for posterior chamber lenses for which little or no separation of the capsule from the IOL exists.

Visually significant pits and cracks can be minimized and avoided through careful techniques, as outlined in Table 37.4. A contact lens such as the Peyman or central Abraham lens stablizes the eye, improves the laser beam optics, and facilitates accurate focusing. Following the usual strategy of beginning the capsulotomy in the 12 o'clock periphery gives an indication of the tendency for IOL markings in a noncritical area. If there is a tendency for unavoidable repeated marks, the usual cruciate pattern should be modified. Instead of progressing from the 12 o'clock to the 6 o'clock positions across the vis-

TABLE 37.3. Posterior capsulotomy technique

Use minimum energy:
- 1 mJ if possible.

Identify and cut across tension lines.

Perform a cruciate opening:
- Begin in 12 o'clock periphery.
- Progress toward 6 o'clock position.
- Cut across at 3 and 9 o'clock positions.
- Clean up any residual tags.
- Avoid freely floating fragments.

TABLE 37.4. Minimizing intraocular lens (IOL) laser marks

Use minimum energy.

Use a contact lens to
- stabilize the eye.
- improve laser beam optics.
- facilitate accurate focusing.

Identify any areas of IOL-capsule separation, and begin treatment there.

If lens marking is occurring, make an opening in the shape of a Christmas tree from the 12 o'clock to the 7:30 o'clock positions without placing any shots in the central optical zone.

Use deep-focus techniques:
- Optical breakdown occurs in the anterior vitreous.
- The shock wave radiates forward and ruptures the capsule.
- Higher energy (2 mJ or more) must be used.

ual axis, the cut should be made nasally and temporally, staying in the periphery of the optical zone. The capsule then can be opened in a "Christmas-tree" fashion, based inferiorly, without any shots in the central visual axis. One other technique is very helpful in avoiding IOL marks. The laser can be intentionally focused posteriorly to the capsule, to cause optical breakdown in the anterior vitreous. The shock wave then radiates forward and ruptures the capsule.

Capsulotomy Size

In the absence of a specific reason for a small opening, such as concern over a patient at high risk for retinal detachment, the capsulotomy should be as large as the pupil in ambient light. A small opening in a dense membrane results in excellent optics, analagous to those of a small pupil. When the capsule is only hazy and transmits images to the retina, however, a small opening is an improvement but is still suboptimal. The hazy membrane continues to transmit a poor-quality image that mixes with the image transmitted through the clear opening. A capsule with residual haze not only impairs vision under standard conditions but also produces glare.

Postoperative Care for Capsulotomy

After laser capsulotomy, protocols for routine administration of topical steroids and cycloplegics vary widely according to the individual surgeon's clinical experience. Many surgeons recommend routine use of topical steroids. The patient is discharged with instructions to apply a strong topical steroid (prednisolone 1% or dexamethasone 0.1%, for example) beginning immediately and continuing four times daily. This application is tapered and discontinued at postoperative visits when the clinical examination discloses an eye without cellular reaction.

An acute increase in pressure in the hours after treatment is common. The patient should be rechecked 1 hour and 4 hours after capsulotomy, and treatment is begun if the pressure has risen 5 or more mm Hg above baseline. If the patient has a baseline pressure greater than 20 mm Hg, or has glaucoma, prophylactic treatment is given. If there is no contraindication such as asthma or congestive heart disease, a drop of timolol 0.5% or betaxolol 0.5% at the conclusion of treatment usually suffices to blunt the pressure rise, since this medication has a maximal effect 2 to 4 hours after administration. Alternative medications are pilocarpine or a carbonic anhydrase inhibitor. The possibility of a delayed pressure elevation after use of these medications must be recognized. An examination on the day following laser treatment is indicated.

For patients already receiving medication for preexisting glaucoma, the level of medication should be increased, using additional or stronger medication. If the patient is already on maximally tolerated medical therapy, a full dose (calculated by weight) of an oral osmotic agent (glycerin or isosorbide dinitrate) should be administered at the conclusion of the treatment and the patient instructed to take another full dose 4 hours after treatment.

Glaucoma patients on intensive therapy, particularly with advanced visual field loss, should be observed closely for at least 4 to 6 hours after treatment. Further options for management of sight-threatening pressure elevation include, progressively, intravenous administration of mannitol, anterior segment paracentesis, anterior chamber washout, and emergency filtration. A case of postcapsulotomy intraocular pressure rise above 80 mm Hg with loss of light perception was successfully treated with anterior chamber paracentesis, and visual recovery to 20/25 was achieved.[11] Treatment of these high-risk patients may be less hazardous if the treatment is divided across multiple sessions, with a few shots given at low energy per session. However, studies of capsulotomy in the general population have not found a consistent correlation of pressure increase with pulse energy, total shots, or total energy.[10,12–14]

Two other causes of acute glaucoma after laser capsulotomy have been reported. Vitreous herniation may cause pupillary block and acute glaucoma.[15] In the absence of a patent peripheral iridectomy, the potential for pupillary block after posterior capsulotomy should be considered unless a posterior chamber lens is present that holds the vitreous in place. An aphakic iridectomy can be readily and safely performed with the Nd:YAG laser. A case of vitreous herniation plugging a filtering bleb with acute pressure increase 10 days after capsulotomy has also been reported.[16]

Results and Complications from Nd:YAG Laser Posterior Capsulotomy

The initial European response to experience with Q-switched and mode-locked Nd:YAG laser secondary capsulotomy in large numbers of patients has been enthusiastic.[1–3] Early short-term American experience has also demonstrated the relative ease of laser capsulotomy with a high rate of visual improvement, but not without complications, including acute transient pressure rise, IOL marking, rupture of the anterior hyaloid face, retinal detachment, and bleeding from diabetic rubeosis iridis.[17–19]

Keates, Steinert, Puliafito, and Maxwell[10] reported the results of a study of 526 patients who underwent Q-switched Nd:YAG laser posterior capsulotomy and were followed a minimum of 6 months by their physicians. These results were compared with observations of a historical control group of 209 pseudophakes who had undergone surgical secondary capsulotomy before the laser became available. The surgical control population had significantly better prediscission visual acuity and lesser preoperative pathology. Nevertheless, 85.7% of the laser-treated pseudophakes achieved 20/40 or better vision compared with 80.2% of the surgically treated group. Excluding patients with preoperative pathology, 90.1% of the laser-treated pseudophakes obtained better vision after treatment, compared with 69.7% of the surgically treated pseudophakes (difference significant at $p < 0.001$).

Of the laser-treated pseudophakes, 3.3% had diminished vision after capsulotomy, compared with 14.8% of the surgical control group ($p < 0.001$). Half of the patients in the laser-treated group with diminished posttreatment acuity at six months were within one line of their pretreatment visual acuity. Cystoid macular edema was diagnosed at any one of the posttreatment visits in 2.3% of the patients, but at 6 months persistent CME was reported in only one patient (0.2%). This was significantly less than the persistent CME rate for the surgical control group of 1.9% ($p < 0.05$). Retinal detachment occurred in two of the laser-treated (0.4%) and in none of the surgically treated patients. Persistent pressure elevation, iritis, vitritis, anterior segment hemorrhage, and IOL dislocation were all reported in fewer than 1% of the patients. IOL marks were reported for 33% of patients with posterior chamber lenses, 4.3% with iris lenses, and 6.5% with anterior chamber lenses. A dissenting report has been made by Knolle. In a retrospective comparison of knife capsulotomies performed at the slit lamp to his early experience with the Nd:YAG laser, Knolle[20] found better restoration of vision with the surgical technique. The patient populations may not have been comparable, however. Nevertheless, Knolle reported that visual recovery was faster and more complete with knife discission.

Posttreatment pressure elevation is now recognized as a common, although usually transient, complication after Nd:YAG laser capsulotomy. In a report of 49 capsulotomies, Terry et al.[17] detected a pressure increase in 37 eyes, with a maximal pressure greater than 30 mm Hg in 16 eyes and greater than 50 mm Hg in four eyes. In most eyes the pressure returned to pretreatment levels within 1 week, but in two eyes it did not normalize until 6 weeks after treatment. When patients were observed carefully after laser capsulotomy, the majority were found to have a pressure peak within 3 hours after the operation. Channell and Beckman[13] found a pressure elevation exceeding 5 mm Hg in 64% of patients and 10 mm Hg in 35% of patients within 4 hours of laser capsulotomy. Persistent pressure elevation after 1 month occurred in 5%.

Richter and co-workers[12] examined the acute elevation of pressure after laser capsulotomy with serial pressure measurements and tonography in 17 patients. The median time to achieve maximal pressure was 3 hours. The higher the pretreatment intraocular pressure and the lower the pretreatment facility of outflow, the greater was the tendency for a large pressure increase. As a consequence, patients with preexisting open angle glaucoma had a higher risk of developing greater pressure elevation. A decline in the facility of outflow paralleled any acute rise in pressure after laser capsulotomy, and the outflow facility returned to baseline level as the pressure normalized.

Mechanistically, the acute pressure rise is thus caused by impaired outflow, and the rapid onset suggests that the reduced outflow may be related to capsular debris, acute inflammatory cells, heavy-molecular-weight protein, or a combination of these mechanisms.[21] An immunologic reaction to liberated lens proteins is unlikely to have such a rapid onset and resolution. Recently, a low-molecular-weight factor from the vitreous has been implicated in the etiology of postcapsulotomy pressure elevation.[22]

Patients with IOL tend to have a smaller elevation in pressure, particularly with posterior chamber lenses. This effect may be related to posterior trapping of capsular debris by the IOL. Alternatively, patients with IOLs may have capsule characteristics different from aphakes, either because of the IOL itself or because of different visual expectations for IOL patients which lead to capsulotomy at an earlier stage, with less fibrotic material or pearl formation.[12,14] Other investigators have not found a significant difference in the extent of pressure elevation in the presence of IOLs.[13]

Prophylaxis of Acute Pressure Elevation

Two studies have prospectively studied the effect of prophylactic administration of antiglaucoma medication after Nd:YAG laser capsulotomy. Brown[23] administered pilocarpine 4% hourly from capsulotomy until bedtime on the day of treatment and markedly reduced the incidence of acute pressure elevation. Richter[24] et al. compared timolol 0.5%, pilocarpine 2%, and a placebo drop in a double-masked study where one drop was given 5 and 30 minutes after capsulotomy. In that study, mean pressure elevation was 8 mm for the placebo control, 5 mm for pilocarpine, and 1 mm for timolol 0.5%. This suggests that acute administration of a beta-blocking agent topically (or perhaps substituting a carbonic anhydrase inhibitor if medically indicated) is the better means of prophylaxis. It should be noted, however, that, even with timolol prophylaxis, one patient experienced a pressure elevation to 40 mm; the protective effect is not absolute, and patients should still be carefully monitored after the laser procedure.

Pupillary Membranectomy

Application of the Q-switched Nd:YAG laser to aphakic pupillary membranes was first described by Fankhauser et al.[3] While less common than posterior capsulotomy, the procedure offers the potential to clear the pupil optically in eyes that frequently have had serious pathology and are either poor candidates for further surgery or, if surgery were to be performed, require major procedures in the operating room with irrigation–suction–cutting instruments.

Several aspects of the treatment of dense membranes must be considered.

Evaluation of Membrane

The density and type of membrane should be evaluated to determine whether laser treatment is appropriate. Dense membranes may require multiple sessions to achieve an adequate opening, and the patient should be informed of this possibility. Lengthy sessions with many pulses and liberation of a large amount of debris seem prone to postlaser inflammation and elevated pressure. Large Elschnig's pearls from old cataracts may liberate protein when opened and result in phacoanaphylactic or phacolytic glaucoma. Such patients may be best served, in the end, by a definitive surgical operation instead of attempted laser membranectomy.

Membranectomy Technique

Unlike posterior capsules, in which each laser shot results in a large opening because the capsule is thin and under tension, membranes may have little or no elastic properties. Treatment with the laser may require high pulse energy, from 4 to 12 mJ. The opening is created by "chipping" away at the edge, in a manner similar to that of a stonemason chipping at marble.

Retained cortical material may be treated with the laser before it condenses into a permanent membrane or to speed its eventual resorption. Early intervention with the laser may be particularly important in pseudophakic patients. The higher energy necessary to open membranes compared to capsules can result in severe IOL marking.

Postoperative Care for Membranectomy

Pressure elevation and inflammation may be more pronounced than with simple capsulotomy. This result should be anticipated, and steroids and glaucoma medications should be administered as indicated.

Aphakic and Pseudophakic Iridectomy and Anterior Hyaloid Vitreolysis

In acute angle closure glaucoma in aphakia and pseudophakia, corneal edema and haze, anterior chamber reaction, and iris congestion may make argon laser iridectomy impossible. Even when a patent opening is created, an argon laser iridectomy may not relieve the glaucoma because of the role of the vitreous. In our opinion the Nd:YAG laser can better treat these conditions, and this is the treatment of choice.[25] The success of the Nd:YAG laser "anterior hyaloidectomy" in curing ciliovitreal block glaucoma, in which surgical and argon iridectomies have failed, demonstrates the pathophysiologic role of the anterior hyaloid face and represents a major advance in treatment.

The role of the hyaloid face in aphakic malignant glaucoma due to posterior diversion of aqueous, rather than pupillary block, is further illustrated by the case shown in Figure 37.2. Three months after complicated cataract extraction and subsequent IOL removal in a pa-

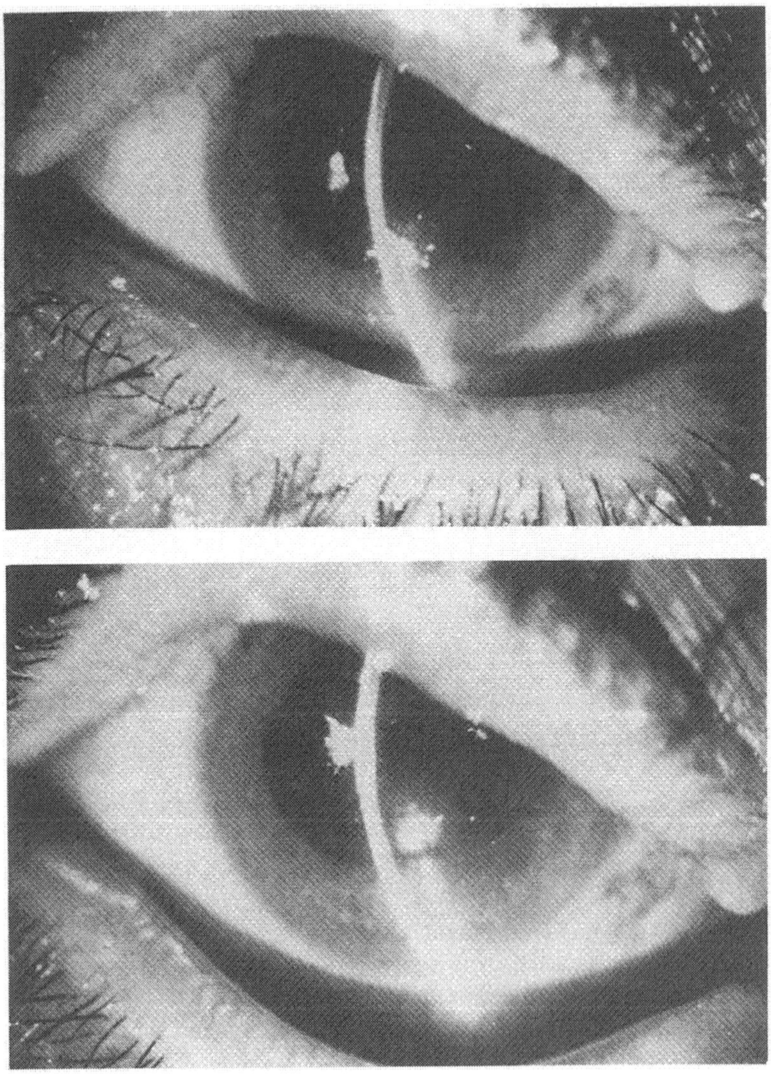

FIGURE 37.2. (*Top*) Aphakic malignant glaucoma with apposition of inferior iris to edematous cornea. (*Bottom*) Depth is restored to the anterior chamber immediately after Nd:YAG laser pulses have opened the anterior hyaloid face.

tient who had had a large superior sector iridectomy, the chamber became shallow and the pressure rose to 34 mm Hg over several days with the onset of deep pain. A thin intact hyaloid face was present. The patient was treated with the Nd:YAG laser, which was focused and fired at 3 mJ on the hyaloid face through mild corneal edema and with less than 1 mm of anterior chamber depth. The chamber deepened immediately.

Procedure for Iridectomy and Hyaloid Vitreolysis

From 4 to 8 mJ is usually adequate to perforate the iris in one shot. Corneal edema or anterior chamber reaction may necessitate higher energy to obtain the same cutting power. At least three iridectomies should be made, if possible, to ensure full relief of aqueous entrapment, which may be localized into sectors, and to increase the chance of maintaining at least one long-term patent iridectomy. Iridectomies tend to shrink as bombe is relieved and the iris falls back. Inflammation also may close iridectomies subsequently.

If the chamber is markedly shallow or flat, the haptic of an anterior chamber pseudophakos, when present, usually provides a small area of clearing from the cornea.

After the iridectomy has been completed or when a patent basal iridectomy is already present, the Nd:YAG laser should be fired into the anterior vitreous through the iridectomy or the pupil. This procedure ruptures the hyaloid face and relieves any malignant glaucoma caused by the intact hyaloid face.

Postoperative Care for Iridectomy

Topical steroids are administered as needed. Cycloplegia, sometimes alternating with miosis, is indicated to prevent formation of synechiae. The patient must be periodically observed to verify patency of the iridectomies.

Synechialysis

Localized synechiae with associated pigment may be broken by photocoagulation with the argon laser. Generally, however, the Nd:YAG laser is more successful than the argon laser in synechialysis because pigmentation of the target is not required and forceful rupture of adhesions can be made.

Synechiae can form around anterior chamber intraocular lens footplates. This condition may lead to pupillary distortion in the absence of tuck. In Figure 37.3 the pupil is seen to be eccentric. The patient complained bitterly of edge glare. Gonioscopy revealed synechia in association with the IOL footplates and haptic struts. Synechialysis through a gonioscopy lens was carried out, requiring four sessions before the pupil moved behind the edge of the IOL and the symptoms were relieved.

Preparation of the Patient for Synechialysis

The patient is told beforehand that multiple sessions are often necessary for complete synechialysis. Prelaser miosis or mydriasis may help by stretching a synechia, which improves both visualization of the abnormality and the pressure wave cutting action of the laser.

Procedure for Synechialysis

Generally the laser is set between 4 and 10 mJ, depending on the stength of the synechia to be lysed. When the abnormality can be directly visualized, the laser is aimed accordingly. Often, however, a gonioscopy lens is necessary to treat synechiae near the limbus and, of course, in the angle. Energy losses and optical aberrations often require higher laser energy settings with a gonioscopy lens in order to achieve the irradiance necessary to cut a synechia.

Postoperative Care for Synechialysis

Strong topical steroids (prednisolone 1%, dexamethasone 0.1%) are used initially at least four times daily and more often if severe inflammation occurs. If there is any tendency for formation of new synechiae the pupil should be moved with intermittent administration of short-acting cycloplegics and mydriatics. Intraocular pressure should be measured and appropriate treatment (using timolol or carbonic anhydrase inhibitors) should be begun when indicated.

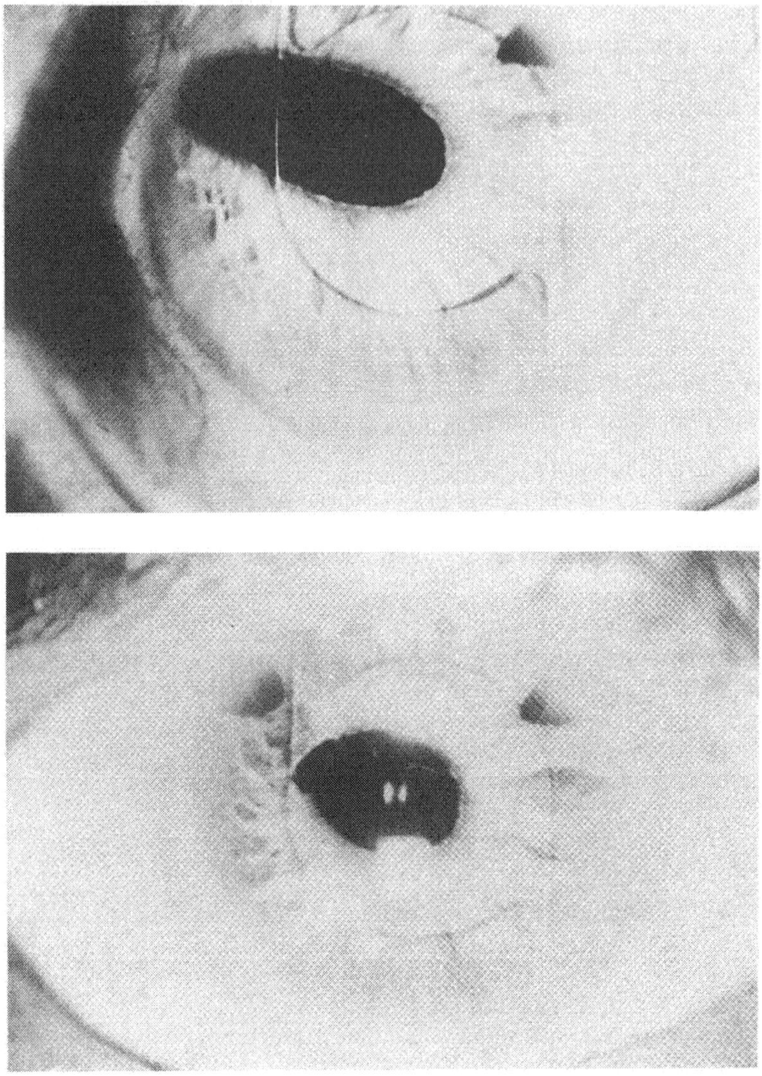

FIGURE 37.3 (*Top*) Eccentric pupil appearing 1 week after intracapsular cataract extraction with anterior chamber intraocular lens. Vitreous loss with iris adherent to the wound occurred at a site of wound leak postoperatively. (*Bottom*) The pupil is now fully behind the area of the intraocular lens optic after lysis of vitreous adhesions to the posterior iris.

Anterior Vitreolysis and Cystoid Macular Edema

Vitreous strands and bands to the wound may cause eccentric pupils and can be associated with cystoid macular edema (Irvine-Gass CME).[26,27] Iliff[28] first reported visual improvement after surgical section of such vitreous bands to the wound.

Katzen and co-workers[29] first reported the use of the Nd:YAG laser to lyse strands of vitreous to cataract wounds. In their series, vision improved by variable degrees in all 14 patients reported. The presence of CME was judged clinically, however, and results of pre- and postlaser fluorescein angiography were not reported for 13 of the eyes.

Because of the unpredictable natural history of aphakic CME, with erratic response to antiinflammatory agents and frequent spontaneous improvement,[30,31] small uncontrolled series cannot unequivocally prove the efficacy of a given technique. However, our initial experience

TABLE 37.5. Fourteen cases of vitreolysis for cystoid macular edema (CME)

Assessment	Patient Data
Interval from cataract surgery to CME	0–3 months
Interval from cataract surgery to laser vitreolysis	1–57 months
Interval from laser vitreolysis to stable visual improvement*	
Range	2–26 weeks
Average	9 weeks
Mode	8 weeks
Fluorescein angiographic change (7 patients evaluated)	
Resolved CME	3 patients
Reduced CME	3 patients
Unchanged	1 patient
Two treatment sessions required	5 patients

*Patient lost to follow-up between 4th and 26th week after vitreolysis.

and that of our colleagues at the Massachusetts Eye and Ear Infirmary has confirmed a high rate of visual improvement after anterior segment vitreolysis. The conditions of 12 of 14 patients improved both objectively and according to the patient's own perception. Each patient had aphakic or pseudophakic CME documented by fluorescein angiography before treatment. The interval between cataract extraction and vitreolysis ranged from 1 to 57 months. The onset of visual loss occurred within 3 months after cataract surgery in all cases. The interval from laser vitreolysis to visual improvement averaged 9 weeks. In our first series, postlaser fluorescein angiograms were obtained for 7 of the 14 patients. Generally, macular edema resolved in those patients who experienced nearly full recovery of vision (20/30 or better). In patients with partial recovery of vision, CME generally persisted, but to a lesser degree. Table 37.5 summarizes these results.

Preoperative Assessment

Because of the high success rate of Nd:YAG laser anterior vitreolysis in the treatment of aphakic and pseudophakic CME, it is particularly important to examine carefully for the presence of a vitreous strand to the wound in any patient with CME. The strand is usually best seen on slit lamp examination with a narrow slit beam in a darkened room, and pigment deposits on the vitreous strand may be visible. In some cases, careful gonioscopy may be necessary to visualize the strand, particularly if the vitreous enters the anterior chamber through the area of a peripheral iridectomy.

Permanent changes in the iris stroma are frequent in long-term cases with decreased but persistent ovalling of the pupil after lysis of a vitreous strand.

Preparation of the Patient for Vitreolysis

When the vitreous strand or band passes through the pupil, treatment is often facilitated by administration of pilocarpine 2% every 15 minutes beginning 2 hours preoperatively. Inducing stretch of the vitreous through miosis facilitates identification of the strand and the cutting action of the laser and shows the release of the tension more definitively.

Procedure for Vitreolysis

The laser can be directed at a vitreous strand in four general areas. The most reliable landmark during vitreolysis is the cataract wound, since the vitreous band or strand has to terminate at that line. The cataract wound is visualized with a gonioscopy lens and the laser is fired at the wound area with a reasonable chance of successful vitreolysis. Because of the contact lens and mirror optics, the energy settings of a Q-switched Nd:YAG laser are usually 4 to 12 mJ in order to obtain adequate cutting power.

If the cornea is clear near the limbus and the vitreous strand can be visualized with some clearance from the iris stroma, direct cutting without a contact lens or with a peripheral button Abraham lens may be successful. Usually, 4 mJ is adequate. Misfocused shots can cause local damage to the underlying iris or overlying cornea.

Occasionally directing the laser at the vitreous passing over the iris collarette can be helpful. This is particularly true when the vitreous has formed adhesions to the collarette, pulling it forward in a tentlike formation. The close proximity of vitreous and iris make damage to the underlying iris stroma likely, but this may be clinically tolerable.

Directing the laser at the vitreous as it passes around the pupil is tempting, but rarely successful. The vitreous traction components are poorly defined as they come around the pupil. The shock wave is ineffective at rupturing vitreous strands except directly at the laser focal point. Firing the laser immediately adjacent to the pupillary border inevitably causes low-grade capillary hemorrhage as well as release of pigment, obscuring further visualization of the area.

Successful treatment releases the tension and converts a discrete strand or band to an amorphous gelatinous appearance. Observation of the change in any iris deformation is the best indicator of successful release of tension. Hundreds of shots may be necessary to cut a large band.

Postoperative Care for Vitreolysis

Strong topical steroids (prednisolone 1%, dexamethsaone 0.1%) are given four times daily until visual improvement occurs, typically in 2 to 3 months.

Pressure rise following vitreolysis has not been well documented. In our experience no patient has been observed to have a pressure increase in excess of 10 mm Hg. A drop of timolol 0.5% at the time of treatment probably provides adequate prophylaxis, if desired.

We consider systemic administration of diflunisal 500 mg twice daily with meals if no visual improvement has occurred in 1 month and no residual traction is present. If the patient cannot tolerate indomethacin, other nonsteroidal antiinflammatory medications can be substituted. A 4-week trial of systemic medication should be adequate to assess the potential for improvement.

Postoperative Anterior Capsular Fragmentation

Retained anterior capsule after extracapsular cataract extraction can become visually significant in several ways. Capsular tags usually retract if they are small. Larger tags may continue to remain in the visual axis and be visually troublesome to the patient. These fragments can be readily severed by the Nd:YAG laser.

Technique for Disruption of Anterior Capsule Fragments

The anterior capsule fragments generally are disrupted with 1 to 4 mJ in only a few pulses. A gonioscopy lens is occasionally useful to properly direct the laser beam to the target.

Postoperative Care

Inflammatory reaction and pressure rise are usually minimal and should be treated as they occur.

References

1. Aron-Rosa D, Aron JJ, Greiseman M, Thyzel R: Use of the neodymium-YAG laser to open the posterior capsule after lens implant surgery. A preliminary report. J Am Intraocul Implant Soc 6:352–354, 1980.
2. Aron-Rosa D, Griesemann JC, Aron JJ: Use of a pulsed neodymium-YAG laser (picosecond) to open the posterior lens capsule in traumatic cataract: A preliminary report. Ophthalmic Surg 12:496–499, 1981.
3. Fankhauser F, Lortscher H, Van der Zypen E: Clinical studies on high and low power laser radiation upon some structures of the anterior and posterior segments of the eye. Int Ophthalmol 5:15–32, 1982.
4. Wilhemus KR, Emery JM: Posterior capsule opacification following phacoemulsification. In Emery JM, Jacobson AC (eds): Current Concepts in Cataract Surgery: Selected Proceedings of the Sixth Biennial Cataract Surgical Congress. Mosby, St. Louis, 1980, pp. 304–308.
5. Emery JM, Wilhemus KR, Rodenberg S: Complications of phacoemulsification. Ophthalmology 85:141–150, 1978.
6. McDonnell PJ, Zarbin MA, Green WR: Posterior capsule opacification in pseudophakic eyes. Ophthalmology 90:1548–1553, 1983.
7. Sinskey RM, Cain W: The posterior capsule and phacoemulsification. J Am Intraocul Implant Soc 4:206–207, 1978.
8. Faulkner W: Laser interferometric prediction of postoperative visual acuity in patients with cataracts. Am J Ophthalmol 95:626–636, 1983.
9. Riggins J, Pedrotti LS, Keates RH: Evaluation of the neodymium-YAG laser for treatment of ocular opacities. Ophthalmic Surg 14:675–682, 1983.
10. Keates RH, Steinert RF, Puliafito CA, Maxwell SK: Long-term followup of Nd-YAG laser posterior capsulotomy. J Am Intraocul Implant Soc 10:164–168, 1984.
11. Vine AK. Ocular hypertension following Nd-YAG laser capsulotomy: A potentially blinding complication. Ophthalmic Surg 15:283–284, 1984.
12. Richter CU, Arzeno G, Pappas H, et al: Intraocular pressure elevation following Nd-YAG laser posterior capsulotomy. Ophthalmology 92:636–640, 1985.

13. Channell MM, Beckman H: Intraocular pressure changes after neodymium-YAG laser posterior capsulotomy. Arch Ophthalmol 102:1024–1026, 1984.
14. Kraff MC, Sanders DR, Lieberman HL: Intraocular pressure and the corneal endothelium after neodymium-YAG laser posterior capsulotomy: Relative effects of aphakia and pseudophakia. Arch Ophthalmol 103:511–514, 1985.
15. Ruderman JM, Mitchell PG, Kraff M: Pupillary block following Nd-YAG capsulotomy. Ophthalmic Surg 14:418–419, 1983.
16. Shrader CE, Belcher CD III, Thomas JV, Simmons RJ: Acute glaucoma following Nd-YAG laser membranectomy. Ophthalmic Surg 14:1015–1016, 1983.
17. Terry AC, Stark WJ, Maumenee AE, Fagadau W: Neodymium-YAG laser for posterior capsulotomy. Am J Ophthalmol 96:716–720, 1983.
18. Fastenberg DM, Schwartz PL, Lin HZ: Retinal detachment following neodymium-YAG laser capsulotomy. Am J Ophthalmol 97:288–291, 1984.
19. Parker WT, Clorfeine GS, Stocklin RD: Marked intraocular pressure rise following Nd-YAG laser capsulotomy. Ophthalmic Surg 15 103–104, 1984.
20. Knolle GE: Knife versus neodymium:YAG laser posterior capsulotomy: A one year follow-up. Am Intraocular Implant Soc J 11:448–455, 1985.
21. Epstein DL, Jedziniak JA, Grant WM: Obstruction of aqueous outflow by lens particles and by heavy molecular-weight soluble lens proteins. Invest Ophthalmol Vis Sci 17:272–277, 1978.
22. Schubert HD, Morris WJ, Trokel SL, Balazs EA: The role of the vitreous in the intraocular pressure rise after neodymium-YAG laser capsulotomy. Arch Ophthalmol 103:1538–1542, 1985.
23. Brown SVL, Thomas JV, Belcher CD, Simmons RJ: Effect of pilocarpine in treatment of intraocular pressure elevation following neodymium:YAG laser posterior capsulotomy. Ophthalmology 92:354–359, 1985.
24. Richter CU, Arzeno G, Pappas HR, et al: Prevention of intraocular pressure elevation following neodymium-YAG laser posterior capsulotomy. Arch Ophthalmol 103:912–915, 1985.
25. Epstein DL, Steinert RF, Puliafito CA: Neodymium-YAG laser therapy to the anterior hyaloid in aphakic malignant (ciliovitreal block) glaucoma. Am J Ophthalmol 98:137–143, 1984.
26. Irvine SR: A newly defined vitreous syndrome following cataract surgery. Am J Ophthalmol 36:599–619, 1953.
27. Gass JDM, Norton EWD: Cystoid macular edema and papilledema following cataract extraction. Arch Ophthalmol 76:646–661, 1966.
28. Iliff CE: Treatment of vitreous-tug syndrome. Am J Ophthalmol 62:856–859, 1966.
29. Katzen LE, Fleishman JA, Trokel S: YAG laser treatment of cystoid macular edema. Am J Ophthalmol 95:589–592, 1983.
30. Gass JDM, Norton EWD: Follow-up study of cystoid macular edema following cataract extraction. Trans Am Acad Ophthalmol Otolaryngol 73:665–682, 1969.
31. Jacobson DR, Dellaporta A: Natural history of cystoid macular edema after cataract extraction. Am J Ophthalmol 77:445–447, 1974.

38
General Anesthesia for Nd:YAG Laser Surgery

Kevin C. Moore

In spite of the high initial costs, an increasing number of medical centers are installing laser facilities. The endoscopic use of the Nd:YAG laser is well documented, and its multidisciplinary application has been described by Joffe et al.[1] A new generation of contact probes are now available that have greatly extended the operative range of the Nd:YAG laser, and its use is currently being explored in a wide variety of open operative procedures. The advantages of these new probes and their possible applications have been highlighted by Joffe.[2]

Anesthesiologists can therefore expect to be increasingly involved in the provision of anesthesia for laser surgery. To date, world anesthesia journals have carried a paucity of articles dedicated to the subject. It is hoped that this chapter will stimulate interest and instigate valuable exchanges of clinical experience.

Laser Biophysics

As with any surgical procedure, a knowledge of surgical technique and effect is of prime importance to the anesthesiologist. For Nd:YAG laser surgery, the anesthesiologist should make himself familiar with the basic biophysics of the Nd:YAG laser including the physical properties of the laser beam and its biologic effect on tissues. All these have been well documented by Fuller[3] and by Carruth and McKenzie.[4]

Laser Safety

Accidents during laser use, although small in number, can be devastating in effect. The Nd:YAG laser with a high power capacity is a class IV device, which attracts strict national safety regulations. In the United Kingdom these are laid down by the Department of Health.[5] All personnel involved in laser therapy should be familiar with the potential hazards and fully conversant with the safety requirements. The anesthesiologist is perhaps ideally placed to supervise the correct operating room procedure.

Anesthesia for Endoscopy

The endoscopic use of the Nd:YAG laser to treat lesions of the bronchial tree, gastrointestinal tract and urinary bladder is expanding. The choice between general or local anesthesia would appear in most cases to depend on user preference, specific laser technique, and the availability of anesthesia services. Whenever general anesthesia is administered for laser surgery the potential fire risk precludes the use of inflammable or explosive anesthetic gas mixtures.

Bronchoscopy

In chest medicine the Nd:YAG laser has primarily been used for the treatment of inoperable malignant lesions of the tracheobronchial tree. In a report of 1000 endobronchial resections, Dumon et al.[6] preferred the use of a rigid bronchoscope under general anesthesia with spontaneous ventilation. The use of the rigid scope ensures proper ventilation, enables the prompt and adequate treatment of hemorrhage, and allows the removal of necrotic debris. The main operative problems include hypoxemia, cardiac arrhythmias, hemorrhage, and airway perforation. Toty et al.[7] also recommend the use of a rigid bronchoscope under general anesthesia and describe their technique of maintaining anesthesia with an intravenous infusion of short-acting agents, while producing muscle relaxation with a suxamethonium infusion and ventilating via a modified Sanders injector using an equal mixture of nitrogen and oxygen. More recently, Dumon and Harrell[8] have described a modification of their general anesthetic technique, introducing the use of jet ventilation.

Other workers, however, prefer the use of a fiberoptic endoscope with topical analgesia and intravenous sedation. Unger and Atkinson[9] reported a series of 30 cases, all using a fiberscope under topical anesthesia. They cite the advantages of useful patient cooperation, avoidance of the risks of general anesthesia, and low procedure cost. McDougall and Cortese[10] also recommend the use of a flexible fiberscope. Hetzel et al.[11] give a detailed account of their method of topical analgesia supplemented by intravenous sedation using diazepam and small doses of diamorphine. A further technique is to introduce the flexible bronchoscope down the endotracheal tube of the anesthetized patient. The problems of obstruction to gas flow during inspiration and expiration caused by this maneuver have been reported by Bunnage and Bennett.[12]

It seems clear that one technique is not suitable for all cases. With careful patient selection many can be treated with the fiberscope as an outpatient procedure under local anesthesia. Conversely, for large obstructive lesions of central airways the method of choice must be general anesthesia with a rigid scope. This is particularly so when the noncontact, high-power method of Nd:YAG delivery is used. Smoke production is excessive, causing severe discomfort with coughing and struggling in the unanesthetized patient. This usually results in the abandonment of the procedure with the need for early retreatment. Heavy intravenous sedation is only partially successful in settling the patient and only serves to produce all the risks of general anesthesia with none of its benefits.

Hetzel et al.[13] now describe a technique combining the use of both the fiberoptic and rigid endoscope. The fiberscope allows the precise control of the Nd:YAG fiber tip for accurate aiming, while the rigid scope promotes effective suction and easy removal of necrotic debris. The technique is performed under general anesthesia, which allows the operator sufficient time to achieve a more complete result at one session, thus obviating the need for frequent initial treatments.

Gastroenterology

The endoscopic use of the Nd:YAG laser for the treatment of acute upper gastrointestinal hemorrhage and for the palliation of obstructive and hemorrhagic tumors of the esophagus, stomach, colon, and rectum is well established. As in bronchoscopy, the choice between general anesthesia or topical analgesia with intravenous sedation seems to be one of user preference. A significant number of users are physician endoscopists with presumably little or no access to regular anesthesia services.

For the treatment of severe upper gastrointestinal hemorrhage, general anesthesia with intubation is recommended to avoid the danger of aspiration and to ensure adequate oxygenation.[14] The one potential problem during anesthesia is caused by the high coaxial CO_2 gas flow down the laser fiber. This can cause rapid overdistension of the abdominal viscera with consequent impairment of respiration. Venting of the gas can be achieved either by using a two channel endoscope or by introducing a small-bore nasogastric tube beside the scope.[15] In practice, neither of these two methods are totally satisfactory, and the answer must be constant vigilance and close cooperation between operator and anesthesiologist. Excepting this, the problems involved in general anesthesia are those mainly associated with the elderly high-risk patient.

In Hira's[16] series of Nd:YAG laser treatment of tumors of the esophagus, stomach, colon, and rectum all patients received general anesthesia. This method allows the operator the necessary time to achieve a complete treatment in one session, thus reducing the need for early reoperation. There were no problems relating to anesthesia and no operative mortality. General anesthesia can be safely administered for these endoscopic procedures to patients otherwise unfit for major operative surgery.

Urology

Several centers now use the Nd:YAG laser for the routine treatment of bladder tumors.

Sacknoff[17] recommends its use on an outpatient basis. Hofstetter et al.[18] describe a large series for the majority of which they employed topical analgesia plus intravenous sedation. The main reported danger during treatment is of bladder perforation with possible damage to adjacent intestinal tissues. All users admit to the production of bladder discomfort during laser treatment. Where this becomes a problem they advocate the use of regional anesthesia or occasionally general anesthesia.

Patient acceptance of laser treatment might be promoted by the greater use of day case anesthesia services which exist in most modern centers.

Anesthesia for Open Surgery

The introduction of contact probes suitable for use with low-power Nd:YAG laser energy has provided laser users with a versatile new tool.[19] The advantages over the noncontact method of usage include greater precision of use, less damage to adjacent tissues, the elimination of laser light backscatter and virtually no smoke plume. The coagulating properties of the Nd:YAG laser are retained at low power. Finally, by attaching the probe to a handpiece the surgeon has a laser scalpel, which he can use in similar fashion to the conventional knife.[2]

The current use of the Nd:YAG laser in all specialties is reviewed by Carruth and McKenzie.[20] Work in some of these is still experimental and requires evaluation. In others, years of experience have demonstrated a positive role for Nd:YAG laser surgery in certain procedures.

In dermatology, the removal of tattoos and the excision of cutaneous lesions by the Nd:YAG laser is performed mainly under topical or local anesthesia. Only the more extensive or deep-seated vascular malformations and hemangiomas require general anesthesia.[21] The anterior segment of eye procedures of posterior capsulotomy and peripheral iridotomy in ophthalmology are carried out under topical anesthesia.[22] In gynecology, endometrial ablation via the hysteroscope under spinal or general anesthesia has been reported by Goldrath and Fuller.[23]

For the remaining specialties using Nd:YAG laser techniques, special reference to anesthesia should be made in neurosurgery, otorhinolaryngology, and general surgery.

Neurosurgery

Takeuchi et al.[24] have described the use of the Nd:YAG laser via a focusing handpiece for debulking large vascular tumors such as meningiomas. A number of hand applicators are available for use with the operating microscope. In 1980 Jain[25] described his techniques for vascular welding using the Nd:YAG laser. General anesthesia is the method of choice for laser neurosurgery. Cerrulo and Koht[26] stress the need for the total immobilization of the patient. All movements should be reduced to a minimum, including the normal physiologic activities such as respiration and myocardial contraction. Their technique involves muscular relaxation, high dosage of potent narcotic analgesics, and ventilation with nitrous oxide and oxygen at a rate of 7 to 8 breaths per minute.

Otorhinolaryngology

More has been written about anesthesia for CO_2 laser surgery of the larynx than about anesthesia for all the other forms of laser surgery put together. It is potentially the most hazardous situation an anesthesiologist will face. Nevertheless, the benefits of laser surgery in the oropharynx and larynx are so great that its use will increase and become standard practice wherever laser facilities exist.[27] The fire hazard that exists is a possible consequence of the impingement of a misdirected laser beam on a combustible endotracheal tube. Several methods have been devised to avoid this catastrophe. Most commonly, a red rubber endotracheal tube is wrapped with an aluminum or copper adhesive-backed metal tape. Inflammable or explosive gas mixtures are avoided, and, wherever possible, the inspired oxygen concentration is maintained between 25 and 30%.

Several metal tubes have been devised that are nonignitable. They have the disadvantage of being uncuffed, and most have a small internal diameter, which may give problems with gas delivery. In addition, they are a potential source of laryngotracheal trauma and do not exclude the possibility of reflective damage. Nevertheless, in experienced hands they have a proven safety record.[28] A laminated cuffed silicone laser-resistant endotracheal tube has been devised by Xomed.[29] Alternatives to endotracheal intubation include the use of a nasopharyngeal airway with spontaneous respiration, which lacks good airway control, or the more popular method of Venturi ventilation.[30] Thode[31] has produced an excellent review of anesthesia for laser surgery of the larynx.

While all the above comments refer to the CO_2 laser it seems reasonable to assume that they would also apply to the use of high-power noncontact Nd:YAG laser energy. However, with the introduction of low-power contact probes for Nd:YAG laser usage the attendant risks may not be so great. There would certainly be a reduction in the danger of both reflective damage and backscatter. Precision of use should be greater. If the contact Nd:YAG probe can match the CO_2 laser for operative ability and postoperative results, then the reduction in the anesthetic risk would be welcomed by anesthesiologists. It is too early to make valid judgments, but initial results on tongue and buccal mucosa are encouraging.[32]

General Surgery

The field of general surgery offers the greatest scope for the use and evaluation of low-power contact Nd:YAG laser surgery. Areas of application include the body surface for such procedures as mastectomy, excision of cutaneous and subcutaneous lesions, herniorrhaphy, hemorrhoidectomy, and the debridement of infected ulcers and bedsores. Within the body cavities its use is postulated for resection of the gastrointestinal tract and for excision of solid organs and tumors.[33] To date, reports of this work are mainly limited to conference presentations.

In their series of gastrointestinal tract surgery, Steger et al.[34] reported the use of contact Nd:YAG laser in bowel resection, cholecystectomy, and on solid vascular organs such as liver, spleen, and pancreas. Sultan et al.[35] used an Nd:YAG focusing handpiece and a combined CO_2 and Nd:YAG delivery system in their series of liver resections. Both reports stress the reduced blood loss and excellent hemostasis achieved when operating on highly vascular organs.

I have studied and reported on the benefits of contact Nd:YAG laser surgery and their effect on the anesthetic management of patients.[36] The increased precision of use, reduced instrumentation, and minimal damage to adjacent tissues resulted in a reduced level of intraoperative trauma. The coagulating effect of the laser greatly reduced the operative blood loss, especially in highly vascular tissues. Because of the foregoing, stable anesthesia was well maintained with minimal need for incremental dosage of analgesic or relaxant drugs. Cardiovascular stability was impressive with little variation in pulse rate and blood pressure, and the need for blood transfusion was virtually eliminated. In this reported series of anesthesia for some 60 laser procedures, more than 50% of the patients were in the 70–90 years age group, with a preponderance of Grades III and IV, according to the American Society of Anesthesiologists classification of physical status. The obvious benefits to these patients of laser surgery can be well appreciated by anesthesiologists. Immediate postoperative recovery was rapid and uncomplicated. As has been reported with CO_2 laser surgery, there appeared to be a definite reduction in initial postoperative pain levels and early mobilization was achieved in most cases.

Further experience in anesthesia for more than 100 laser operations has supported these impressions, which are currently being evaluated by prospective comparative studies of laser versus conventional operating techniques. With this in mind, I reported on a standard anesthetic technique suitable for the majority of laser and conventional operative procedures.[37] Following premedication with lorazepam, anesthesia is induced with sodium thiopentone, muscular relaxation with alcuronium, and analgesia with fentanyl (or alfentanil in short procedures). Ventilation is by intermittent positive pressure with a gas mixture of oxygen and nitrous oxide. Incremental doses of muscle relaxant and analgesic are given when clinically indicated. Vital parameters are monitored and recorded. Blood loss is measured. All anesthesia is administered by the same anesthesiologist. Postoperatively, recovery, analgesic requirements, mobilization, morbidity, and hospital stay are also recorded.

The results of a small trial involving simple mastectomy for malignancy and following this methodology is shown in Table 38.1. This

TABLE 38.1. Comparison of contact Nd:YAG laser and conventional surgery: Breast surgery

Factor	Laser	Nonlaser
No. of cases	10	10
Age range (years)	49–92	49–84
Blood loss (average in ml)	34	208
Wound drainage	None	All
Postoperative analgesia (no. of cases requiring)		
Papaveretum	2	6
Paracetamol	6	3
Nil	2	1
Mobilization		
<12 hours	3	0
<24 hours	5	5
<48 hours	2	5
Complications	1	1
Inpatient stay (average in days)	5.5	8.5

showed reduced blood loss, reduced analgesic requirement, earlier mobilization, and shorter hospitalization in the contact Nd:YAG laser group.[38]

Conclusion

The anesthesiologist's contribution to endoscopic laser therapy varies according to user preference. Nevertheless, general anesthesia is safe and gives the operator and the patient the advantage of completing initial treatment in a single session.

In open surgery there is clear evidence that technologic advances have initiated the use of contact Nd:YAG laser surgery in many specialties and extended its use in others. Anesthesiologists will therefore be called upon to provide general anesthesia with increasing frequency. The opportunity exists to contribute to the assessment and evaluation of new laser procedures by the application of their own specialized skills and experience.

Currently the only clear conclusion is that for the high-risk elderly patient requiring anesthesia and surgery the contact Nd:YAG laser is the method of choice for both surgeon and anesthesiologist.

References

1. Joffe SN, Muckerheide MC, Goldman L: Neodymium-YAG Laser in Medicine and Surgery. Elsevier, New York, 1983.
2. Joffe SN: Contact neodymium: YAG laser surgery in gastroenterology: A preliminary report. Lasers Surg Med 6:155–157, 1986.
3. Fuller TA: Fundamentals of lasers in surgery and medicine. In Dixon JA (ed): Surgical Application of Lasers. Year Book Medical Publishers, Chicago, 1983, pp 11–28.
4. Carruth JAS, McKenzie AL: Medical Lasers, Science and Clinical Practice. Adam Hilger, Bristol and Boston, 1986, pp. 36–38, 56–70.
5. Department of Health and Social Security: Guidance on the Safe use of Lasers in Medical Practice. HMSO, London, 1984.
6. Dumon JF, Bourcereau J, Meric B, et al: Report of 1000 YAG laser endobronchial resections. In Joffe SN, Muckerheide MC (eds): Neodymium-YAG Laser in Medicine and Surgery. Elsevier, New York, 1983, pp. 60–69.
7. Toty L, Personne C, Colchen A, Vourc'h G: Brochoscopic management of tracheal lesions using the neodymium yttrium aluminum garnet laser. Thorax 36:175–178, 1981.
8. Dumon JF, Harrell J: A universal rigid bronchoscope. (Abstract 244). Lasers Surg Med 6:196–197, 1986.
9. Unger M, Atkinson GW: Nd:YAG Laser Applications in Pulmonary and Endobronchial Lesions. In Joffe SN, Muckerheide MC (eds): Neodymium-YAG Laser in Medicine and Surgery. Elsevier, New York, 1983. pp 71–81.
10. McDougall JC, Cortese DA: Neodymium YAG laser therapy of malignant airway obstruction. Mayo Clin Proc 58:35, 1983.
11. Hetzel MR, Millard FJC, Ayesh R, et al: Laser treatment for carcinoma of the bronchus. Br Med J 286:12–16, 1983.
12. Bunnage SM, Bennett MJ: Nd:YAG laser airway surgery: Resistance of tracheal tubes partially occluded by flexible bronchoscope. (Abstract 162). Anesthesiology 63:3A, 1985.
13. Hetzel MR, Nixon C, Edmonstone WM, et al: Laser therapy in 100 tracheobronchial tumors. Thorax 40:341–345, 1985.
14. Keifhaber P, Kiefhaber K, Huber F, Nath G: Endoscopic applications of Neodymium-YAG laser radiation in the gastrointestinal tract. In Joffe SN, Muckerheide MC (eds): Neodymium-YAG Laser in Medicine and Surgery. Elsevier, New York. 1983, pp. 5–14.
15. Swain CP: Endoscopic Nd:YAG laser control of gastrointestinal bleeding. In Joffe SN, Muckerheide MC (eds): Neodymium-YAG Laser in Medicine and Surgery. Elsevier, New York, 1983, pp 15–28.
16. Steger A, Hira N, Moore KC: Inoperable gastrointestinal tract tumors. (Abstract 286). Lasers Surg Med 6:278, 1986.
17. Sacknoff EJ: Neodymium-YAG laser in urology.

In Joffe SN, Muckerheide MC (eds): Neodymium-YAG Laser in Medicine and Surgery. Elsevier, New York, 1983, pp 105–117.
18. Hofstetter A, Frank F, Keiditsch E, Bowering R: Endoscopic neodymium-YAG laser application for destroying bladder tumors. Eur Urol 7:278–282, 1981.
19. Joffe SN, Daikuzono N: Multidisciplinary applications of contact Nd:YAG laser surgery. (Abstract 39). Lasers Surg Med 6:217, 1986.
20. Carruth JAS, McKenzie AL: Medical Lasers, Science and Clinical Practice. Adam Hilger, Bristol and Boston, 1986.
21. Rosenfeld H, Sherman R: Treatment of cutaneous and deep vascular lesions with the Nd:YAG laser. Lasers Surg Med 6:20–23, 1986.
22. Jagger J, Dhillon BJ: Nd:YAG laser therapy for the anterior segment of the eye. Lasers Med Sci 1:139–142, 1986.
23. Goldrath MH, Fuller TA: Hysteroscopic ablation of the endometrium using Nd:YAG laser. Lasers Surg Med 3:186, 1983.
24. Takeuchi J, Handa H, Taki W, Yamagami T: The Nd:YAG laser in neurological surgery. Surg Neurol 18:140–142, 1982.
25. Jain KK: Sutureless microvascular repair with neodymium-YAG laser. J Microsurg 1:436, 1980.
26. Cerrulo LJ, Koht A: Anesthesiological considerations in laser neurosurgery. Lasers Surg Med 3:1–35, 1983.
27. Carruth JAS, McKenzie AL: Medical Lasers, Science and Clinical Practice. Adam Hilger, Bristol and Boston, 1986, pp 164–179.
28. Anand VK, Herbert J, Robbett WF, Zellman W: Safe anesthesia for endoscopic laryngeal laser surgery. (Abstract 27). Lasers Surg Med 6:203, 1986.
29. Xomed Inc: Laser Shield Endotracheal Tube. Product Literature, Jacksonville, FL, 1983.
30. Norton ML, Strong MS, Vaughn CW, et al: Endotracheal intubation and venturi (jet) ventilation for laser microsurgery of the larynx. Ann Otol Rhinol Laryngol 87:554–557, 1978.
31. Thode SA: Laryngo-tracheal laser surgery and general anesthesia. Lasers Surg Med 6:369–372, 1986.
32. Hira N: Personal communication, 1986.
33. Joffe SN, Daikuzono N: Contact laser surgery in gastroenterology—An update on the endoscopic and open surgical applications. (Abstract 20). Lasers Surg Med 6:200, 1986.
34. Steger A, Hira N, Moore KC: Use of laser in gastrointestinal disease and lasers in gastrointestinal surgery. (Abstract 287:288). Lasers Surg Med 6:279, 1986.
35. Sultan RA, Fallouh H, Lefebvre-Vilardebo M, Ladouch-Badre A: Separate and combined use of Nd:YAG and carbon dioxide lasers in liver resections: A preliminary report. Lasers Med Sci 1:101–105, 1986.
36. Moore KC: Anesthesia for Nd:YAG laser surgery. Todays Anaesthesiol 1:6–7, 1986.
37. Steger A, Moore KC, Hira N: Anesthesia for laser surgery. (Abstract 290). Lasers Surg Med 6:280, 1986.
38. Steger A, Hira N, Moore KC: Contact laser surgery. (Abstract 289). Lasers Surg Med 6:279–280, 1986.

39 The Variable-Function Fiberoptic Laser Apparatus Using Nd:YAG and Carbon Monoxide Lasers

Tsunenori Arai, and Makoto Kikuchi

For laser apparatus used in medical treatments, there are two major requirements that have not been completely met. One of them is the use of a flexible optical transmitting line by which endoscopic medical applications will be possible. The other is the possession of a variable function of cutting/coagulating performance similar to the electrical surgical unit. By solving these problems, laser apparatus will be adaptable to treat complex medical conditions. The former requirement has been partially solved using Nd:YAG or argon laser deliveries by a silica glass fiber. Both of the interactions of the argon and Nd:YAG lasers essentially indicate thermal coagulation. The latter requirement has been partially met using the combined irradiation of Nd:YAG and CO_2 lasers.[1] The variable function was realized by the power-ratio control of these lasers, since the strong cutting interaction occurs by the CO_2 laser radiation. However, the laser apparatus that simultaneously satisfies all of these requirements has not been realized yet. One cause of this non-establishment is due to a lack of flexible optical fibers for the CO_2 laser radiation, which indicates a strong cutting function.

In this chapter we describe our own novel method for fulfilling these requirements. In order to solve the lack of flexible fibers for cutting lasers, CO lasers of oscillation wavelength 5-μm band have been employed as cutting lasers.[2] At this wavelength, chalcogenides and fluorides of infrared glass materials are available to make the flexible optical fibers. Moreover, even Nd:YAG lasers can transmit some types of fibers made from these glasses. Thus the combination of Nd:YAG and CO lasers with infrared glass fibers will realize a variable-function fiberoptic laser apparatus for medical treatments. Figure 39.1 shows a schematic conceptual illustration of the variable-function fiberoptic laser apparatus.[3] The power delivery of CO and Nd:YAG lasers and the variable tissue interaction by the power-ratio control of CO and Nd:YAG lasers are presented in this chapter. The characteristics of the CO laser irradiation on the living tissue is described in Chapter 42 of this book.

Principles of the Variable-Function Fiberoptic Laser Apparatus

The Variable Function and Fiber Delivery

The Variable Function by Combined Irradiation

The variable function to medical treatments, that is cutting/coagulating capacity change, will be completely obtained by a wavelength change of laser light source due to a change of the tissue interaction between a laser light and tissue. In order to establish this function, it is necessary to change the wavelength of a high-power laser from at least 1 to 3 μm. Although the tunability of lasers has been attained in this region, they have reached neither high-power nor compact. The employment of the tunable laser to medical treatment equipment is impossible. A unique method to practically obtain the variable function has been by the employment of simulta-

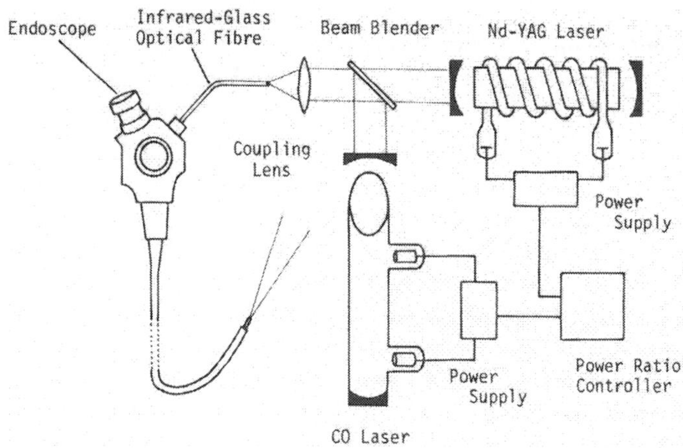

FIGURE 39.1. A schematic conceptual illustration of the variable-function fiberoptic laser apparatus. [From Arai T, Kikuchi M, Sakuragi S, Saito M, Takizawa M, CO laser power delivery by As_2S_3 IR glass fiber with Teflon cladding. In Katzir A (ed): Optical Fibers in Medicine and Biology, SPIE, Bellingham, 1985, pp 24–31, with permission.]

neous irradiation of coagulating and cutting lasers. A practical system using this method has been realized by the combined irradiation of Nd:YAG and CO_2 lasers. The variable function is realized by the power-ratio control of these lasers. The usefulness of this system has been particularly demonstrated in neurosurgery by this new tissue interaction.[1] However, its applications are quite limited since the manipulator arms (i.e., reflector array) must be used to deliver the laser beams in this system. Despite the fact that endoscopic applications of laser treatments have a great necessity for precise control of the laser interaction, , the use of the system for this application is impossible. The cause of this defect of the system is not only a lack of flexible optical fibers for the CO_2 laser light, but also the difficulty of the combined delivery to two different wavelength lasers. The flexible optical delivery should be preferentially considered to design laser apparatus for endoscopic application.

The Combined Power Delivery

The power delivery of laser beams by optical fibers has been reported by many authors,[4] almost all of them of the delivery of Nd:YAG lasers or CO_2 lasers. In all these reports, a certain kind of the fiber was selected for a certain kind of laser. Thus following, the variable-function laser apparatus, which uses two different laser beams, should employ two different power fibers. However, in the endoscopic application, it should be pointed out that the diameter of the biopsy hole (1.5 to 3 mm) is too small to insert two power fibers simultaneously. It would seem that the combined power delivery of two different laser beams by a single power fiber is necessary to develop the fiberoptic variable-function apparatus.

The wavelength of a coagulating laser is from visible to 1.5 μm. The wavelength of a cutting laser is over 3 μm. There are many crystalline fiber materials that cover both wavelengths. However, the optical transmission of crystalline fibers is decreased by repetitive bendings due to the increase of the scattering.[5] This growth of scattering is attributed to the production of scatterings by the destruction of the crystal structures from plastic strain. Since the Rayleigh scattering intensity is inversely proportional to the fourth power of the wavelength, the transmission of the crystalline fiber for the coagulating laser is strongly affected by this scattering. The medical fiber should resist tight repetitive bendings, so that the practical use of the crystalline fiber for the combined power delivery will be impossible. The brittle glass fiber is useful to prevent this scattering promotion by repetitive bendings.

Infrared glass materials have been studied to make an ultra-low-loss fiber for optical communications.[6] These materials have high mechanical strength with brittleness. Their transmission range extends from 1 to 8 μm, in general. However, they have not covered the CO_2 laser wavelength. Therefore, it is necessary to employ a new cutting laser that has a shorter wavelength than the CO_2 laser. CO lasers of wavelength 5 μm band have been selected as cutting laser radiation. The power delivery of CO lasers by the infrared glass fiber has already been successfully demonstrated by the authors.[7] This laser is a unique practical laser within cutting range of infrared wavelengths. Please refer to our Chapter concerning both the choice of CO lasers and the interaction of CO lasers.

Components of the Variable-Function Fiberoptic Laser Apparatus

Infrared Glass Fibers

The transmission loss of the fiber made from infrared glass has still been greater than desired for optical communications. However, since the practical transmission length of the medical fiber is only up to 2 m, the transmission loss of up to 3 dB/m is allowable without considering the heat-up of the fiber. The fibers made from these materials have thus already been adapted for medical applications as concerns the attenuation of the fiber.

The infrared glass materials are classified into three kinds of glasses, chalcogenides, fluorides, and oxides. Their optimum transmission wavelength becomes longer in the order: oxides, fluorides, and chalcogenides glasses. Figure 39.2 shows their transmission spectrum reported with the silica glass fiber.[8–11] The most typical glass systems are selected in the figure. As shown in Figure 39.2, chalcogenide glasses in particular, have a wide transmission range. Its transmission range generally extends from 1 to 8 μm. The combined power delivery of CO and Nd:YAG lasers is enabled by the wide transmission wavelength range of chalcogenide glass fibers. In general, the bonding energy of optical transmission materials is related to a transmission cutoff of a long wavelength side, so that chalcogenide glasses have a low mechanical strength within infrared glasses. However, the fibers made from them indicate further flexibility than crystalline glass fibers. In the near future, a fiber made from the fluoride glasses will be important candidates for CO laser delivery by their high mechanical characteristics

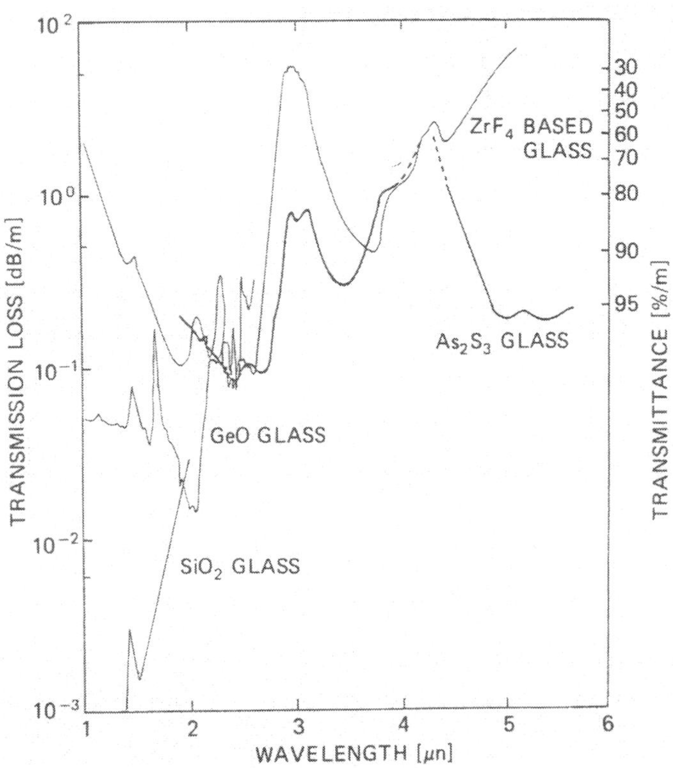

FIGURE 39.2. Transmission spectrum of typical infrared glass fibers reported with the silica glass fiber.

in spite of the discrepancy of wavelengths between their optimum transmission and CO laser radiation.

Infrared glasses are advantageous in mass production, since the normal drawing method for production of the silica glass fiber is adaptable to manufacturing the infrared glass fiber to reduce its cost. Hence, disposable use of the infrared glass fiber might be possible, so that the disinfection of the medical fiber may be eliminated.

Carbon Monoxide Lasers

Performance of CO Lasers

The CO laser, a kind of electrically excited gas laser, was discovered by Patel in 1964 using the same apparatus that was used for the first CO_2 laser.[12] The quantum efficiency which indicates the maximum theoretical efficiency is estimated at as high as 98.8% in spite of the impossibility of a precise definition of the efficiency of CO lasers. The cause of this high efficiency originated from the small friction of CO molecules. CO lasers are characterized by this high efficiency. Electrical efficiencies of 47 and 63% are reported in continuous and pulse mode operations, respectively.[13,14] However, in general it appears only when the temperature of the laser mixture is kept at a low value (for example, liquid nitrogen temperature), since the pumping process of this laser is strongly dependent on the gas temperature.

Room-Temperature CO Lasers

Room-temperature operations of CO lasers have been reported by many authors using a xenon additive in the laser mixture. The room-temperature operation is extremely important due to its usefulness for easy handling and maintenance, which are necessary for medical equipment. The role of xenon in CO laser kinetics is estimated to optimize electrical excitation efficiency to cover the low pumping speed at room temperature.[15] The room-temperature CO laser is less efficient than CO_2 lasers, so that the room-temperature CO laser is not popular in the market. The room-temperature CO laser was developed for use with spectroscopic applications, so that there was little interest in the improvement of the power and efficiency of of this kind of laser.[16] Currently, research of the room-temperature CO laser has focused on its sealed-off type.[17]

We have improved the performances of the room-temperature CO laser by high gas flow.[18] The gas flow (i.e., gas convection) extracts the heat generated by the waste energy of the laser kinetics to outside of the laser discharge region, so that the temperature of the laser mixture is decreased. This effect promotes excitation by the internal vibrational transfer of CO molecules and restricts the relaxation of CO molecules. The performances of our CO laser were at the maximum power of 40.7 W, the maximum efficiency of 20.3% from the laser tube of 1.06 m in length.[19] They indicated a 30% improvement in performance against previous reports.

There are few production models of CO lasers available in the world. Almost all of them are not immediately adaptable for medical treatment. However, since CO lasers can be manufactured by the same technique as CO_2 lasers, it will be easy to manufacture practical CO lasers to satisfy the medical application needs.

Fundamental Experiments of the Variable-Function Fiberoptic Laser Apparatus

Experiments of the Combined Power Delivery

Experimental Setup for the Combined Power Delivery

As_2S_3 Chalcogenide Glass Fiber

The chalcogenide glass fiber used in this experiment has been made by As_2S_3 glass, 400 μm in core diameter. The cladding is made of FEP Teflon resin, which protects the core surface from scratching. The core and the cladding are optically attached to form a core-clad structure. The allowable bending radius of this fiber is less than 30 mm. The transmission losses of this fiber for CO and Nd:YAG laser radiation are less than 1 dB/m.[20] The refractive index of the core material is 2.41 at 5 μm, so that approximately 30% of incident laser energy is reflected backward. In other words, the coupling efficiency is limited to 70%. To improve the coupling efficiency in the future, antireflection coatings will be available. The refractive index of cladding material is 1.3. This fiber transmits all incident light collimated on the incident surface. The solubility for water of As_2S_3 is 6×10^{-5} g/100 gH_2O. This solubility suggests a low toxicity of As_2S_3. The termination of the fiber was polished using fine-grade sandpaper, so to suppress the scattering of measured data for maximum power delivery.

Setup of Optical Components

We have demonstrated the combined power delivery of CO and Nd:YAG lasers by As_2S_3. The setup for the combined power delivery of the CO and Nd:YAG laser is illustrated in Figure 39.3.[21] The chalcogenide glass fiber made from As_2S_3 used in the experiment is as described above. Two laser beams were aligned into one beam on a ZnSe plate. The ZnSe plate was set at the Brewster angle for a liner polarized CO laser beam. The Nd:YAG laser beam reflected on the ZnSe plate was combined with the CO laser beam. The coupling efficiencies were 100% and 30% for CO and Nd:YAG lasers, respectively. This combined technique is appropriate only for laboratory use. In the actual application, multicoated dielectric beamblenders will be available to improve the coupling efficiency of both lasers. The combined beam was collimated into the incident end of the fiber by a CaF_2 lens of 75 mm of focal length. The beam diameter of the combined beam was 6 mm, so that the numerical aperture of incident optics was approximately 0.1. The fiber output was measured by a thermal power meter.

Results and Discussion of the Combined Power Delivery

The transmission loss under the power delivery was measured by an angle of line inclination, in a graph of the dependence of the fiber length on the fiber transmittance. The transmission loss for the Nd:YAG laser delivery was measured to 2.6 dB/m. The transmission loss for the CO laser delivery was 1.2 dB/m. Since the wavelength of the Nd:YAG laser, 1.06 μm, is near the low-wavelength cutoff for this fiber, the attenuation for Nd:YAG lasers is larger than that for CO lasers.

In order to determine the capacity of the power delivery, the incident laser power was increased until the fiber was destroyed. This experiment was undergone at various combined ratios of the Nd:YAG and CO lasers. In a previous paper[3] we revealed that the maximum capacity of the power delivery for a CO laser by the same As_2S_3 glass fiber was over 15 W. The light intensity at the output end of the fiber was in excess of 12 kW/cm^2.[3] By the experiment of the combined power delivery, it is evident that the maximum delivered power is decreased by increasing the Nd:YAG laser power ratio. Since the destruction of the fiber by the laser power results by melting down the fiber, it is well understood by the measured transmission loss which induces the heat generation. Nevertheless, the fiber could transmit over 8 W laser power with an output intensity of 6.4 kW/cm^2, even though the entire delivered light power

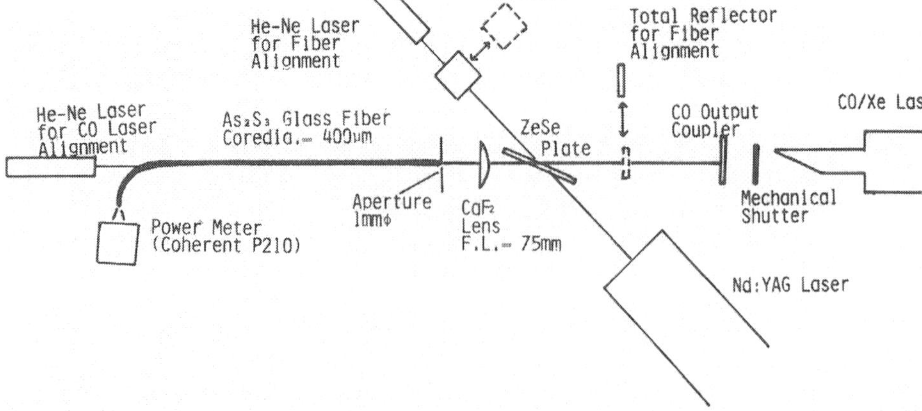

FIGURE 39.3. Schematic illustration of the setup for the combined power delivery of CO and Nd:YAG laser.

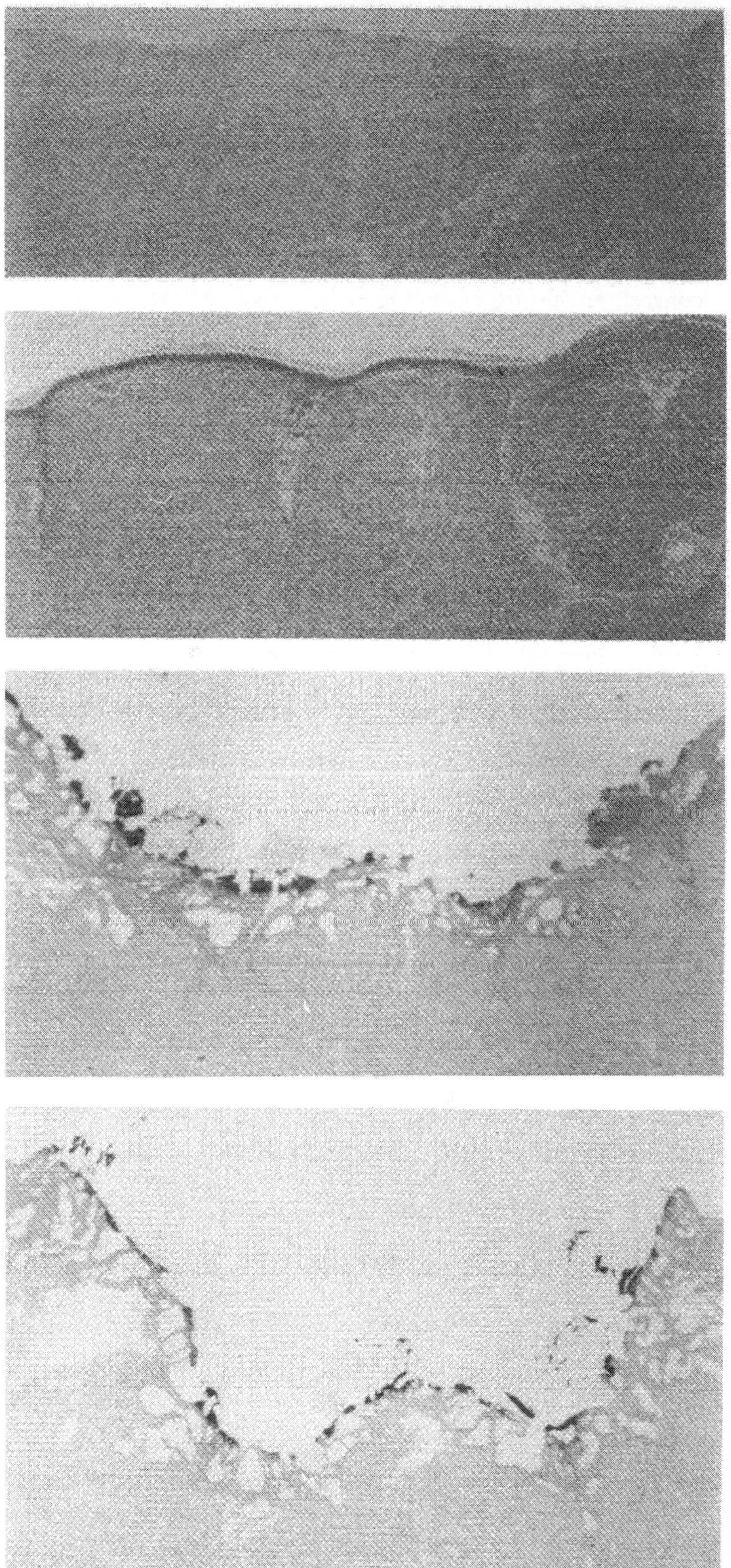

A

B

C

D

FIGURE 39.4. Microphotographs of manufactured specimens of combined irradiation samples. Irradiation power ratio (CO/Nd:YAG): (A) 0/100, (B) 5/95, (C) 10/90, (D) 25/75. Average light intensity: 1.2 kW/cm^2. Irradiation time: 15 seconds. Sample: cow liver.

consisted of a Nd:YAG laser.[21] It is noted that these performances were carried out by the 400 μm diameter fiber without any cooling of the fiber. This capability for power delivery will be sufficient to realize the variable-function fiber-optic laser apparatus. When forced cooling by air convection was applied to the ends of the fiber, the maximum delivered power was increased. However, since in practical endoscopic applications there are many geometric restrictions to attain forced cooling of the fiber, the power delivery fiber should be used without the cooling.

The Variable Function by the Power Ratio Control of the Nd:YAG and CO Lasers

Experimental Setup

The tissue interactions by the combined irradiation of CO and Nd:YAG lasers were experimentally measured in vitro. To demonstrate the usefulness of the simultaneous delivery by the fiber, the fiber output beam was used in this investigation. The exsanguinated livers of pigs were used as subjects. The total fiber output was fixed to 5 W. The fiber which was bent down to the sample in 80 mm of curvature was approximately 400 mm in length. A preliminary experiment was done to indicate that the fiber output originating two different lasers was constructed in a concentric configuration. The fiber output was directly irradiated on the liver sample of which the surface was separated 5 mm from the fiber termination. The averaged light intensity on the sample was 1.2 kW/cm^2. The power ratio of the CO and Nd:YAG laser was varied five steps within from 0/100 to 50/50. The irradiated livers were manufactured to tissue specimens.

Results and Discussion

Figure 39.4 shows microphotographs of manufactured specimens of irradiated samples. The irradiation power ratio (CO/Nd:YAG) increases from Figure 39.4A–D.[22] Despite the interaction of the thermal coagulation not being obviously indicated in the microphotographs, the cutting interaction was completely investigated. Figure 39.4A,B show the increase in temperature on the sample surface; still there was no cutting. Figure 39.4C,D show the strong cutting interaction. It is evident that the function variability is easily attained by the power ratio control of lasers. The depths of the cutting grooves in this experiment were not proportional to the CO laser power. In other words, the tissue interaction was sensitively varied to the addition of cutting laser power. This result may be attributed to a rapid change in the composition of the tissue surface by cutting laser irradiations. This fact suggests that the power of the CO laser which is necessary for the combined laser apparatus might be smaller than that of the Nd:YAG laser.

Summary

The variable-function fiberoptic laser apparatus for medical treatment was described in this chapter. The discussion of its conceptual design was described. The laser apparatus for medical treatment should be designed from a standpoint of flexible optical delivery, since endoscopic applications of the laser apparatus are both unique and the most important laser treatments. In addition, variable-function similar to the electrical surgical unit will be necessary. The employment of a new cutting laser and an infrared fiber made of new material make it possible to construct this apparatus. A brief explanation of the infrared glass fiber and the room-temperature CO laser was given. The experimental results of the fundamental combined power delivery of the Nd:YAG and CO laser by the flexible As_2S_3 glass fiber appealed to the validity of our approach. The tissue interactions by combined irradiation with a varying power ratio successfully demonstrated the variability of the function of this system. This apparatus will be useful for entire endoscopic applications including vascular recanalizations. The authors believe that this apparatus will be manufactured for actual application in the near future.

References

1. Tsuyumu M, Yamazaki S, Takei H, Suzuki K, et al: Experimental study of combined coaxial irradiation by high-peaked pulse wave form CO_2 and Nd:YAG laser on the brain. J Jpn Soc Laser Med 4:141–142, 1984.

2. Arai T, Kikuchi M: A study for development of CO laser scalpel (1) Investigation of the effect of CO laser light on living tissue. J Jpn Soc Laser Med 3:223–230, 1982.
3. Arai T, Kikuchi M, Sakuragi S, et al: CO laser power delivery by As_2S_3 IR glass fiber with Teflon cladding. In Katzir A (ed): Optical Fibers in Medicine and Biology. SPIE, Bellingham, 1985, pp 24–31.
4. Pinnow DA, Gentile L, Standlee AG, Timper AJ: Polycrystalline fiber optical waveguides for infrared transmission. Appl Phys Lett 33:28–29, 1978.
5. Mimura Y, Ota C: Transmission of CO_2 laser power by single-crystal CsBr fibers. Appl Phys Lett 40:773–775, 1982.
6. Miyashita T, Manabe T: Infrared optical fibers. IEEE J Quant Electron QE-18:1432–1450, 1982.
7. Arai T, Kikuchi M: Carbon monoxide laser power delivery with an As_2S_3 infrared glass fiber. Appl Opt 23:3017–3019, 1984.
8. Horiguchi M, Osanai H: Spectral losses of low-OH-content optical fibers. Electron Lett 12:310–312, 1976.
9. Takahashi H, Sugimoto I, Sato T: Germanium-oxide glass optical fiber prepared by VAD method. Electron Lett 18:398–399, 1982.
10. Mitachi S, Miyashita T: Preparation of low-loss fluoride glass fiber. Electron Lett 18:170–171, 1982.
11. Miyashita T, Terunuma Y: Optical transmission loss of As-S glass fiber in 1.0–5.5 μm wavelength region. Jpn J Appl Phys 21:L75–L76, 1982.
12. Patel CKN, Kerl RJ: Laser oscillation on $X^1\Sigma+$ vibrational-rotational transitions of CO. Appl Phys Lett 5:81–83, 1964.
13. Bhaumik ML, Lacina WB, Mann MM: Characteristics of CO laser. IEEE J Quant Electron QE-8:150–160, 1972.
14. Mann MM, Rice DK, Eguchi RG: An experimental investigation of high energy CO lasers. IEEE J Quant Electron QE-10:682–683, 1974.
15. Murray GA, Smith ALS: The efficacy of xenon as an additive gas in carbon monoxide lasers. J Phys D 11:2477–2487, 1978.
16. Peters PJM, Witteman WJ, Zuidema RJ: Efficient simple sealed-off CO laser at room temperature. Appl Phys Lett 32:119–121, 1980.
17. Browne PG, Smith ALS: Efficient long life sealed CO lasers at room temperature. J Phys E 8:870, 1975.
18. Arai T, Kikuchi M: High power coaxial-flow room-temperature CO laser. In Kaye AS, Walker AC (eds): Gas Flow and Chemical Lasers. Adam Hilger, Bristol, 1984, pp 29–34.
19. Arai T, Kikuchi M: High-power room-temperature CO laser. Appl Phys Lett 45:362–364, 1984.
20. Saito M, Takizawa M: Teflon clad As-S glass IR fiber with low absorption loss. J Appl Phys 59:1450–1452, 1986.
21. Arai T, Kikuchi M, Tomita Y, et al: Combined laser power delivery of CO laser and Nd:YAG laser by IR glass fiber. J Jpn Soc Laser Med 6:355–358, 1986.
22. Arai T, Kikuchi M, Tomita Y, et al: Simultaneous laser irradiation of fiber delivered CO and Nd:YAG laser on living tissue. J Jpn Soc Laser Med 6:283–286, 1986.

40

Computer-Controlled Contact Nd:YAG Laser System for Interstitial Local Hyperthermia

Norio Daikuzono, Masaru Ohyama, Stephen N. Joffe, Soutaro Suzuki, Hisao Tajiri, and Hiroshi Tsunekawa

Contact Nd:YAG laser surgery is assuming a greater importance in endoscopic and open surgery, allowing coagulation, cutting, and vaporization with greater precision and safety. A new contact probe allows a wider angle of irradiation and diffusion of low-power laser energy (< 5 W) using the interstitial technique for local hyperthermia. Continuously monitoring temperature sensors are placed directly into the surrounding tissue or tumor. Using a computer program interfaced with the laser and sensors, a controlled and stable temperature (e.g., 42°C) can be produced in a known volume of tissue over a prolonged period of time (e.g., 20–40 minutes).

Several kinds of energy resources have been used for hyperthermia.

1. Heat flow	Hot water
2. Electromagnetic energy	RF, Microwave
3. Sonic energy	Ultrasonic induction
4. Scattered light	Infrared light
5. Laser	Nd:YAG Laser

For hyperthermia, greater and more uniform heating, easier and more precise control for temperature, and no invasive methods are desired. For certain clinical purposes, localized hyperthermia and a means of transmitting energy are very important. The Nd:YAG Laser can be transmitted by a flexible optical fiber; it can penetrate tissue deeper than other kinds of medical lasers.

S.G. Bown[1] tried to use the Nd:YAG Laser for hyperthermia by the interstitial method—sticking bare fiber into a tumor. However, high-power density at the distal end of the fiber causes damage at the tip of the fiber and vaporizes the tissue. Burnt tissue, including char, absorbs laser energy and causes a very limited localized high temperature, which is difficult to control properly and is too unstable for use in hyperthermia. We have introduced several kinds of sapphire contact probes[2,3] for attachment to the Nd:YAG laser optical fiber (Figure 40.1 and 40.2). Contact probes delivering different kinds of beam patterns can be used for coagulating, vaporizing, and cutting tissue with much lower power than conventional noncontact methods (Figure 40.3). The interstitial contact probe has

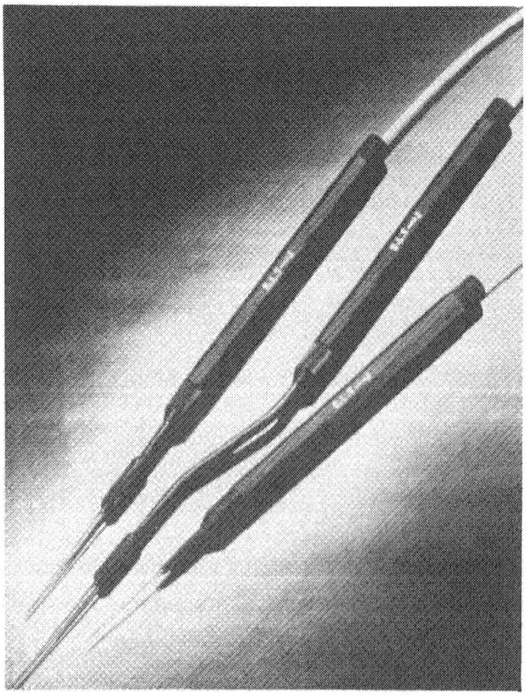

FIGURE 40.1 Contact laser scalpel.

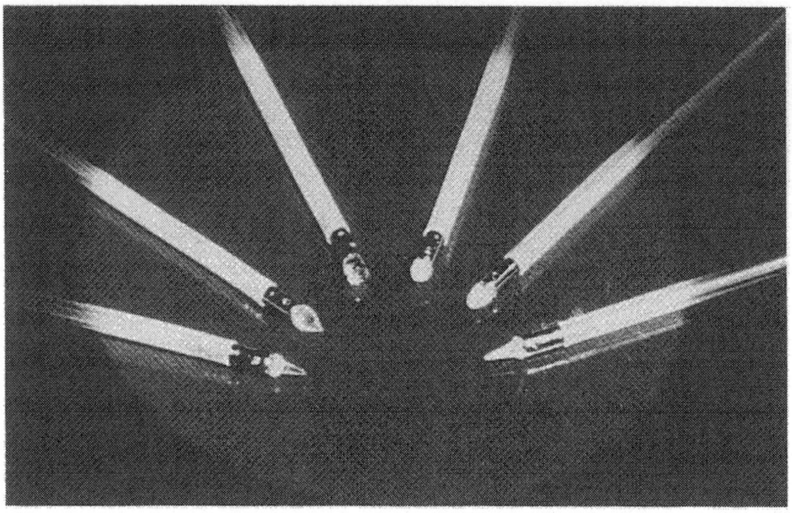

FIGURE 40.2. Contact endoprobes.

the ability to diffuse the laser beam on the probe surface because of its optical design (Figure 40.4). It can withstand higher temperature and is much harder than the bare quartz fiber, which assures thermal and mechanical stability. In this chapter, we will describe local hyperthermia controlled by a computer, using a thermocouple as monitor for temperature and an interstitial probe to transmit diffuse low power through the Nd:YAG laser. We call this method laserthermia® which is a registered trademark of Surgical Laser Technologies Inc. (Malvern, PA)

Interstitial Probes

Noncontact laser irradiation can lose 30–40% of beam energy to backscatter. The contact method, especially the interstitial method, can deliver the laser beam more effectively and quantitatively into tissue. This is very important for clinical procedures requiring a total dose of laser energy. The probe's conical shape facilitates mechanical penetration of the tumor (Table 40.1). Diffused laser light on the surface of the probe has lower power density, less than 0.05

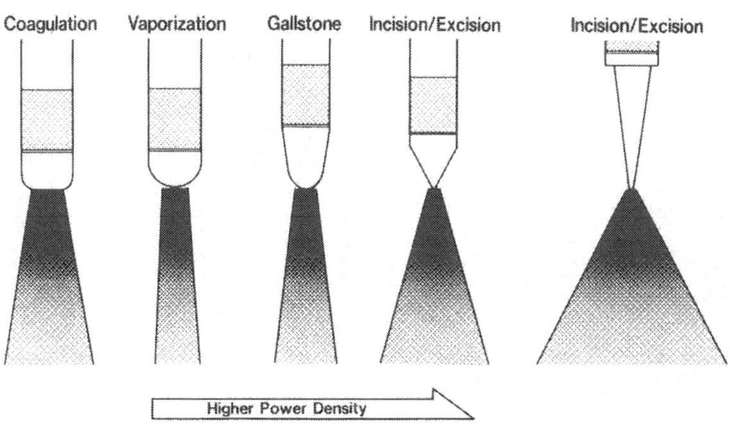

FIGURE 40.3 Beam divergence of endoprobe.

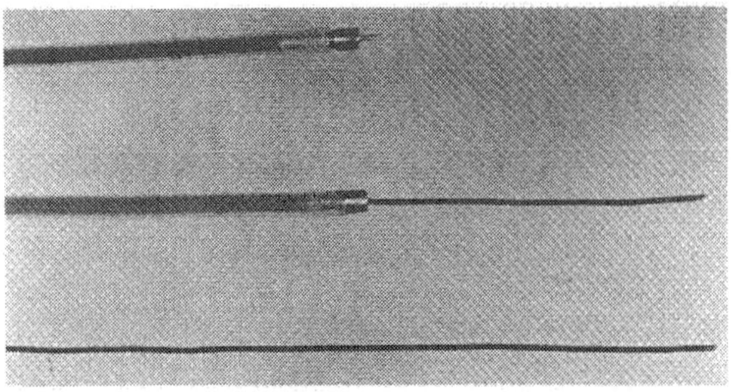

FIGURE 40.4 Interstitial endoprobe local hyperthermia/Photodynamic therapy: Distribution of power density.

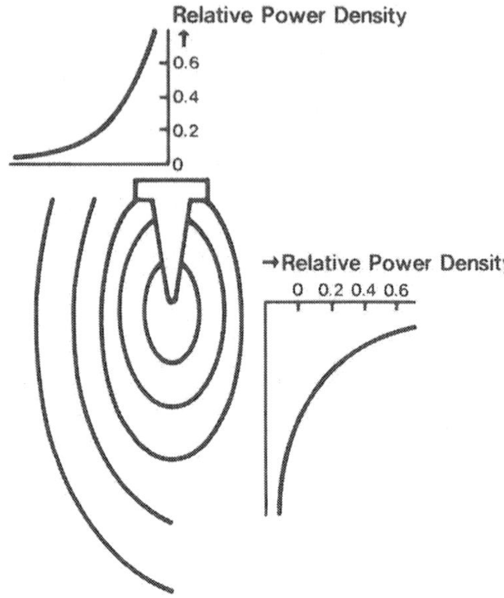

FIGURE 40.5 Thermocouples.

W/cm² for 1 W of total irradiation from the probe, having 3 mm length, in contrast to the bare fiber, 3.6 W/cm² for 1 W of 600 μm. With a longer probe it is possible to have longer irradiation time so that different probe lengths can be applied based on the tumor volume. Due to low power density on the surface and characteristics of the probe, the probe has less damage than bare fiber under more energy delivery.

Thermocouple

For the practical purpose of inserting the thermocouple into the tumor, the needle-shaped stainless steel thermocouple has stopperlike flange to control the depth of insertion. The surface of the needle is well polished for laser beam reflectance. Different length of needles are available for different clinical cases (Figure 40.5). It was confirmed by a comparison of measured temperatures from the thermocouple and thermograms that there was no temperature interference from exposure of the laser beam directly onto the thermocouple during low-power laser irradiation from the probe in the tissue (Figure 40.6).

TABLE 40.1. Characteristics of single crystal artificial sapphire

Property	Sapphire	Quartz
Material/formula	Al_2O	S10
Melting point	2030–2050°C	1600°C
Specific heat	0.18 (25°C)	0.17 (25°C)
Thermal Conductivity (g°cal. cm s)	0.0016–0.0034 (40°C)	0.0158 0.0299 (40°C)
Coefficient of thermal expansion (10 cm/°C)	50–67	80
Elastic Coefficient (10 kg/cm)	5.0	0.76
Specific gravity	4.0	2.2
Hardness (mohs)	9	7
Compressive strength (kg/cm)	28000	20000
Tensile strength	2000	900 1200
Index of refraction	1.76	1.54
Absorption degree of water	0.00	0.00
Chemical characterstic appearance	Acid- and bace-proof clear	Acid- and base-proof clear
Crystal form	hexagonal system	hexagonal system
Transmittance for YAG laser	More 90%	More 90%

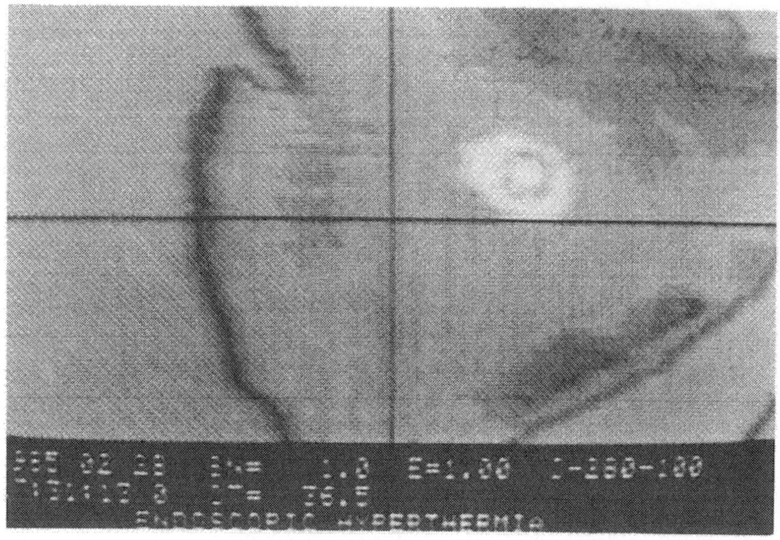

FIGURE 40.6 Thermogram during laserthermia.

Computer System

The delivery of laser energy from the probe to increase the temperature of tumor is controlled by computer, monitoring one representative temperature at the certain distance from the probe to the thermocouple. Feedback system of measured temperature to laser delivery is possible to keep the programmed temperature at the point where the thermocouple is located (Figures 40.7 and 40.8). Currently the medical laser gen-

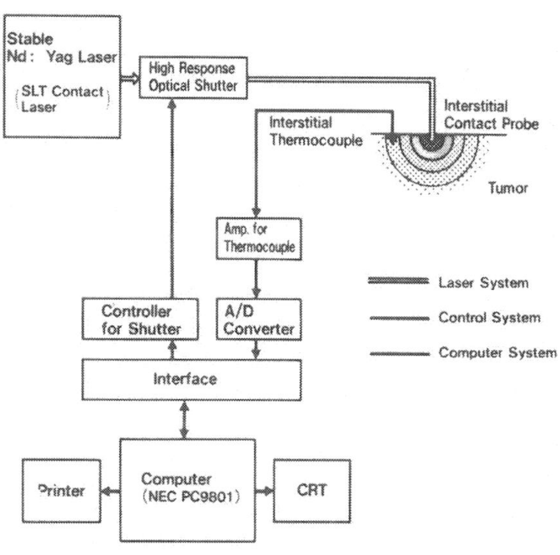

FIGURE 40.7 Computer-controlled Laserthermia system—single channel.

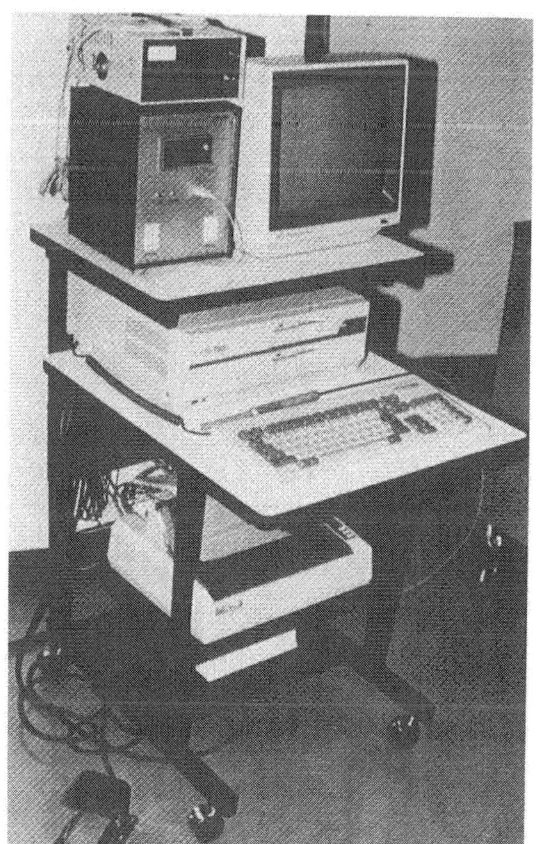

FIGURE 40.8 Single-channel control system.

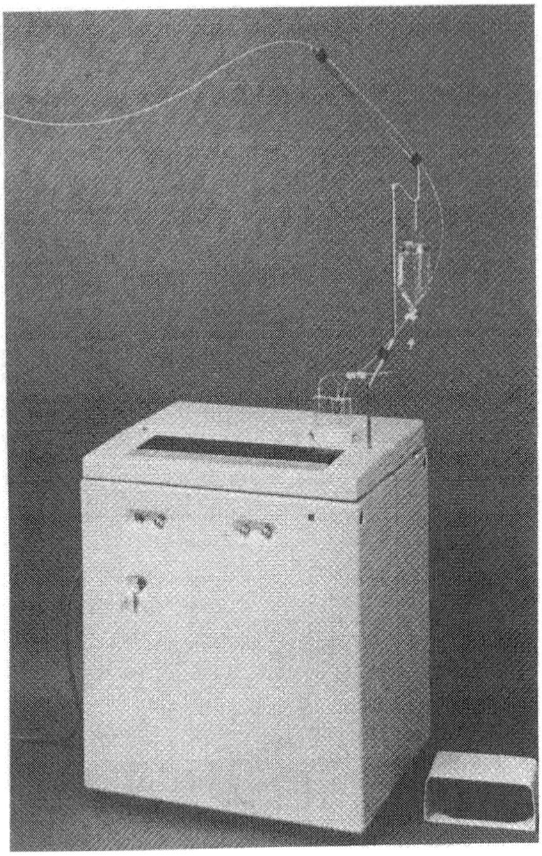

FIGURE 40.9 SLT Contact Laser.

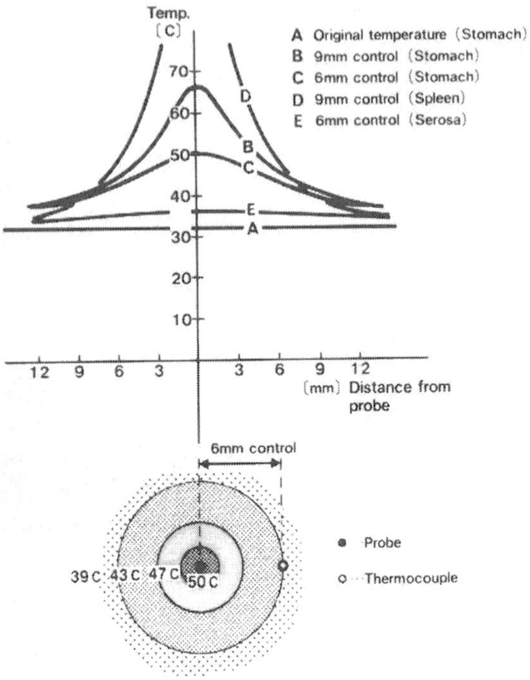

FIGURE 40.10 Temperature distribution in canine stomach and spleen.

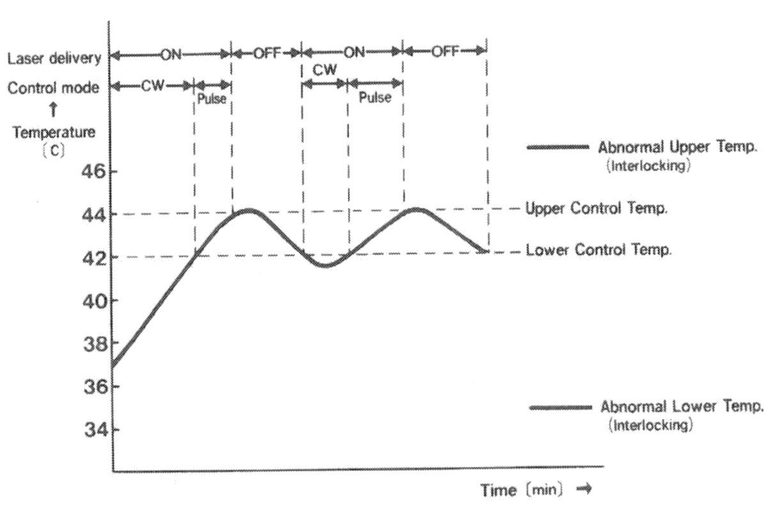

FIGURE 40.11 Control method for temperature with laser delivery.

erator is manufactured for the purpose of high power and noncontact methods, so we require a very stable laser generator such as the SLT Contact Laser, especially using low powers (Figure 40.9). If the probe is not changed, the temperature distribution will differ with the color of the tissue and the distance between the probe and the thermocouple. The temperature on the surface of the probe has the highest temperature. But to get wider heating and controllable temperature, it is important not to obtain more than 100°C on the surface of the probe. Otherwise burning of the tissue occurs with a great energy loss leading to damage of the probe. For this reason, in this method a suitable power level is required, normally less than 5 W. This depends on the duty cycle of laser delivery and also limits the heated area to a 1–2 cm diameter (Figure 40.10). A cross sectional view of temperature distribution is almost semicircular, so that it is possible be easily get a known volume of tissue heated adequately.

Control Method for Temperature

At the beginning of the laserthermia procedure, laser energy must be delivered rapidly in a continuous mode, since the tissue temperature is lower than "lower control temperature" set at 42°C (Figure 40.11). However, if the tissue temperature is within the control range between the "lower control temperature" and the "upper control temperature" such as 44°C, the system delivers the laser energy slowly, which is possible by using the pulse mode. If the temperature is over the "upper control temperature," it will stop the delivery of laser energy. For safety considerations, the system will stop delivering laser energy if the temperature is over the "abnormal upper temperature," suggesting local overheating, or lower than "abnormal lower temperature," suggesting disconnection of thermocouple from tissue. The system allows various input ranges and conditions for controlling the system so that it has versatility for a wide variety of clinical purposes (Table 40.2 and Figure 40.12).

TABLE 40.2. Input ranges for controlling system

1. Input power	; 0.1–100 w
2. Total time	; 0.01–30 min
3. Total joules	; 0.1–10,000 J
4. Upper temperature (Upper temperature controlled)	; 35.1–55.0°C
5. Lower temperature (Lower temperature controlled)	; 35.0–49.9°C
6. Ab.-Up. temp. (Abnormal upper temperature)	; 35.1–55.0°C
7. Ab.-Lo. temp. (Abnormal lower temperature)	; 30.0–49.9°C
8. Laser output mode (Control mode)	; Continuous or pulse
8-1.C (Continuous)	; 0–30 min
8-2. P (Pulse)	; Programmable
8-2-1. Pulse on (Pulse width)	; 0.1–5.0 sec
8-2-2. Pulse off (No pulse width)	; 0.1–5.0 sec

```
Operating data           (Data Input End => f·5 key enter)
  Date - - - - - - - :;  85/04/25
  Time - - - - - - - :;  12:48:00
  Patient  - - - - - :;
    Number - - - - - :;  00000001
    Name - - - - - - :;  H.OHASHI/////////////
    Birthday - - - - :;  23/Aug/1949////
    Sex  - - - - - - :;  Female
Doctor Name- - - - - :;  =====================================
Nurse Name - - - - - :;  ------------------------------
Operation
 Input Power(w)- - - :;  10.0
 Total Joule(j)- - - :;  10000.0
 Total Time (m)- - - :;  20.00
 Upper Temp.(°C) - - :;  44.5
 Lower Temp.(°C) - - :;  43.5
 Ab.-Up Temp.(°C)- - :;  45.5
 Ab.-Lo Temp.(°C)- - :;  35.0
Laser Output Mode- - :;  Continuous
```

FIGURE 40.12 Operating data input.

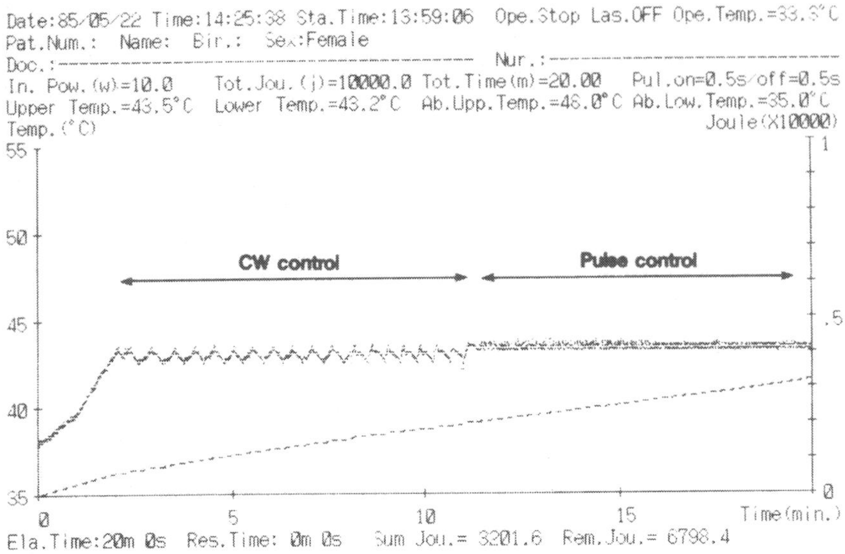

FIGURE 40.13 Data output.

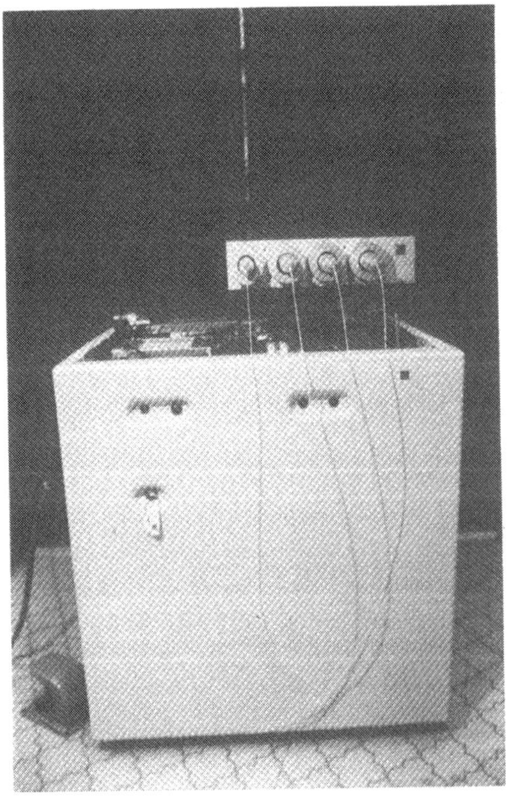

FIGURE 40.14 Multiple-channel laser system.

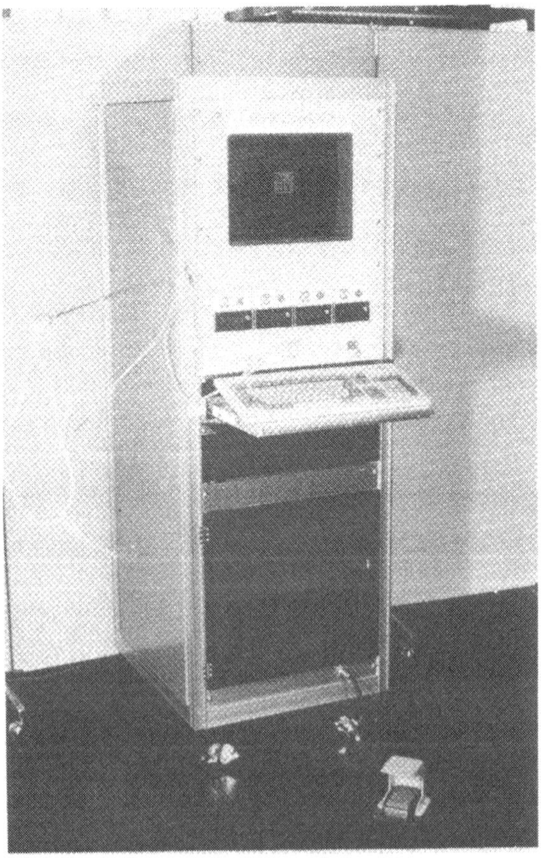

FIGURE 40.15 Multiple-channel control system for Laserthermia.

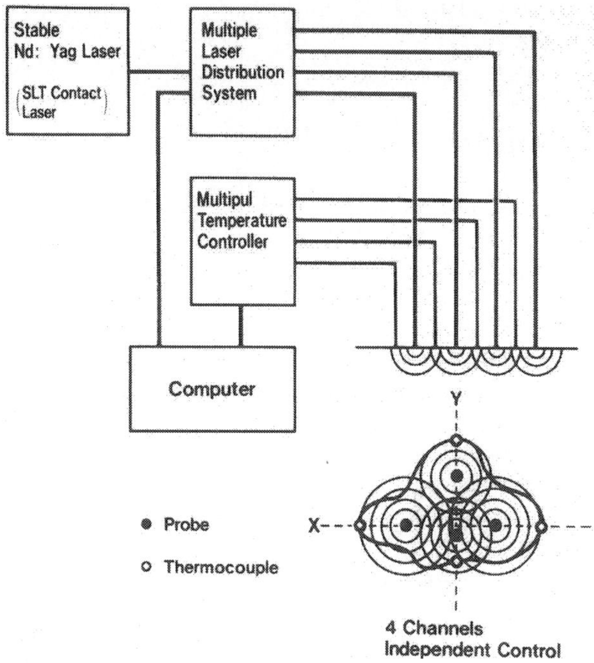

FIGURE 40.16 Computer-controlled Laserthermia system—multiple channels.

Suitable Power Ranges and Pulse Delivery

From experiments in vivo it is clear that higher power causes overshooting the "upper control temperature" so the controlled range of temperature is wider and not precise. Contrary to that, lower power takes a longer time to increase the temperature with less flexibility to respond the change of tissue conditions such as blood flow. The suitable power range seems to be from 1 to 5 W. This will be clearer with more experiments. The system allows the use of continuous wave or pulse mode for laser delivery during the raising of temperature between "lower and upper control temperature." But the proper condition with the pulse mode makes more pre-

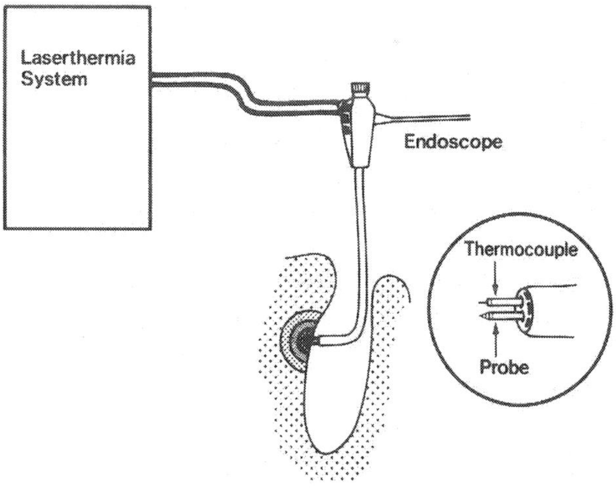

FIGURE 40.17 Endoscopic Laserthermia.

cise control than the continuous wave mode (Figure 40.13).

Multiple Laserthermia System

The single-probe Laserthermia System is limited for heating a large volume of tissue. To get larger tissue volumes with more uniform temperature heating we have developed Multiple Laserthermia system,® consisting of a SLT contact laser with multiple laser distribution system (Figure 40.14) and a computer (Figure 40.15). Considering the rapid localized change of temperature in the tumor, each probe is independently controlled by its own thermocouple. In this report a four-channel system is shown. There are no known technical problems to using more channels, which would be determined by the volume of tissue to be treated. The temperature around the probe in the tumor is higher. This is not of much concern as long as the probe does not cause tissue vaporization. The temperature should be controlled strictly and precisely at the border between normal tissue and tumor. A monitoring thermocouple should be placed at this junction and the probes should be directed to the center of the tumor (Figure 40.16).

Conclusion

We have successfully developed both a Single and Multiple Laserthermia System, which make it possible to control temperature precisely. These therapeutic modalities are very easier to operate, safer and have more precise temperature control than currently used laser system with their high power and short therapeutic durations. The single system is useful for endoscopic Laserthermia,[4] using a two-channel endoscope (Figure 40.17). Obviously, a multiple Laserthermia system will be used for larger tumor located on an open surgical field. Recent biomedical and clinical studies of Laserthermia shows that in addition to normal efficacy of hyperthermia, it may have additional advantages based on the interaction between laser energy and cancer cell with a direct effect with laser light on the cancer cells.[5] Damage to normal tissue with Laserthermia is minimum as shown by studies measuring arachidonic acid metabolites in vivo. This method has been evaluated by different specialties.[6] Further study will be focused on this point and on the influence of Laserthermia, especially on normal tissue.

Reference

1. Brown SG: Tumor therapy with the Nd:YAG laser. In Joffe SN, Muckerheide M, Goldman L. (eds): Neodymium-YAG Laser in Medicine and Surgery Elsevier, New York, 1983, pp. 59–70.
2. Daikuzono N: Introduction of a newly developed contact ceramic probe connected to a laser optical quartz fiber for wide applications in medicine and surgery. Proceedings for 2nd International Nd:YAG Laser Conference in Springer-Verlag, Munich, 1985. pp 302–306.
3. Daikuzono N: Artificial sapphire probe for contact photocoagulation and tissue vaporization with the Nd:YAG laser. Med Instrum 19(4):173–178, 1985.
4. Suzuki S: Endoscopic local hyperthermia with Nd-YAG laser. Gastroentererology (Japan) 4(4):363–370, 1986.
5. Tajiri H: Experimental studies of local hyperthermia using Nd-YAG laser. Oncologia 17:161–163, 1986.
6. Ohyama M: Treatment of head and neck tumors by contact Nd-YAG laser surgery. Auris Nasus Larynx (Tokyo) 12 (Suppl 11):S138–S142, 1985.

41
Safety Procedures for Nd:YAG Laser Surgery

R. James Rockwell, Jr.

Understanding the specifics of laser safety is absolutely essential to the medical community. In the past there has been uncertainty over the regulations that apply in laser surgery. This can create unnecessary concerns, particularly at the time the first laser is acquired. Therefore, it is the goal of this chapter to provide a review of the various hazards associated with the surgical use of lasers and an understanding of the applicable standards, with suggestions for several specific safety procedures that can be applied when using the Nd:YAG laser in a surgical setting.

Some of the primary factors that must be considered when implementing the Nd:YAG laser in surgery are (1) the operational characteristics of the specific Nd:YAG laser; (2) the adaptability to desired accessories (e.g., endoscopes, fiber optics, sapphire tips, handpieces); (3) education and training, including inservice training; (4) ongoing service and maintenance of the equipment; and (5) the level of anticipated use.

It should not be surprising that there are safety considerations involved in each of these areas. In fact, virtually *all* aspects of activity associated with medical laser usage involve some safety factors that require continuing attention. For example, it is often desirable to purchase the most advanced laser system design to meet the changing needs of multiple discipline use. This may mean that one surgical team uses the laser in an open-beam configuration, which usually requires the maximum safety requirements. Others may use the same laser endoscopically with no "open-beam" hazards during the procedure. The *same* laser system is used in *both* cases but there are significant differences in the potential hazards. Safe use of lasers—in particular, Nd:YAG lasers—requires procedures and practices based on knowledge and understanding.

Laser Hazards to the Eye

The hazards of lasers that represent a potential for injury to the eye generally depend upon the wavelength of the laser and which part of the eye absorbs the most radiant energy per unit volume of tissue at that wavelength. *Retinal* effects are generally considered the most serious and are possible when the laser wavelength falls in the visible and near-infrared spectral regions (0.4–1.4 μm). Hence the Nd:YAG laser with emission at 1.064 μm (or 1.32 μm in some experimental systems) represents a definite retinal hazard.

The Nd:YAG laser beam entering the eye either directly from the laser, or from a specular (mirror), or diffuse (scattered) reflection can be focused to an extremely small spot-image on the retina. This causes an excessive irradiance (W/cm^2) or radiant exposure (J/cm^2) incident on the retinal tissues even for modest corneal exposure levels. The absorbed energy is converted into heat, and, if the incident laser energy is too great, it causes an irreversible retinal burn. The process is due to tissue proteins being denatured by the rise in tissue temperature following absorption of laser energy (Figure 41.1).

The principal thermal effects of laser expo-

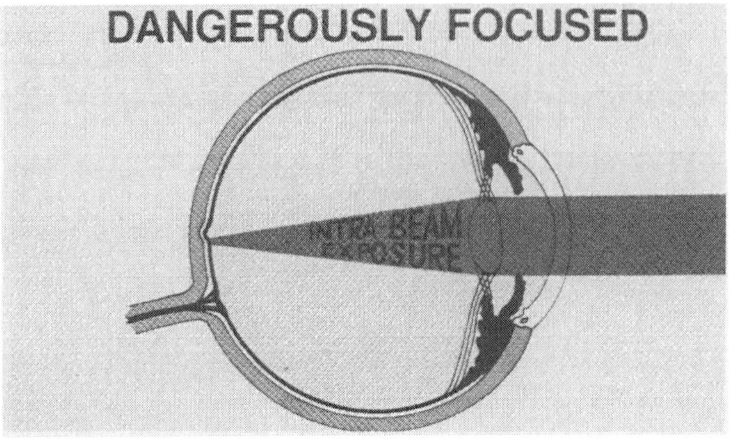

FIGURE 41.1. Focused intrabeam condition. Focused spot can be 20 μm or smaller. Retinal irradiance will be approximately 140,000 times greater than irradiance at the cornea. For example, the retinal irradiance produced by a 1-mW laser, just filling the worst-case 7 mm pupil size, will be about 440 W/cm^2.

sure, therefore, depend upon the following factors:

1. Absorption and scattering coefficients of the tissues at the 1.064-μm Nd:YAG laser wavelength
2. Irradiance or radiant exposure of the laser beam
3. Exposure duration and pulse repetition characteristics
4. Local vascular blood flow
5. Size of the irradiated area

The mechanism of tissue damage caused by repetitively pulsed or scanned Nd:YAG laser exposures is still being investigated. The current evidence indicates that the major mechanism is a thermal process with an additive effect related to the accumulated energy of the individual pulses.

Tissue damage may also be caused by thermally induced acoustic-shock waves and/or photodissociation (electric field effects) following exposures to submicrosecond Q-switched or mode-locked Nd:YAG laser pulses.

Other mechanisms of tissue damage have also been demonstrated for other specific wavelength ranges and/or exposure times. For example, photochemical reactions are the principal cause of tissue damage following exposures to either actinic ultraviolet radiation (0.200–0.315 μm) for any exposure time or "short-wave" visible radiation (0.4–0.55 μm) when exposures are greater than 10 seconds.

Intrabeam Viewing

A retinal injury occurring in the macular region is very serious, since the visual functions are most highly developed in this area. Blindness can result from a laser exposure that lasts only an infinitesimal fraction of a second. Similar damage, on the other hand, in the periphery of the retina will often have minimal effect, usually without functional significance.

A macular burn would probably result if the individual is viewing the beam under conditions where the eye is resolving the laser source or a diffuse reflection. The latter could occur, for example, while viewing the focused spot without protective filters either directly or through a binocular microscope or endoscope. A peripheral burn might occur through an accidental exposure when the eye is not directly viewing the beam and the eye is not "relaxed" but rather focused on something other than the laser point source.

Diffuse Reflections

Viewing a large beam area which has been reflected from a diffuse surface will usually produce a much larger retinal image spot size than direct (intrabeam) viewing. This provides, at first consideration, some degree of protection, since, at distances close to the reflecting surface, the retinal irradiance can be significantly lower due to the larger spot size.

Most surgical Nd:YAG lasers are, however, of sufficient power (Class IV) as to be diffuse reflection hazards. The resulting degree of retinal damage would be significant due to the larger retinal spot sizes associated with a typical extended source viewing condition. Also, larger image sizes (typically 100 μm or greater) of longer exposure times (>10 seconds) do not dissipate the heat buildup as rapidly as smaller image sizes. Consequently, the retinal *irradiance* threshold level that produces a minimal burn on the retina will be about 10–20 times *lower* for larger image sizes than for the smaller (20 μm) point-source image sizes. Hence different safety limits are needed for the two different exposure conditions resulting from point and extended sources.

Eye Exposure to Infrared Wavelengths

A transition zone between retinal effects and effects on the front segments of the eye (cornea, lens, aqueous media) begins at the far end of the visible spectrum and extends into the infrared "A" region (0.700–1.4 μm). The Nd:YAG laser operates in this so-called near-infrared region. Although the 1.064-μm wavelength does not evoke a visual response, this frequency still transmits back to the retinal surface. There will be some significant absorption and scattering losses and the laws of physical optics dictates that the eye of the lens will not focus a longer invisible wavelength to as small a spot as a visible frequency. Nonetheless, the Nd:YAG laser must still be considered one of the most dangerous laser types simply because of the high power (typically 100 W in a surgical laser) and also because the beam is not visible. These two factors present a situation where even a small reflection can cause irreversible retinal damage.

In the infrared "B" region (1.4–3.0 μm) damage is observed to both the lens and cornea. The ocular media becomes opaque to radiation in the infrared "C" region (3.0 μm–1 mm), as the absorption by water (a major portion of all body cells) is high in this region. In the infrared "C" region, as in the ultraviolet "A" and "B" regions, the threshold for damage to the cornea is comparable to that of the skin. Damage to the cornea, however, is much more disabling and of much greater concern.

Maximum Permissible Exposure Limits

The safe exposure limits provided in the various standards seem to be set about a factor of 10 or more *lower* than the actual retinal damage threshold levels reported in the biologic literature. This factor of 10 is sometimes erroneously referred to as a "safety factor." In fact, the values called thresholds are actually so-called "ED_{50}" doses; that is, doses where 50% of the exposures *resulted* in injury and 50% of the exposures *did not result* in changes which were visible by an ophthalmoscope. Obviously, safety limits must be concerned with whether there may be permanent or delayed visual loss or tissue damage, and not whether damage is simply ophthalmoscopically visible.

Many studies have been performed to determine at what levels below the so-called ED_{50} dose some loss of visual function or morphologic change in the retinal tissue will be encountered. These studies generally suggest that for exposure durations of 10 microseconds to 10 seconds, changes are still observed by histologic evaluation at power/energy levels reduced from the ED_{50} value by a factor in the range of 2 to 5. Hence the apparent safety factor of 10 based on ophthalmoscopic visible burn criteria is, in reality, only a value of 2 above the level of actual morphologic or histologic change.

The most accepted safety limits are the maximum permissible exposure (MPE) limits obtained from the Z-136.1 (1986) standard published by the American National Standards Institute (ANSI); an organization for which expert volunteers participate on committees to determine industry consensus standards in various fields. The MPE limits are determined as a function of laser wavelength, exposure time, and pulse repetition frequency (prf). Table 41.1 gives MPE limits for various Nd:YAG laser exposure criteria and compares them to other laser types.

TABLE 41.1. Maximum permissible exposure (MPE) levels

Laser	Wavelength (μm)	Exposure time (s)	MPE
Helium-neon	0.633	cw: 3×10^4	17 μW/cm^2
Helium-neon	0.633	cw: 0.25[a]	2.5 mW/cm^2
Argon	0.514	cw: 3×10^4	1.0 μW/cm^2
Nd:YAG	1.064	cw: 3×10^4	1.6 mW/cm^2
Nd:YAG	1.064	pulsed: 1×10^{-8}	5.0 μJ/cm^2
Ruby	0.694	pulsed: 1×10^{-8}	0.5 μJ/cm^2
Carbon dioxide	10.6[b]	3×10^4	100 mW/cm^2

cw = continuous wave.
[a]0.25 second is considered aversion response time.
[b]Far-infrared radiation is not a retinal hazard.

Safety Controls for Laser Surgery

Laser safety practices are commonly effected in laser surgery by implementing specific safety procedures that are designed to either eliminate ocular and skin exposures to direct or scattered laser radiation. In cases where a hazard analysis has been done, controls can be implemented to reduce potentially hazardous laser exposures to acceptable levels.

Safety controls are also needed for the hazards associated with toxic fumes, electrical power supplies, laser induced-plasma by-products, and fire, which are often associated with the laser devices. Important in this area are the problems associated with anesthesia and, particularly, fires produced by an accidental laser exposure of a tube supporting high oxygen levels.

Four basic categories of safety controls are useful in laser environments. These are engineering, personal protective equipment, administrative and procedural controls, and special controls.

The recommendations in this chapter are based on the contents of the recently revised Z-136.1 (1986) standard of the American National Standards Institute (ANSI). It should be noted that the existing Federal Laser Product Performance Standard (FLPPS) of the FDA that regulates laser manufacturers (CFR: Part 1040.10 and 1040.11), and the Suggested State Regulation for Lasers (SSRL), which is being considered for adoption at this time by several states, have terminology and concepts nearly identical to the ANSI Z-136.1 standard.

An ANSI standard *specific* to the medical environment is also in preparation. This standard will be designated ANSI Z-136.3 "Safe Use of Lasers in Health Care Facilities" (1987). This document will provide guidance specific to the medical use of lasers but will be based upon specific requirements of the Z-136.1 (1986) "parent" standard as detailed in this chapter.

The ANSI Z-136.1 standard has been universally adopted by industry, medicine, and government departments as the "user requirements" of lasers. The requirements are easily implemented by the designated Laser Safety Officer (LSO) of the facility.

The Laser Hazard Classes

Both the ANSI and FDA standards divide all lasers into four major hazard categories called the laser classifications. These are summarized as follows:

Class I: Cannot emit laser radiation at known hazard levels (typically cw: 0.4 mW). Users of a Class I laser are generally exempt from radiation hazard controls during operation and maintenance (but not necessarily during service). Since lasers are not classified on beam access during service, most all Class I lasers will consist of a higher class (high-power) laser *enclosed* in a properly interlocked and labeled protective enclosure.

Class II: Low-power visible lasers that emit above Class I levels, but not above 1 mW. The concept is that the human aversion reaction to bright light will protect a person. (Note: Class IIA is a special designation that is based upon a 1000-second exposure and applies to lasers that are "not intended for viewing.")

Class IIIA: Intermediate-power lasers (cw: 1–5 mW). Only hazardous for chronic intrabeam viewing. Some limited controls are usually recommended.

Class IIIB: Moderate-power lasers (cw: 5–500 mW, pulsed: 10 J/cm^2: or the diffuse reflection limit). In general, Class IIIB lasers will not produce a hazardous diffuse reflection unless intentional staring is done at close distances. Specific controls are recommended.

Class IV: High-power lasers (cw: >500 mW) are hazardous to view under any condition (directly or diffusely scattered). Significant controls are required of Class IV laser facilities.

Important in the classification and implementation of safety controls is the distinction between the functions of operation, maintenance and service. First, most laser systems are classified on the basis of the laser radiation accessible during operation and maintenance, where the latter is considered as those tasks required to maintain routine system operation (e.g., cleaning a lens, changing gas bottles). Service functions are usually performed with far less frequency than maintenance functions (e.g., replacing the laser resonator mirrors, repair of faulty components) and often will require access to the laser beam.

The Federal Government does *not* "approve" laser systems. The *manufacturer* of the laser system first *classifies* the laser and then *certifies* that it meets all performance requirements of the FLPPS. This is reviewed by the laser division within the Center for Devices and Radiological Health (CDRH) of the Food and Drug Administration (FDA). One of the first responsibilities, then, of the hospital's Laser Safety Officer (LSO) is to assure that the lasers are, in fact, manufacturer-certified and classified.

In addition, the CDRH also has the responsibility for enforcing compliance of the Medical Device Regulations. All surgical laser manufacturers must, therefore, obtain premarket approval of their laser surgical devices from CDRH before they can be sold. The CDRH sanctions the investigational use of lasers for specific surgical procedures through a process referred to as an Investigational Device Exemption (IDE). Approval of an IDE allows the limited use of a laser expressly for the purpose of conducting an investigation of the laser's "safety and effectiveness." Once an IDE has been done and approved, the manufacturer may market the device for that specific use only.

Nominal Hazard Zone

There are some laser uses, such as surgery, where it is useful to define the area where the possibility exists for potentially hazardous exposure. The nominal hazard zone (NHZ), by definition, describes the space within which the level of direct, reflected, or scattered radiation *exceeds* the level of the applicable maximum permissible exposure (MPE). Consequently, persons *outside* the NHZ boundry would be exposed *below* the MPE level and are considered to be in a "safe" location. The NHZ boundry may be defined by direct laser beams, diffusely scattered laser beams, and beams transmitted from fiberoptics and/or lenses, special contact tips, etc. The NHZ perimeter is the envelope of MPE exposure levels from any laser in a given application or installation geometry (Figure 41.2).

The principal use of the NHZ evaluation is to define that region where control measures are required. Thus, as the scope of surgical laser has expanded, the classic method of controlling lasers in an interlocked room has become limiting and, in many instances, can be an overreaction to the real hazards present.

Intrabeam Nominal Hazard Zone

The intrabeam nominal hazard zone can be determined by the so-called laser range equation. This is useful in calculating the distance the beam must travel before the beam size has grown large enough so that the irradiance is reduced to the maximum permissible exposure (MPE) level. In this case, the range (r) is expressed as

$$r = \frac{1}{\phi}\left[\left(\frac{4\Phi}{\pi E_s}\right)^{0.5} - a\right], \qquad (1)$$

where

ϕ = the laser beam divergence (rad),
Φ = the laser power (W),

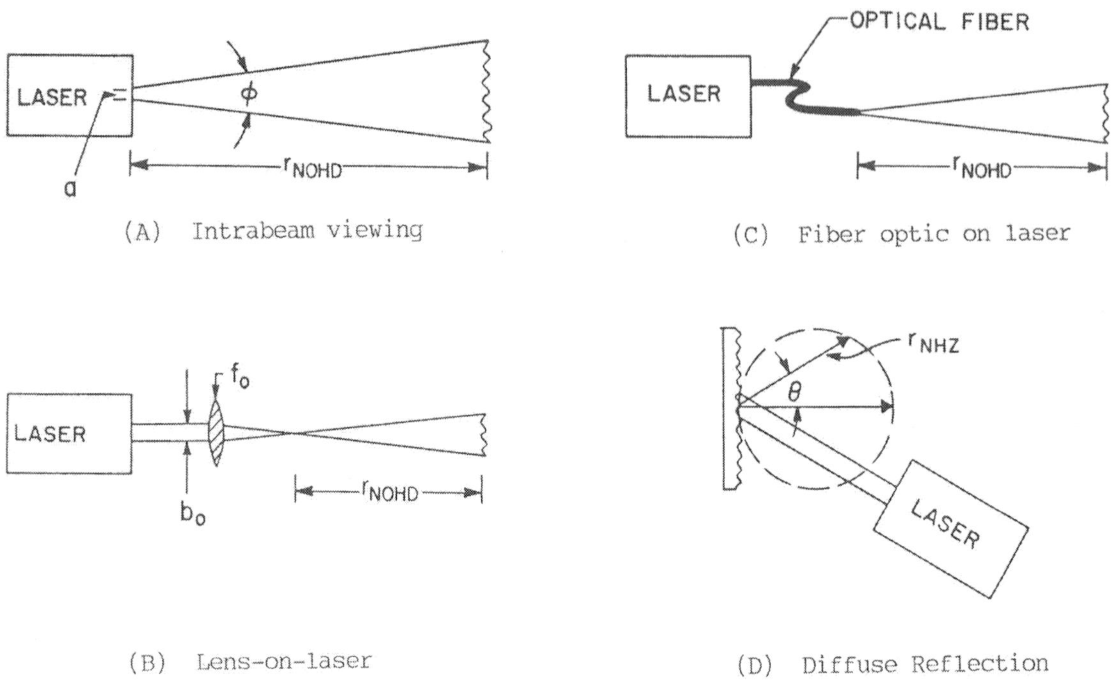

FIGURE 41.2. Nominal hazard zone (NHZ) geometry. (A) Intrabeam (direct) viewing condition. NHZ range (nominal ocular hazard distance) measured from laser to point where beam has grown large enough so that MPE irradiance is attained. (B) Lens-on-laser condition. NHZ range measured from focal plane of lens. (C) Fiberoptic on laser condition. NHZ range is measured from fiber tip. (D) Diffuse reflection condition. NHZ range is measured from target point on diffuse surface.

E_s = the irradiance at the range (r) (W/cm^2), and
r = range from the laser to target (cm).

If the value of the irradiance at a distance (r) away from the laser is maintained at (or below) the MPE, then the distance is considered the intrabeam nominal hazard zone range (R^{IB}_{NHZ}) or "safe range" value. That is, substituting E_s = MPE in Equation 1 we have

$$R^{IB}_{NHZ} = \frac{1}{\phi}\left[\left(\frac{4\Phi}{\pi(\text{MPE})}\right)^{0.5} - a\right]. \quad (2)$$

For example, consider the case of a typical 100-W Nd:YAG surgical laser with a beam divergence of 2.0 m rad and an exit beam diameter of 0.2 cm. Using Equation 1 and assuming the "worst-case" (8-hour) MPE = 1.6 mW/cm^2, we find that

$$R^{IB}_{NHZ} = \frac{1}{2 \times 10^{-3}} \left[\left(\frac{4 \times 100}{3.14 \times (1.6 \times 10^{-3})}\right)^{0.5} - 0.2\right] = 1.41 \times 10^3 \text{ meters.}$$

The intrabeam hazard extends to a distance of 1.4 km from the laser, and certainly extends beyond the surgical operating-room limits. This implies, therefore, that uses of a Nd:YAG laser in this "natural" state may require entryway and personnel controls more detailed than in those cases where the delivery optics, fibers, or fiber tips cause rapid beam expansion.

Diffuse Reflections

In practice, most partially roughened nonglossy surfaces act as diffusing surfaces to incident visible or near-infrared laser beams. Tissues, for example, are an excellent diffuse reflecting media. Such a diffusing "rough" surface acts as a plane of very small scattering sites that reflect the beam in a radially symmetric manner. The roughness of the surface is such that the scattering sites are larger than the laser wavelength. Consequently, the reflected radiant intensity (power per unit solid angle), denoted by I(θ), can be shown to be dependent upon the cosine of the viewing angle (θ) as measured from the normal to the surface. That is,

$$I(\theta) = I_0 \cos(\theta), \quad (3)$$

where

$I(\theta)$ = radiant intensity occurring at an angle from the normal [W/sr],
I_0 = radiant intensity [W/sr] reflected along the normal to the surface, and
θ = angle measured from the normal to the surface.

This relationship is known as Lambert's Cosine Law. A surface behaving in this manner is usually referred to as a lambertian surface. This relationship defines an ideal plane diffuse reflector (Figure 41.3).

It should be stressed that "rough" surfaces do not act as diffuse reflectors at all wavelengths. For example, brushed aluminum (which is partially diffuse for visible wavelength laser radiation) is a good specular mirrorlike reflector for far-infrared wavelength lasers such as the CO_2 laser (10.6 μm). Nonpolished metals such as brushed aluminum and stainless steel, as would be found in some "sand-blasted" surgical instruments, will produce a more diffuse reflection than polished metals. The average surface roughness should be larger than the laser wavelength; which for the Nd:YAG laser is just over 1 μm.

Most partially roughened surfaces may still have properties that contribute specular reflection. This may occur when a low percentage of the incident radiation is specularly reflected and the remainder diffusely reflected. This behavior is generally the rule, and not the exception, for most common surfaces. As a result, the reflected radiation is not exactly radially symmetric, but skews toward the specularly reflected component.

Inverse Square Law and Diffuse Reflections from Point Sources

The diffusely reflected irradiance (E) or radiant exposure (H) resulting when a point source beam is incident upon a lambertian surface, which is inversely related to the square of the distance (r) from the surface, is expressed by the following equation for continuous wave sources:

$$E(r,\theta) = \frac{\rho\Phi \cos\theta}{\pi r^2} \quad [\text{W/cm}^2], \quad (4)$$

or for pulsed lasers by

$$H(r,\theta) = \frac{\rho Q \cos\theta}{\pi r^2} \quad [\text{J/cm}^2],$$

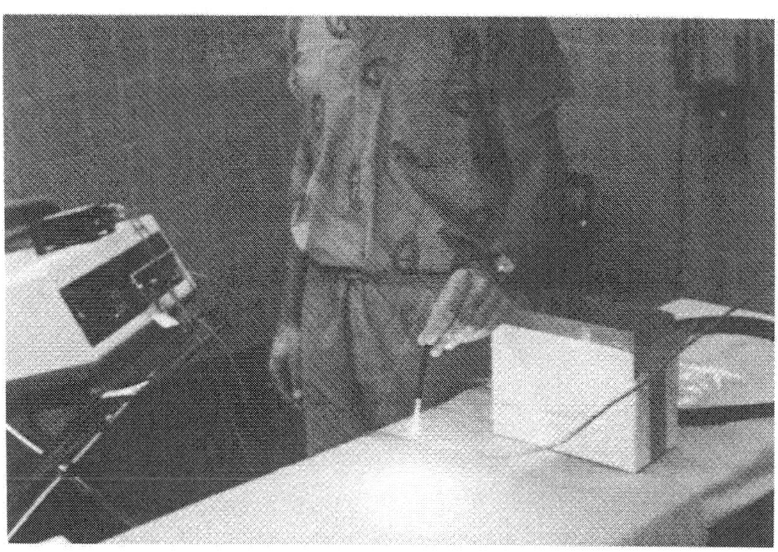

FIGURE 41.3. Diffuse reflection of laser beam emitted from fiberoptic. System shown with visible argon laser to depict situation produced by invisible Nd:YAG laser under similar conditions. Spot produced can be an extended source to retina and for Class IV lasers (>0.5 W) can produce a condition of hazardous diffuse reflection viewing throughout the diffuse nominal hazard zone. This can include an entire surgical room.

where

Q = the energy incident upon the surface (J),
ρ = the surface reflectivity (fraction),
θ = viewing angle measured relative to the normal to the reflecting surface (degrees), and
r = distance from diffusing surface to viewer (cm).

All other terms are as previously defined.

The inverse square distance relationship is valid, provided the distance (r) is much greater than the spot diameter D_L. Consequently, a diffuse surface acts as a distance-dependent attenuator that permits indirect viewing of some low-powered laser beams when the reflecting spot is small. If the laser power is sufficient, that is, >0.5 W, even a diffuse reflection is hazardous to view. This is an important consideration for those working with high-powered visible or near-infrared Class IV lasers.

Diffuse Reflection Nominal Hazard Zone Range

There are some instances where it is useful to calculate the distance away from a "point source" diffuse reflector at which a specific irradiance occurs. Solving Equation 4 for distance, we find that the diffuse reflection nominal hazard zone (R_{NHZ}^{DR}) can be written as

$$R_{NHZ}^{DR} = \left(\frac{\rho\Phi\cos\theta}{\pi(\mathrm{MPE})}\right)^{0.5}. \qquad (5)$$

For example, assume a normal ($\theta = 0°$) viewing of a 100-W Nd:YAG surgical laser directed upon a surface with a 100% reflectance. At what distance does the MPE irradiance of 1.6 mW/cm^2 occur? Solving Equation 5 and inserting numerical values, we find that

$$R_{NHZ}^{DR} = \left(\frac{1.0 \times 100 \times 1.0}{3.14 \times (1.6 \times 10^{-3})}\right)^{0.5}$$
$$= 1.41 \text{ meters.}$$

Thus, the maximum NHZ range for a 100% point-source diffuse reflection from a Nd:YAG laser will be only 141 cm or about 4.6 ft! The diffuse hazard exists around the laser surgical operating site and eye protection, for example, would be required in this zone.

Extended Source Diffuse Reflections

In cases where the laser creates large spot diameters on the diffuse target relative to the viewing distance, the diffuse surface is said to create an "extended source" relative to the eye. In this case, the retinal image size of the focused laser light will usually exceed 100 μm, and the viewer can resolve the details of the diffuse target source. Such larger area retinal images are of special concern because the threshold for biologic damage for the larger retinal images is at least ten times lower than for point-source images.

A laser beam reflected from a diffuser is often expressed in radiant energy units, which combine the reflected radiant power or energy with the geometry of a solid angle "cone" and the reflecting "source" area. This is referred to as the radiance (L) of a plane diffuse lambertian surface, and it is related to the irradiance incident on the surface by the equation

$$L = \frac{\rho E_s}{\pi} = \frac{4\rho\Phi}{(\pi D_L)^2}, \qquad (6)$$

where

L = radiance of the diffuse reflector [W cm^{-2} sr^{-1}],
E_s = irradiance incident upon the surface [W/cm^2], and
ρ = reflectivity of the surface.

Equation 6 allows us to calculate the radiance of a diffusely reflected laser beam while knowing only the irradiance incident upon the surface and the reflectivity of the surface.

For example, assume that a 100-W Nd:YAG surgical laser beam is expanded to a size of 1.0 cm onto a nearby 100% diffusely reflecting surface. The irradiance incident on the surface will be 127 W/cm^2. Assuming the reflectivity of the surface to be 100% (ρ = 1.0), we find from Equation 6 that the radiance of the reflected beam (L) is

$$L = \frac{1.0 \times 127}{3.14}$$
$$= 40.5 \text{ W cm}^{-2}\text{ sr}^{-1}.$$

Note that this term is given in units of radiance, expressed in terms of the power (watts) reflected from the source area (cm^2) into a solid-angle cone (steradian).

For comparative purposes, note that staring directly at a standard 100-W frosted light bulb at close range is equivalent to viewing a diffuse light source with a radiance of about 0.04 W cm^{-2} sr^{-1}. Hence the radiance from the diffuse reflection of the 100-W Nd:YAG laser is over *1000 times greater* than *directly* viewing a 100-W diffused light bulb!

Since the ANSI Z-136.1 long-term (8-hour) MPE for Nd:YAG laser extended sources is 3.2 W cm^{-2} sr^{-1}, the 100-W laser produces an extended source diffuse reflection that is over 12 times greater than the allowed extended source exposure. Note that the dividing point between hazardous and nonhazardous diffuse reflections is considered to be at 0.5 W, the cuttoff between continuous wave Class IIIB and Class IV lasers).

Also important is fact that the resulting retinal irradiance produced while viewing an extended source at close range is *independent* of the distance between the source and viewer. This is due to the fact that, as one moves away from such an extended source, the inverse square law reduces the amount of irradiance incident upon the cornea but, at the same time, the spot size of the focused beam gets proportionally smaller. The result is a retinal irradiance that remains constant and is independent of the distance from the diffuser to the eye. In general, Equation 6 applies up to that point where the source is sufficiently close that it can still be resolved by the viewer. Beyond that point, point-source characteristics apply as described by Equations 4 and 5.

In practice, the evaluation of the point source/extended source dilemma has been addressed in the ANSI Z-136 standard by requiring an evaluation of the subtense angle (α) between the viewer and the extended source target. For lambertian (diffuse) viewing, this angle is also a measure of the resultant retinal image size ($d_r = f\alpha$) and may be expressed in terms of the so-called viewing angle (θ_V) and the extended source diameter (D_L) by the relationship

$$\alpha = \frac{D_L \cos \theta_v}{R}. \tag{7}$$

The cutoff between point source and extended source occurs at a defined "minimum" viewing angle, called α_{min} which corresponds to the maximum viewing distance (R_{max}) for which extended source MPE values apply. In this case, R_{max} is given by

$$R_{max} = \frac{D_L \cos \theta_v}{\alpha_{min}}. \tag{8}$$

For example, the ANSI Z-136 standard indicates that for exposures of 10 seconds or more, the value of α_{min} is 24 mrad. Hence, for the diffused beam spot diameter of 1 cm in the previous example, the extended source criteria will apply for a distance of $R_{max} = 1.0 \times 1.0 / (24 \times 10^{-3}) = 41.7$ cm or nearly 1.4 ft. In this range, a 10-second MPE of 10.8 W cm^{-2} sr^{-1} applies and, at 1.4 ft, produces a *corneal* irradiance of 5 mW/cm^2. Beyond 1.4 ft, point-source criteria apply.

Lens-on-Laser Nominal Hazard Zone Range

Most surgical Nd:YAG lasers incorporate a lens as the final component in the beam path. This not only provides the increased irradiance in the focal plane of the lens to do the work intended of the laser, but it also forces the beam to spread with an angle usually many times larger than the beam divergence angle in the space *beyond* the focal plane. The result is that the MPE irradiance is reached in a distance much less than the intrabeam nominal hazard zone range. This can be referred to as the lens-on-the-laser nominal hazard zone range (R_{NHZ}^{LL}):

$$R_{NHZ}^{LL} = \frac{f_0}{b} \times \left(\frac{4\Phi}{\pi(\mathrm{MPE})}\right)^{0.5}, \tag{9}$$

where

f_0 = the lens focal length (cm), and
b = the diameter of the beam at the lens (cm).

For example, consider a 100-W surgical Nd:YAG laser with a 2.54-cm focal length lens in the beam path and a 6.3-mm beam size as the beam strikes the lens. Substituting into Equation 9, we have

$$R_{NHZ}^{LL} = \frac{2.54}{0.63} \times \left(\frac{4 \times 100}{3.14 \times (1.6 \times 10^{-3})}\right)^{0.5}$$
$$= 11.4 \text{ meters.}$$

Thus, in the direction defined by the cone of laser light directed through the lens, the hazard

TABLE 41.2. Nominal hazard zone distance values for typical surgical lasers

Laser type	Exposure criteria	Hazard range (m)		
		Diffuse	Lens-on-laser	Direct
Nd:YAG	8 h	1.4	11.4	1410
	10 s	0.8	6.3	792
CO_2	8 h	0.18	2.4	168
	10 s	0.18	2.4	168
Argon	8 h	12.6	1.7×10^3	25.2×10^3
	0.25 s	0.25	33.3	240

zone extends up to a distance of 11.4m, at which point the beam has expanded to a diameter of 282 cm or slightly over 9 ft. At that distance, the irradiance will be 1.6×10^{-3} W/cm^2, which is the MPE level. Thus, addition of a lens in the beam path reduced the hazard range from 1.4 km to about 38 ft.

Fiberoptic-on-Laser Nominal Hazard Zone Range

Similar to the lens-on-laser example, a multimode fiber optic attached in the beam path also provides a beam expanding element that shrinks the hazard range depending upon the characteristics of the fiber. For a typical multimode fiber, such as would be used in laser endoscopy, the fiberoptic nominal hazard zone range (R_{NHZ}^{FO}) is given by

$$R_{NHZ}^{FO} = \frac{1.7}{NA} \times \left(\frac{\Phi}{\pi(MPE)}\right)^{0.5}, \qquad (10)$$

where

NA = the fiberoptics numerical aperture (typically in the range of 0.20).

The NHZ for a multimode fiberoptic with a numerical aperture (NA) of 0.20 attached to a 100-W Nd:YAG laser can be computed as

$$R_{NHZ}^{FO} = \frac{1.7}{0.2} \times \left(\frac{100}{3.14 \times (1.6 \times 10^{-3})}\right)^{0.5}$$
$$= 12 \text{ meters}.$$

Thus, the fiberoptic hazard range is nearly optically equivalent to a system with a lens in the beam path.

A summary of all of the NHZ distances is given in Table 41.2 and 41.3 for the Nd:YAG laser. In addition, comparative values are also given for a 100-W CO_2 and a 5-W argon laser, which are two commonly used surgical laser units.

Beam-Path Controls

Class IIIB and IV lasers are sometimes used in situations where the entire beam path is totally

TABLE 41.3. Laser criteria used for nominal hazard zone distance calculations

Laser parameter	Nd:YAG	CO_2	Argon
Wavelength (μm)	1.064	10.6	0.488
Beam power (W)	100.0	100.0	5.0
Beam divergence (mrad)	2.0	2.0	1.0
Beam size at aperture (mm)	2.0	20.0	2.0
Beam size at lens (mm)	6.3	30.0	3.0
Lens focal length (mm)	25.4	200.0	200.0
MPE: 8 h (μW/cm^2)	1.6×10^3	1.0×10^5	1.0
MPE: 10 s (μW/cm^2)	5.1×10^3	1.0×10^5	—
MPE: 0.25 s (μW/cm^2)	—	—	2.5×10^3

MPE = maximum permissible exposure.

enclosed. Other uses may find a beam path with extremely limited access. In some uses, such as surgery, the beam path is totally open. In each case, the controls required will vary.

Totally Enclosed Beam Path

Perhaps the most common form of a Class I laser system is a high-power laser that has been totally enclosed (embedded) inside a protective enclosure equipped with appropriate interlocks on all removable panels and access doors. This prevents beam access during operation and maintenance. Such a completely enclosed system, if properly labeled and safeguarded with protective housing interlocks and all other applicable engineering controls, will fulfill all requirements for a Class I laser and may be operated in the enclosed manner without the requirement for additional controls for the operator. For example, during actual operation, a Nd:YAG laser used endoscopically could be considered operationally a Class I system. During use the laser beam can be contained within the laser, the fiber delivery system, the endoscope and, finally, the patient. If the system were designed to *preclude* operation except when the system was completely enclosed and the endoscope placed within the patient, it could be considered a Class I device by FDA. Endoscopic systems manufactured to date do not have such a classification due to the difficulty and expense of assuring such a Class I condition.

However, the Laser Safety Officer (LSO) could decide, using the ANSI Z-136.1 standard, that an endoscopic Nd:YAG laser was Class I operationally, provided certain procedural controls were met. This would eliminate many of the Class IV controls that would be required for this system. The major concern would be related to assuring that the fiber does not break during the procedure.

It should be noted that during periods of service, controls appropriate to the class of the embedded laser are required, perhaps on a temporary basis, when the beam enclosures are removed and beam access is possible. Beam access during service will *not change* the Class I status of the laser during operation.

Limited Open-Beam Path

Some surgical laser uses, particularly those using fiberoptic intrapatient delivery may, in fact, enclose the immediate area of beam delivery *almost completely*. Such a system would not meet, perhaps, the stringent "human access" requirements of the FLPPS for a Class I laser, but the real laser hazards are well confined.

Such a design provides what can be called a limited open-beam path. In this situation, the ANSI Z-136.1 standard recommends that the LSO shall effect a laser hazard analysis and establish the extent of the nominal hazard zone (NHZ). In many system designs, such as described above, the NHZ will be extremely limited and procedural controls rather than elaborate engineering controls will be sufficient.

Protective equipment (eye protection, temporary barriers, clothing and/or gloves, respirators, etc.) would be recommended, for example, only if the hazard analysis indicated a need or if the Standard Operating Procedure (SOP) required periods of beam access, such as during setup or infrequent maintenance activities. Temporary protective measures would be handled in a manner similar to operation of any Class IV surgical laser.

Totally Unenclosed Beam Path

Most surgical laser uses are used in an unenclosed beam condition. Such laser uses will require that a complete hazard analysis and NHZ assessment be effected by the LSO if such information is not furnished by the manufacturer of the laser. Then, the controls implemented will reflect the magnitude and extent of the accessible beam.

A 100-W Nd:YAG surgical laser system will require beam path controls during surgical use. As summarized in Table 41.2, the intrabeam (direct) hazard extends from 792 to 1410 m, depending upon whether the 10-second or 8-hour MPE criteria are used during the NHZ calculations. Simularly, with a lens on the laser, the hazard exists over a range from 6.3 to 11.4 m. The diffuse reflection zone is, however, markedly smaller, ranging from 0.8 to 1.4 m. This suggests that surgeons and support staff close to the operative site would still need laser eye protection, even for diffuse reflections from the surgical area.

If the LSO provides a detailed procedural control to limit the "beam on" condition only to situations where the lens was in place and the beam was focused only onto the surgical site, then the zone of potential beam hazard would be limited to that resulting from diffuse reflections and, in an absolute "worst-case" scenario, to the specular reflections of the focused beam. This implies a maximum hazard region that extends no greater than about 30 ft. This certainly would project outside a surgical room. The LSO would be correct to require a barrier be placed just *inside* the entrance way to prevent an unlikely stray beam from going out a doorway. Although entryway interlocking is also an alternative, it is limiting in most surgical settings. Entryway controls such as interlocking may, however, be more strongly considered by the LSO in areas such as outpatient clinics and research laboratories where one cannot closely monitor personnel flow in and out of the laser area.

Similar analyses are provided in Tables 41.2 and 41.3 for a 100-W CO_2 laser and a 5-W argon laser. Note that the NHZ distances do not vary for the CO_2 laser (because the MPE values are nearly identical for the 10-second and 8-hour exposure times). Also note that the diffuse reflection NHZ distances are very small except for the 8-hour criteria for the argon laser. In most cases, the 0.25-second criteria can be used with visible frequency lasers unless intentional staring is possible.

Laser-Controlled Area

When the entire beam path from a Class IIIB or IV laser is not sufficiently enclosed and/or baffled such that access to radiation above the MPE is possible, a "laser-controlled area" is required. During periods of service, the controlled area is established on a temporary basis. The controlled area will encompass the NHZ. Those controls required for *both* Class IIIB and Class IV installations are as follows:

1. *Posting with appropriate laser warning signs:* Class IIIA (beam irradiance >2.5 mW/cm^2), Class IIIB and Class IV lasers require the DANGER sign format: white background, red laser symbol with black outline and black lettering. Note that area posting is *required* only for Class IIIB and Class IV lasers and laser systems (Figure 41.4).

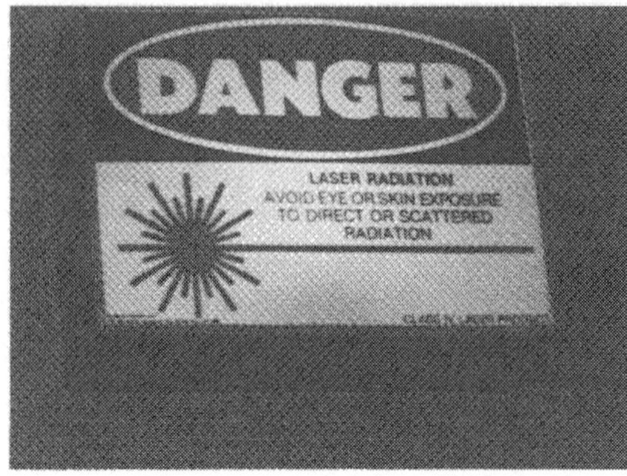
DANGER
LASER RADIATION
AVOID EYE OR SKIN EXPOSURE
TO DIRECT OR SCATTERED
RADIATION

FIGURE 41.4. Laser danger warning sign. Typical posting for a medical laser installation. Signs are recommended for Class IIIB and Class IV lasers. Lighted sign is connected to laser system so that light is on when laser is activated. Some facilities install flashing light capability. Design and colors are specified in ANSI-Z136 standard.

   If the LSO chooses to post Class II or Class IIIA areas, then all signs (and labels) associated with these lasers (when the beam irradiance for Class IIIA does not exceed 2.5 mW/cm^2) will use the CAUTION format: yellow background, with black laser symbol and letters.
2. *Operation by qualified and authorized personnel:* This includes appropriate training of the individuals in aspects of laser safety.
3. *Transmission from indoor controlled area:* The beams shall not, under any circumstances, be transmitted from an indoor laser controlled area unless for specific purposes (such as atmospheric testing). In such cases, the operator and the LSO must assure that the beam path is limited to controlled air space.

Those items recommended for Class IIIB but *required* for Class IV lasers are as follows:

1. Supervised directly by of an individual knowledgeable in laser safety.
2. Require approved entry of any noninvolved personnel.
3. Terminate all potentially hazardous beams in a beam stop of an appropriate material.
4. Use diffusely reflecting materials near the beam, where appropriate.

5. Personnel within the laser controlled area are provided with appropriate laser protective eyewear.
6. Secure and locate the laser such that the beam path is above or below eye level in any standing or seated position.
7. Have all windows, doorways, open portals, and so on from an indoor facility covered or restricted thus reducing transmitted beams below the appropriate ocular MPE level.
8. Require storage or disabling of lasers when not in use.

In addition, there are specific controls required at the entryway to a Class IV laser controlled area. These can be summarized as follows:

1. All personnel entering a Class IV area shall be adequately trained and given proper laser protective eyewear.
2. All personnel shall follow all applicable administrative and procedural controls.
3. All Class IV area area/entryway controls shall allow both rapid entrance and exit under all conditions.
4. The controlled area shall have a clearly marked "Panic Button" (disconnect switch) that allows rapid deactivation of the laser.

In addition, Class IV areas also require some form of area/entryway controls. In the past, doorway interlocking was required for all Class IV installations. In the revised ANSI Z-136.1 (1986) standard, a set of options is provided that allow the LSO to provide an entryway control suited for the installation. The options include:

1. *Nondefeatable entryway controls:*
   Controls such as a magnetic switch built into the entryway door. In this case, training is required *only* for those persons who *regularly* require access into the laser area.
2. *Defeatable entryway controls:*
   Controls such as may be required, for example, in long-term testing in a laser area or for some surgical laser environments. In this case the controls may be overridden if it is clearly evident that there is no hazard at the point of entry. Training is required for all personnel who may require entry into the area.

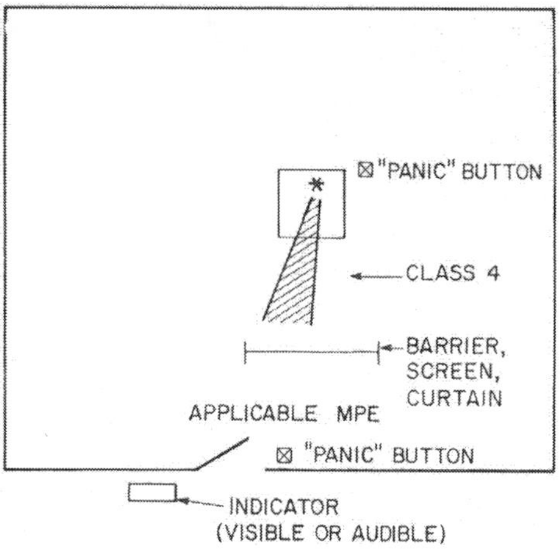

FIGURE 41.5. Procedural entryway control. A barrier can be used to prevent beam from exiting laser room. Barrier design should be such as to withstand direct, lens-on-laser and/or scattered laser light for a specified period (nominally 60 seconds) and not produce a fire hazard.

3. *Procedural entryway controls:*
   Controls such as blocking barrier, or screen, or curtain which can block or filter the laser beam at the entryway may be used *inside* the controlled area to prevent the laser light from exiting the area at levels above the applicable MPE level. In this case, a warning light or sound is required *outside* the entryway that operates when the laser is energized and operating. In addition, *all personnel* shall receive training (Figure 41.5).

Administrative and Procedural Controls

One of the more important of the so-called administrative and procedural controls is the Standard Operating Procedure (SOP). This is required for a Class IV laser and is recommended for a Class IIIB laser.

The key to a written SOP is that those individuals who operate, maintain, and service the equipment should be involved in the preparation with guidance from the LSO. Most laser equipment will be provided with instructions for safe operation by the manufacturer. However, sometimes these are not well suited to a specific use due to special conditions of use.

Other administrative and procedural controls include:

1. *Alignment procedures:*
   One of the highest rates of laser eye accidents occurs during laser alignment. Such procedures must be done with extreme caution. A written procedure is recommended for recurring alignment tasks.
2. *Limitations on spectators:*
   Persons unnecessary to the laser operation should be kept away. For those who do enter the laser area, appropriate eye protection and instruction is recommended.

As mentioned, the overall laser safety program is administered by the LSO. Some of the main LSO duties are to monitor and enforce the control of laser hazards and, when needed, effect the knowledgeable evaluation and control of laser hazards. In addition, the LSO establishes and periodically reviews appropriate control measures, avoids needless duplication of controls in cases where several alternate but equally effective means may be used to limit exposure, and effects laser safety training, when appropriate.

Laser Factors

In the selection of any laser, one must consider the applications intended by the *various specialties*. The more versatile laser can be used by many of the hospital services and, therefore, justify the initial financial investment. This usually requires SOP's for each specialty, since different delivery systems and procedures are required.

The safety protocols will usually be *adapted to the different delivery systems* such as handpieces, microscopes, endoscopic couplers, and fiberoptic couplers.

Mobility is also important in permitting increased usage. Although it is best to move any laser system as infrequently as possible, the requirement for mobility should be considered when developing the SOP's, since a *complete* system checkout will be required prior to use to assure optimum performance. Laser systems include delicate optics that are sensitive to moving.

Education and Training

Frequent presentations to the medical staff on laser applications and the correct safety procedures are recommended, especially when new procedures are introduced. These are in addition to the detailed initial laser inservice training.

An extensive hands-on and theory training of the Medical Laser Specialists to run and be responsible for laser equipment and procedures is also recommended.

Availability of a dealer's or manufacturer's agent for technical assistance is important to the purchase decision as is the availability for ongoing educational presentations for the staff and/or medical community.

Service and Maintenance

All lasers malfunction. Even the best instrument is of little value when it is not working properly. The availability of a dependable, qualified service team is essential.

The quality of education and service personnel must be considered with the same emphasis that is given to choosing laser technology. In a rapidly evolving technological field, the ability to modify equipment, adjust to new developments, and learn the new scientific material is very important.

In order to assure a smooth implementation of new laser technology, several steps should be taken before initiating the clinical use of the laser. A laser safety committee should be established, nurses appointed to receive training as Laser Medical Specialists, and educational presentations planned.

Laser Safety Committee

A laser safety committee should be established even before a laser is delivered to the hospital. This committee is essential for planning, legal, and safety purposes. The committee is often comprised of physicians from various specialties, chief of surgery, operating room director and head nurse, primary laser nurse, and an administrator. This committee will establish written guidelines for laser procedures, protocol on its use, and credentials standards for laser privileges. The purpose of this committee is to promote the safe and frequent use of the laser.

Medical Laser Specialists

It is essential that the responsibilities for operating and controlling the laser be limited to a few well-trained individuals. A minimum of two or three nurses or technicians should receive thorough training in lasers in general and the hospital's unit in particular. A manufacturer's inservice program on how to "push the button and turn the dials" is not sufficient to make the unit operative and ensure safe use.

Inservice and Trial Run

A trial laser case should be scheduled if the laser is a new piece of equipment. This procedure would involve the primary physician, laser nurse, and operating room personnel. All other equipment such as microscopes, bipolars, video equipment, and so on that will be used in the laser case should also be activated. Such a trial procedure allows one to learn beforehand the best physical setup of the room, how to appropriately drape the new equipment, whether there are ample electrical outlets, and whether sufficient current is available in the operating area. All safety protocols should be developed and practiced at this session.

A general inservice session should be scheduled for the entire surgical staff. This is an introductory session designed to acquaint all personnel with the new instrumentation. A medical presentation on the medical applications of lasers may enhance interest and promote increased use of the instrument by diverse physicians.

Continuing Education

Periodic refresher courses are recommended for all laser personnel. Emphasis should be placed on new techniques, procedures, and methods to assure safety. The laser safety personnel, laser nurses, and technicians should undergo continuing training on at least a biyearly basis.

Patient Concerns and Safety

A medical laser safety discussion would not be complete without some comments about patients who undergo treatment. Medical personnel should not dismiss psychological concerns or fears their patients could have when faced with laser surgery. For patients, the concern over "Star Wars" may be difficult to resolve. In addition, sounds and smells of laser surgery can be very frightening. Moreover, since everyone in the room may be wearing safety glasses (Figure 41.6), the impact can be potentially upsetting, since such safety equipment and procedures implies a dangerous procedure. In order to reduce such fears, medical personnel can do the following:

1. Take the patient step-by-step through the procedure and carefully explain what to expect.
2. Explain what a laser is, how it works, and how it is used.
3. Remind the patient about smells and sounds, and the need for safety glasses.
4. Help patients understand the concerns about having "excessive expectations" of laser treatments.

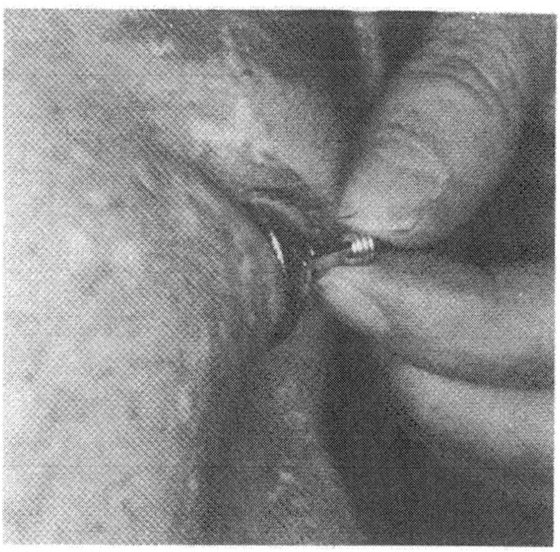

FIGURE 41.6. Patient eyeshields. Special reflecting eyeshields can be applied to completely cover eye. Such protection is especially important in dermatologic procedures around the eye, such as port-wine nevi treatment.

Personal Protective Equipment

Personal protective equipment for laser safety generally means eye protection in the form of goggles or spectacles. This can include special prescription eyewear using special high optical density filter materials or reflective coatings to reduce the potential ocular exposure below MPE limits. Some applications, such as use of high-power excimer lasers operating in the ultraviolet, may also dictate the use of a skin cover if chronic repeated exposures are anticipated at exposure levels at or near the maximum permissible exposure (MPE) limits for skin.

In general, it is recommended that, if possible, other means of controls be employed rather than reliance specifically on the use of protective eyewear. This argument is predicated on the fact that so many accidents have occurred when eyewear was available but not worn. There are many reasons for this lack of use, but the most common are, most probably, that the eyewear is dark and uncomfortable to wear and limits vision.

Laser protective eyewear filters are specified in terms of the logarithmic units of optical density (usually referred to as "OD"). Optical density (OD) is a logarithmic function defined by the equation

$$\mathrm{OD} = \log_{10}\left(\frac{H_0}{\mathrm{MPE}}\right), \tag{11}$$

where

H_0 = anticipated worst-case exposure (J/cm^2 or W/cm^2), and

MPE = maximum permissible exposure level expressed in same units as H_0.

It should be noted that, since the MPE values have, in effect, been normalized to the area of the so-called limiting aperture, which is the 7-mm pupil size for visible and near-infrared, the calculation for H_0 for beams *smaller* than the limiting aperture requires that the limiting aperture be used *instead of* the smaller beam size. Thus, the calculation is made *as though* the beam were spread over the limiting aperture.

As an example, consider the case of a 100-W Nd:YAG laser emitted in a 2-mm beam diameter. This would be a Class IV laser with an MPE = 1.6 mW/cm^2. Thus the OD is calculated by first determining the value of H_0. From the above, we calculate the worst-case exposure spread over the 7-mm limiting aperture and *not* the 2-mm laser beam diameter. Thus the effective "area" is found: $A = \pi d^2/4 = \pi(0.7)^2/4 = 0.385$ cm^2. The radiant exposure $H_0 = 100/0.385 = 259.7$ W/cm^2. Calculation for the OD is done as follows:

$$\mathrm{OD} = \log_{10}\left(\frac{259.7}{1.6 \times 10^{-3}}\right) = 5.2.$$

Thus a filter with OD = 5.2 for the 1.064-μm Nd:YAG laser wavelength would provide adequate protection.

Optical Density When a Fiber is Used

A hazard analysis of a typical Nd:YAG surgical laser (1.06 μm) with a fiberoptic delivery could be based upon the following parameters using a maximum of 100 W of continuous wave laser power with a beam divergence of 210 mrad (12 degrees) from the fiber tip and an exposure time of 10 seconds.

Using these parameters, a mathematical hazard analysis can be done to estimate the general region around the surgical site where hazardous exposures may be possible. The following analysis is representative of Nd:YAG surgical lasers.

The worst-case MPE value for a direct intrabeam or point source diffuse reflection with a Nd:YAG laser exposure of 10 seconds is 50.6 mJ/cm^2. The MPE for a long-term (>8-hour) extended source diffuse reflection of this laser is 3.2 W cm^{-2} sr^{-1} contained within an apparent visual angle (α_{min}) which is not smaller than 24 mrad. The 10-second MPE value for skin exposure is 10.5 J/cm^2.

To estimate a diffuse reflection from the site, one must first estimate the approximate scattering distance from the target site on the tissues to the surgeon's eye. This is about 40 cm (approximately 16 in.). The ANSI Z-136.1 point-source MPE criterion is used in this case because, using Equation 7 and applying an α_{min} of 24 mrad, one can show that point-source conditions exist when the laser spot size is less than 1 cm diameter (e.g., $D_L = 40 \times 24 \times 10^{-3} = 0.96$ cm). Since beam diameters less than 1 cm are anticipated in the fiberoptic procedure, the beam acts as a point source. Solving Equation 4, the irradiance at the eye will be 19.9 mW/cm^2. This produces a radiant exposure of nearly 200 mJ/cm^2 during a 10-second exposure.

Based upon these typical exposure conditions, the optical density required for a suitable filter can be determined. Using a worst-case exposure condition outlined above, one can determine the optical density recommended to provide adequate eye protection for this laser. Using Equation 11, the minimum optical density at the 1.064 μm Nd:YAG laser wavelength for a 10-second direct intrabeam exposure (MPE = 50.6 mJ/cm^2) to the 100-W maximum laser output (H_o = 2597 J/cm^2) would be OD = 4.7.

The more conservative approach reviewed previously would be to consider the full-day 8-hour occupational exposure. In this case, (MPE = 1.6 mW/cm^2, H_o = 259.7 W/cm^2) the optical density at 1.06 μm is OD = 5.2 for the 100-Watt intrabeam viewing condition.

The optical density required for safe viewing of the diffuse reflection off tissues is substantially reduced from the 100 W intrabeam case. Using the 40-cm "viewing distance" described above, the required optical density at 1.06 μm (H_o = 200 mJ/cm^2, MPE = 50.6 mJ/cm^2) would be OD = 0.6 for a 10-second exposure and (H_o = 19.9 mW/cm^2, MPE = 1.6 mW/cm^2) an OD = 1.1 for the occupational 8-hour exposure.

These worst-case conditions suggest that an optical density in the range from 4.7 to 5.2 at the 1.064-μm wavelength is recommended for 100-W Nd:YAG laser surgical situations using an open beam fiberoptic. Diffuse viewing will require optical density values of 1.1 or smaller, depending on viewing time and beam spot size.

A wide variety of commercially available optical absorbing filter materials either of glass or plastic and various coated reflecting "filters," including dielectric coatings and some experimental holographic designs, are available for laser eye protection. Some are available in spectacles ground to prescription specifications. One filter type may be applicable to more than one wavelength. Some filters have a high optical density below a certain "cutoff" wavelength, usually limiting overall visibility (Figure 41.7).

One of the more superior eye protection filters for the Nd:YAG laser is the near-infrared absorbing glass designated KG-3 or KG-5 from the Schott Optical Company. These two glass types have optical density values sufficient to meet almost all surgical Nd:YAG situations and yet has nearly 95% luminous (visible light) transmission.

The typical optical density and internal transmittance values for various filter thickness values from 1 to 5 mm for the KG-3 and KG-5 are given in Table 41.4. Eye protection usually is done with filter thickness no less than 3 mm. Unless the glass is thermally treated, eye protection using KG-3 and KG-5 filters will require additional clear coverage to provide impact resistance using, for example, a high-impact resistant plastic.

The need for protection for multiple laser wavelengths is becoming more common in the

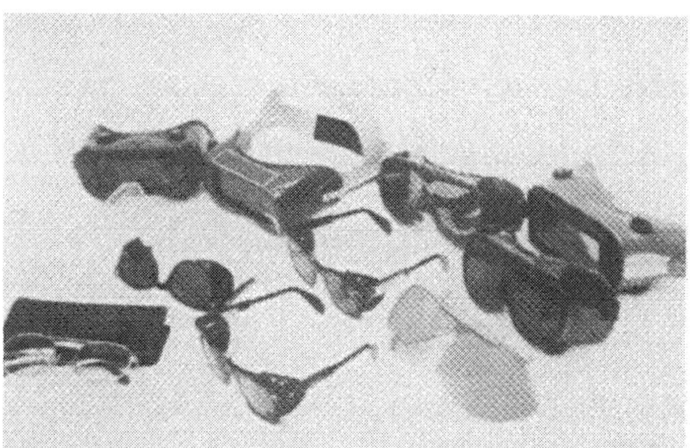

FIGURE 41.7. Laser protective eyewear. Protective filters can be obtained in a range of designs, including prescription spectacles and traditional goggles. Filters have high optical density values at the laser wavelength and reduce worst-case exposure to the MPE level.

TABLE 41.4. Optical density and internal transmittance for Schott KG-3 and KG-5 glass as a function of glass thickness

Glass type	Thickness (mm)	Transmission at 1060 nm	Optical density
KG-3	1.0	0.24E-01	1.6
	1.5	0.38E-02	2.4
	2.0	0.60E-03	3.2
	2.5	0.94E-04	4.0
	3.0	0.15E-04	4.8
	3.5	0.23E-05	5.6
	4.0	0.36E-06	6.4
	4.5	0.56E-07	7.2
	5.0	0.88E-08	8.1
KG-5	1.0	0.55E-02	2.3
	1.5	0.41E-03	3.4
	2.0	0.30E-04	4.5
	2.5	0.22E-05	5.7
	3.0	0.16E-06	6.8
	3.5	0.12E-07	7.9
	4.0	0.90E-09	9.0
	4.5	0.67E-10	10.2
	5.0	0.49E-11	11.3

surgical environment, as procedures may involve several laser wavelengths or different laser types. In this case, dual filters are often the design of choice, frequently mounted in a "flip-up"-style goggle or spectacle frame.

Of special concern is the management of eye protection in such multiple laser environments to assure that proper protection is being used for each laser type and wavelength. Some medical facilities have color-coded the eyewear to aid in proper selection. Then the LSO or nurse responsible for safety practices during a procedure can quickly check that proper eyewear is being used.

Invisible Beam Control

Infrared (0.7–10^3 μm) and ultraviolet (0.2—0.4 μm) laser radiation are "invisible" radiations, and special controls are often necessary. For example; The beams from Class IIIB and Class IV lasers should be terminated in highly absorbent, nonspecular reflecting materials wherever practicable. Many metal surfaces that appear "dull" visually can act as a specular reflector of infrared radiation. All secondary beams from reflections should be appropriately terminated in an absorbent material. Periodic inspection is required of the absorbent materials, since they degrade with use.

Firebrick materials containing beryllium or other hazardous substances should not be used. An optical-wedge absorber is recommended for beam termination.

Engineering Controls

The most universal controls are referred to as engineering controls. Usually, these are items built into the laser equipment that provide for safety. In most instances, these will be included on the equipment provided by the laser manufacturer as so-called "Performance Requirements" mandated by the FDA. The systems will have, for example, built-in beam shutters, laser power monitors, maintenance panel interlocks, "beam-on" indicator lights or tones, key-operated control switches, and numerous labels related to safety (Figure 41.8).

All of these features do provide a baseline for safe operation, but do not replace the need for evaluation of the hazards during use and the implementation of adequate area and personal controls and adopting proper standard operating procedures (SOP's) for each type of surgical procedure.

DANGER

INVISIBLE LASER RADIATION WHEN OPEN
AVOID EYE OR SKIN EXPOSURE TO
DIRECT OR SCATTERED RADIATION

FIGURE 41.8. Laser protective housing label. Required by FDA and ANSI standards for portions of the laser housing that, when removed for servicing, permit access to the beam.

Training Programs

Detailed training is recommended for those working with Class III and Class IV lasers, including the technical support staff and technicians. The training should provide a complete understanding of the requirements of a safe laser environment. Emphasis should be placed on practical, safe laser techniques and procedures, as well as safety devices that provide an overall safe environment.

The need for frequent update training sessions, particularly for the laser professional, was well shown in a published account by an individual who lost the sight of one eye when protective eyewear was not used. This article concluded: "But more important than the actual event is the idea that this incident could have been avoided. Don't let it happen to you or a coworker. Take time to assess safety conditions, and do it again in 6 months or a year; additional hazards arise in an ever-changing research environment. Safety deserves your thoughtful considerations, now, before your accident."

Often each training session will need to be tailored for the different groups working with specific lasers in the facility. The type of laser(s) and locations will impact the content of the training program. For example, the hazards and controls recommended for the far-infrared carbon dioxide lasers are usually different than those for a near-infrared Nd:YAG laser or a visible argon laser.

In addition, the use of several laser types at the same facility will require review of each system in the training sessions. Special analysis will be necessary in the event that two or more lasers are used in the same location at one time. In this event, the protective eyewear and operational precautions may need to be adjusted for the presence of multiple laser wavelengths.

Conclusions

The Nd:YAG laser used in surgery has the potential of providing hazards to the eye and skin of the surgeon, support staff, and patient. The hazard evaluation methods described can allow for analysis of the zone within the surgical area where direct and scattered beam hazards exist. Implementation of the protective procedures and use of proper safety equipment can provide adequate safety to all involved in the surgical procedure.

Bibliography

American National Standard for the Safe Use of Lasers. ANSI Z-136.1 (1986). Laser Institute of America, Toledo, OH, 1986.

Comment: It could happen to you. Laser Focus p 10, Apr 1982.

Goldman L, Rockwell R Jr: Lasers in Medicine. Gordon & Breach, New York, 1971.

Ham WT Jr: The eye problem in laser safety. Arch Environ Health 20:156, 1970.

Laser Safety Guide, 6th ed. The Laser Institute of America, Toledo, OH, 1986.

Meyer Arendt JR: Radiometry and photometry units and conversion factors. Appl Opt 7:2081, 1968.

Performance Standard for Laser Products. Center for Devices and Radiological Health, Food and Drug Administration (DHHS), CFR 50 (161):33682–33702 Tuesday, Aug 20, 1985.

Rockwell RJ Jr: Ensuring safety in laser robotics. Lasers Applications 3(11):65–70, Nov 1984.

Rockwell RJ Jr (ed): Laser Safety in Surgery and Medicine, 2nd ed. Rockwell Associates, Cincinnati, OH, 1985.

Rockwell RJ Jr: Analyzing laser hazards. Lasers Applications 5(5):97–103, May 1986.

Rockwell RJ Jr: Controlling laser hazards. Lasers Applications, 5(9):93–99, Sep 1986.

Rockwell RJ Jr, Moss CE: Optical radiation hazards in laser welding processes. Part I: Neodymium-YAG Industrr Hyg Assoc 44(8):572–579, Aug 1983.

Safety of Lasers and Other Optical Radiation Source. Rockwell Associates, Cincinnati, OH, 1986.

Sliney DH, Freazier BC: The evaluation of optical radiation hazards. Appl Opt 12:1, 1973.

Sliney DH, Wolbarsh ML: Safety Manual for Lasers and Other Optical Sources. Plenum, New York, 1978.

42
Tissue Interactions of Carbon Monoxide and Carbon Dioxide Lasers

Tsunenori Arai, and Makoto Kikuchi

The principle and the practical experimental results for the tissue interaction of CO and CO_2 lasers are described in this chapter. The high-intensity irradiation of these lasers indicates strong cutting to the living tissue. Despite the fact CO_2 lasers have been used as the unique light source for the laser scalpel, one problem remaining unsolved is the lack of available flexible optical fibers that can deliver CO_2 laser radiation of 10.6 μm in wavelength. The CO laser radiation of wavelength 5 μm indicates similar tissue interaction to the CO_2 laser radiation. Moreover, the flexible glass fibers made from infrared glasses can be available for CO laser delivery. We have recommended using CO lasers for cutting instead of CO_2 lasers.

Principles of Cutting Interactions to Living Tissue

General Principles

The tissue interaction against an incident laser beam can be essentially explained by the absorption and the scattering characteristics of the living tissue. A light that is strongly absorbed by the tissue indicates cutting capacity as the tissue interaction. On the other hand, a light that is weakly absorbed by the tissue induces strong coagulation capacity to the tissue. The scattering process is not dominant for the cutting phenomenon so that the extinction length of the tissue for the cutting laser light is extremely short. Moreover, the scattering process may be weak since the diameter of the scatterer in the living tissue is generally small compared with the cutting laser wavelength.

Since the tissue optical characteristics and the irradiation conditions have been continuously changed by the irradiation, a definite statement about tissue interaction cannot be made. For instance, even Nd:YAG laser irradiation can be used for cutting and vaporizing, in spite of this radiation essentially indicating strong coagulation. The low intensity with long-term irradiation of CO_2 lasers coagulates the surface of the tissue. Moreover, a contact irradiation method was currently developed as an irradiation technique of the Nd:YAG laser.[1] This contact irradiation of Nd:YAG laser using the sapphire tip attachment indicates fine cutting injuries, due to high heat deposition on the boundary between the tip and the tissue and/or mechanical pushing by the tip.

In this chapter the essential interaction of tissue is only described in order to present the fundamental characteristics of CO and CO_2 irradiations to the tissue.

Tissue Light Absorption

The absorption characteristics are particularly important in describing the cutting phenomenon to tissue. The absorption characteristics of the living tissue in the light region of electromagnetic waves is characterized mainly by water, hemoglobin, and protein absorption.

Tissue Light Absorption by Water

Water is the major constituent of living tissue, the maximum component excluding the fat and bone. Approximately 50 to 60% of the whole human body in weight consists of water. In the muscle, this rate is increased to 75%. The strong absorption of water appears in the wide wavelength region of the electromagnetic wave. Figure 42.1 shows the absorption spectrum of liquid water in the infrared.[2] In general, this absorption within the light region decreases with the wavelength in spite of the existence of some absorption peaks. In the visible and ultraviolet region, the absorption coefficient is less than 10^{-1} cm^{-1}; in other words, the extinction length which is defined as a length at one-tenth of the attenuation of light intensity is in excess of 23 cm. Therefore, water is almost transmitting material for visible and ultraviolet light, and the water absorption is merely important for infrared light to discuss the cutting interaction. For wavelengths over 2.3 μm, water indicates a strong absorption of which the coefficient is over 10^2 cm^{-1}. The extinction length h of this wavelength region is less than 230 μm. The kinetics of this absorption range is attributed to the stimulated absorption of the vibrational mode of water, for instance, as in a strong absorption peak of approximately 3 μm ascribed to the vibrational absorption of OH radical. In the liquid phase, a certain internal energy mode can be strongly affected by the interaction force, so that it forms a broad absorption band. Particularly as water is composed by hydrogen bonds, this tendency is obviously enhanced.

Tissue Light Absorption by Proteins

Living tissue contains less than 10% protein on an average. This content is as high as 12% in muscles. Despite absorption by proteins appearing from ultraviolet to far-infrared, they play an important role at ultraviolet and mid-infrared regions. In the ultraviolet, since water is almost a window material, the protein absorption will be effective. Protein absorption near 280 nm is due to the electronic state of aromatic amino acids. Currently, excimer lasers that oscillate ultraviolet laser radiation with high average power are used for preliminary medical applications to obtain nonthermal cutting by destruction of the structure of proteins.[3] This cutting has a useful advantage for the restriction of thermal injuries; however, simultaneously it has harmful cytotoxicity and mutagenicity due to the destruction of the inherited information in the cell. In mid-infrared, proteins have strong absorption peaks caused by amino acids which are the fundamental component of proteins. These peaks appear 1660–1610 cm^{-1} and 1550–1485 cm^{-1}, generally called amino acid I and amino

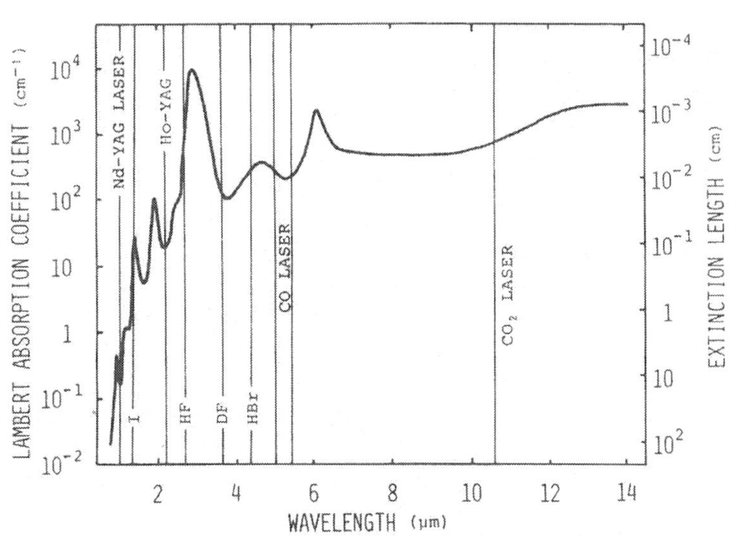

FIGURE 42.1. Absorption spectrum of liquid water in infrared with the oscillation wavelength of infrared high-power lasers. The extinction length (Le) is expressed as; Le = 1/0.434μm, where μm is the absorption coefficient.

acid II, respectively. These peaks are attributed to the vibrational state of the NH_3^+ bending mode.

Tissue Light Absorption by Dyes

Dyes in the living tissue strongly affect tissue absorption in the visible and near-infrared regions. Dyes have efficient kinetics for light absorption, and the existence of small amounts of dyes indicates strong absorption. The most important dye in living tissue is hemoglobin, which composes a third of the red blood cell in weight. Melanin in the skin is effective when discussing the surface optical characteristics of black skin. The absorption spectrum of hemoglobin is changed by oxidation.[4] If the tissue contains a density of 2×10^{-3} mol/L oxyhemoglobin (over estimation), the absorption by oxyhemoglobin becomes larger than by water at least from 1 μm of wavelength. The absorption of the oxyhemoglobin is important in describing tissue interaction by argon and Nd:YAG lasers. However, in normal tissue, absorption by oxyhemoglobin is not effective for cutting lasers, that is, CO and CO_2 lasers.

Mechanism of Tissue Cutting

The absorbed light energy is delivered into the internal mode (vibrational or electrical) of molecules, then it rapidly relaxes to the lowest internal mode within a few microseconds. The energy of the lowest mode, that is, the translational mode, is called thermal energy. The increase of the thermal energy is characterized by an increase of translational temperature which can be directly measured by a thermometer. By irradiation of high absorption light to the tissue, the rapid increase of the temperature in the tissue induces the evaporation of water. The irradiated portion of the tissue disappears with this evaporation. The evaporation heat is extracted from the irradiated portion by the evaporation. The heat conduction also stimulates heat extraction from the irradiated portion. However, since the rate of the heat generation by the light irradiation is set extremely higher than this heat extraction, the continuous evaporation by the radiation is steadily kept. In addition, under the high temperature condition, proteins of which the tissue is composed burns with the existence of air. This burning enhances the disappearance of the tissue. These descriptions are general explanations of the tissue cutting by light irradiation which is strongly absorbed by the tissue. Since the complex processes simultaneously occurred under the light irradiation, the precise estimation method of cutting interaction has not been reported.

The resulting damaged layer aside from the cutting groove is thinner than other cutting methods due to the short extinction length of the irradiated light and the short time period of cutting. This thin damaged layer induces an advantage in the healing of injuries. Moreover, an advantage against infection is this noncontact process of cutting. However, the thin damaged layer can also imply a poor capacity of hemostasis. The high rate of heat generation in a small volume is necessary for this cutting, produced by the high intensity of light irradiation and/or strong absorption of the tissue. To obtain such high light intensity, the use of the coherent laser source is necessary. That is the reason why mid-infrared lasers are employed for the noncontact tissue cutting.

Tissue Interaction of CO and CO_2 Lasers

Available Infrared Lasers

Since lasers are oscillators that use the interaction between the internal energy mode of molecules/atoms and the electromagnetic field, lasers have essentially a poor tunability of oscillation wavelength. Moreover, there are few lasers which can extract high power with practical efficiency. In the wavelength range over 2.3 μm, they are CO_2, CO, HBr, DF, and HF lasers. HBr, DF, and HF lasers being chemically pumped lasers, are not practical because of the problem of the treatment of exhaust gases. CO and CO_2 lasers are electrically excited (i.e., discharge excited) lasers with high efficiencies.[5,6] The sealed-off operation of laser gases has been established in these lasers.[7,8] Therefore these lasers are extremely useful for cutting applications.

To apply cutting lasers to endoscopic applications, it is important to select a wavelength with a transmission range of flexible fibers. Despite CO_2 lasers having been applied to a laser scalpel, the optical transmission line of all production models of the CO_2 laser scalpel have been made by a series of reflectors in the manipulator. It was not until recently that an inflexible crystalline fiber was equipped in the production model of the CO_2 laser scalpel for the first time.[9] This defect of the CO_2 laser scalpel is due to the lack of available glass materials with long oscillation wavelengths of CO_2 lasers. CO lasers have not been applied in practical use, however they have an attractive wavelength for light delivery by flexible optical fibers. The authors predict that CO lasers might be used as cutting lasers instead of CO_2 lasers. Please refer to Chapter 39 for further details.

Experimental Setup

The interaction of the cutting laser should be determined by this experimental investigation because of the difficulty of giving a precise description of the laser cutting.[10] The interactions of CO and CO_2 laser irradiations to the tissue were experimentally investigated.[11,12] The interaction of the CO laser has been preliminarily reported by Karbe et al.,[13] however the authors could not find quantitative information from the prior report. A small laser device was constructed for this purpose. This laser device had a laser tube of 7 mm inside diameter and 60 cm in length. By changing laser gases, optical components, and cryogens, the device could oscillate both CO and CO_2 lasers. The oscillation transverse mode was TEM_{oo} with a spot diameter of 3.5 mm. The oscillation wavelengths were measured by a grating monochrometer. The measured wavelength of the CO laser was distributed from 5.0 μm to 5.4 μm (5.2 μm in an average). The measured wavelength of the CO_2 laser was approximately 10.6 μm [the branches of P(16), P(20), or P(22)]. All laser irradiations were carried out in vitro. The samples for laser irradiations were exsanguinated dog and cow livers. Since the interactions by CO and CO_2 irradiations are mainly attributed to water absorption in the tissue, the content of blood (i.e., hemoglobin) does not seriously affect the interaction.

To irradiate a high-intensity laser beam, a gold concave mirror of 250 mm in curvature was used to collimate the laser beam. The diameter of the collimated laser beam at a focal point was 0.2 mm with a focal depth of 16 mm. The refractive optics were used for collimation, so that the collimated beam geometry was slightly changed. However, since the incident angle to the concave mirror was limited up to 10° this transformation was quite small. In order to express the intensity of the light beam, the average light intensity was defined to use;

$$I_{av} = P/\pi \times R_s^2$$

where

I_{av} = the average light intensity;

P = the beam power; and

R_s = the spot radius.

I_{av} is half the intensity as the peak intensity within the beam at TEM_{oo} transverse mode. The sample surface was aligned at 120 mm from the concave mirror, so the spot diameter on the sample surface was 0.5 mm. The irradiated area was scanned automatically by moving the sample by a servo mechanism. This action was coordinated to move the collimated beam in actual applications to cut the tissue. In the case of the low-intensity irradiation, the laser beam oscillated was directly delivered to irradiate on the sample. The sample position was fixed in this case.

Results and Discussion

High-Intensity Irradiation

The high-intensity laser beams of CO and CO_2 lasers irradiated on the surface of the moving samples. The average light intensity was set to 2.6 kW/cm^2. The moving speed was varied within 0.1 to 10 mm/second. These results are shown in Figure 42.2.[11,12] The results show that the high-intensity irradiation of these lasers indicates strong cutting performance, although the cutting depth by the CO laser irradiation is slightly less than that by the CO_2 laser irradiation. The incised depth is proportional to the incision speed (i.e., the movement speed of the sample). In the case of 1.3 kW/cm^2 irradiation, the incised depth was decreased to a half of that of 2.6 kW/cm^2 for both lasers.

To investigate the damage of the tissue by

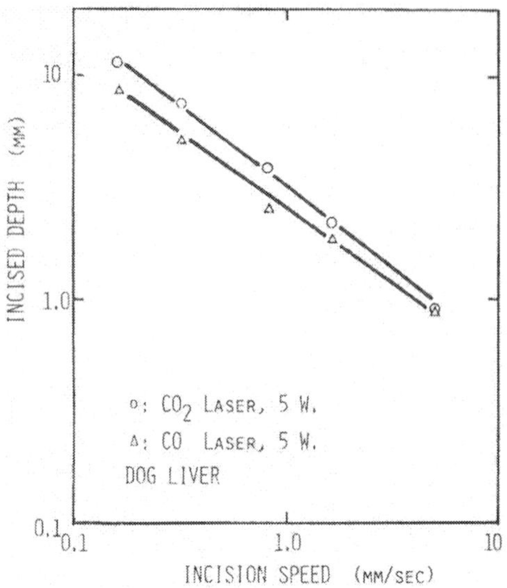

FIGURE 42.2. Dependence of the incision depth on the incision speed of high-intensity CO and CO_2 laser beams. Average light intensity: 2.6 kW/cm^2. △: CO laser irradiation. ○: CO_2 laser irradiation. Sample: dog liver. [From Arai T, Kikuchi M, Sakuragi S, Saito M, Takizawa M: CO laser power delivery by As_2S_3 IR glass fiber with Teflon cladding. In Katzir A (ed): Optical Fibers in Medicine and Biology. SPIE, Bellingham, 1985, pp 24–31, with permission.]

laser cutting, specimens of the sectional view of the cutting samples were made. The light intensity and the beam scanning speed were 2.6 kW/cm^2 and 0.33 mm/second, respectively. Figure 42.3A,B shows the groove specimens for CO and CO_2 lasers.[11] The thermal necrotic layer beside the cutting groove by CO laser irradiation is 50% thicker than that by CO_2 irradiation. That is because the extinction length of the CO laser light by water absorption is 0.1 mm, three times larger than that of the CO_2 laser light. Moreover, the scattering of vaporized debris (i.e., smoke) under the CO laser irradiation with high intensity was stronger than that by the CO_2 laser irradiation due to the wavelength dependence of the Rayleigh and/or Mie scattering process. This effect might promote this tendency. This promoted thermal necrotic layer might be available for hemostasis bleeding from the cutting injuries. Despite the enhanced thickness of the thermal necrotic layer to the CO laser cutting, the thickness is still thinner than the injuries by the electrosurgical unit.

Low-Intensity Irradiation

To investigate the interaction for the low-intensity irradiation, a 10 to 45 W/cm^2 laser beam was irradiated on the sample. This intensity corresponds to the laser hemostasis by cutting laser irradiation for liver and/or kidney hemorrhages. The thermal coagulated layer and carbonized layer thicknesses were measured as a function of the average light intensity and the irradiation duration time. The result of this experiment is shown in Figure 42.4.[11,12] Since the difference of the extinction length of the CO and CO_2 lasers is approximately 100 μm, for the irradiation time

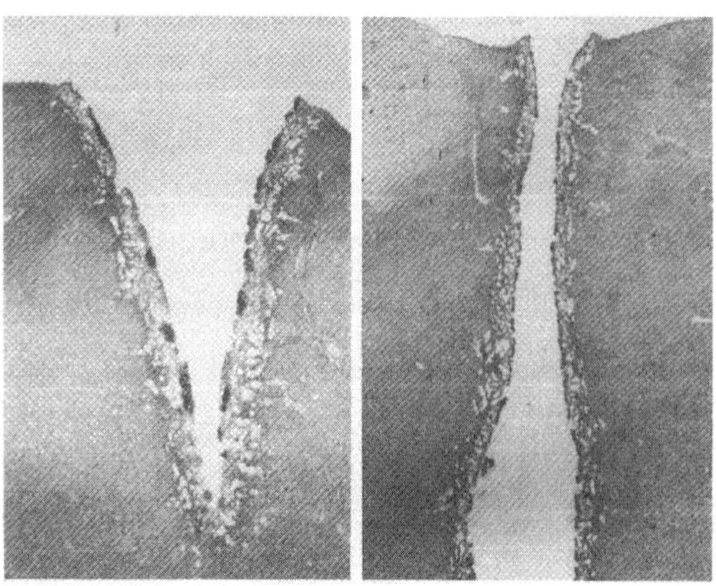

FIGURE 42.3. The sectional view of the specimens of the cutting samples. Average light intensity: 2.6 kW/cm^2. Beam scanning speed: 0.33 mm/second. Sample: dog liver. (*Top*) For CO laser cutting. (*Bottom*) For CO_2 laser cutting.

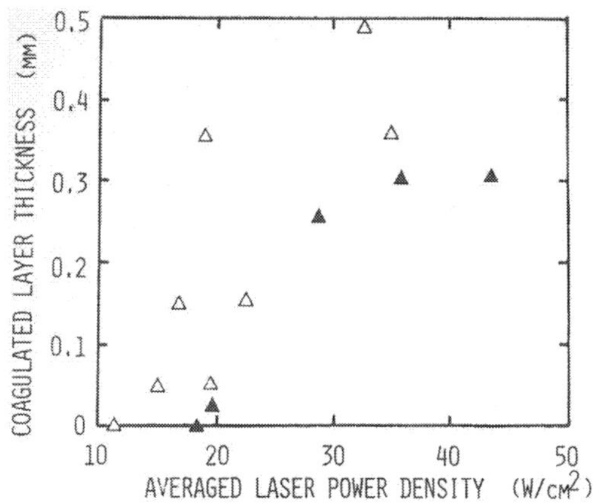

FIGURE 42.4. The thermal coagulated layer thickness on the sample surface for low-intensity irradiation of CO and CO_2 lasers as a function of the average light intensity. △: CO laser irradiation. ▲: CO_2 laser irradiation. Irradiation time: 2 seconds. Sample: cow liver. [From Arai T, Kikuchi M, Sakuragi S, Saito M, Takizawa M: CO laser power delivery by As_2S_3 IR glass fiber with Teflon cladding, In Katzir A (ed): Optical Fibers in Medicine and Biology. SPIE, Bellingham, 1985, pp 24–31, with permission.]

over 2 seconds, the coagulated and carbonized layer thicknesses of these lasers were the same due to the thermal conduction. The interaction difference was then studied under 2 seconds duration. The measured thickness of the thermal coagulation layer by the CO laser irradiation is 0.2 to 0.3 mm thinner than that by the CO_2 laser.

Summary

In general, the cutting process by the light irradiation is essentially explained by the thermal process. The optical process affected the cutting mainly by the absorption of light by the material of the tissue. Thus, the absorption coefficient and the intensity of the irradiation beam are important for cutting. The incision had been easily controlled by the light intensity and the movement speed of the beam with the great advantages by noncontact cutting. The interactions of the CO and CO_2 lasers applied to living tissue were experimentally investigated. CO_2 lasers are the most popular and unique lasers for cutting applications. However, as they do not have a method of optical delivery by flexible fibers, endoscopic applications via soft endoscopes are impossible. In this chapter, we showed the similarity of the tissue interaction of the CO laser and CO_2 laser. The CO laser is a profitable candidate for the cutting and vaporizing laser for endoscopic applications in the near future.

References

1. Joffe SN, Daikuzono N, Osborn J, et al: Contact probes for the Nd:YAG laser. In Katzir A (ed): Optical Fibers in Medicine and Biology. SPIE, Bellingham, 1985, pp 42–50.
2. Downing HD, Williams D: Optical properties of water in the infrared. J Geophys Res 80:1656–1661, 1975.
3. Trokel SL, Srinivasan R, Braren B: Excimer laser surgery of the cornea. Am J Opthalmol 96:710–715, 1983.
4. Gordy E, Drabkin DL: Determination of the oxygen saturation of blood by a simplified technique, applicable to standard equipment. J Biol Chem 227:285–299, 1957.
5. Bhaumik ML, Lacina WB, Mann MM: Characteristics of CO laser. IEEE J Quant Electron QE-8:150–160, 1972.
6. Cheo PK: CO_2 lasers. In DeMaria AJ (ed): Lasers. Marcel Dekker, New York, 1971, pp 111–267.
7. Browne PG, Smith ALS: Efficient long life sealed CO lasers at room temperature. J Phys E 8:870, 1975.
8. Witteman WJ: High-output and long lifetimes of sealed-off CO_2 lasers. Appl Phys Lett 11:337–338, 1967.
9. Ikedo M, Ishiwatari H, Watari M, et al: Infrared optical fiber for energy transmission. Rev Laser Eng (Jpn) 11:834–841, 1983.
10. Halldorsson T, Langerhole J: Thermodynamic analysis of laser irradiation of biological tissue. Appl Opt 17:3948–3952, 1978.
11. Arai T, Kikuchi M: A study for development of CO laser scalpel (1) Investigation of the effect of CO laser light on living tissue. J Jpn Soc Laser Med 3:223–230, 1982.
12. Arai T, Kikuchi M, Sakuragi S, et al: CO laser power delivery by As_2S_3 IR glass fiber with Teflon cladding. In Katzir A (ed): Optical Fibers in Medicine and Biology. SPIE, Bellingham, 1985, pp 24–31.
13. Karbe E, Beck R, English W, Experimental surgery with neodymium, holmium, CO and CO_2 lasers. In Kaplan I (ed): Laser Surgery. Jerusalem Academic Press, Jerusalem, 1976. pp 174–177.

43
Tissue Interactions of Nd:YAG Lasers

Kim A. Brackett

The primary mechanism of action of the standard 1064-nm wavelength Nd:YAG laser on biologic tissue is dependent upon the conversion of radiant optical energy into thermal energy. However, there are some exceptions to this rule. The major exception to the thermal mechanism is the Q-switched or mode-locked laser, which is capable of producing short bursts (10^{-9} to 10^{-12} seconds) of high power levels, inducing mechanical as well as thermal damage to the tissue, as will be briefly described later. There is also some evidence of a reduction in collagen synthesis by fibroblasts exposed to Nd:YAG laser irradiation in vitro, which was not duplicated by equal heating of cultures with an alternative light source.[1] The mechanism behind this inhibition and whether it is wavelength-specific remains to be elucidated. This chapter will be mainly concerned with the primary thermal effects.

Theoretical Considerations

The conversion of light energy to thermal energy depends upon absorption and scattering of the beam within the tissue. Halldorsson et al.[2] have established an absorption coefficient (α) of 0.11 and a scattering coefficient (β) of 9.89 per centimeter of tissue traversed by the beam. Thus, if absorption alone were responsible for dissipating the energy of the beam, penetration would reach approximately 9 cm, as is the case with a sample composed of water. However, the complex and nonhomogeneous three-dimensional array of proteins within the cells and intercellular matrix causes a high degree of scattering within a relatively short distance below the surface of the tissue, making this the more significant parameter. Scattering converts the coherent column of photons into a diffuse oblate spheroid of radiation[2,3] in agreement with the results of the Monte Carlo method of calculation of multiple scattering events within a solid. A significant proportion of these events results in backscattered energy from the incident surface toward the source and operator. In a hollow viscus with a wall thickness of 2 to 3 mm, 30 to 40% of the power applied will be backscattered, compared to 25 to 30% scattered forward through the opposite surface of the wall.[2] This scattering within a thin-walled viscus causes a doubling of beam diameter at the incident surface and a fourfold increase at the rear wall. Thus, the area irradiated is 4 and 16 times as great, respectively, as that of the original beam profile.[2] The forward-scattered energy is very diffuse, with a resultant low-power density due to the multiple scattering events within the tissue.

The magnitude of the absorption and scattering coefficients is dependent upon wavelength and duration of exposure. As the wavelength of the laser decreases, its absorption increases, accompanied by a decrease in scattering. This phenomenon offers possibilities for the use of the 532- and 266-nm harmonics of the Nd:YAG laser to achieve effects for which the fundamental 1064-nm wavelength is not well suited. The coefficient of scattering, in particular, also changes with increasing exposure time due to changes in the optical properties of the tissue as necrosis proceeds. Initially, coagulation of tissue proteins causes an increase in scattering.[2] This increase in the value of β results in a rising proportion of backscattered energy, with an accompanying decrease in forward scatter. As the temperature of the tissue reaches 100°C, there is a sharp increase in backscattering, which remains at this elevated level until tissue water is boiled off. At the point of tissue dehydration and carbonization there is a sharp decrease in backscattering and an increase in forward transmission of beam energy.

Correlation of Temperature Rise With Tissue Damage

The initial phase of absorption of energy raises the tissue temperature from 37°C to approximately 60°C, with some accompanying hyperemia and swelling but no permanent structural damage. As the temperature increases beyond 60°C, protein denaturation and coagulation occur.[3,4] This phase is signaled by blanching of the exposure site and an increase in the scattering properties of the tissue, as previously described. At this point, shrinkage of the tissue is also observed. Further absorption of energy raises the tissue temperature to 100°C and begins to boil the water in the cells and intercellular matrix. The conversion of water to steam has two effects. The first is related to the thousandfold increase in volume of the water as it changes from a liquid to a gas, with resultant rupturing of cells and cavitation of the tissue as this expansion occurs. The second effect is the action of water as a heat sink because of its high latent heat of vaporization during this phase transition. Once all the water has been driven out, a rapid rise in temperature occurs. Carbonization takes place when the temperature has reached a level between 300 and 400°C. This stage is made evident by the production of smoke. Absorption of energy increases as the tissue blackens, and if temperatures exceed 500°C the tissue can ignite. This increased absorption of energy with attendant scattering and thermal conduction, before the ignition point is reached, will greatly extend the total volume of tissue affected around the area of beam contact.

Acute Effects of 1064-nm Exposure

When tissue that has been subjected to laser irradiation is examined histologically immediately after exposure, one finds the development of zones of tissue damage, which is in agreement with the described theoretical considerations (Figure 43.1). The degree of tissue effect is dependent upon both the power level applied and the duration of application. Short pulses of higher power will cause a narrower, deeper, and more localized effect than the same total energy applied as longer pulses at a lower power level.[3] In other words, the defect caused by high power levels is more dependent on the distribution of beam energy within the tissue, while lower power, longer duration exposure allows more time for thermal conduction to adjacent cells and produces a shallower but wider defect.

At very low energies temporary hyperemia and mild edema of the tissue may occur. As more energy is applied, the tissue temperature increases, with the greatest rise occurring below the surface at a depth of 0.7 to 1.3 mm, as determined by Marchesini et al.[5] Thus subsurface coagulation is achieved before surface damage

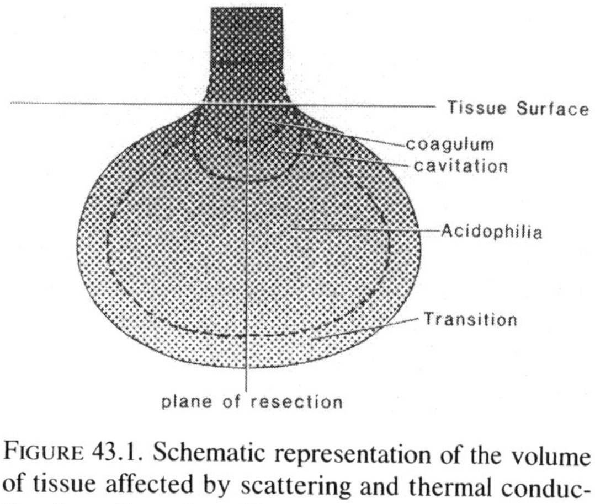

FIGURE 43.1. Schematic representation of the volume of tissue affected by scattering and thermal conduction from the point of beam contact. Zones of tissue damage corresponding to the amount of energy absorbed are indicated but not drawn to scale. (From Brackett KA, Sankar MY, Joffe SN: Effects of Nd:YAG laser photoradiation on intra-abdominal tissues: A histological study of tissue damage versus power density applied. Lasers Surg Med 6:123–130, 1986. With permission.)

is visible. In a highly cellular organ such as the liver, stained with azure-eosin, a small spheroid of acidophilic, necrosed cells will be seen below a surface minimally affected by the beam (Figure 43.2). Tissue with a thin epithelium or mucosa often shows a condensation of collagen in the submucosa, accompanied by swelling, again under a normal-appearing surface. Such tissues stained with Masson's Trichrome sometimes show a homogeneous analine blue staining of the submucosa, resulting in a vitrified appearance. These connective tissue effects are important in the mechanism of Nd:YAG laser-induced hemostasis. Swelling of the matrix surrounding small blood vessels provides occlusive pressure. The total energy required to achieve this effect varies with technique and the volume of blood flow to the tissue, which acts as a thermal sink. Higher power densities (up to approximately 2500 J/cm^2) are required to increase the depth of this effect up to 3 mm, which is about the limit after which vaporization of superficial layers of cells begins.[5] However, this maximum depth may be increased into the range of 4 to 6 mm by artificial cooling of the surface of the tissue with saline irrigation.[6,7] Here, water acts as a heat sink at the surface without affecting the thermal characteristics of the deeper layers of the tissue.

Application of increasing amounts of energy until vaporization of the superficial layers occurs results in the appearance of distinct zones of damage related to the proportional intensity of energy absorbed at that point in the tissue.[8] Again using liver as an example, four zones can be distinguished (Figure 43.3). The most super-

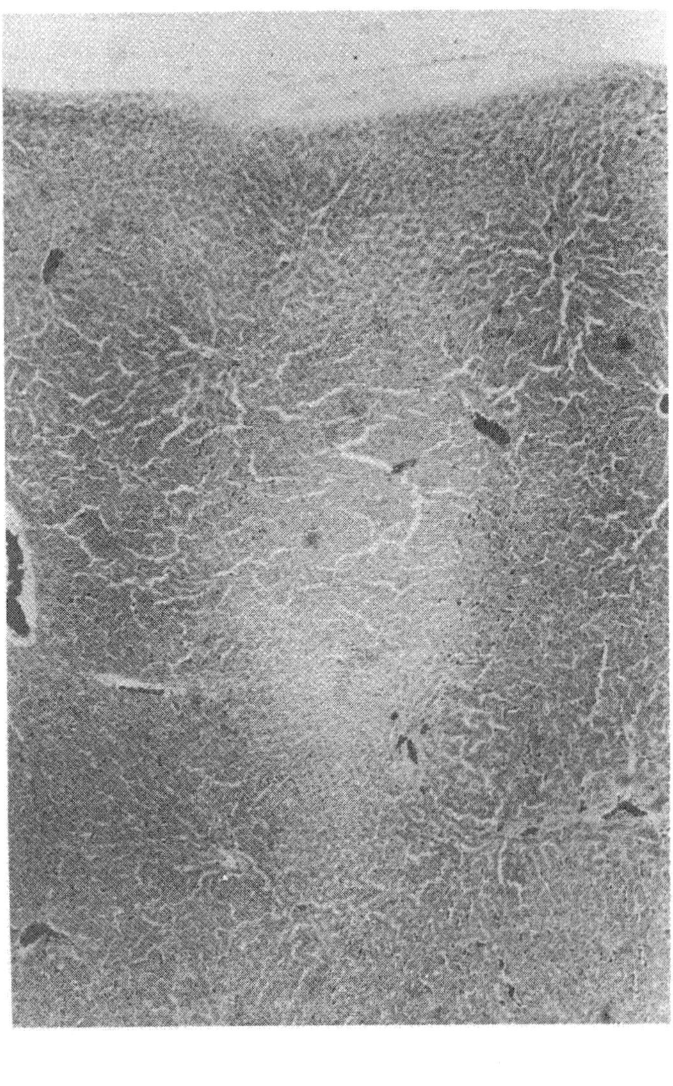

FIGURE 43.2. Liver subjected to low dosage of noncontact Nd:YAG laser irradiation. Tissue in the center of the field displays heat necrosis and coagulation, while the overlying hepatocytes are normal. Dosage was sufficient to cause capsular swelling at the surface. Azure-eosin, ×90.

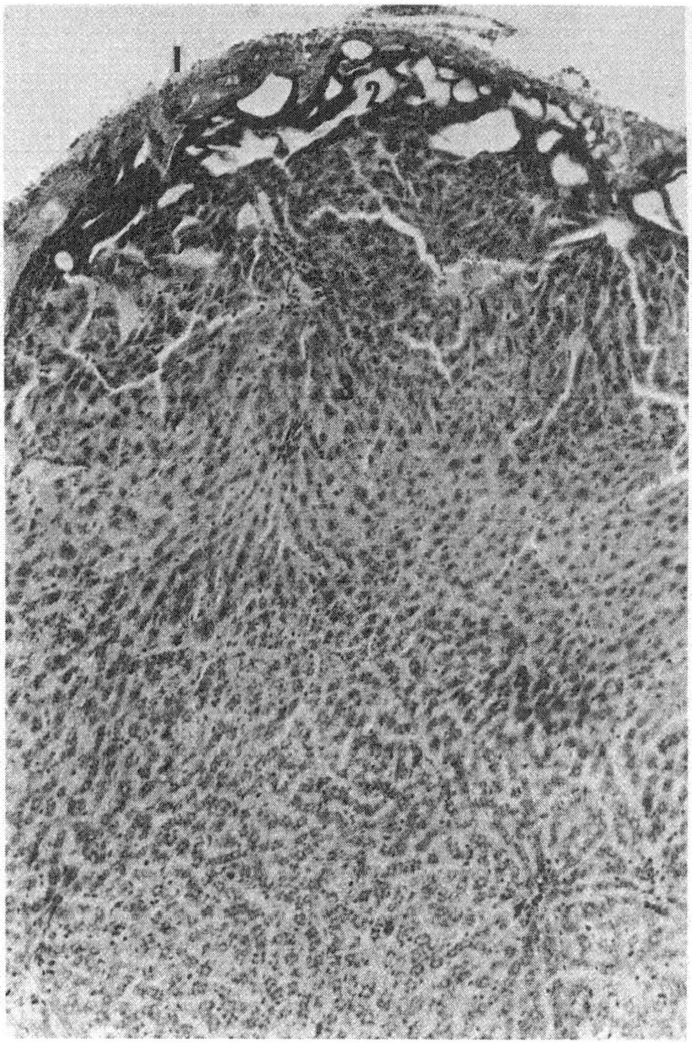

FIGURE 43.3. Liver resected by SLT contact Nd:YAG laser probe. Four zones of tissue damage can be observed. *1*, surface coagulum; *2*, cavitation; *3*, acidophilia; *4*, transition. Noncontact resected liver would demonstrate the same four zones, but the acidophilic zone would occupy 3 to 5 times the volume of tissue affected here. Azure-eosin, ×180.

ficial zone is composed of a thin (<100 μm) layer of intensely stained coagulated proteins and islands of carbonized debris. Beneath this layer, cavitation occurs from the formation of steam within the tissue. The depth to which cavitation can occur is variable but is usually restricted to the upper 500 μm. The bulk of the tissue affected by the laser lies under the cavitation layer. Here cells are characterized by acidophilic cytoplasm with nuclei varying from densely pyknotic near the surface to normal or slightly swollen as the transition to normal tissue is approached. Many of these cells do not appear to be structurally damaged, but coagulation and heat inactivation of the basophilic cytoplasmic ribosomal nucleoproteins have rendered them nonviable. This zone can extend up to 5 mm into the tissue and corresponds to the spheroid exposed to scattered photons and thermal diffusion. A transition zone, located between the acidophilic cells and normal tissue, in which the cytoplasm of the cells is more acidophilic than normal but retains the basophilic staining of the rough endoplasmic reticulum, is generally present but often difficult to distinguish. These cells appear to have swollen mitochondria and activated lysosomes when examined with the electron microscope. This layer represents the minimum detectable structural effect of the laser and/or thermal energy on the cells. The normal tissue below this level is hyperemic. Similar zones are identifiable in other, more heterogeneous, organs as well. When the stomach is exposed to a power density high enough to vaporize the mucosa, the defect is surrounded by a coagulum, a thin layer of cavitation and a broader zone of condensed necrotic cells and connective tissue (Figure 43.4). The smooth muscle of the wall responds with shrinkage of individual fibers, pyknosis of the nuclei, and the formation of intercellular clefts. These zones are analogous to those seen in the liver. Generally, no specifically identifiable transition zone can be recognized. A raised ring can often be found on the surface surrounding the site of laser application, caused by swelling of the surrounding vital tissue. Often the adjacent normal tissue is hyperemic and focal hemorrhages are common.

This broad spheroid of damage caused by the low absorption and high degree of scattering makes the Nd:YAG laser less than ideal for creating a precise incision when used in the conventional noncontact mode. Such incisions are accompanied by a band of necrotic tissue showing the described zones of damage arrayed parallel to the plane of resection. The width of the zone of necrosis (acidophilic cells) appears to be independent of the power applied when operating in the range of 50 to 100 W.[8] The primary reason for this independence is the reduction in the amount of time the beam is in contact with any unit volume of tissue as a result of the higher rate of excavation with increased power, thus allowing less thermal diffusion.

The recent development of a variety of SLT contact sapphire laser probes permits the use of 1064-nm radiation to be used to create a much more precisely localized coagulation and/or

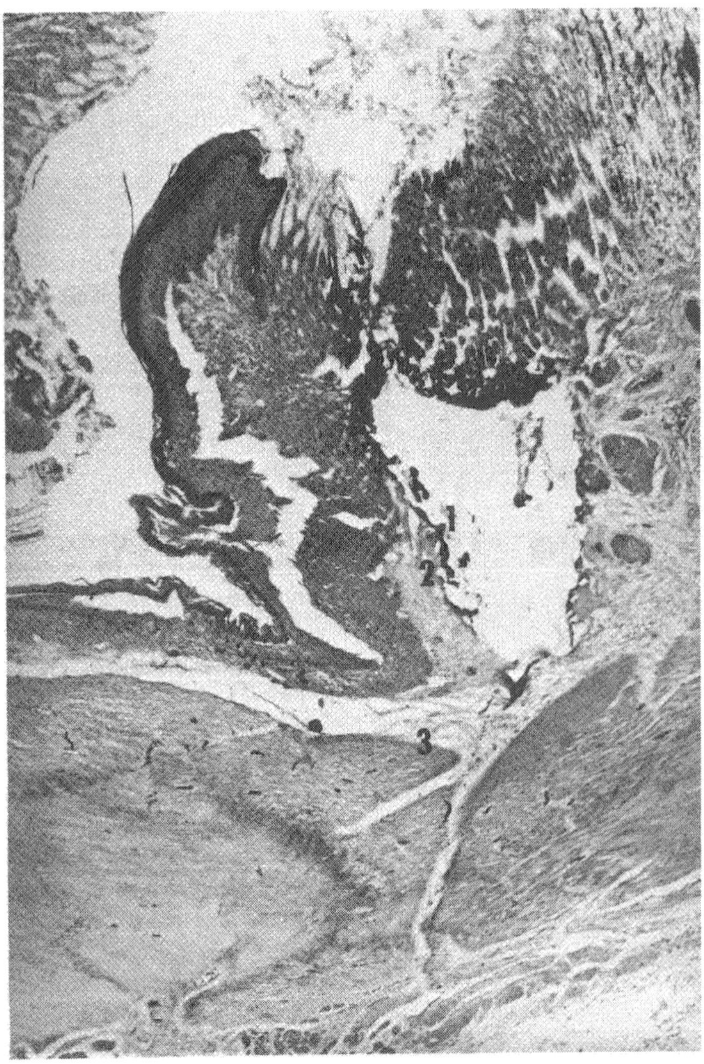

FIGURE 43.4. Gastric wall exposed to Nd:YAG laser radiation. Zones of damage include regions corresponding to *1*, surface coagulum; *2*, cavitation; *3*, acidophilia. Damage extends through the smooth muscle of the externa. Masson's Trichrome, ×90.

cutting effect than was previously possible. Contact techniques are effective at greatly reduced power levels, typically between 5 and 25 W, and result in an average fivefold decrease in the volume of tissue damaged when used for cutting.[9] This tissue damage is qualitatively similar to that seen with the noncontact mode, but is reduced quantitatively to the range typically encountered with the CO_2 laser or Bovie electrocautery. An additional difference seen in preliminary studies is the reduction, or complete elimination, of the raised ring of tissue surrounding the exposed area. Scanning electron-microscopic examination of contact versus noncontact lesions in the trachea shows an abrupt transition to normal tissue at the edge of the crater, in contrast to coagulated debris interposed in the noncontact lesions (Figure 43.5). Early measurements also indicate a reduction in backscattering when the contact probe is used, which may be related to this phenomenon as well as to the use of lower power densities.[10]

Acute Effects of Alternate Modes and Wavelengths

The use of Q-switched or mode-locked Nd:YAG lasers allows the storage of high levels of energy during optical pumping, which is then released in extremely short pulses.[11] This high-density energy has an explosive effect on atoms within the target tissue.[12] Electrons are inelastically scattered from the atoms and form a plasma shield that helps to screen deeper structures from the beam. After the pulse, released electrons are recaptured, giving off the energy which they gained from the photon pulse. This microdischarge of energy creates a shock wave that disrupts and vaporizes the local tissue. This technique is often employed in ophthalmologic surgery for penetrating and incising the nonpigmented structures such as the cornea and lens.

The alternative Nd:YAG laser wavelengths investigated thus far include 1340 nm and the second (532 nm) and fourth (266 nm) harmonics of the 1064-nm wavelength. The 1340-nm radiation has been found to result in increased depth of penetration and tissue damage, particularly in hemoglobin-rich tissue.[13] As tested on retinal tissue, 532 nm causes mechanical disruption of tissue subjected to a single pulse.[14] The disruption appears to be caused by the creation of a bubble of vapor at the site, or possibly by the propagation of a nonlinear shock wave. A train of lower energy pulses at this wavelength results in thermal damage to the photoreceptors and pigmented epithelium of the retina whose cells were highly vacuolated with accompanying nuclear pyknosis. Rapidly pulsed 266-nm photoradiation has been used experimentally to produce fine, precisely controlled cuts in cadaver corneas.[15] At this wavelength the tissue absorbs most of the energy with greatly reduced scattering. Further study of this wavelength is necessary, but scanning electron microscopy demonstrated minimal coagulation and carbonization along the incision. The 260-nm ultraviolet radiation has long been known to have mutagenic effects on DNA, and the carcinogenic effects of 266-nm radiation and what degree of thermal spread may occur remain to be investigated.

A fourth area of laser-tissue interaction that remains to be developed involves the use of one or more of the available Nd:YAG wavelengths in photodynamic therapy. Such applications await the development of suitable photochemically active substances responsive to Nd:YAG laser radiation.

Healing of Nd:YAG Laser-Induced Lesions

The pattern of healing following Nd:YAG laser exposure is typical of that seen following any thermal injury. Subsurface areas of photocoagulation following low exposure levels are rapidly invaded by fibroblasts, macrophages, and capillary buds from adjacent tissues and heal with the formation of a connective tissue scar. Craters and resected surfaces undergo a slightly more complex process, which can result in the formation of a scar or in segregation of the damaged area by connective tissue encapsulation with eventual sloughing or resorption of the necrotic mass, depending upon the extent of the original injury. The connective tissue arises from the capsule of the organ, its stroma, or perivascular connective tissue sheath, and invades the mass along the transition zone. Regeneration of normal tissue occurs concurrently in those

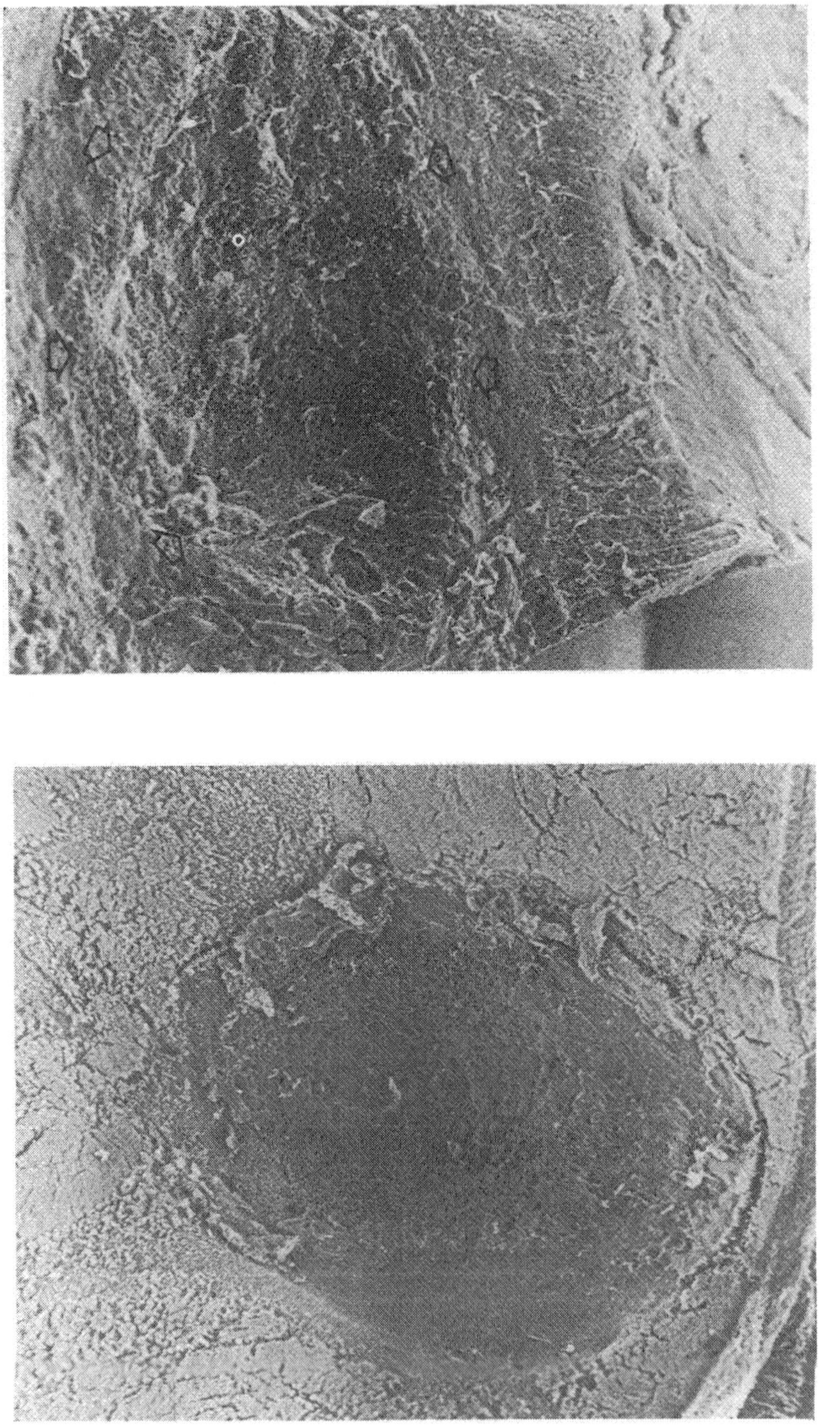

A

B

FIGURE 43.5. (A) Scanning electron micrograph (SEM) of tracheal mucosa, 100-W, noncontact laser lesion. Crater is surrounded by a raised ring of coagulated, necrotic tissue (*arrows*). ×50. (B) SEM of tracheal mucosa, 15-W SLT contact probe laser lesion. Transition from normal surface mucosa to crater is abrupt, lacking the coagulated rim seen in noncontact lesions. ×50.

organs capable of regeneration. In most instances, little inflammatory cell infiltrate is observed. Presumably, the creation of a sterile area, coinciding with the necrotic zone as a result of absorption of thermal energy, eliminates exogenous stimulation of inflammation. By the same token, heat denaturation of cellular enzymes and other proteins suppresses endogenous stimulation.

One exception to the pattern of healing has been found in experimental pancreatic resections. Resections involving the use of noncontact and contact techniques have been found to produce acute and chronic pancreatitis in rats and dogs.[16] However, similar results were obtained using Bovie electrocautery, indicating that the results were not necessarily related to the instrumentation and are probably related to leakage of pancreatic secretions into the surrounding parenchyma and into the abdominal cavity from unclosed ducts. Further refinements in operating technique should eliminate this problem.

Thus, current investigations hold promise for the development of a highly versatile system of multimode Nd:YAG lasers capable of producing a variety of complementary tissue effects.

References

1. Abergel RP, Meeker CA, Dwyer RM, et al: Nonthermal effects of Nd:YAG laser on biological functions of human skin fibroblasts in culture. Lasers Surg Med 3:279–284, 1984.
2. Halldorsson Th, Rother W, Langerholc J, Frank F: Theoretical and experimental investigations prove Nd:YAG laser treatment to be safe. Lasers Surg Med 1:253–262, 1981.
3. McKenzie AL, Carruth JAS: Lasers in surgery and medicine. Phys Med Biol 29(6):619–641, 1984.
4. Sacknoff EJ: Neodymium-YAG laser surgery in urology. In Joffe SN, Muckerheide MC, Goldman L (eds): Neodymium-YAG Laser in Medicine and Surgery. Elsevier, New York, 1983, pp 106–117.
5. Marchesini R, Andreola S, Emanuelli H, et al: Temperature rise in biological tissue during Nd:YAG laser irradiation. Lasers Surg Med 5:75–82, 1985.
6. Kroy W, Halldorsson Th, Langerholc J: Practical advice in laser coagulation from a theoretical viewpoint. Appl Opt 196:6–9, 1980.
7. Frank F, Keiditsch E, Hofstetter A, et al: Various effects of the CO_2−, the neodymium:YAG-, and the argon-laser irradiation on bladder tissue. Lasers Surg Med 2:89–96, 1982.
8. Brackett KA, Sankar MY, Joffe SN: Effects of Nd:YAG laser photoradiation on intra-abdominal tissues: A histological study of tissue damage versus power density applied. Lasers Surg Med 6:123–130, 1986.
9. Joffe SN, Brackett KA, Sankar MY, Daikuzono N: Liver resection with the Nd:YAG laser. A comparison of a new contact probe, the laser scalpel, with the conventional non-contact method. Surg Gynecol Obstet 163:437–442, 1986.
10. Daikuzono N, Joffe SN: Artificial sapphire probe for contact photocoagulation and tissue vaporization with the Nd:YAG laser. Med Instrum 19.173–178, 1985.
11. Fuller TA: The physics of surgical lasers. Lasers Surg Med 1:5–14, 1980.
12. Osher RH: The neodymium:YAG laser in ophthalmology. In Joffe SN, Muckerheide MC, Goldman L (eds): Neodymium-YAG Laser in Medicine and Surgery. Elsevier, New York, 1983, pp 164–169.
13. Stokes LF, Auth DC, Tanaka D, et al: Biomedical utility of 1.34 μm Nd:YAG laser radiation. IEEE Trans Biomed Eng BME-28(3):297–299, 1981.
14. Mosier MA, Champion J, Liaw L-H, Berns MW: Retinal effects of the frequency-doubled (532 nm) YAG laser: Histopathological comparison with argon laser. Lasers Surg Med 5:377–404, 1985.
15. Berns MW, Gaster RN: Corneal incisions produced with the fourth harmonic (266 nm) of the YAG laser. Lasers Surg Med 5:371–375, 1985.
16. Schröder T, Brackett K, Joffe SN: Proximal pancreatectomy: A comparison of electrocautery with the contact and non-contact Nd:YAG laser techniques in the dog. Am J Surg (In Press), 1987.

44
Setting Up Ambulatory Laser Centers

Carolyn J. Mackety

As cost-effective, multidisciplinary laser centers become a strategic goal for many health care facilities, many elements must be taken into consideration during the development.

Types of Laser Centers

Conceptually, a "Laser Center" is a cluster of laser systems used for outpatient treatment. General anesthesia is not required. There are three types of laser centers:

1. A contained unit; a space within a hospital but not contiguous to an operating room or ambulatory surgery clinic
2. A unit integrated into an operating room or ambulatory surgery clinic or contiguous to them in a medical facility, with the laser center reporting to the administrative manager of the parent department
3. A free-standing building that is owned and operated by a medical facility or in a joint venture with the facility and a group of physician users

Contained Unit

The contained unit is constructed as a "mini" ambulatory surgery department, where patients are scheduled to have their laser treatment and are admitted to the unit in a prescribed manner. The admission process is expedited, as these patients require little or no preadmission testing or assessment. They are usually in good health and will require little or no anesthesia for their procedure. The patients usually do not have to change their clothes, and they can leave shortly after their laser treatment is completed. This unit has its own personnel and may administratively report to the ambulatory services or chief operating officer of the facility. This unit can be set up either as a for-profit department or as a part of the hospital's not-for-profit structure. An example of a contained unit is the Grant Hospital Laser Center, Columbus, OH.

Integrated Unit

The integrated unit is physically contiguous to, or is a part of, an operating room or ambulatory surgery unit. Since the operating room department and the ambulatory surgery clinic have their own laser-trained staff, the laser center that is within these departments can schedule and use all the laser systems as they are needed. The laser center can be designed as treatment rooms in an area that is contiguous to the OR or the ASC, and in this setting the unit can provide outpatient laser treatment without general anesthesia. This type of laser center has its own personnel, however, and when the laser is used in the main operating room or ambulatory surgery, the laser center personnel must be available during laser treatment. In view of the fact that staff, and the scheduling of patients for the laser center is integrated with the regular operative schedule, the laser equipment, accessories are used in both surgical units, as well as the laser center. This type of center is very cost-effective, as there is minimal duplication of equipment or personnel. The patients treated in this unit are low-risk outpatients who do not require general anesthesia and can be discharged immediately after treatment. An example of the integrated unit is the Wenske Laser Center, Ravenswood Hospital Medical Center, Chicago, IL.

Free-Standing Center

The free-standing laser center is a separate building that contains all types of laser systems, with related accessories, supplies, and personnel to administer laser treatments to all indicated patients. The facility is designed and constructed to meet all ambulatory surgical care guidelines, including general anesthesia, if required, and postoperative recovery. Physicians must apply for privileges as described in the bylaws of the center, and nursing and ancillary staff are available for patient care and the general management of the center. Administratively, the center has a manager who reports to a board of directors or the chief executive officer of the corporation. Inasmuch as this center owns all of its laser systems and related equipment and has its own personnel, it is usually run as a for-profit organization. An example of a free standing laser center is the Beckman Institute, Irvine, CA.

Development of Ambulatory Laser Centers

This section will discuss the following topics that should be considered in the development of ambulatory laser centers (ALC):

1. Task force
2. Feasibility Study
3. Construction parameters
4. Policies and procedures
5. Staffing
6. Marketing strategies

Each element should be addressed in relation to implementing the laser center concept, to optimize the overall success of the program.

Task Force

A laser task force should be appointed as a basic work group to expedite the coordination and management of the overall program. If the facility has an ongoing laser program with a Laser Committee in place, the work group can be an ad hoc committee reporting to the Laser Committee. The composition of this task force should be physicians who use lasers, laser nurses, hospital administrators (C.O.O. or V.P. for Ambulatory Services), planners, marketing directors, and biomedical engineers. Other experts can be asked to participate on the task force as needed during the design, development, and implementation phase. The task force should set realistic goals and workable time frames. Meetings should be held frequently at first; then as the ALC develops, a regular schedule should be maintained. The task force should have an agenda and the responsibility and authority to make decisions and recommendations.

Feasibility Study

The feasibility study, to ensure a successful program, will have multiple components:

Medical staff commitment
Case-mix (medical/surgical) analysis
Financial considerations
- Acquisition
- Evaluation
- Reimbursement factors
- Operating budget

When these elements have been considered, a go–no go decision is made and the implementation phase commences.

Medical Staff Commitment

A survey form should be devised and sent to the medical staff to assess interest, motivation, and commitment to use lasers in their daily practice. Why survey the medical staff? The survey analysis will document interest and commitment, identify laser-specific patient populations, ascertain the extent of attendance in laser education programs, and it will generate interest where it may have been minimal. Physician commitment to significant use of the laser ensures maximum laser usage.

Case-Mix Analysis

The case-mix analysis will give the facility a potential utilization base and case load projection. There are three methods to analyze this information:

1. Identify types of procedures that could be converted into laser cases.

2. Review those procedures in relation to the ICD-9-CM codes within the DRG's.
3. Compare those codes and DRG's with each physician's profile indicating those potential "gainers or loss leaders."

Most facilities have their case-mix information computerized and readily available for data and current trends analysis. There are several ways to request this information from the computer: physician, procedure, DRG, ICD-9-CM code, inpatient, and outpatient. Experience shows that, after identifying procedures from the case-mix of the facility, approximately 10% of the yearly operative base can convert to laser procedures.

After all these data are collected and analyzed, the appropriate laser systems and accessories will be recommended for acquisition. There are many laser manufacturers in the medical industry today, with laser systems varying in power, mode, type, and installation requirements. Lasers are available across the broad spectrum of wavelengths to meet most of the medical indications for laser usage in today's medicine.

Once the facility makes the decision to purchase the lasers recommended the acquisition process begins.

Financial Considerations

Acquisition

It would be advantageous to add the Materials Manager or Purchasing Agent to the laser task force at this time. Bid letters are sent to the vendors with specifications for each laser system noted. Within a specific time period after the quotations are returned, the bids are reviewed to negotiate the "best deal" for the facility. As the ALC may or may not be a specific geographic location, the Materials Manager may need to purchase contracts for new construction or renovation, equipment, and accessories needed as the program expands to continually meet the needs of the physicians and community. During this process the biomedical department should become involved in a discussion of installation requirements.

In today's health care economy, creative methods of acquisition will become necessary. Outright purchase of the laser systems gives the facility the opportunity to immediately capitalize and depreciate the equipment. At current interest rates, leasing equipment, using revenue to pay the lease rates would be advantageous. The option to purchase by the pay-per-use method initially seems advantageous; however, the vendor usually profits excessively from this arrangement. A suggestion would be to have a portion of the payment put in escrow as an equity investment and at the end of a specific time period convert the "deal" to purchase or, if there is not enough use, return the product. Although current tax advantages are in a state of flux, joint ventures with physicians are still a viable option. Entering into a joint venture with physicians represents a commitment for utilization.

Evaluation

Lasers represent significant capital outlay for the facility and as the market for lasers is changing it becomes very competitive. An evaluation process should be developed, considering the following elements:

System type and power to meet needs
Advantages/reliability/cost
Manufacturing history
Technical services available
Education process for physicians and nurses

The evaluation process should be structured so each laser system is on site, usually no longer than a week. The evaluation process should take place in an area that can accommodate a safe demonstration, that is accessible for physicians, and that can be reached by the greatest number of potential laser users at convenient times. Completion of the evaluation process is important. Documentation of the evaluation will be summarized for the decision-making process.

When the evaluation process is complete, the decision made, the price negotiated, accessories identified, and delivery date decided, all policies and procedures should be developed and be approved to provide the facility with the appropriate medical-legal standards for laser practice.

Reimbursement Factors

To identify reimbursement factors, all financial data should be reviewed, including medicare, third-party payors, other payors, bad-debt factors, and any other financial information that will affect income and the operation of the center.

The development of laser usage charges will be based on all those factors, to include reimbursement under the DRG's. Other factors taken into consideration will be the facility's demographic information for their core and service area. Looking at the demographics will have other ramifications, such as age groups, which will affect patient population, potential laser procedures, and the types of lasers needed.

Next, the operation proforma will need to be developed for budgetary purposes. The elements for developing laser usage are as follows:

1. How the local third-party payors will handle charges for laser procedures.
2. Can equipment be charged to the patient in a particular state.
3. Develop cost/charge ratios that are realistic.
4. Develop ongoing budgetary information for the center.
5. Make sure all procedures have the correct codes assigned (both ICD-9-CM and DRG).
6. Charges for outpatient surgery should be developed as procedural charges that are reasonably competitive in the community marketplace.
7. A flat-rate user charge can be developed using the facility's usual formula for equipment charging. An alternative is pricing on an incremental cost base, that is, based on volume and competitive cost using the center vs office pricing.

Again, using the case-mix history, the procedure analysis by physicians should give the overall average time for all procedures. Based on yearly potential patient population, amortization time, and profit margin, an incremental cost base can be established.

Operating Budget

The operating budget of the center is simultaneously developed and is crucial to the cost:charge ratio. The factors to be addressed in this process are as follows:

Construction/renovation
Equipment/furniture
Wage/salaries/benefits
Consumable supplies/maintenance costs
Marketing/education materials
Utilities/environmental services
Service contracts/insurance

When this proforma is complete the facility will be able to establish an incremental charge (see Table 44.1).

Construction Parameters

This section will discuss the parameters for the development of an integrated and self-contained unit. There are similar considerations, so this information should be read in that context. The laser task force should now be expanded to include the construction project engineer, architects, and the significant persons involved with administration to plan, design, and develop the center.

Financing the project is an administrative decision; however, the following options can be considered:

1. Use of operational funds: Develop the ALC as a center of excellence and a for profit department. Enter into joint ventures with the facility and the physicians.
2. Venture capitalization: This decision is based on the strategic goals of the facility and the support of the Board of Trustees.

The design phase will be important for the efficient operation of the center and the following should be considered:

Location
- Convenient for patients and physicians
- Parking/access to the facility
- Adequate space to accommodate all the equipment
- Logistics for patient flow
- Access to needed utilities
- Patient comfort area

Space Planning
- Patient waiting/reception
- Patient/staff/lockers/toilet facilities
- Treatment rooms
- Recovery rooms
- Instrument clean/set-up areas
- Office/conference space
- Nursing stations
- Reception/scheduling area
- Storage space

Access to the building should be convenient for patients and physicians. The parking or drop-off area should have accommodations for handicapped patients. The signs should be easy to

TABLE 44.1. Cost of gynecological laser surgery

Service	ICD-9-CM	Cost ($)
Gynecological procedures by DRG		
DRG 360 Reimbursement	$1691.00	
LOS		
1982	4.2	
1985	1.8	
Excision cervical lesion	67.39	
Hymenotomy	70.31	
Marsupialization Bartholin cyst	71.24	
Partial vulvectomy	71.61	
Ablation herpes lesion	70.33	
Excision vaginal septum	70.33	
Excision vaginal warts/condyloma	70.33	
Inpatient consumption		
OR Time		375
Anesthesia supplies		82
Pharmacy		24
Suture		40
Laser drape pack		53
Miscellaneous		20
Laser (flat fee)		269
Recovery		100
Total		963
Per diem 1.8		754
Nursing care 1.8		484
Total cost		2201
Loss		−510
Outpatient Procedure DRG 360/above codes		
Procedure charge		375
Facility fee		100
Laboratory		30
Recovery		50
Laser*(incremental)		180
Total		735
Reimbursement		+956

*First 15 m = $100.000; each subsequent 15 m $80.00.

read, as many patients may be visually impaired. The patient treatment areas should be semirestricted to allow patients to have their procedure in a clean environment without crossover of sterile and nonsterile techniques.

Patient flow through the ALC may present logistical problems. The patient should fall within the anesthesia classification I and II, be healthy, or have minor health problems under control. Access and egress through a common admitting and discharge area conserves space. Patient mix in a common change area with lockers and toilet facilities does not present a problem. Toilet facilities should have panic hardware installed.

Utilities will have to be identified to include electricity, water, heating, and air contidioning. All laser systems will need to be identified to adequately meet the installation requirements. Most CO_2 lasers have no added requirements. Continuous wave Nd:YAG lasers have special requirements such as 208 three-phase electricity and flowing water at 45 psi. The newer cw Nd:YAG lasers are air-cooled; however, air exchanges in the treatment rooms should be at least 12 to 15 exchanges per hour. Argon lasers can be fixed or mobile. The pulsed Nd:YAG for ophthalmology does not have additional installation requirements.

The patient and family waiting area should be comfortable, and soft lighting and warm colors will assist in reducing anxiety. For diversion there should be light music, television, patient education information, and current quick reading material. Personnel should be available to answer questions. A nourishment station should be provided for patients and family, as many of them may have come from a distance and may have been on restricted fluids prior to their procedure.

The treatment rooms will need sufficient space to accommodate the laser systems, treatment tables, modular storage, and emergency equipment. Treatment rooms should be approximately 200 square feet and should have the functional capacity to accommodate all laser systems, including installation. The ophthalmologic laser center is a good example of how the center can be set up.

Supplies needed for each room can be stored in modular units, either as an exchange cart or "topped-out" by the staff or central supply. All drugs used in the unit can be consumed and replaced or availability can be on an exchange basis with the pharmacy.

The physicians' offices and conference rooms can be combined by using modular office concepts. The Scheduling/Receptions area can be planned in a modular concept, able to be expanded as needed. Space should include a computer station for data entry and retrieval.

Nursing work stations should be installed in each treatment room; however, a central nursing work area should be considered for intraoperative documentation, care planning, discharge summaries, and preoperative assessment.

Stations for decontamination and setting up of accessories and instruments for reprocessing will be necessary. Some laser accessories are cleaned immediately and stored appropriately.

Policies and Procedures

For medico-legal purposes, policies and procedures should be developed, approved, and implemented for safe laser practice. There is no bureaucratic body that has dictated what these should state; however, the American National Standards Institute will be publishing their Z136.3 addendum for "Safety in Medical Facilities", soon. The following is a suggested list that should be developed prior to laser program implementation:

1. Function of the Laser Committee
2. Job descriptions for laser personnel
3. Education criteria
4. Accident and malfunction report
5. Troubleshooting and maintenance documentation
6. Education for laser support personnel
7. Orientation of personnel to laser safety
9. Operational safety procedures:
   a. Eye protection
   b. Controlled access
   c. Signage
   d. Endotracheal tube safety
   e. Instrumentation
   f. Laser shutdown
   g. Smoke evacuation
   h. Care of all laser accessories
9. Setup and Shutdown procedures
10. Moving the lasers
11. Consent forms
12. Documentation
13. Laser safety officer

These policies and procedures are developed and approved in accordance to institutional protocol.

Staffing

Whatever type of ALC is developed, staff selection is important for the ongoing management and viability of the center. The person selected to direct the program must demonstrate effective management skills, for both people and material, and he or she must have basic understanding of all medical and surgical procedures, as well as the motivation and dedication to expend considerable energy to participate in the growth of the center.

The general staff will include nurses, ancillary personnel (e.g., secretary/receptionist), and technicians, both clinical and biomedical (Table 44.2). Staffing decisions will be depend on the following:

Number of laser systems
Where the lasers are geographically placed
Number of procedures
Number of credentialed physicians
ALC staff utilization
Patient/staff education
Marketing

The director's responsibilities will depend on how the department is developed within the organizational structure.

TABLE 44.2. Recommended staff for a typical laser center

Position	FTE	Salary (K)
Director	1	35–40
RN	2	25–28
Technician	1	18–22
Secretary/Receptionist	1	12–15
Biomedical technician	.5	8–12
Marketing	.25	5–8

Integrated Laser Unit

The director of the integrated unit would report to the Vice-President of Operations of Ambulatory Care as a middle manager. The duties of the director would be, however, not all-inclusive:

Direct daily activities of the ALC
Budget maintenance
Liaison between physicians and administration
Designated Laser Safety Officer
Responsibility for all equipment and accessories
Marketing liaison
Educational activities to include, hands-on training, inservice and continuing education

Self-Contained/Free-Standing Laser Unit

The director of the free-standing unit, as a part of independent departments and for-profit centers, would have added responsibilities, including all the duties listed for the director of the integrated unit, and the following additional activities:

Trends analysis
Statistical utilization
Revenue tracking
Community education
Laser research

Job Descriptions

CLINICAL NURSE SPECIALIST/LASER

Responsibility

To the Head Nurse, Assistant Supervisor or Director of Operating Room Service or the designated Director of the Laser Program:

Typical Responsibilities

1. Participates in the planning and implementation of nursing care for the laser patients.
2. Assumes the perioperative role.
3. Day-to-day management of the Laser Support team.
4. Assists in the development and implementation of continuing education laser programs.
5. Participates in the orientation of new employees regarding laser safety and laser policy and procedures.
6. May assume responsibility for the laser during the surgical procedure.
7. Monitors safe laser practice.
8. Maintains the lasers and the laser accessories.
9. Documents all laser procedures.
10. Participates in clinical laser research projects.
11. Participates in nonlaser procedures as assigned.

LASER SAFETY TECHNICIAN

Responsibility

To the Clinical Nurse/Laser, or to the appropriate designated person in the area where laser treatments are being performed.

Typical Responsibilities

1. Sets the laser up and does the check procedure prior to each laser case.
2. Assumes responsibility for the laser and accessories during each laser procedure.
3. Assists in the orientation of new employees with regard to laser safety and policy and procedures.
4. Assists in the monitoring of safe laser practice.
5. Assists in the documentation of all laser procedures.
6. Assists in research projects as needed.
7. Performs other duties as requested or assigned.

Note

The above statements are intended to describe the general nature and level of the persons assigned to the job classification. They are not to be considered as an exhaustive list of all job duties performed by personnel in this classification.

BIOLASER TECHNICIAN

Responsibility

To the Clinical Nurse/Laser, Director of Operating Room services or the designated supervisor where laser treatments are being performed, or the Medical Director of the Laser Program.

Typical Responsibilities

1. Operates, maintains, and troubleshoots all laser and assessories.
2. Has the responsibility, with approval, to call the manufactures service representative.
3. Performs preventive maintenance on a prescribed schedule an all lasers and related equipment.
4. May assume responsibility for the operation of the laser and assessories during laser procedures.
5. Assists in the orientation and continuing education of the employees.
6. Remains current in the field of all laser modalities and equipment.
7. Participates in clinical laser research projects.
8. Assists in the evaluation of laser and related equipment for upgrade in the current available laser modalities
9. Performs other duties as assigned or requested.

SECRETARY/RECEPTIONIST

Responsibility

Major responsibilities will be scheduling, admission, logistic patient flow, record keeping, and following through with patient appointments. This person should be efficient and personable, with excellent secretarial skills, telephone personality, and ability to use the computer and word processor. Her organizational skills should be equal to an office manager.

Marketing Strategies

A percentage of the marketing position should be allocated to the ALC. Marketing of the ALC will have a two-pronged attack: physicians and community. Marketing to the physicians will be essential for the viability of the center, a referral base will need to be established. A laser "hotline" can be the connection from the center to the community, information should be available, a speaker's bureau established, local media informed regarding the efficacy of laser procedures, and publication in various journals and other media.

Marketing attempts to identify first the needs of consumers and then to provide a product or service that so closely matches these needs that the exchange process is made from the consumer's perspective. Selling is concerned with helping the potential consumers understand their needs, and then to provide support to facilitate the purchase decision.

Marketing and selling are not mutually exclusive, but there is a difference in their orientation. Marketing identifies potential users of a product or services, while selling focuses on the purchase transaction. In the marketing and selling of health care services, both must be market-driven, that is, allowing consumers' needs to determine what services will be provided and the levels of usage.

The goal of marketing the Laser Center is to track the changing needs and desires of consumers and constantly adjust the hospital's mix of services to meet these needs. The marketing program will continue to produce value for the consumers through the services provided.

Another critical factor in marketing of the services provided by the Laser Center is to correctly identify the persons who play a key role in the purchase decision. It is at this point that the marketing of health care services differs from the marketing of the other professional services.

The unique feature of marketing health care services is created by the role of the physician as the key actor in the purchase decision. Consumers can purchase medical and surgical services provided by the Laser Center only through the physician.

Today the masses can be easily reached by the media and therefore the customer can be the consumer. The physician can decide who will purchase these services, the amount of services that may be purchased, and in some instances when they will be purchased.

Elements of Patient Satisfaction

The elements that are needed for patient satisfaction of the laser center may include the following factors:

Friendliness of the nursing staff
Quality of care
Attention to patient needs
Waiting time
Physical environment
Confidence in physician
Cost of procedure
Ambiance of the facility

There has been significant increase in awareness both in the consumer and customer market of the advantages of lasers in medicine and surgery; however, the laser market is still underdeveloped as a service in the hospital market place.

This demand is created by

1. A growing awareness among consumers of the most cost-effective health care services
2. The prospective payment system
3. The concern of corporations to use modalities of health care that are less costly

The Laser Center must provide quality services (high tech) that are consumer-centered (high touch) at a reasonable cost with a high convenience factor for the consumer.

Summary

Ambulatory Laser Centers, whatever the geographic location, present a challenge for the facility. Most health care facilities will face a variety of issues that include determining the feasibility of laser usage, assessment of specific laser needs, evaluation, selection, and acquisition of equipment, establishing laser safety rules, policies and procedures, training and credentialing of personnel, and determination of laser usage charge structure. For a majority of institutions, these issues provide a challenge, presenting difficulties and opportunities for administration and staff.

A decision as to whether or not the "ideal" program or center is feasible for the facility must take several factors into consideration. After these factors have been weighed, a determination of the feasible program or center for the hospital can be made.

With the proliferation of lasers in all aspects of medicine and surgery, eventually to enter the diagnostic departments, lasers will be everywhere. What does the future hold? Oncology centers will implement photodynamic therapy as an alternative treatment for various types of cancer. Vascular laboratories will begin using laser diagnostic tools, such as laser dopplers. Cardiac catheter laboratories will expand their services to include laser angioplasty. The invasive radiologists are exploring various types of lasers to add to their armamentarium. Lasers already are in the laboratory, separating blood cells and products.

Technology is impacting our practice as physicians and nurses, expanding our horizons with new, exciting practice techniques. Cost-effective delivery of health care is a prime concern, and technology assists in this process. It is predicted that the growth for lasers in medicine and surgery will be 26% per year until the end of this century. Are we as health care professionals ready to meet this growth potential in the delivery of quality patient care?

45
The Laser Industry: Present and Future

Arthur A. Bertolero

The laser industry, is more than 15 years old. While the first medical lasers were developed and used in the mid-1960s, it was not until the mid-1970s that published reports established the laser as a useful surgical tool. The argon laser has been used clinically in ophthalmology and in plastic surgery since 1976. The CO_2 laser has been used in ENT surgery since 1972, in gynecology since 1973, and in neurosurgery since 1976. The surgical Nd:YAG laser was first used in gastroenterology and urology in 1977, and the ophthalmic pulsed Nd:YAG laser in 1980.[1-3]

By 1986, the equipment segment of the worldwide medical laser business represented a $200 million market. The method of marketing medical lasers has changed little over the last ten years. Lasers continue to be sold by specialty-directed marketing, with lasers being sold for primary use by a single specialty. It is this type of marketing and utilization that gives laser critics their case against lasers. With the exception of ophthalmology, lasers used by a single specialty are often underutilized, and therefore are not cost-effective. With a few qualifications, the critics are correct. However, in the last ten years, there have been hundreds of papers presented and published that prove, well enough for most physicians, that lasers can do many procedures significantly better than conventional methods. Thus we can conclude that the surgical benefits and better quality of care provided by the laser, rather than its cost-effectiveness, are responsible for the esteem this technique currently enjoys.

Ten years of laser research and applications development have led to considerable overlap in regard to matching lasers to applications expediently. Argon, CO_2, Nd:YAG, and other wavelengths are all capable of performing many of today's laser procedures. This fact is substantiated by clinicians every day, as they choose laser wavelengths in much the same way as they choose scalpel blades or electrosurgical devices. These decisions are based on training, experience, ease of use, availablity, and personal preference as much as they are based on wavelength.[4,5]

The ability for a laser to be used in more than one specialty gives the laser the potential to be a more highly utilized, more cost-effective in strument. Unfortunately, this potential has yet to be fully realized. However, in the area of prospective reimbursement, the laser has emerged as the most often-mentioned factor in converting inpatients to outpatients and in reducing the length of stay in hospital. In this way alone, many lasers are justifying their expense.

Today the laser industry is at its most critical phase since the introduction of lasers to the medical community. Of the dozens of laser companies, less than a handful are profitable. At the same time, fierce competition is driving laser prices down, and customers are demanding more services. The confusion in the marketplace about the specific therapeutic applications of each laser, and about how to choose a laser manufacturer most advantageously, has lengthened the decision-making process and increased the cost of selling lasers. The only certain fact is, that the financial numbers do not add up for most laser companies, and, as a result, there will be a major shakeout in the laser industry in the next few years similar to that which has occurred in the computer industry.

The worldwide medical laser equipment market is forecasted to grow to more than $400 million by 1990. Several factors indicate that even a market that is twice the size of today's market will have a difficult time providing a return to investors in medical laser equipment companies.[6]

There is, however, a bright side. Medical lasers are no longer the "concept sell" they once were. Effective marketeers will be able to shorten the buying cycle substantially and thereby increase profits. An emerging disposables segment offers the promise of a higher profit aftermarket. Finally, the inevitable shakeout will leave a few major companies with enough volume to gain profitability.

The Present-Day Laser Industry

The laser industry today is in one of its most dynamic stages. Rapid growth and fierce competition in a confused marketplace have made difficult financial times for a large number of laser companies. Before we discuss this issue, we will analyze the relatively small market for which too many are competing (Table 45.1).

There are at least five major companies selling surgical Nd:YAG lasers and five times as many selling ophthalmic Nd:YAG lasers. There are more than ten companies selling CO_2 lasers. In all, there are more than 30 companies competing for a market that is big enough for no more than 12 companies at the most. The shakeout and consolidation that will take place over the next few years will leave no more than six to seven major companies. In addition, there will be four or five minor companies selling specialty or low-price "generic" lasers.[6]

TABLE 45.1. The medical laser equipment market (in million $, worldwide)

Type of laser	1986	1987	1988	1989	1990
Nd:YAG	39.0	50.7	65.9	85.7	121.4
CO_2	62.6	78.3	97.90	122.4	135.0
Argon	11.5	13.2	15.2	17.5	20.1
Ophthalmic	82.0	92.5	105.2	119.5	135.5
Other	2.0	4.3	7.0	12.5	16.0
Total	197.1	239.0	291.2	357.6	428.0

Source: Surgical Laser Technologies and industry estimates.

The various types of lasers are at different stages in their adoption. Figures 45.1 to 45.7 show the hospital and office market penetration in the United States, with estimates for the total size of each segment worldwide.

The CO_2 laser hospital market is entering the "late majority" phase, characterized by acceptance by nearly 50% of the market (Figure 45.1). This market is now mature. The number of applications has increased, prices have come down, and the size of this market segment has grown. Now, smaller hospitals are entering the market, and larger hospitals are buying their second and third CO_2 lasers, so that by 1990 this market segment should represent over 8000 lasers worldwide.

The office CO_2 market is in the "early adopter" phase, with the market still under development (Figure 45.2). The office applications and CO_2 lasers designed and priced for this market will increase the size of this market. This market represents at least 4000 lasers worldwide by 1990.

The Nd:YAG laser hospital market segment is in the "early adopter" phase (Figure 45.3). This market is still in development, and several potential applications could substantially increase its size. This market will represent 6000 lasers worldwide by 1990. Some market analysts feel this segment will be the fastest-growing segment in the next two to three years.

The Nd:YAG laser office market segment is in the "innovator" phase (Figure 45.4), characterized by purchases by a small group of innovative physicians who will prove the profit potential for "office YAG" lasers. If the office Nd:YAG laser is viable, then smaller, less expensive, Nd:YAG lasers could expand the potential of this market. With the products currently available, and with the limited number of applications, the office Nd:YAG market will represent 2000 lasers worldwide by 1990.

The argon and KTP-532 (potassium titanyl phosphate) lasers are in the "early adopter" phase, with some well-proven applications that, unfortunately, offer only limited market potential (Figure 45.5). However, the development of new applications could expand the market for these products. Currently, the market for these products represents 2000 lasers worldwide.

The ophthalmic laser market includes argon, krypton, and short-pulsed Nd:YAG lasers (Fig-

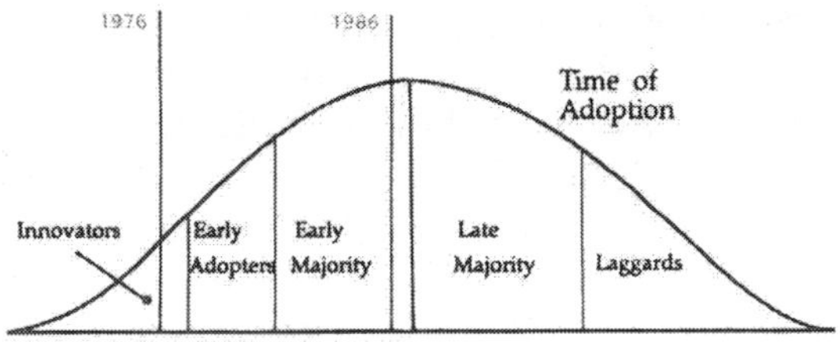

FIGURE 45.1. The CO_2 laser hospital market.

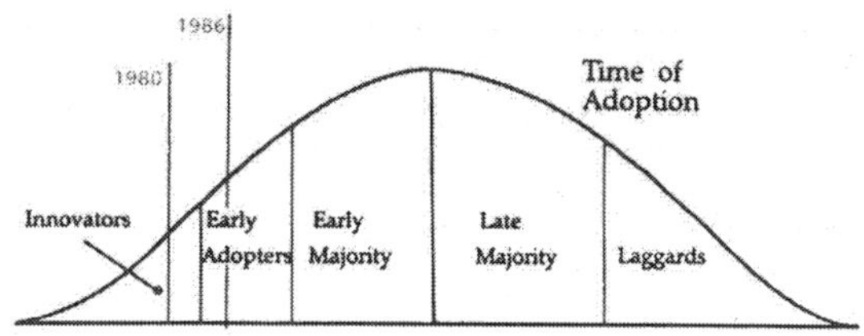

FIGURE 45.2. The CO_2 laser office market.

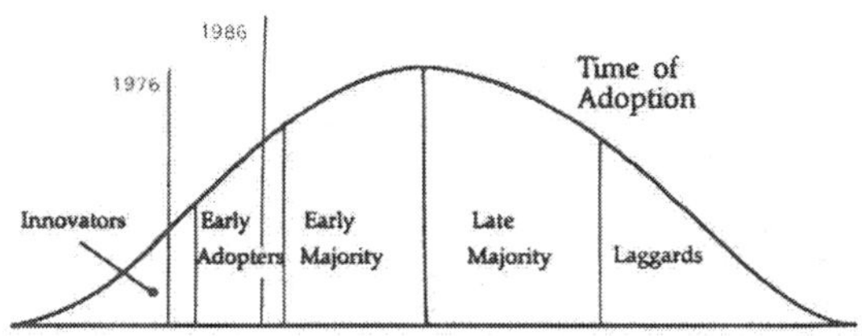

FIGURE 45.3. The surgical Nd:YAG laser hospital market.

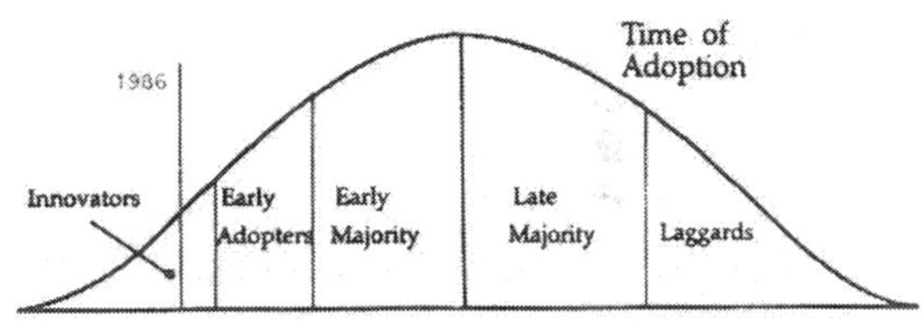

FIGURE 45.4. The surgical Nd:YAG laser office market.

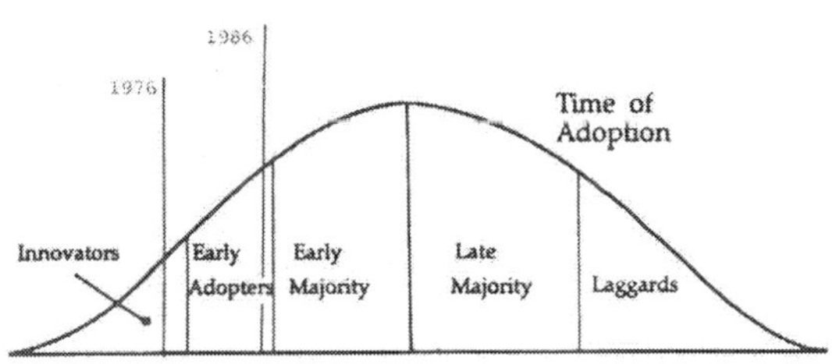

FIGURE 45.5. The argon and KTP-532 (potassium titanyl phosphate) lasers hospital and office markets.

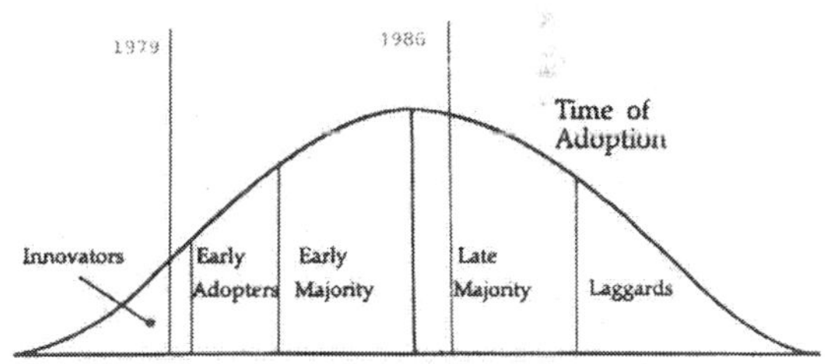

FIGURE 45.6. The ophthalmic laser hospital and office markets.

ure 45.6). This market is in the "late majority" stage and is the most mature of all of the segments. This market may provide a model for all the other segments. One example of this is that the price of ophthalmic lasers has decreased and the market size has increased. This seems to be holding true for the CO_2 office market, also. However, making too many comparisons to the ophthalmic market may not be wise. No other segment has yet to produce an application that is near the frequency of posterior capsulotomy or retinal coagulation procedure. This market is estimated to represent 8000 lasers worldwide.

Present-Day Laser Users

Figure 45.7 exhibits the current mix of laser users. Table 45.2 shows the varying degrees of usage by the major medical specialties in 1986.

Laser Applications

Table 45.3 shows the various types of lasers and their applications. It is reassuring to see the multitude of applications that certain lasers

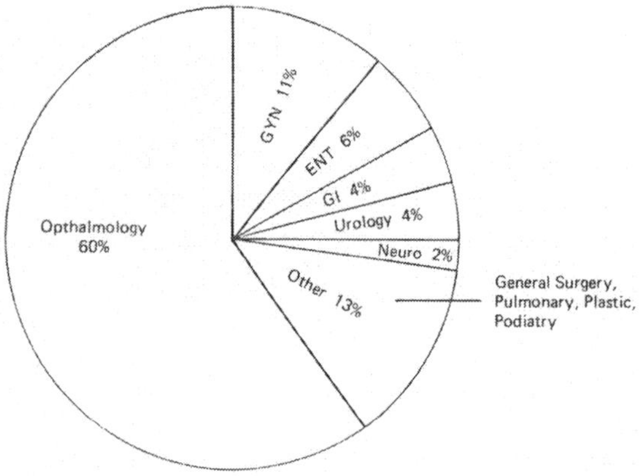

FIGURE 45.7. Laser user mix: Percent of total laser procedures performed. (Estimates from the industry and Surgical Laser Technologies, Inc.)

have. However, the overlap in applications has caused a great deal of confusion for the potential laser buyer. It is not as simple as a CO_2 for this procedure and a YAG for that operation. For certain procedures, it is possible to have one physician who prefers CO_2, one physician who prefers YAG and one physician who prefers Argon. However, the challenge for the hospital administrator is almost always the same: Choose a laser that will provide the highest utilization.[4,7] Utilization can be adequate to justify purchase with one or two procedures being performed frequently. However, as smaller hospitals or outpatient clinics justify laser purchases, they may make determinations based not only on the primary uses but on the range of applications any one laser offers their physician mix.

TABLE 45.2. Access to lasers by laser type

	Percent of specialists with access to laser		
Clinical Specialty	Argon	CO_2	Nd:YAG
Neurosurgery	<3	70	10
Ophthalmology	40	N/A	65*
ENT surgery	5	60	<5
Gynecologic surgery	15	40	10
Gastroenterologic surgery	<2	N/A	25
Plastic surgery	10	15	<5
Urology	N/A	5	10
Pulmonary surgery	N/A	<5	10
General surgery	N/A	10	<3

The Marketplace for Medical Laser Meeting, Boston; May, 1986, Roger Guidi, sponsored by Laser Focus Magazine.
*Pulsed Nd:YAG.

The Profitability Problem

Many people find it beyond belief that laser companies have a hard time making a profit. Yet, the fact remains, there are only a few profitable laser companies. A closer examination of the typical laser sale explains the dilemma most laser companies face.

Average laser selling price	\$ 75,000
Typical cost of selling and marketing	−16,000
Typical cost of first-year warranty	− 3,000
Typical cost of installation	− 1,000
Typical cost of inservice	− 3,000
Typical cost of physician training	− 2,000
Typical cost of manufacturing/ overhead	−45,000
Typical cost of inventory and debt	− 1,000
Typical cost of research and development	− 4,000
Total cost =	\$ 75,000
Profit =	0

Laser prices are being forced down by competition, and confused buyers are demanding costly on-site demonstrations, causing selling costs to increase. It is easy to see why laser companies are struggling to make a profit. The revenue that most companies generate from service contracts rarely produces profit. It is this dilemma that makes a shakeout in the laser industry inevitable.

The Future of the Laser Industry

There will be fewer laser companies to deal with in the next few years. Those that weather the storm will be left with a market that is big enough to produce profits for well-positioned companies. Several laser companies may try to ride out the storm under the umbrella provided by a large parent corporation. While a few companies may survive with help from a parent company, they will do no more than survive unless they establish a viable position in the market.

TABLE 45.3. Current applications for laser surgery* (September 30, 1986)

			Type of laser					
Clinical Specialty	Application	ICD-9	Argon	Argon/ Krypton	CO_2	Dye	Nd:YAG	Contact Nd:YAG**
Dermatology and Plastic surgery	Excision/destruction of lesion of skin and subcutaneous tissue						X	X
	Port-wine nevi (birthmarks)	86.3	X		X			
	Tattoos	86.3	X		X		X	X
	Warts	86.3			X		X	X
	Keloids (acne)	86.3			X			
	Excision of eyelid wart	08.22			X			
	Excision of lesion or tissue of lip	27.43			X			X
	Excision of soft tissue	83.49			X			X
	Photodynamic therapy	—				X		
ENT (Otolaryngology) surgery	Excision/destruction of lesions/tissue of							
	External ear	18.29			X			X
	Nose	21.30–21.32		X			X	
	Lips	27.43			X			X
	Oral cavity	27.49			X			X
	Tongue	25.1		X			X	
	Pharynx	29.3			X			X
	Larynx (vocal cord)	30.09			X			
	Stapedectomy	19.1	X					
	Myringotomy	20.1, 20.09	X					
Gastroenterologic surgery	Excision/destruction of lesion/tissue of							
	Esophagus	42.39					X	X
	Stomach	43.41–43.49					X	X
	Duodenum	45.31, 45.32					X	X
	Small intestine	45.33, 45.34					X	X
	Large intestine	45.4					X	X
	Rectum	48.33, 48.35					X	X
	Hemorrhoids	49.46			X		X	X
General and Oncologic surgery	Excision/destruction of lesion of							
	Pancreas	52.2			X		X	X
	Liver	50.21, 50.29			X		X	X
	Abdominal wall	54.3					X	X
	Pancreatectomy, partial	52.59			X		X	X
	Hepatectomy, partial	50.22			X		X	X
Gynecologic surgery	Excision/destruction of lesions of							
	Cervix	67.3			X			X
	Vulva	71.3			X			X
	Uterus/intrauterine	69.19			X		X	X
	Vagina	70.33		X			X	
	Urethra	58.3			X			X
	Perirectal tissue (warts)	48.82			X		X	X

TABLE 45.3. Continued

Clinical Specialty	Application	ICD-9	Type of laser					
			Argon	Argon/ Krypton	CO_2	Dye	Nd:YAG	Contact Nd:YAG**
	Surgical procedures, including							
	Celiotomy	54.11			X			
	Conization, cervix	67.2			X			X
	Endometrial ablation						X	X
	Intrauterine septae/ adhesiolysis						X	X
	Myomectomy	68.29			X			X
	Oophororrhaphy	65.71			X			X
	Oophorcystectomy	65.29			X			X
	Oophorotomy	65.0			X			X
	Salpingolysis	68.29			X			X
	Salpingoplasty	66.79			X			X
	Salpingostomy	66.73			X			X
	Treatment of endometriosis		X		X		X	X
	Tubal ligation	66.2, 66.3			X			X
	Vaginectomy	70.4			X			X
	Vulvectomy	71.5, 71.61, 71.62			X			X
Neurosurgery	Excision/destruction of							
	Brain tissue & lesions	01.51, 01.59			X		X	X
	skull lesions	01.6	X					
	Spinal cord lesions	03.4			X			X
	Cranial and peripheral nerves	04.07			X			X
	Division of intraspinal nerve root	03.1			X			
	Partial excision of pituitary gland	07.62					X	X
	Endarterectomy, intracranial vessels	38.11			X		X	X
Ophthalmology	Excision/destruction of							
	Eyelid lesion	08.20, 08.25			X			
	Retina & choroid lesion	14.24, 14.25	X					
	Iridotomy	12.12	X				X	
	Iridoplasty	12.39	X					X
	Trabeculoplasty	12.79	X					
	Discission and excision of secondary cataract	13.64, 13.65, 13.69			X			
	Repair of retinal tear	14.34, 14.35	X					
	Endophotoincision (removal of vitreous strands)	14.79						X
Orthopedic surgery	Osteotomy (division of bone)	77.3			X			
	Excision of lesion or tissue of bone	77.6			X			
	Arthroscopy	80.2			X			X

TABLE 45.3. Continued

Clinical Specialty	Application	ICD-9	Argon	Argon/ Krypton	CO_2	Dye	Nd:YAG	Contact Nd:YAG**
	Soft tissue, ganglion neurolysis				X			X
Thoracic surgery	Thoracotomy	34.09			X			X
	Excision or destruction of lesion of lung	32.29			X			X
	Bronchial dilation	33.91			X		X	X
	Dilation of larynx	31.98			X			
	Dilation of trachea	31.99			X		X	X
Urology	Partial nephrectomy	55.4			X		X	X
	Excision of bladder lesion (transurethral)	57.59	X				X	X
	Excision or destruction of urethral tissue	58.3				X	X	X
	Exxcision of lesion of ureter	56.41					X	
	Excision of perirectal tissue (condylomas, warts)	48.82			X		X	X
	Excision/destruction of lesion of penis	64.2			X			X

Source: Hospital Technical Series, Vol. 5, No. 9, Guideline Report. Implementing Laser Technology in the Community Hospital. 1986 American Hospital Association, Division of Technology Management and Policy, 840 North Lake Shore Drive, Chicago, IL 60611

*This table lists several of the major clinical applications that can be enhanced through the use of surgical lasers. While every attempt has been made to include the most common laser applications, the table is not meant to be comprehensive or exhaustive. Its purpose is to illustrate the diversity of various surgical lasers.

**Based on data supplied to Surgical Laser Technologies, Inc. in conjunction with clinical investigations. These data were not included in the original work. Also, this material is intended to describe clinical applications, *not* FDA market clearances. Current market clearance status should be obtained directly from the regulatory affairs department of the laser manufacturer.

See references 8–10 for further discussion.

There will only be room for one or two full-line manufacturers who offer all the currently used wavelengths. The rest of the market will be made up of well-positioned specialty companies. There will likely be companies specializing in CO_2 office products, laser lithotripsy, laser angioplasty, and laser hyperthermia. There will be successful specialty companies due to technology advances aided by the ability to gain FDA market clearance well in advance of other competitors, thus enabling the specialty company to establish a position in a market niche before the full-line manufacturer can enter.

The most exciting prospect for the future is the potential size of the accessory market. In 1986, the accessory market, comprised of protective eyewear, smoke evacuators, micromanipulators and handpieces, was no larger than a $5 million market. With the introduction of disposable Nd:YAG fibers, CO_2 waveguides, Contact Laser Probes and Laser Scalpels, and other consumables, the size of the accessory market could grow to more than $100 million in 1990. Numerous market observers have felt that the single factor most relentlessly holding back the development of lasers has been the lack of adequate delivery systems. The further development of delivery systems could make the accessory segment of the market one of the industry's most important market segments.[6]

In any discussion of the future, photodynamic therapy (PDT) and new wavelengths must be discussed. The current restrictions imposed by the FDA, requiring lengthy clinical trials and extended follow-up, have helped to protect the laser industry from itself—like it or not. However, this process means that any new drug-enhanced therapy or any new wavelength will take two to three years before it is cleared for marketing by the FDA. Therefore, new wavelengths will play only a minor role in the next five years.

The Future is Now

In the last few years, the laser has moved from a device that still had many detractors to a device that is widely accepted as a tool that enables physicians to do better, more cost-effective surgery and endoscopy.

Today, the future is being shaped by clinicians using lasers to do more and more of their surgery and therapeutic endoscopy. The techniques they are developing today will not be published for some time. The products they want today will not be ready soon enough. The laser industry is struggling to keep up. When industry listens to those who use the lasers, they realize—the future is happening right now.

References

1. Dixon JA: Surgical Application of Lasers. Year Book Medical Publishers, Chicago, 1983.
2. Joffe SN: Neodymium-YAG Laser in Medicine and Surgery. Elsevier, New York, 1983.
3. March WF: Ophthalmic Lasers: Current Clinical Uses. Slack Inc., Thorofare, NJ, 1984.
4. Surgical Practice News. Lasers in surgery come of age. May 1986.
5. Alder HC: 1986 Guideline Report. Implementing laser technology in the community hospital. Hosp Tech Ser 5(9), 1986.
6. In Vivo: The Business and Medicine Report, July/Aug, No 17, 1986.
7. Lasers in Surgery and Medicine, Vol 6, No 4, 1986.
8. Goldman L: Current and future development in laser surgery. Surg Clin North Am 61(5), 1984.
9. Lobraico R, Bellina JH, et al: Guide to Laser Surgery. 1982.
10. Mackety C: Beyond your first laser. Paper presented at the First National Conference on Clinical Lasers—Practical Management and Utilization Strategies, Aug. 15, 1984.

Index

SPRINGER NATURE

GPSR Compliance

The European Union's (EU) General Product Safety Regulation (GPSR) is a set of rules that requires consumer products to be safe and our obligations to ensure this.

If you have any concerns about our products, you can contact us on ProductSafety@springernature.com

In case Publisher is established outside the EU, the EU authorized representative is:

Springer Nature Customer Service Center GmbH
Europaplatz 3
69115 Heidelberg, Germany

FSC
www.fsc.org
MIX
Papier | Fördert gute Waldnutzung
FSC® C083411

Kolibri 360 GmbH
Ferdinand-Jühlke-Straße 7
99095 Erfurt, Deutschland
produktsicherheit@kolibri360.de